11263

D1496294

Blood Stem Cell Transplantation

Cancer Treatment and Research

Steven T. Rosen MD, *Series Editor*

Nathanson L (ed): Malignant Melanoma: Biology, Diagnosis, and Therapy. 1988. ISBN 0-89838-384-6.
Pinedo HM, Verweij J (eds): Treatment of Soft Tissue Sarcomas. 1989. ISBN 0-89838-391-9.
Hansen HH (ed): Basic and Clinical Concepts of Lung Cancer. 1989. ISBN 0-7923-0153-6.
Lepor H, Ratliff TL (eds): Urologic Oncology. 1989. ISBN 0-7923-0161-7.
Benz C, Liu E (eds): Oncogenes. 1989. ISBN 0-7923-0237-0.
Ozols RF (ed): Drug Resistance in Cancer Therapy. 1989. ISBN 0-7923-0244-3.
Surwit EA, Alberts DS (eds): Endometrial Cancer. 1989. ISBN 0-7923-0286-9.
Champlin R (ed): Bone Marrow Transplantation. 1990. ISBN 0-7923-0612-0.
Goldenberg D (ed): Cancer Imaging with Radiolabeled Antibodies. 1990. ISBN 0-7923-0631-7.
Jacobs C (ed): Carcinomas of the Head and Neck. 1990. ISBN 0-7923-0668-6.
Lippman ME, Dickson R (eds): Regulatory Mechanisms in Breast Cancer: Advances in Cellular and
    Molecular Biology of Breast Cancer. 1990. ISBN 0-7923-0868-9.
Nathanson L (ed): Malignant Melanoma: Genetics, Growth Factors, Metastases, and Antigens. 1991.
    ISBN 0-7923-0895-6.
Sugarbaker PH (ed): Management of Gastric Cancer. 1991. ISBN 0-7923-1102-7.
Pinedo HM, Verweij J, Suit HD (eds): Soft Tissue Sarcomas: New Developments in the Multidisciplinary
    Approach to Treatment. 1991. ISBN 0-7923-1139-6.
Ozols RF (ed): Molecular and Clinical Advances in Anticancer Drug Resistance. 1991. ISBN 0-7923-1212-0.
Muggia FM (ed): New Drugs, Concepts and Results in Cancer Chemotherapy. 1991. ISBN 0-7923-1253-8.
Dickson RB, Lippman ME (eds): Genes, Oncogenes and Hormones: Advances in Cellular and Molecular
    Biology of Breast Cancer. 1992. ISBN 0-7923-1748-3.
Humphrey G, Bennett Schraffordt Koops H. Molenaar WM, Postma A (eds): Osteosarcoma in Adolescents
    and Young Adults: New Developments and Controversies. 1993. ISBN 0-7923-1905-2.
Benz CC, Liu ET (eds): Oncogenes and Tumor Suppressor Genes in Human Malignancies. 1993.
    ISBN 0-7923-1960-5.
Freireich EJ, Kantarjian H (eds): Leukemia: Advances in Research and Treatment. 1993.
    ISBN 0-7923-1967-2.
Dana BW (ed): Malignant Lymphomas, Including Hodgkin's Disease: Diagnosis, Management, and Special
    Problems. 1993. ISBN 0-7923-2171-5.
Nathanson L (ed): Current Research and Clinical Management of Melanoma. 1993. ISBN 0-7923-2152-9.
Verweij J, Pinedo HM, Suit HD (eds): Multidisciplinary Treatment of Soft Tissue Sarcomas. 1993.
    ISBN 0-7923-2183-9.
Rosen ST, Kuzel TM (eds): Immunoconjugate Therapy of Hematologic Malignancies. 1993.
    ISBN 0-7923-2270-3.
Sugarbaker PH (ed): Hepatobiliary Cancer. 1994. ISBN 0-7923-2501-X.
Rothenberg ML (ed): Gynecologic Oncology: Controversies and New Developments. 1994.
    ISBN 0-7923-2634-2.
Dickson RB, Lippman ME (eds): Mammary Tumorigenesis and Malignant Progression. 1994.
    ISBN 0-7923-2647-4.
Hansen HH (ed): Lung Cancer. Advances in Basic and Clinical Research. 1994. ISBN 0-7923-2835-3.
Goldstein LJ, Ozols RF (eds.): Anticancer Drug Resistance. Advances in Molecular and Clinical Research.
    1994. ISBN 0-7923-2836-1.
Hong WK, Weber RS (eds): Head and Neck Cancer. Basic and Clinical Aspects. 1994. ISBN 0-7923-3015-3.
Thall PF (ed): Recent Advances in Clinical Trial Design and Analysis. 1995. ISBN 0-7923-3235-0.
Buckner CD (ed): Technical and Biological Components of Marrow Transplantation. 1995.
    ISBN 0-7923-3394-2.
Muggia FM (ed): Concepts, Mechanisms, and New Targets for Chemotherapy. 1995. ISBN 0-7923-3525-2.
Klastersky J (ed): Infectious Complications of Cancer. 1995. ISBN 0-7923-3598-8.
Kurzrock R, Talpaz M (eds): Cytokines: Interleukins and Their Receptors. 1995. ISBN 0-7923-3636-4.
Sugarbaker P (ed): Peritoneal Carcinomatosis: Drugs and Diseases. 1995. ISBN 0-7923-3726-3.
Sugarbaker P (ed): Peritoneal Carcinomatosis: Principles of Management. 1995. ISBN 0-7923-3727-1.
Dickson RB, Lippman ME (eds): Mammary Tumor Cell Cycle, Differentiation and Metastasis. 1995.
    ISBN 0-7923-3905-3.
Freireich EJ, Kantarjian H (eds): Molecular Genetics and Therapy of Leukemia. 1995. ISBN 0-7923-3912-6.
Cabanillas F, Rodriguez MA (eds): Advances in Lymphoma Research. 1996. ISBN 0-7923-3929-0.

Blood Stem Cell Transplantation

edited by

Jane N. Winter, M.D.
Northwestern Memorial Hospital and Northwestern University
Robert H. Lurie Cancer Center
Chicago, Illinois

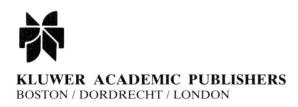

KLUWER ACADEMIC PUBLISHERS
BOSTON / DORDRECHT / LONDON

Distributors for North America:
Kluwer Academic Publishers
101 Philip Drive
Assinippi Park
Norwell, Massachusetts 02061 USA

Distributors for all other countries:
Kluwer Academic Publishers Group
Distribution Centre
Post Office Box 322
3300 AH Dordrecht, THE NETHERLANDS

Library of Congress Cataloging-in-Publication Data

Blood stem cell transplantation / edited by Jane N. Winter.
    p.   cm. — (Cancer treatment and research; CTAR 77)
    Includes index.
    ISBN 0–7923–4260–7 (alk. paper)
    1. Hematopoietic stem cells—Transplantation.   2. Cancer-
Immunotherapy. I. Winter, Jane N. II. Series.
    [DNLM: 1. Hematopoietic Stem Cell Transplantation. 2. Bone
    Marrow
Transplantation. W1 CA693 v.77 1996/WH 380 B6547 1996]
RC271.B59B566 1996
617.4′4—dc20
DNLM/DLC
for Library of Congress   96–35387
                                                          CIP

Printed on acid-free paper.

PRINTED IN THE UNITED STATES OF AMERICA

Contents

Contributing Authors   ix

Preface   xiii
JANE N. WINTER

I.   Developments in Immuno-, Molecular, and Cell Biology:
     Implications for Clinical Stem Cell Transplantation   1

     1. Gene therapy of solid tumors and hematopoietic neoplasms. . .   3
        CARLOS R. BACHIER and ALBERT B. DEISSEROTH

     2. Post-bone marrow transplant use of immunotherapy   27
        UDIT N. VERMA, KENNETH R. MEEHAN,
        and AMITABHA MAZUMDER

     3. Graft-versus-leukemia effect of allogeneic bone marrow
        transplantation and donor mononuclear cell infusions   57
        DAVID L. PORTER and JOSEPH H. ANTIN

     4. Graft-versus-host disease: implications from basic
        immunology for prophylaxis and treatment   87
        GEORGIA B. VOGELSANG

     5. The detection of minimal residual disease: implications for
        bone marrow transplantation   99
        JOHN G. GRIBBEN and JOACHIM L. SCHULTZE

     6. The use of radiolabeled antibodies in bone marrow
        transplantation for hematologic malignancies.   121
        DANA C. MATTHEWS, FREDERICK R. APPELBAUM,
        OLIVER W. PRESS, JANET F. EARY, and
        IRWIN D. BERNSTEIN

II. Sources of Hematopoietic Stem Cells and
     Their Ex Vivo Expansion   141

7. Peripheral blood stem cell harvesting and CD34-positive
   cell selection 143
   ELIZABETH J. SHPALL, PABLO J. CAGNONI,
   SCOTT I. BEARMAN, MAUREEN ROSS, YAGO NIETO,
   and ROY B. JONES

8. Ex vivo expansion of hematopoietic stem and progenitor
   cells for transplantation 159
   JENNIFER A. LAIUPPA, E. TERRY PAPOUTSAKIS,
   and WILLIAM M. MILLER

9. Allogeneic umbilical cord blood transplantation 187
   JOHN E. WAGNER

10. The use of unrelated donors for bone marrow
    transplantation 217
    GUIDO TRICOT

III. Reducing the Toxicity Associated with Hematopoietic Stem
Cell Transplantation 229

11. Supportive care in bone marrow transplantation: pulmonary
    complications... 231
    STEPHEN W. CRAWFORD

12. Recombinant cytokines and hematopoietic growth factors in
    allogeneic and autologous bone marrow transplantation 255
    HILLARD M. LAZARUS

IV. Clinical Applications: Continued Progress and New Frontiers.... 303

13. Bone marrow transplantation in thalassemia 305
    GUIDO LUCARELLI, CLAUDIO GIARDINI, and
    EMANUELE ANGELUCCI

14. Immune ablation and hematopoietic stem cell rescue for
    severe autoimmune diseases (SADS) 317
    RICHARD K. BURT

15. Autologous bone marrow transplantation in pediatric
    solid tumors 333
    MORRIS KLETZEL and AE RANG KIM

16. Autologous stem cell transplantation for the treatment of
    chronic myelogenous leukemia......................... 357
    RAVI BHATIA and PHILIP B. MCGLAVE

V. A New Challenge for the Field of Stem Cell Transplantation:
    Financial Constraints..................................... 375

    17. Health care economics and bone marrow transplantation 377
        ILANA WESTERMAN, TERESA WATERS,
        and CHARLES BENNETT

Contributing Authors

EMANUELE ANGELUCCI, Divisione di Ematologia e Centro Trapianto Midollo Osseo di Muraglia, Azienda Ospedaliera di Pesaro, 61100 Pesaro, Italy

JOSEPH H. ANTIN, Hematology Oncology Division and Department of Medicine, Brigham and Women's Hospital, Boston, MA 02115

FREDERICK R. APPELBAUM, Fred Hutchinson Cancer Research Center and the Department of Medicine, University of Washington, Seattle, WA 98104

CARLOS BACHIER, Adult Blood and Marrow Transplantation, South Texas cancer Institute, San Antonio, Texas 78229

SCOTT I. BEARMAN, University of Colorado Bone Marrow Transplant Program, University of Colorado, University Hospital, Denver, CO 80262

CHARLES BENNETT, Department of Medicine, Northwestern University Medical School and VA Lakeside Medical Center, Chicago, IL 60611

IRWIN D. BERNSTEIN, Fred Hutchinson Cancer Research Center and Department of Pediatrics, University of Washington, Seattle, WA 98104

RAVI BHATIA, Department of Hematology and Bone Marrow Transplantation City of Hope National Medical Center, Duarte, CA 91010

RICHARD K. BURT, Bone Marrow Transplant Program, Northwestern University Medical School, Robert H. Lurie Cancer Center, Chicago, IL 60611

PABLO J. CAGNONI, University of Colorado Bone Marrow Transplant Program, University of Colorado, Denver, CO 80262

STEPHEN W. CRAWFORD, Program in Pulmonary and Critical Care Medicine, Fred Hutchinson Cancer Research Center, University of Washington, Seattle, WA 98104

ALBERT B. DEISSEROTH, Department of Hematology, Box 24, The University of Texas M.D. Anderson Cancer Center, Houston, Texas, and the Department of Internal Medicine, Section of Medical Oncology, Yale University School of Medicine, New Haven, CT 06520

JANET F. EARY, Department of Radiology, University of Washington, Seattle, WA 98195

CLAUDIO GIARDINI, Divisione di Ematologia e Centro Trapianto Midollo Ossco di Muraglia, Azienda Ospedaliera di Pesaro, 61100 Pesaro, Italy

JOHN G. GRIBBEN, Division of Hematologic Malignancies, Dana-Farber cancer institute, Department of Medicine, Harvard Medical School, Boston, MA 02115

ROY B. JONES, University of Colorado Bone Marrow Transplant Program, University of Colorado, University Hospital, Denver, CO 80262

AE RANG KIM, Northwestern University Medical School, Chicago, IL 60611

MORRIS KLETZEL, Division of Oncology and Hematology and Bone Marrow Transplantation, Children's Memorial Hospital and Northwestern University Medical School, Chicago, IL 60614

JENNIFER A. LAIUPPA, Department of Chemical Engineering, Northwestern University, Evanston, IL 60208; Present address: Baxter Healthcare, Renal Division, McGaw Park, IL 60085

HILLARD M. LAZARUS, Ireland Cancer Center, University Hospitals of Cleveland, Case Western Reserve University Cleveland, OH 44106

GUIDO LUCARELLI, Divisione di Ematologia e Centro Trapianto Midollo Osseo di Muraglia, Azienda Ospedaliera di Pesaro, 61100 Pesaro, Italy

DANA C. MATTHEWS, Division of Clinical Research, Fred Hutchinson Cancer Research Center and Department of Pediatrics, University of Washington, Seattle WA 98104

AMITABHA MAZUMDER, Bone Marrow Transplantation Program, Georgetown University Medical Center, Washington, DC 20007

PHILIP B. MCGLAVE, Division of Hematology, Department of Medicine and Bone Marrow Transplantation Program, University of Minnesota Health System, Minneapolis, MN 55455

KENNETH R. MEEHAN, Bone Marrow Transplantation Program, Georgetown University Medical Center, Washington, DC 20007

WILLIAM M. MILLER, Department of Chemical Engineering, Northwestern University, Evanston, IL 60208

YAGO NIETO, University of Colorado Bone Marrow Transplant Program, University Hospital, Denver CO 80262

DAVID L. PORTER, Hematology-Oncology Division and Department of Medicine, University of Pennsylvania School of Medicine, Philadelphia, PA 19104

E. TERRY PAPOUTSAKIS, Department of Chemical Engineering, Northwestern University, Evanston, IL 60208

OLIVER W. PRESS, Fred Hutchinson Cancer Research Center and the Department of Medicine, University of Washington, Seattle, WA 98195

MAUREEN ROSS, University of Colorado Bone Marrow Transplant Program, University of Colorado, University Hospital, Denver, CO 80262

JOACHIM L. SCHULTZE, Division of Hematologic Malignancies, Dana-Farber Cancer Institute, Department of Medicine, Harvard Medical School, Boston, MA 02115

ELIZABETH J. SHPALL, University of Colorado Bone Marrow Transplant Program, University Hospital, Denver, CO 80262

GUIDO TRICOT, Division of Hematology/Oncology and Department of Medicine, University of Arkansas for Medical Sciences, Little Rock, AR 72205

UDIT N. VERMA, Bone Marrow Transplantation Program, Georgetown University Medical Center, Washington, DC 20007

GEORGIA B. VOGELSANG, The Johns Hopkins University School of Medicine, Bone Marrow Transplant Unit, Baltimore, Maryland 21287

JOHN E. WAGNER, Department of Pediatrics, Division of Bone Marrow Transplantation of the University of Minnesota School of Medicine, Minneapolis, Minnesota 55455

TERSESA WATERS, Center for Health Services and Policy Research, Northwestern University, Evanston, IL 60208

ILANA WESTERMAN, Robert H. Lurie Cancer Center, Northwestern University, Chicago, IL 60611

JANE N. WINTER, Bone Marrow Transplant Program, Robert H. Lurie Cancer Center, Northwestern University, Chicago, IL 60611

Preface

The chapters that constitute this volume convey the excitement that accompanies the newest developments in hematopoietic stem cell transplantation. Some of the applications that stand to impact this field most significantly are based on recent advances in the biological sciences, as demonstrated by the chapters on gene therapy (Bachier and Deisseroth), on the detection of minimal residual disease using molecular techniques (Gribben and Schultze), and on the use of radioimmunoconjugates targeting lymphoma and leukemia-associated antigens (Matthews and colleagues). Others are the results of clinical observations — e.g., the association between graft-versus-host disease (GVHD) and durable remissions — that have led to creative clinical experiments such as donor leukocyte infusions (DLIs) (see the chapter by Porter and Antin). Attempts to unravel the biological events that underlie the responses seen in patients with relapsed chronic myelogenous leukemia treated with DLI are likely to provide the basis for future refinements in this clinical approach. Hopefully, improved response rates and reduced toxicity will result. The power of the immunologic response in controlling malignant disease is further underscored by Verma, Meehan, and Mazumder in their chapter on post-transplant immunotherapy. It is becoming evident that the complex immunologic process that results in clinical GVHD may be dissected and engineered to provide clinical benefits that include — in addition to its antineoplastic effects — the amelioration of its clinical manifestations. As discussed by Vogelsang in her chapter on GVHD, better control of GVHD with less global immunosuppression will facilitate the use of mismatched and unrelated donors as summarized in the chapter by Tricot. This area of investigation perfectly illustrates the continued interplay between the laboratory and the clinic. The continued cross-fertilization of ideas between immunologists, molecular biologists, and clinical investigators is likely to yield important advances in this field for years to come.

The possible applications of stem cell transplantation continue to grow with the identification of alternative sources of stem cells and the potential to engineer and/or expand the graft. Although the use of unrelated and mismatched donors continues to increase, the possibilities associated with umbilical cord blood transplantation described by Wagner are legion, especially if stem cells can be expanded ex vivo to provide grafts for full-sized adults. LaIuppa and colleagues describe recent efforts to achieve this goal. Using techniques reviewed by Shpall et al., in which contaminating malignant cells may be eliminated from autografts through positive selection, autologous transplantation may prove highly effective, especially when coupled with post-transplant immunotherapy. Some of these same methodologies have helped facilitate the use of autologous grafts for transplantation in patients with chronic myelogenous leukemia without allogeneic donors. This promising alternative is reviewed by Bhatia and McGlave.

Advances in the supportive care of transplant patients, including the pretransplant identification of those at risk from pulmonary complications (see Crawford) and the use of cytokines (reviewed in exquisite detail in the chapter by Lazarus) to speed engraftment, have reduced morbidity and mortality to such a degree that it is appropriate to consider high-dose therapy and stem cell reconstitution in patients with nonmalignant diseases. The impressive advances that have occurred in transplantation for thalassemia are described by the pioneers in this area of investigation, Lucarelli and colleagues. The burgeoning field of transplantation for autoimmune disorders, including its immunobiological basis and soon-to-be realized clinical potential, is summarized by Burt. Continued progress in the use of high-dose therapy with stem cell rescue for the treatment of pediatric tumors — which derives in part from improved supportive care — is documented by Kletzel and Kim.

The sobering voice of the health care economists (Westerman, Waters, and Bennett) brings us down to reality, underscoring the necessary limitations to our seemingly unbridled imagination. Cost-consciousness and financial savvy will need to be reflected in future study designs. Given the seemingly endless applications to our technology, strategies to ensure its cost-effectiveness will be necessary. Continued financial support for laboratory investigations and for the clinical experiments they generate will be required if we are to go forward. The foundation for many future advances has already been laid, as described in this volume, and it is incumbent upon us all to ensure their realization.

—Jane N. Winter

Blood Stem Cell Transplantation

Developments in Immuno-, Molecular, and Cell Biology: Implications for Clinical Stem Cell Transplantation

1. Gene therapy of solid tumors and hematopoietic neoplasms

Carlos R. Bachier and Albert B. Deisseroth

The ultimate goal in cancer treatment is to identify and correct at the molecular level the derangements that cause the various human malignancies. Important scientific discoveries about the mechanisms through which cancer develops are increasing the likelihood that the introduction of foreign genetic material into mammalian cells may be used as a primary method of therapy. Genetic modification of malignant and nonmalignant cells can be performed on the patient (in vivo) or on cells removed from the body (ex vivo) with subsequent reinfusion into the patient. Delivery systems in gene therapy strategies have included transduction mediated by retrovirus, adenovirus, liposomes, and direct injection of DNA (table 1). Genetic manipulations aimed at correcting disease processes at the molecular level have already been introduced into clinical trials. There are now over 100 cancer treatment trials involving gene transfer or antisense treatment, according to the records of regulatory committees worldwide. These trials involve both gene marking trials and trials based on the use of genetic modification designed for activation of the immune system, chemoprotection of hematopoietic cells, or chemosensitization of tumor cells. The major obstacles to gene therapy in cancer have been selectivity, transduction frequencies, stability of transduction, and effectiveness due to the complexity of genetic alterations found in human tumors. In this chapter, we will discuss the various delivery systems used in gene therapy strategies and the early results of clinical trials with these strategies, with emphasis on their application to high-dose chemotherapy approaches.

Viral vector systems

Retroviral vectors

Initial gene therapy trials have utilized retroviral vector systems as a means of introducing foreign genetic material into normal and malignant cells. The first of these vectors was used in 1990 [1] for the treatment of a patient with severe combined immunodeficiency disease (SCID). This disease arises from the

Jane N. Winter (ed.) BLOOD STEM CELL TRANSPLANTATION. 1997. Kluwer Academic Publishers. ISBN 0-7923-4260-7. All rights reserved.

Table 1. Characteristics of delivery systems

Vector	Advantages	Disadvantages
Retrovirus	1%–30% transduction frequency; permanent modification; infects hematopoietic cells and epithelial cells	Unstable; low titre; must integrate into dividing cell for expansion; 9–12-kb limit
Adenovirus	Infects epithelial cells at high frequency; cellular proliferation not required	Does not infect marrow; immunogenic; temporary in its effect
Adeno-associated virus	Stable; integrates into nondividing cells at a low frequency	Small capacity for DNA (5 Kb); low titres; good for small scale only
Herpes simplex virus type I	Infects wide range of cell types; very high titers; relatively prolonged expression of foreign genes	No integration into genome of infected cells; cytotoxic; difficult to develop due to complexity
'Naked' DNA	No viruses involved; easy to use and develop	Low integration frequency; temporary expression
Liposome	No proliferation required No viruses involved	Low frequency of modification; cytotoxic to certain cells

Abbreviation: kb = kilobase.

absence of the adenosine deaminase gene, and the therapy was based on strategies designed to replace the missing gene [2]. Although the transduction efficiency was low, the percentage of genetically modified lymphocytes appeared to increase, perhaps due in part to the fact that the adenosine deaminase cDNA conferred a selective growth advantage over the SCID peripheral blood lymphocytes. The therapy consisted of monthly infusions of the genetically modified cells. The transduction methods used were based on the incubation of the cell-free retroviral vector supernatants with the target cells for only six hours. Recent modifications in transduction conditions, which now involve cultivation of the target cells with the vector markers in the presence of hematopoietic growth factors and stromal cell monolayers, have increased transduction efficiencies. It is not yet known what effect these new transduction conditions will have on the self-renewal capability of the genetically modified hematopoietic stem cells.

Structure and replication cycle of wild-type retroviruses. The retrovirus has an envelope composed of an outer lipid membrane derived from the cell in which the vector is produced. This viral coat carries and maintains the viral genetic information composed of double-stranded RNA strands. Although retroviral vectors are composed of RNA, once inside a host cell this RNA is reverse transcribed into a complementary DNA copy. This 'cDNA' double-stranded product is then integrated into the host chromosomal DNA, where it is referred to as a provirus [3] (figure 1).

In these replication-competent retroviruses, the provirus encodes three viral proteins, namely, gag, pol, and env, which are responsible for stabiliza-

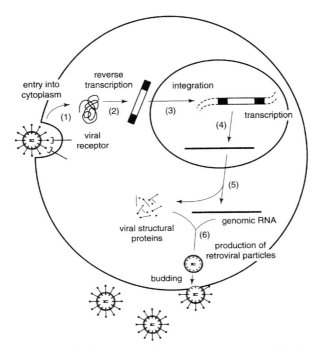

Figure 1. Replication cycle of wild-type retroviruses. Steps in retroviral infection and replication include 1) receptor-mediated entry into the cytoplasm; 2) unfolding and reverse transcription of sRNA into dsDNA; 3) entry into nucleus and integration into the host DNA. The provirus then encodes genomic RNA and transcription of viral structure proteins (4,5). Retroviral particles are then assembled in the cytoplasm and exit the host cell to start a new cycle (6).

tion of the viral RNA, the intraconversion of the RNA into cDNA, and the synthesis of outer proteins that form the coat of the virus. The provirus also contains the nontranscribed encapsidation sequence ψ. This sequence is recognized by the packaging proteins to allow encapsidations into a viral particle. Finally, the proviral DNA is flanked by long terminal repeats (LTRs) that provide functions necessary for synthesis of the full-length viral genome. Once encapsidated, the infectious virus exits the cell to begin another cycle in other host cells [3].

Replication-incompetent retroviral vectors. Partial deletion of retroviral gag, pol, and env replicative sequences has made it possible to insert genetic material into target cells and has prevented the synthesis of infectious retroviral competent particles [4]. Several viral components necessary for replication of the provirus are provided by producer cell lines. These include the ψ packaging sequence necessary for viral RNA recognition and encapsidation into viral particles, reverse transcriptase, integration signals, and viral promoters. These components are provided in trans to the provirus.

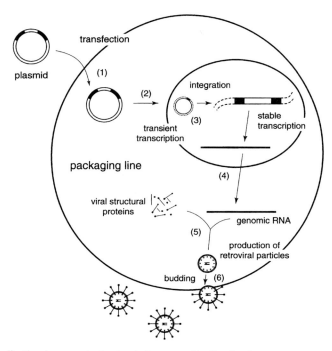

Figure 2. Replication-incompetent retroviral vectors. Replication-incompetent retroviral vectors are produced by transfection into producing cell lines of retroviral plasmids in which gag, pol, and env sequences are replaced with the gene of interest. Producing or packaging cell lines contain the missing structural genes but lack encapsidation sequences required for production of replication competent retrovirus. Plasmids with the gene of interest and a selectable marker are introduced (1) into packaging cell lines through different mechanical methods (electroporation, calcium–chloride transfection, or lipofection). Then the viral RNA is reverse transcribed and integrated into the producer cell line genome (2,3). Transcription of RNA sequences follows with production of retroviral vector particles accomplished by incorporation of packaging-cell-line-transcribed viral structural proteins (4,5). Finally, complete retroviral vector particles exit the cell.

Commonly, the central structural genes (gag, pol, env) are replaced by the therapeutic gene of interest plus a marker gene that allows selection with drugs such as aminoglycoside analogues. Various modifications of the basic structure of these vectors, such as inducible and noninducible nonviral promoters, expression of the gene of interest in the reverse orientation, and use of modified LTRs, have increased the utility of these vectors [3–8]. The viral vector is then introduced into a packaging cell line containing the missing structural genes in the chromosomal DNA, but lacking the RNA molecules capable of producing complete retroviral sequences. These producer cell lines make replication-incompetent vector particles capable of introducing genes into target cells (figure 2).

Pitfalls and limitations. Drawbacks of retroviral vectors include the following:

6

1. Retroviral vectors have the potential to give rise to replication-competent retroviruses (RCRs) after homologous recombination. Modifications such as removal of LTR and replacement with heterologous promoters, separation of gag-pol and env genes, and alteration of the cellular background of packaging and producing cell lines have decreased the incidence of RCRs [9].

2. Retroviral vectors can integrate the transgenes only into actively replicating cells. Modifications aimed at increasing retroviral transduction efficiency are under investigation. These include the creation of pseudotype vectors in which the best elements of different viruses are combined into one vector [10].

3. Retroviral transduction systems are not effective in introducing large DNA fragments (>8 kb) into target cells.

4. The retroviral coat proteins are unstable in the presence of serum proteins at 37°C. This limits the ability to achieve high-titre viral preparations.

5. The ecotrophic and amphotrophic receptors for the retroviral coat proteins are present at low density on the plasma membrane. This also limits the transduction frequency.

Adenoviral vectors

The adenoviral vector is under investigation as a delivery system. It is possible to produce higher vector titres than is the case with retroviral vectors. Adenoviral vectors can infect and express their transgenes in quiescent, nondividing cells without integration [11]. There are approximately 40 adenovirus subtypes, and in immunocompetent humans these cause only benign respiratory tract infections [12]. A concern with the use of adenoviral vectors in the immunodeficient host is that a replication-competent adenoviral vector could lead to an infection that would result in lethal hemorrhagic cystitis, hepatitis, or pneumonitis [13,14]. However, this process does not occur in the immunocompetent host, where hypersensitivity reactions to the adenoviral coat proteins are more prevalent.

Wild-type adenoviral structure and cell cycle. Adenoviruses are icosohedral double-stranded DNA viruses, which do not contain a plasma membrane envelop like the retrovirus. Absence of a plasma membrane envelope makes them more stable than a retrovirus and less prone to complement-mediated lysis. The viral genome encodes approximately 30 mRNA. Transcription products include the early (E1–E4) and late (E5) protein involved in the control of DNA replication, transcription, and structural protein synthesis, including capsid polypeptides and proteins that allow recognition of host cells [3]. After binding to host cells through its capsid fiber, the Penton protein, adenoviruses are internalized into endosomes (figure 3). Only cells with the $\alpha V\beta 3$ integrin receptor can take up the adenovirus. Notably, this integrin is not commonly found among hematopoietic cells with the capacity for self-renewal, perhaps

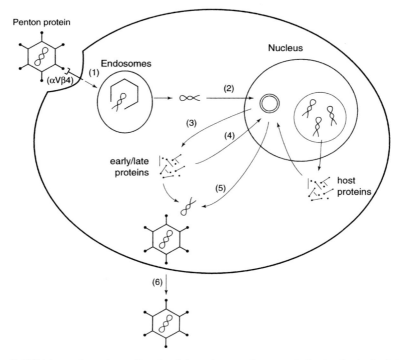

Figure 3. Wild-type adenovirus cell cycle. Adenoviruses gain access to host cells via the integrin receptor αVβ4 (1). Acidic endosomes in the cytoplasms unfold and release the adenoviral DNA. The virion DNA then travels into the nucleus where transcription occurs without integration (2). Transcription and replication of early and late viral proteins and viral DNA are mediated by viral and host transcribed proteins (3,4,5). After a few hours from entry into the host cell, infectious virions are assembled, and the cells die releasing infectious particles (6).

accounting for the difficulty in introducing the adenoviral genes into these early hematopoietic cells. The acidic pH of the endosome unfolds the capsid proteins, thus releasing the DNA [15]. The virion DNA travels into the nucleus, where transcription occurs without integration of the virus into the host chromosomal DNA. DNA replication is promoted through the expression of both viral and cellular genes, including early and late viral proteins such as E1a and E1b. The adenovirus then controls the synthesis of cellular proteins in the infected cells; after a few hours, infectious virions are assembled into their capsids, and the cells die, releasing infectious particles [3]. Some of the proteins of the adenovirus are toxic to the cells, perhaps due in part to the suppression of endogenous gene expression.

Adenoviral vectors. Within the adenovirus family, adenoviral types 2 and 5 are the most extensively characterized [16]. Therefore, most adenoviral vectors have been constructed based on the backbone structure of these two subtypes. Deletion of part of the E1 sequence has allowed the construction of

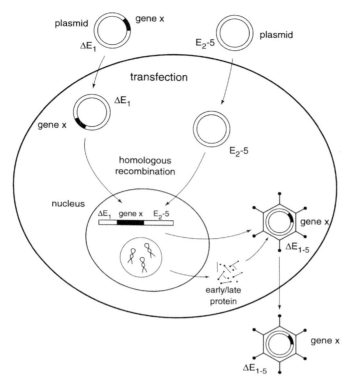

Figure 4. Adenoviral vectors. Adenoviral vectors can be produced by homologous recombination. Two defective plasmids, one of them with the gene of interest, are transfected into a producer cell line. They travel into the nucleus, and by homologous recombination, an adenoviral defective vector is produced. The desired recombinants are then identified by plaquing on 293 cells and screening for the presence of the gene of interest.

replication-defective adenoviral vectors. These vectors are then grown in packaging cell lines, most notably the embryonic-kidney-derived cell line 293 [3], which contain the E1 replicative functions in trans to the vectors. The gene of interest is typically cloned into a plasmid composed of an E1 deleted virus (Ad5 or Ad3). This plasmid is then transfected into 293 cells containing E1 sequences in which the recombinant DNA is replicated and packaged into infective adenoviral particles [17]. Alternatively, a plasmid carrying the gene of interest and E1 sequences is cotransfected into cells infected with adenoviral vectors [18]. Homologous recombination between the plasmid and the adenoviral vector will produce adenoviral defective vectors with the gene of interest (figure 4).

Pitfalls and limitations. Although adenoviral vectors can infect quiescent cells and although the transfection efficiency of these vectors is usually higher than that of retroviral vectors, expression is short-lived for at least three reasons: 1) the adenoviral vector is not integrated into host DNA; 2) the viral proteins stimulate an immune response against the cells infected by the vector; and 3) the vectors are directly toxic to the infected cells [19,20]. Thus, adenoviral vectors will be most suitable for genetic therapy programs that require only short-term expression, as in the case of chemosensitization. Offsetting this disadvantage is the very high frequency of infection and the high level of expression of adenoviral transgenes. Replacement strategies involving adenoviral vectors will require repeated exposure to the adenoviral vector.

Adeno-associated viral vectors

Adeno-associated viral vectors are attractive for use in gene treatment because of their long-term expression, especially in quiescent cells. However, this expression may arise from extrachromosomal vectors. In contrast to the adenovirus itself, which does not integrate into the host chromosomal DNA, the adeno-associated virus (AAV) integrates preferentially into chromosome 19 [21]. The recombinant adeno-associated viral vector from which the REP and CAP genes have been removed randomly integrates into DNA but at very low frequency. Some controversy exists as to whether the integration frequency is as high as once thought; this apparent high frequency of integration, if not measured directly, may be due to long-term episomal expression of the transgene. Most authors report production lots with a low titre. Another limitation of the adenoviral vectors is the small capacity (5 kb) of these vectors for foreign DNA.

Wild-type adeno-associated viral structure and replication. The wild-type adeno-associated virus type 2 has been extensively studied and characterized for use as a vector for genetic therapy. It does not belong to the adenovirus family, but to the parvovirus family. It requires cotransfection with a helper virus such as the adeno or herpes viruses, along with a plasmid that contains the AAV replicative functions, REP and CAP. The DNA viral wild-type genome is composed of two inverted terminal repeats (ITRs), three internal promoters (p3, p19, p40) and two open-reading frames (REP and CAP). CAP encodes viral protein, while REP directs viral replication [22] (figure 5).

In the absence of a helper virus, AAV will integrate into host cells and remain latent. When provided with a helper virus, infectious particles are produced, and the virus enters a lytic cycle. E1A sequences from adenoviruses usually serve helper functions during replication and prior to exit from the host.

AAV vectors. AAV vectors are constructed by deletion of the REP and CAP genes, followed by insertion of the gene of interest into this region. Similar to other vector systems, the modified AAV is transfected into packaging cell lines that provide the required CAP and REP sequences [22].

10

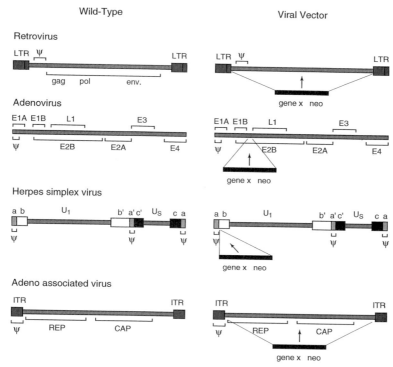

Wild-Type   Viral Vector

Figure 5. Wild-type and viral vector particles. Viral vectors are produced by modification either by replacement (retroviral, adeno-associated virus) or intercalation (herpes simplex, adenovirus) of the gene of interest into the wild-type virus.

Pitfalls and limitations. The major drawback in the use of AAV vectors is the cytolytic activity of REP protein when it is continuously expressed [22]. Furthermore, 40% to 80% of human adults have immunity to AAV, and expression may be limited by a reduction in the numbers of infected cells resulting from immune destruction [23]. Finally, there are reports of modifications of host cells after infection with wild-type AAV strains [24].

Herpes simplex viral vectors

Herpes simplex viral (HSV) vectors have been extensively studied for their potential application in the treatment of neurological disorders due to their tropism for central nervous system (CNS) tissue. The capacity for long-term expression in quiescent neuronal cells has made it an attractive delivery system for the CNS [25]. As in other viral systems, HSV molecular biology and structure is well known, facilitating construction of vectors and helper viruses. Finally, HSV vectors can integrate large sequences of DNA.

Wild-type herpes simplex viral structure and replication. HSV is a double-stranded DNA virus. It is icosahedral and has a surrounding protein layer (tegament) [26]. It has a large (>15 kb) genome encoding approximately 70 genes [25]. The genome is composed of two sequences (Ul Us), flanked by inverted repeats. Wild-type replication of HSV occurs through the sequential transcription of early and late genes. Both lytic and latent phases exist. The latent state is unique to neuronal tissues. The maintenance of the latent state involves downregulation in the transcription of early genes [27].

Herpes simplex vector. Herpes simplex vectors can be constructed by engineering defective viruses or by homologous recombination. Defective viral vectors are constructed by cloning the gene of interest into an HSV amplicon plasmid containing sequences required for replication and packaging, the HSV origin of replication, and a packaging signal [28]. This plasmid is then used to infect a packaging cell line containing regulatory and structural genes required for viral replications. Both defective and helper virions are produced. The defective virions can be incorporated into host cells but cannot replicate in the absence of a helper virion. The defective and helper viruses cannot be physically separated. Alternatively, recombinant HSV vectors are constructed by inserting the gene of interest into a fragment of HSV [29]. This plasmid and wild-type HSV are cotransfected into a permissive cell line. Homologous recombination yields progeny virus consisting of parental wild-type virus and recombinant virions containing the gene of interest. The yield of recombinant virus is increased by using an excess of plasmid over viral DNA.

Pitfalls and limitations. Drawbacks of HSV vectors include the potential for recombination between plasmid and viral sequences. In addition, there are potentially lethal and oncogenic effects of encoding toxic sequences and transcription factors.

Cancer gene therapy

Isolation of hematopoietic stem cells, genetic modification, and reinfusion after high-dose chemotherapy is at present the only way of achieving long-term systemic expression of genetically modified cells in humans. Therefore, stem cell transplantation forms the basis for many of the current clinical approaches to gene therapy. Several stem cell transplant gene therapy trials are currently underway. The goals of these trials are as follows: 1) chemoprotection of stem cells with potential applications for the delivery of missing factors and cytotoxic agents; 2) evaluation of the role of contaminating cells in the graft as a source of relapse; 3) modulation of graft-vs.-host disease and graft-vs.-tumor effects; and 4) investigation of the local delivery of suicide genes for genetic chemosensitization and gene-mediated immune activation.

12

Gene marking trials

The first clinical trials using genetically modified human cells studied the trafficking and persistence of various malignant and nonmalignant cells after in vitro retroviral transduction. The aims of these studies were 1) to determine whether contamination of the infused autologous stem cell transplant with tumor or leukemia cells contributes to relapse; 2) to evaluate the reconstitutive capacity of blood vs. bone marrow stem cells following autologous stem cell transplant; and 3) to test whether tumor-infiltrating lymphocyte (TIL) infused for therapy selectively home to the tumor tissue.

Gene marking trials to determine the origin of relapse after peripheral blood or marrow autologous transplant. The delivery of high-dose chemotherapy regimens followed by autologous transplant have increased the disease-free survival and overall survival in some hematologic malignancies and solid tumors. In some of these malignancies, the bone marrow can itself become infiltrated with tumor cells. Neoplastic involvement of the bone marrow has prevented the use of high-dose chemotherapy and stem cell rescue due to concerns regarding the role of the graft in relapse posttransplant. In follicular lymphomas, for example, Gribben and collaborators have shown that patients whose autografts are positive for the indolent lymphoma marker t(14;18) after immunopurging have a shorter disease-free survival following transplant than do patients in whom no residual lymphoma cells were detectable [30]. At the time of relapse, it is impossible to determine whether systemic therapy failed to eradicate all of the systemic disease, or whether infusion of neoplastic cells contributed to relapse. Gene marking trials are being used to tag or mark the infused cells so that at the time of relapse, the neoplastic cells can be tested for the retroviral transgenes. Positive tests for such cells would suggest that the relapse arises at least in part from the infused cells. Data concerning the origin of relapse after autologous transplants are available from five marking trials: two for acute myeloblastic leukemia (AML) [31–33], one for chronic myelogenous leukemia (CML) [34–37], one for neuroblastoma [38], and one for multiple myeloma and breast cancer [39].

Transduction systems used in gene marking trials. The vectors in gene marking trials have utilized the murine Moloney leukemia virus long terminal repeat as a promoter and the neomycin phosphotransferase gene to mark normal hematopoietic and malignant cells. This protein is absent in human cells and confers upon the infected cells resistance to the antibiotic neomycin and some of its analogues. As explained earlier, partial deletion of retroviral sequences makes these retroviruses replication incompetent, thus permitting their safe use in the introduction of foreign genetic material into mammalian cells. Most if not all of the transductions in these marking trials involved incubation of bone marrow stem cells in cell-free retroviral supernatants for six hours. These cells were then frozen until the day of the transplant when they were thawed and infused back into the recipient to generate hematopoietic reconstitution. Transduction efficiencies were determined by polymerase chain reaction (PCR) amplification of retroviral sequences in blood and bone marrow after hematopoietic recovery and by measuring the number of colonies grown in semi-solid media after exposure to neomycin. Transduction efficiencies in these trials averaged between 1% and 5%. Results from the trials of Brenner in AML and Deisseroth in CML showed that the relapsed cells contained the Neo viral marker, suggesting that the relapse arose, at least in part, from the infused cells. A similar result was also shown for autografts in neuroblastoma patients [38]. In addition, genetically modified cells have persisted in the normal hematopoietic population, suggesting that cells with significant proliferative potential have been genetically modified in these trials. More recently, in an attempt at increasing transduction efficiencies, Dunbar and collaborators at the National Cancer Institute have used hematopoietic growth factors and a longer retroviral supernatant incubation period [39]. They analyzed the role of marrow and peripheral blood stem cells in relapse and their hematopoietic reconstitutive capacity following high-dose chemotherapy. Patients with breast cancer and multiple myeloma underwent peripheral blood progenitor cell and bone marrow collection. A fraction of these cells underwent CD34-positive selection using the CellPro column. CD34-positive cells from the bone marrow and the peripheral blood were then incubated with either G_1Na or LNL6 retroviral vectors for 72 hours in the presence of growth factors. Differences in the sequences of G_1Na and LNL6 allowed for semiquantification of marked cells after hematopoietic reconstitution.

The authors were able to show that both peripheral blood and bone marrow stem cells can contribute to hematopoietic reconstitution. However, the frequency of the transduced cells that contained the neomycin marker was low and short-lived. Furthermore, the authors have not yet been able to document marker sequences in malignant cells at the time of relapse. It is possible that the use of hematopoietic growth factors could have driven cells into a differentiation pathway, thereby limiting their long-term reconstitutive capacity. Other factors determining the transduction efficiencies in these trials include damage to the stem cells' reconstitutive capability due to previous exposure to alkylating-agent chemotherapy. It can be concluded from these trials that bone marrow transplants may contribute at least in part to relapse in patients with CML, AML, and neuroblastoma. The degree to which malignant cells that are infused with the autograft rather than residual tumor cells surviving intensive systemic therapy contribute to relapse is unclear.

These studies also showed that retroviral vectors are present in normal hematopoietic cells of all lineages, including myeloid and lymphoid cells, for up to 18 months, suggesting that an early hematopoietic progenitor was transduced. Additional gene marking trials, which are designed to test this question of origin of relapse, are ongoing in other malignancies, including non-Hodgkin's lymphoma, acute lymphoblastic leukemia, and breast cancer (table 2).

14

Table 2. Trials of replication-incompetent retroviruses for marking hematopoietic cells

Goal	Investigator (Institution)	Disease
Identification of the origin of relapse and evaluation of hematopoietic reconstitution of the autologous transplant, and the evaluation of purging	Brenner (St. Jude)	AML
	Brenner (St. Jude)	Neuroblastoma
	Deisseroth (M.D. Anderson)	CML
	Deisseroth (M.D. Anderson)	CLL
	Deisseroth (M.D. Anderson)	NHL
	Schüning (Fred Hutchinson)	Isograft
	Schüning (Fred Hutchinson)	HD/NHL
	Schüning (Fred Hutchinson)	Breast
	Dunbar (NIH)	Myeloma
	Dunbar (NIH)	CML
	O'Shaughnessy (NIH)	Breast
	Cornetta (Univ. of Indiana)	AML, ALL
In vivo trafficking of lymphocytes	Rosenberg (NIH)	TILs (cancer)
	Lotze (Univ. of Pittsburgh)	TILs (melanoma)
	Economou (UCLA)	TILs (renal cell, melanoma)
	Favrot, Merrouche (France)	TILs (cancer)
	Heslop (St. Jude)	Cytotoxic T lymphocytes
	Freedman (M.D. Anderson)	TILs (ovarian)
Comparison of the reconstitutive capability of peripheral blood and marrow	Deisseroth (M.D. Anderson)	CML
	Brenner (St. Jude)	AML; breast
	Dunbar (NIH)	Metastatic breast; myeloma
	O'Shaughnessy (NIH)	Breast
	Schüning (Fred Hutchinson)	Breast; HD lymphoid malignancies
	Douer/Norris (USC)	Breast; lymphoma
	Bjorkstrand/Gahrton (Sweden)	Myeloma

Abbreviations: TILs, tumor infiltrating lymphocytes; ALL, acute lymphocytic leukemia; NHL, non-Hodgkin's lymphoma; HD, Hodgkin's disease; CLL, chronic lymphocytic leukemia; CML, chronic myelogenous leukemia; AML, acute myelogenous leukemia.

Tumor-infiltrating lymphocyte marking trials

Novel treatment approaches in cancer include the ex vivo activation of lymphocytes against malignant cells. Tumor cells express antigens including the MHC 1 molecules recognized by cytotoxic T-cells. Through recognition of these antigens, T-cells become activated, resulting in cytotoxic activity against tumor cells in part due to an increase in IL-2 production. If either the cellular cytoadhesion molecules CD28 or the T-cell receptor is not expressed by the lymphocytes, and if the B_7 antigen is not present at sufficient density on the antigen-presenting (tumor) cells, the activated lymphocytes undergo apoptosis. This abrogates the lymphocyte response, possibly by eliminating the lymphocyte's capacity to recognize tumor cells, thus producing a state of anergy.

Thus, cancer cells that have defective antigen presentation proteins or inadequate levels may produce a state of anergy, crippling the immune system's capacity to kill cancer cells. Studies have shown that MHC 1 antigens and B_7 costimulatory molecules are present in tumor cells in suboptimal concentrations for immune activation. Several workers have proposed the use of genetic modification to enhance the cellular immune response to cancer cells. These techniques have included isolation of lymphocytes infiltrating tumors, their expansion through exposure to IL-2, and reinfusion of these cells into patients with various malignancies.

Cancer vaccine gene therapy trials

Since the current vector systems modify only a percentage of the target cells, genetic modification of somatic cells for cancer control should ideally generate a durable systemic immune response on the basis of modification of a few cells. Examples of such strategies include 1) immunoenhancement based on tumor-specific and anti-idiotypic antibodies or through immune activation after exposure of effector cells to autologous tumors; and 2) subcutaneous inoculation of irradiated tumor cells that have been transfected with cytokines, costimulatory molecules, or MHC antigens [40,41]. Only minor responses were seen initially in a small fraction of the patients treated by Nabel who directly transferred DNA to the tumor cells. Therefore, alternative delivery systems are currently under study.

Animal studies have shown that naked plasmid DNA containing neoantigens can elicit an immune response [42,43]. The mechanisms of uptake and internalization of plasmid DNA are not well known. At least in muscle cells, the process seems to be energy dependent. After uptake, plasmid DNA is internalized through T-tubules and delivered to the nucleus. Once in the nucleus, plasmid DNA persists as a nonepisomal molecule leading to dose-dependent and long-lived expression [44]. The mechanism by which plasmid DNA can elicit an immune response is even less well understood. It appears to involve coexpression of transcribed proteins with MHC and costimulatory proteins. Tumor antigens such as carcinoembryonic antigen (CEA) or prostatic-specific antigen (PSA) could be used to enhance immune responses. This methodology may be a way of increasing host immune responses against tumor cells and is currently under study.

Other strategies designed to enhance immune responses include the use of genetically modified tumor cells with viral vectors containing cytokines known to stimulate cytotoxic T-cells. There are now more than ten ongoing clinical trials in which cytokines such as IL-2, TNF, and interferon are overexpressed in tumor cells through the use of retroviral vectors [45–50] (table 3). These strategies produce local concentrations of proteins that promote the recruitment of accessory cells in the immune response.

Chemotherapy sensitization genes

Genes coding for proteins that activate chemotherapeutic agents may be used to increase the selectivity required to kill cancer cells without damaging normal cells. A number of prodrugs that are nontoxic unless metabolized to toxic

16

Table 3. Immunotherapy clinical trials

Disease	Gene	Investigator (Institution)
Advanced Cancer	HLA-B7	Nabel (U. Michigan)
	IL-2	Rosenberg (NIH)
		Hersh (Arizona Cancer Center)
	GM-CSF	Dranoff (Dana Farber)
	IL-4	Lotze (Univ. of Pittsburgh)
	IL-12	Lotze/Tahara(Univ. Pittsburgh)
	TNF	Rosenberg (NIH)
Brain	IL-2	Sobol/Royston (San Diego)
	IL-2/TGF-β2	Black/Fakhrai (UCLA)
	IGF-1 Antisense	Ilan (Case Western Reserve)
Colon	IL-2	Sobol/Royston (San Diego)
	CEA	Curiel (Univ. of Alabama)
	HLA-B7	Rubin (Mayo Clinic)
Breast	IL-2	Kim Lyerly (Duke University)
Prostate	GM-CSF	Simons (Johns Hopkins)
Lung	IL-2	Mao (China)
		Cassileth (Univ. of Miami)
Melanoma	IL-2	Economou (UC Medical Center)
		Gansbacher (Sloan-Kettering)
		Osanto (Netherlands)
		Das Gupta (Univ. of Illinois)
		Cascinelli/Foa (Italy)
	IL-4	Chang (Univ. of Michigan)
		Cascinelli/Fao (Italy)
	HLA-B7	Sznol/Fenton (NIH)
		Hersh (Arizona Cancer Center)
	IFNγ	Seigler (Duke University)
Renal	IL-2	Gansbacher (Sloan-Kettering)
	HLA-B7	Vogelzang (Univ. Chicago)
	GM-CSF	Simons (John Hopkins)
Colon/renal melanoma	IL-7	Schmidt-Wolf (Germany)
Neuroblastoma	IL-2	Brenner (St. Jude)
	IFN	Rosenblatt/Seeger (UCLA)

Abbreviations: HLA, human leukocyte antigen; IL, interleuken; TNF, tumor necorsis factor; TGF, tumor growth factor; CEA, carcinoembryonic antigen; GM-CSF, granulocyte-macrophage colony stimulating factor; IFNγ, interferon-gamma; IFN, interferon.

intermediates by various enzymes are available for use. Some of the required enzymes are absent in both malignant and nonmalignant mammalian cells. Gene therapy approaches aimed at introducing these drug-converting or -activating enzymes into malignant cells could selectively sensitize cells without damaging normal cells that lack these genes. To achieve selectivity, these genes must be transfected so that only the malignant cells express the converting enzyme. To date, most centers are exploring the use of herpes virus thymidine kinase and the bacterial cytosine deaminase genes in clinical trials

Table 4. Herpes virus thymidine kinase gene sensitization in cancer

Disease	Investigator (Institution)
Brain tumor	Eck/Alavi (Univ. of Pennsylvania Medical Center)
	Grossman (Baylor College of Medicine)
	Raffel/Culver (Children's Hospital Los Angeles)
	Kun (St. Jude Children Hospital)
	Oldfield (NINDS, DHHS)
	Culver/Van Gilder (Iowa Methodist Medical Center)
Head and neck	Gluckman/Stambrook (U. Cincinnati Medical Center)
Melanoma	Klatzmann (France)
Carcinoma	Oldfield (NINDS, DHHS)
Mesothelioma	Albelda (Univ. of Pennsylvania Medical Center)
Ovary	Freeman (Tulane University)

involving drug sensitization (table 4). Both of these enzymes are from nonmammalian sources. A number of other prodrug sensitization strategies are under development in several centers.

Thymidine kinase

Thymidine kinase phosphorylates thymidine, providing enough substrate for DNA synthesis. The herpes-virus-family thymidine kinase phosphorylates not only thymidine but also guanosine analogues such as acyclovir and gancyclovir, which inhibit viral replication through the incorporation of a variant nucleotide into viral DNA. These drugs are commonly used in the treatment and prevention of viral infection. The phosphorylated substrates can mimic endogenous guanosine and are utilized for DNA synthesis. Although they can be incorporated into DNA, they prevent further elongation of DNA chains by DNA polymerase [51]. Administration of gancyclovir at low doses to cells transfected with HSV-TK genes is associated with a selective cytotoxic effect [52]. Furthermore, animal models in which HSV-TK-transfected tumors are systematically exposed to gancyclovir have shown significant reduction in tumor volume and prolongation of survival [53]. Interestingly, it has been shown that in a cell population composed of a mixture of cells expressing the HSV-TK and cells not expressing the HSV-TK, the cells lacking HSV-TK sequences also die after exposure to gancyclovir. This phenomenon has been termed the 'bystander effect.' Phosphorylated gancyclovir from neighboring cells can gain access to HSV-TK-negative cells either through uptake from the extracellular space or directly via intracellular gap junctions. The exact mechanism for this bystander effect is unknown.

18

Cytosine deaminase

The enzyme cytosine deaminase deaminates cytosine to uracil. It also converts the relatively nontoxic 5-fluorocytosine (5-FC) into the cytotoxic compound 5-fluorouracil. This enzyme is present in some fungi and bacteria but is absent in mammalian cells. Thus, 5-FC is used as a therapeutic agent to treat yeast and fungal infections. Introduction of cytosine deaminase into pancreatic and colon cancer cell lines sensitizes them to the toxic effects of 5-FC [54]. Using this strategy, enhanced cytotoxic activity has been demonstrated in animal models of xenograft tumors transfected with cytosine deaminase [55]. A trial of cytosine deaminase in colon cancer metastatic to liver, developed by Dr. Ronald Crystal, has been approved by the National Institutes of Health Recombinant DNA Advisory Committee.

Suicide gene therapy trials

Due to the difficulty in delivering viral vectors to different sites of metastasis, genetic chemosensitization approaches have been developed for the treatment of localized tumors at single primary sites. Primary CNS tumors are ideal candidates, since 1) they are restricted to the brain and are usually unresectable due to their location; 2) adjacent, normal CNS cells are quiescent and therefore unlikely to be transduced by retroviral vectors or affected by gancyclovir; and 3) not all tumor cells need to be transduced, since the bystander effect may allow for untransduced cells to be eradicated. In fact, this bystander effect was first demonstrated in an animal model of brain gliomas [56]. The method of delivery in early trials using HSV-TK suicide genes for brain tumors included direct injection of producer cell lines containing the HSV-TK vector or infusion of retroviral or adenoviral vectors into the tumor bed to allow for increased and prolonged exposure to viral particles. Preliminary results of HSV-TK gene therapy trials for brain tumors have shown partial tumor responses in some but not all patients, but a cure has not yet been achieved [57].

Other malignancies in which suicide HSV-TK gene therapy is undergoing clinical evaluation include ovarian cancer, melanoma, head and neck cancer, and mesotheliomas. At the University of Texas M.D. Anderson Cancer Center, we are evaluating, in collaboration with Dr. Ronald Crystal, an adenoviral vector containing cytosine deaminase as a purging reagent to eradicate malignant epithelial cancer cells from stem cell autografts from breast cancer patients. Since nonhematopoietic cells, but not hematopoietic cells, can be infected with adenoviral vectors, this system ensures that only malignant cells will be transduced with the HSV-TK vector. In vitro experiments show that this system can kill transduced MCF-7 breast cancer cells after exposure to 5-FC. Untransduced controls are unaffected by the exposure to the prodrug.

Severe acute and chronic graft-vs.-host disease (GVHD) occurs in approximately 20% to 40% of matched HLA identical siblings. Prophylaxis and treatment consists mainly of ex vivo T-cell depletion of the marrow graft and posttransplant immunosuppression. The former is associated with an increased risk of graft rejection and a decrease in graft-vs.-leukemia effect (GVL), while the latter increases the risk of infections. Suicide genes are under investigation as modulators of GVL and GVHD. T-cells, expanded ex vivo and transduced with an HSV-TK/neo retrovirus, can be enriched by incubation in neomycin [58]. Exposure of these expanded and transduced cells to gancyclovir not only abolishes 80% of their growth but also completely inhibits allogeneic reactivity in vitro. This approach could allow for more effective treatment of GVHD while maintaining a GVL effect if patients receiving allografts with genetically modified T-cells are exposed to gancyclovir at the onset of acute or chronic GVHD.

Antisense cancer gene therapy

Disruption of translation or processing of mRNA transcripts from genes implicated in carcinogenesis forms the basis for antisense approaches to cancer gene therapy. The expression of mRNA implicated in malignant transformation, such as c-myc, bcr-abl, bcl-2, p53, can be blocked by the binding of mRNA oligonucleotides to endogenously synthesized mRNA. Two approaches have been developed: 1) direct infusion of antisense oligomers [59] or 2) transfection of vector systems encoding the antisense sequences [60] (table 5). Several obstacles must be overcome before antisense oligonucleotides become clinically applicable for the treatment of human disease.

DNA degradation. Mammalian cells protect themselves against foreign DNA and RNA with nucleases that degrade cytosolic phosphodiesters. Methods to render antisense sequences resistant to nucleases include phosphodiester backbone substitutions. Oligodeoxynucleotide analogues that substitute one of the phosphate oxygens, forming a resistant bond, are now available.

Delivery and cell uptake. Antisense oligonucleotides delivered systematically must be water soluble, reach significantly high serum concentrations, and

Table 5. Anti-oncogenes/antisense clinical trials

Disease	Gene	Investigator (Institution)
Lung	p53/K-ras (Antisense)	Roth (M.D. Anderson Cancer Center)
Head and neck	p53	Clayman (M.D. Anderson Cancer Center)
Colorectal/liver	p53	Venook/Warren (UCSF)
Breast	c-fos/c-myc (Antisense)	Holt/Arteaga (Vanderbilt University)
CML	bcr/abl (Antisense) c-myb (Antisense)	Bishop (Univ. of Nebraska Medical Center) Luger/Gewirtz (Univ. of Pennsylvania)

Abbreviation: CML, chronic myelogenous leukemia.

gain access to tumor cells. Several studies on the pharmacokinetics of oligodeoxynucleotides have been reported in animal models. Some of the analogues previously mentioned are water soluble, and sufficient tissue concentrations have been achieved after intravenous injection. The mean half-life in these animal models is 34 hours [61]. Other means of delivery includes direct infusion into tumors and systemic delivery via liposomal complexes.

Tumor resistance. Even if antisense oligonucleotides bind and inhibit expression of target mRNA, tumor growth may not be inhibited if multiple genetic lesions contribute to malignant transformation. For this reason, antisense approaches should be directed when possible to downstream regulators of oncogenic products. For example, c-fos acts downstream to regulate known proto-oncogene products such as c-src, c-vas, or c-raf. The potential application of c-fos inhibition has been demonstrated in an in vitro model. In this model, c-fos antisense was able to decrease c-fos mRNA and protein, to restore density-dependent growth arrest, and to reduce tumorigenicity on simian sarcoma-virus-infected NIH-3T3 cells [64]. Stimulation of this cell line with PDGF-like molecules leads to c-fos expression, which is necessary for the expression of the transformed phenotype.

Hematopoietic chemoprotection

Ex vivo expansion of hematopoietic progenitors and reinfusion after myeloblative chemotherapy may allow repetitive cycles of dose-intensive chemotherapy to be administered without the potential risk of permanent bone marrow aplasia. This approach may favorably impact the outcome of tumors with steep dose–response curves. A similar approach is under investigation whereby hematopoietic progenitors are made resistant to the effects of chemotherapy.

The multiple drug resistant (MDR) gene encodes an energy-dependent 170-kDa glycoprotein (p-glycoprotein) that transports chemotherapeutic agents out of cells. Expression of this glycoprotein is but one of many mechanisms by which cancer cells become resistant to the effects of chemotherapeutic agents such as anthracyclines, vinca alkaloids, and epipodophylotoxins. P-glycoprotein has also been shown to be expressed at high levels in CD34+ bone marrow stem cells [63]. If this MDR gene can be further overexpressed in hematopoietic stem cells, these cells may become resistant to the effect of increasing doses of chemotherapeutic drugs. An animal model has already shown the potential benefits of this approach. Serial transplantation studies in mice transplanted with stem cells transduced with retroviral MDR vectors followed by several cycles of treatment with Taxol have shown that the number of progenitors containing the transgene increase with each cycle of chemotherapy. At the same time, their sensitivity to chemotherapy increased to the point of becoming virtually resistant to this agent. These early reports have stimulated the use of MDR retroviral chemoprotection in phase I clinical trials

Table 6. Chemoprotection for breast or ovarian cancer

Tissue modified	Investigators (Institution)
Bone marrow	Kavanagh/Hanania/Deisseroth (M.D. Anderson Cancer Center) Hanania/Rahman/Holmes/Hortobagyi/Deisseroth (M.D. Anderson Cancer Center)
Peripheral blood stem cells	O'Shaughnessy (NIH) Bank/Hesdorffer/Antman (Columbia University)

in ovarian and breast cancer by groups in the United States and one in The Netherlands (table 6). With this strategy, women with advanced ovarian and breast cancer will undergo CD34-positive selection and transduction of these marrow or peripheral blood cells with a retroviral vector containing the MDR sequence. After high-dose myeloblative chemotherapy and reinfusion of modified hematopoietic progenitors, these patients will be exposed to increasing doses of Taxol, a drug active in breast and ovarian cancer. Treatment with chemotherapy in the early posttransplant stage is usually not well tolerated due to a decreased stem cell pool posttransplant. It is hoped that by protecting and enriching these modified stem cells, hematopoietic resistance will ensue. Other genetic strategies to increase resistance of hematopoietic cells include retroviral transduction of a mutated dihydrofolate reductase gene to confer resistance to methotrexate or retroviral transduction of the enzyme alkyltransferase for resistance to nitrosureas [64,65]. No clinical trials using these two approaches have been submitted to NIH regulatory committees. Genetic chemosensitization, if successful, could be applied to the replacement of important proteins such as coagulation factors and to the delivery of therapeutic molecules by genetically modified hematopoietic cells followed by enrichment of these cells with agents such as Taxol, methotrexate, or alkylating agents.

Future directions

Although important advances have been made in the use of genetic modifications for use in clinical trials, there are important obstacles that must be overcome before this strategy can be available for general use. Transduction efficiency must be improved. Newer systems including use of stromal cell monolayers, liposomal particles, and more efficient retroviral constructs may bring about higher transduction efficiencies. The problem of tumor selectivity and systemic delivery must be overcome to allow specific and widespread delivery of target sequences to tumor sites. Finally, gene therapy must be made accessible and economically feasible for general use, especially in these days of economic stringency. There has been significant controversy regarding the rapid proliferation of gene therapy clinical trials and the large amount of money spent in these trials. This issue prompted the creation of an NIH-sponsored panel to evaluate present results and future directions of gene therapy studies. It is clear that more work needs to be done in the basic science of gene therapy. Nevertheless, the advances already achieved merit the continuous investigation of certain gene therapy approaches in well-designed clinical studies.

References

1. Wei CM, Gibson M, Spear PG, et al. Construction and isolation of transmissible retrovirus containing the src gene of Harvey murine sarcoma virus and thymidine kinase gene of herpes simplex virus type 1. J Virol 39:935–944, 1981.
2. Anderson WF, Blaese RM, Culver K. The ADA human gene therapy clinical protocol. Human Gene Ther 1:331–362, 1990.
3. Coffin JM. Retroviridae and their replication. In Fields BN, Knipe DM (eds), Virology, 2nd ed. New York: Raven Press, 1990, pp. 1437–1489.
4. Miller AD, Miller DG, Garcia JV, et al. Use of retroviral vectors for gene transfer and expression. Methods Enzymol 217:581–599, 1993.
5. Miller AD, Jolly DJ, Friedman T, et al. A transmissible retrovirus expressing human hypoxanthine phosphoribosyltransferase (HPRT) gene transfer into cells obtained from humans deficient in HPRT. Proc Natl Acad Sci USA 80:4709–4713, 1983.
6. Hock RA, Miller AD, Osborne WRA. Expression of a human adenosine deaminase from various strong promoters after gene transfer into human hematopoietic cell lines. Blood 74:876–881, 1989.
7. Overell RW, Weisser KE, Cosman D. Stably transmitted triple-promoter retroviral vectors and their use in transformation of primary mammalian cells. Mol Cell Biol 8:1803–1808, 1988.
8. Dzierzak EA, Papayannopoulou T, Mulligan RC. Lineage-specific expression of a human β-globin gene in murine bone marrow transplant recipients reconstituted with retrovirus-transduced stem cells. Nature 331:35–41, 1988.
9. Jolly DJ, Barber JR, Respess JG, et al. 'Packaging cells' patent application PCT WO 92/05266, 1992.
10. Burns JC, Friedman T, Driever W, et al. Vesicular stomatitis virus glycoprotein pseudotyped retroviral vectors: concentration to very high titer and efficient gene transfer into mammalian and non-mammalian cells. Proc Natl Acad Sci USA 90:8033–8037, 1993.
11. Horwitz MS. Adenoviridae and their replication. In Fields BN, Knipe DM (eds), Virology, 2nd ed. New York: Raven Press, 1990, pp. 1679–1712.
12. Meiklejohn G. Viral respiratory disease at Lowry Air Force Base in Denver, 1952–1982. J Infect Dis 148:775–784, 1983.
13. Shields AF, Hackman RC, Fife KH, et al. Adenovirus infections in patients undergoing bone marrow transplantation. N Engl J Med 312:529–533, 1985.
14. Zahradnik JM, Spencer MJ, Porter DD. Adenovirus infection in the immunocompromised patient. Am J Med 68:725–732, 1980.
15. Michael SI, Curiel DT. Strategies to achieve targeted gene delivery via the receptor mediated endocytosis pathway. Gene Ther 1:223–232, 1994.
16. Chroboczek J, Bieber F, Jacrot B. The sequence of the genome of adenovirus type 5 and its comparison with the genome of adenovirus type 2. Virology 186:280–285, 1992.
17. Stratford LD, Levero M, Chase JF, et al. Evaluation of the transfer and expression of mice of an enzyme-encoding gene using human adenovirus vector. Human Gene Ther 1:241–256, 1990.
18. Graham FL, Prevec L. Manipulation of adenovirus vectors. In Murray EJ (ed), Methods in Molecular Biology. Clifton, NJ: Humana Press, 1991, pp. 109–128.

19. Rich DP, Berger HA, Chen SH, et al. Development and analysis of recombinant adenoviruses for gene therapy of cystic fibrosis. Human Gene Ther 4:461–476, 1993.
20. Yang Y, Nunes FA, Berencsi K, et al. Cellular immunity to viral antigens limits E1-deleted adenoviruses for gene therapy. Proc Natl Acad Sci USA 91:4407–4411, 1994.
21. Kotin RM, Linden RM, Berns KI. Characterization of a preferred site on chromosome 19q for integration of adeno-associated virus DNA by non-homologous recombination. EMBO J 11:5071–5078, 1992.
22. McLaughlin SK, Collis P, Hermonat PL, et al. Adeno-associated virus general transduction vectors: analysis of proviral structures. J Virol 62:1963–1973, 1988.
23. Muzyczka N. Use of adeno-associated virus as a general transduction vector for mammalian cells. Current Topics Microbiol Immunol 158:97–129, 1992.
24. Grossman Z, Mendelson E, Brok-Simoni F, et al. Detection of adeno-associated virus type 2 in human peripheral blood cells. J Gen Virol 73:961–966, 1992.
25. Geller AL, Keyomarski K, Bryan J, et al. An efficient deletion mutant packaging system for defective HSV-1 vectors; potential applications to neuronal physiology and human gene therapy. Proc Natl Acad Sci USA 87:8950–8954, 1990.
26. Harris RA, Everett RD, Zhu X, et al. Herpes simplex virus type 1 immediate-early protein Vmw 110 reactivates latent herpes simplex virus type 2 in an in-vitro latency system. J Virol 63:3513–3515, 1989.
27. Spivack JG, Fraser NW. Detection of herpes simplex virus type 1 transcripts during latent infection in mice. J Virol 61:3841–3847, 1987.
28. Palella TD, Hidaka Y, Silverman LJ, et al. Expression of human HPRT mRNA in brains of mice infected with a recombinant herpes simplex virus-1 vector. Gene 80:137–144, 1989.
29. Geller AI, Keyomarsi K, Bryan J, et al. An efficient deletion mutant packaging system for defective herpes simplex virus vectors: potential applications to human gene therapy and neuronal physiology. Proc Natl Acad Sci USA 87:8950–8954, 1990.
30. Gribben JG, Neuberg D, Freedman AS, et al. Detection by polymerase chain reaction of residual cells with the bcl-2 translocation is associated with increased risk of relapse after autologous bone marrow transplantation for B-cell lymphoma. Blood 81:3449, 1993.
31. Rill DR, Moen RC, Buschle M, et al. An approach for the analysis of relapse and marrow reconstitution after autologous marrow transplantation using retrovirusmediated gene transfer. Blood 79:2694–2700, 1992.
32. Brenner M, Rill D, Moen RC, et al. Gene marking to origin of relapse after autologous bone marrow transplantation. Lancet 341:85–86, 1993.
33. Brenner MK, Rill DR, Holladay MS, et al. Gene marking to determine whether autologous marrow infusion restores long-term hematopoiesis in cancer patients. Lancet 342:1134–1137, 1993.
34. Deisseroth AB. Autologous bone marrow transplantation for CML in which retroviral markers are used to discriminate between relapse which arises from systemic disease remaining after preparative therapy versus relapse due to residual leukemia cells in autologous marrow: a pilot trial. Human Gene Ther 2:359–376, 1991.
35. Claxton D, Suh S-P, Filaccio M, et al. Molecular analysis of retroviral transduction in chronic myelogenous leukemia. Human Gene Ther 2:317–321, 1991.
36. Etkin M, Filaccio M, Ellerson D, et al. Use of cell-free retroviral vector preparations for transduction of cells from the marrow of chronic phase and blast crisis chronic myelogenous leukemia patients and from normal individuals. Human Gene Ther 3:137–145, 1992.
37. Deisseroth AB, Zu Z, Claxton D, et al. Gene marking shows that Ph+ cells present in autologous transplants of chronic myelogenous leukemia contribute to relapse after autologous bone marrow in CML. Blood 83:3068–3076, 1994.
38. Rill DR, Buschle M, Foreman NK, et al. Retrovirus-mediated gene transfer as an approach to analyze neuroblastoma relapse after autologous bone marrow transplantation. Human Gene Ther 3:129–136, 1992.
39. Dunbar CE, Cotler Fox M, O'Shaughnessy JA, et al. Retrovirally marked CD34-enriched

24

peripheral blood and bone marrow cells contribute to long-term engraftment after autologous transplantation. Blood 85:3048–3057, 1995.

40. Pardoll DM. Cancer vaccines. Immunol Today 14:310–316, 1993.
41. Dalgleish AG. Cancer vaccines. Eur J Cancer 30:1029–1035, 1994.
42. Tang D, DeWit M, Johnston SA. Genetic immunization is a simple method for eliciting an immune response. Nature 356:152–154, 1992.
43. Cox GJ, Zaub TL, Babiuk LA. Bovine herpes virus I: immune responses in mice and cattle injected with plasmid DNA. J Virol 67:5664–5667, 1993.
44. Wolff JA, et al. Long-term persistence of plasmid DNA and foreign gene expression in mouse muscle. Human Mol Gen 1:363–369, 1992.
45. Aebersold P, Kasid A, Rosenberg SA. Selection of gene marked tumor infiltration lymphocytes from post treatment biopsies: a case study. Human Gene Ther 1:373–384, 1990.
46. Schendel DJ, Gansbacher B, Oberneder R, et al. Tumor-specific lysis of human renal cell carcinomas by tumor-infiltrating lymphocytes I. HLA-A2-restricted recognition of autologous and allogeneic tumor lines. J Immunol 151:4209–4220, 1993.
47. Chen L, Ashe S, Brady WA, et al. Costimulation of antitumor immunity by the B7 counterreceptor for the T lymphocyte molecules CD28 and CTLA-4. Cell 71:1093–1102, 1992.
48. Nabel GJ. Immunotherapy of malignancy by in vivo gene transfer into tumors. Human Gene Ther 3:399–410, 1992.
49. Mulligan R. The basic science of gene therapy. Science 260:926–932, 1993.
50. Schendel DJ, Gansbacher B. Tumor-specific lysis of human renal cell carcinomas by tumor infiltrating lymphocytes: modulation of recognition through retroviral transduction of tumor cells with interleukin 2 complementary DNA and exogenous alpha-interferon treatment. Cancer Res 53:4020–4025, 1993.
51. Reid R, Eng-Chun M, Eng Shang H, et al. Insertion and extension of acyclic, dideoxy, and ara nucleotides by herpesviridae, human alpha and human beta polymerases. J Biol Chem 263:3898–3904, 1988.
52. Freeman SM, Abboud CN, Whartenby KA, et al. The 'bystander effect': tumor regression when a fraction of the tumor mass is genetically modified. Cancer Res 53:5274–5283, 1993.
53. Ram Z, Culver KW, Wallbridge S, et al. In situ retroviral-mediated gene transfer for the treatment of brain tumors in rats. Cancer Res 53:83–88, 1993.
54. Huber BE, Austin EA, Good SS, et al. In vivo antitumor activity of 5-fluorocytosine on human colorectal carcinoma cells genetically modified to express cytosine deaminase. Cancer Res 53:4619–4626, 1993.
55. Harris JD, Gutierrez AA, Hurst HC, et al. Gene therapy for cancer using tumour-specific prodrug activation. Gene Ther 1:170–175, 1994.
56. Culver KW, Ram Z, Wallbridge S, et al. In vivo gene transfer with retroviral vector producer cells for treatment of experimental brain tumors. Science 256:1550–1552, 1992.
57. Fairbairn LJ, Cross MA, Arrand JR. Meeting report. Paterson Symposium 1993 — gene therapy. Br J Cancer 69:972–975, 1994.
58. Tiberghien P, Reynolds CW, Keller J, et al. Gancyclovir treatment of herpes simplex thymidine kinase-transduced primary T lymphocytes: an approach for specific in vivo donor T-cell depletion after bone marrow transplantation. Blood 84:1333–1341, 1994.
59. Steele C, Sacks PG, Adler SK, et al. Effect on cancer cells of plasmids that express antisense RNA of human papilloma virus 18. Cancer Res 52:4706–4711, 1992.
60. Colobretta B, Sims RR, Valtieri M, et al. Normal and leukemic hematopoietic cells manifest differential sensitivity to inhibitory effects of c-myb antisense oligonucleotides: an in-vitro study with relevance to bone marrow purging. Proc Natl Acad Sci USA 88:2351–2355, 1991.
61. Iversen P, Mata, J, Zon G. The single-injection pharmacokinetics of an antisense phosphorothioate oligodeoxynucleotide against rev (art/trs) from the human immunodeficiency virus (HIV) in the adult male rat. Antisense Res Dev 4:43–52, 1994.
62. Mercola D, Westwick J, Rundell AY, et al. Analysis of a transformed cell line using antisense c-fos RNA. Gene 72:253–265, 1988.

63. Chaudhary PM, Roninson IB. Expression and activity of p-glycoprotein, a multidrug efflux pump in human hematopoietic stem cells. Cell 66:85–94, 1991.
64. Flosshove M, Banerjee D, Mineishi S, et al. Ex-vivo expansion and selection of human CD34+ peripheral blood progenitor cells after introduction of a mutated dihydrofolate reductase cDNA via retroviral gene transfer. Blood 85:566–574, 1995.
65. Allay JA, Dumenco LL, Koc DN, et al. Retroviral transduction and expression of the human alkyl-transferase cDNA provides nitrosourea resistance to hematopoietic cells. Blood 85:3342–3351, 1995.

2. Post-bone marrow transplant use of immunotherapy

Udit N. Verma, Kenneth R. Meehan, and Amitabha Mazumder

A wealth of information demonstrating the graft-vs.-leukemia (GVL) or graft-vs.-tumor (GVT) effect following allogeneic bone marrow transplant (BMT) has accumulated over the past few decades and suggests that immune mechanisms are important for eradication of residual disease in the recipient [1–3]. The lack of GVT effect after autologous BMT (ABMT), along with reinfusion of clonogenic tumor cells with the autologous graft, may be responsible for the increased relapse rate seen after ABMT as compared to allogeneic BMT [4]. Due to dose-limiting nonhematological toxicities of current autologous BMT preparative regimens, innovative therapeutic modalities are needed. Posttransplant immunotherapy provides an attractive strategy.

Both tumor-specific and -nonspecific immunotherapeutic approaches have been evaluated for treatment of neoplastic disorders in experimental models and clinical trials, with variable results. The definition of oncogenes and their products and the discovery of several other antigenic molecules on tumor cells that are either aberrantly expressed or are products of mutated genes have paved the way for differentiating the tumor cell from 'self' [5–9]. This has led to renewed interest in the area of tumor-specific immunotherapy.

In this chapter, we will review laboratory and clinical immunotherapeutic approaches pursued in bone marrow transplant settings to treat different neoplastic disorders, including solid tumors and hematological malignancies.

Nonspecific immunotherapy

Innate immune defense mechanisms include cells, such as macrophages, non-MHC-restricted killer cells of either natural killer (NK) cell or T-cell origin, and activated NK (A-NK) or lymphokine activated killer (LAK) cells. In addition, several cytokines secreted by these cells, such as interferon-γ (IFN-γ) and tumor necrosis factor (TNF), demonstrate prominent antitumor activity. Antitumor responses have been generated in various tumor models by 1) in vitro activation of lymphoid cells with cytokines, antibodies (CD3), or lectins, 2) direct in vivo administration of cytokines to stimulate antitumor effectors in

Jane N. Winter (ed.) BLOOD STEM CELL TRANSPLANTATION. 1997. Kluwer Academic Publishers. ISBN 0-7923-4260-7. All rights reserved.

vivo, or 3) a combination of these two approaches [10–16]. These strategies have demonstrated encouraging results in patients with melanoma and renal cell carcinoma in the nontransplant setting [17]. Currently, these approaches are being evaluated following both allogeneic and autologous bone marrow transplantation.

The GVL effect observed after allogeneic bone marrow transplantation is well recognized. However, its full impact has only been recently appreciated due to the prevalence of T-cell depletion for the prevention of graft-vs.-host disease (GVHD) [18–20]. GVHD and GVL effects are caused by immunocompetent cells contained in the graft that recognize major or minor histocompatibility antigens [21]. The mechanism for these processes has not been fully elucidated, but this has not precluded the development of clinical trials to obtain GVL activity by infusion of donor-specific leukocytes following allogeneic BMT [3,22]. It is conceivable that induction of autologous GVHD following ABMT may lead to GVL/GVT effect. Attempts to induce this autoimmune state (autologous GVHD/syngeneic GVHD) following ABMT to obtain preferential lysis of tumor cells are in progress [23].

Most of the immunotherapeutic trials following BMT have focused on augmentation of antigen nonspecific defenses and are discussed below.

Interleukin-2 with or without LAK cells

Human IL-2 is a 133-amino-acid-long 15.4-kD peptide primarily secreted by T cells [24]. The cytokine acts via a specific IL-2 receptor, consisting of α, β, γ subunits [25]. In addition to T-cell proliferation, IL-2 leads to activation and proliferation of NK cells, increasing their tumoricidal activity (A-NK/LAK cells) [26]. Other actions of IL-2 include augmentation of B-cell growth and immunoglobulin production, enhancement of IFN-γ and TNF-β production from T cells, IL-6 production by monocytes, modulation of histamine release by basophils, and upregulation of IL-2 receptors.

LAK cells, induced by incubation of peripheral blood mononuclear cells with IL-2, lyse a variety of tumor cells, both in vitro and in vivo in an MHC unrestricted manner [26,27]. LAK cell activity mainly resides in activated NK cells with variable contribution from T cells and other cell types [28]. In vivo administration of LAK cells has demonstrated efficacy in several experimental models and clinical trials, particularly in patients with renal cell carcinoma and melanoma [29]. IL-2 alone may be effective due to induction of endogenous LAK activity and elaboration of tumor-inhibitory cytokines, such as IFN-γ and TNF [30]. Murine studies suggest that IL-2 therapy is most effective in a situation of low tumor burden [31]. Due to the minimal residual disease status after transplantation, BMT offers an attractive setting for evaluation of IL-2 therapy. The administration of IL-2 with or without LAK cell infusion is being evaluated both in the setting of autologous and allogeneic transplantation, with results summarized below.

28

Autologous BMT. Early anecdotal reports suggested that IL-2 administered after BMT induced responses in patients with advanced malignancies [32]. Since then, early results from several phase I/II clinical trials have bee published [33–36]. The dose and schedule of IL-2 therapy in these trials were variable. However, these results suggest that a lower dose of IL-2 therapy was well tolerated. At moderate to high dosages, toxicity was common but manageable in a nonintensive care setting. The spectrum of toxic effects was similar to that observed in nontransplant settings. Although profound immune stimulation has been seen in these patients following treatment with IL-2, antitumor activity is still unproven.

Gottlieb et al. administered IL-2 to patients with acute myeloid leukemia (AML) or multiple myeloma in a phase I dose-escalation protocol [33]. IL-2 was started at $1.5 \times 10^6 \, \text{IU/m}^2\text{/day}$, infused over six hours with doubling of the dose every 48 hours, until the maximum tolerated dose was determined. In one patient with AML, IL-2 therapy was started immediately after BMT resulting in severe toxicities requiring the cessation of treatment. In the subsequent nine treatment courses, IL-2 infusion was initiated after the neutrophil count reached 0.5×10^9/l. Mild to moderate toxicities were observed, which were manageable in a nonintensive care setting, with the dose up to $1.4–10.5 \times 10^6 \, \text{IU}$ per patient. Dose-limiting toxicity included hypotension, which responded rapidly to cessation of IL-2. Blaise et al. administered IL-2 to a cohort of 10 patients undergoing ABMT for various neoplastic disorders, including acute lymphocytic leukemia (ALL), AML, non-Hodgkins lymphoma (NHL), carcinomas of ovary or breast, and malignant thymoma [34]. Conditioning regimens included high-dose chemotherapy or chemoradiotherapy. IL-2 was administered at $18 \times 10^6 \, \text{U/m}^2\text{/day}$ as a continuous infusion for six days, beginning a median 79 ± 12 days after BMT. Moderate toxicities occurred in all patients but were well tolerated. The predominant toxicities included involvement of skin, gastrointestinal tract, and liver. Changes in hemodynamic parameters necessitated cessation of treatment on a few occasions. Ninety-one percent of the planned dose was administered. There were no toxic deaths. Although the study was small and with limited follow-up, at the time of reporting, five patients were in continuous CR at 8 to 10 months after BMT. Higuchi et al. [35] examined the role of IL-2 in inducing immunological changes in 16 patients undergoing ABMT for hematologic malignancies after high-dose chemotherapy or chemoradiotherapy. IL-2 was administered at a dose of $0.3–4.5 \times 10^6$ Hoffman La Roche Units (RU) (specific activity 1.2–1.5 units/mg protein)/m^2/day as a continuous infusion for five days beginning 14 to 91 (median 33) days posttransplant. After five days of rest, a ten-day maintenance course $(0.3 \times 10^6 \, \text{RU/m}^2\text{/day})$ was administered. Most of the patients developed mild to moderate toxicities, including fever, rash, nausea, diarrhea, dyspnea, and weight gain. Toxicities were related to dose and rapidly reversed after completion of treatment. There was no mortality from IL-2-induced toxicities, and all patients received the prescribed IL-2 maintenance therapy. At the time of reporting, 9 of the 16 patients were in continuous CR for 7 to

23 months after BMT. Soiffer et al. have examined the role of prolonged infusion of low-dose IL-2 in inducing immunological changes with the aim of producing a GVT effect after ABMT for ALL, NHL, and carcinomas of breast and ovary [36]. IL-2 was initiated once engraftment was established, usually several months after BMT, at a dose of 2×10^5 RU/m^2/day as a continuous IV infusion for 90 days. Toxicities were mild and included rash, dyspnea, weight gain, and hypothyroidism. Sixty-nine percent of the patients completed the full course of therapy, and most developed immunological changes suggestive of a GVT effect in vitro.

Weisdorf et al. evaluated the role of IL-2 instituted immediately after BMT in phase I trial in 14 patients with ALL undergoing ABMT following cyclophosphamide (Cy) and total body irradiation (TBI) [37]. IL-2 was started on day +1 and administered by continuous IV infusion in a dose of 0.5 to 2.0×10^6 RU/m^2/day for four days a week for three weeks. Ten patients received IL-2 therapy as planned, while four did not due to fever or respiratory distress. Serious toxicities occurred at the highest dose level of IL-2. Overall, patients treated with IL-2 experienced a shorter hospital stay (median 38 days) when compared to a control group of similar patients not receiving IL-2 (median 63 days). However, two patients in this cohort of 14 patients died of toxicity attributed to IL-2 therapy.

Preclinical and clinical studies have shown that the combination of IL-2 and LAK cells is associated with greater antitumor responses than treatment with either modality alone [29,38,39]. Significant endogenous LAK cell activity can be generated only with high doses of IL-2, which are toxic and poorly tolerated. Animal studies have demonstrated that the increase in cure rate achieved by high-dose IL-2 therapy can be offset by an increased toxic mortality [39]. In the transplant setting, animal models show that a combination of IL-2 and LAK cells did not interfere with engraftment and induced a GVT effect in a syngeneic model of BMT for AML [31]. Thus, treatment with a combination of IL-2 and LAK cells may be more effective in eradicating minimal residual disease (MRD) and reducing relapse rates following autologous BMT.

Fefer et al. recently reported the results of a phase Ib trial using IL-2 with or without LAK cells in 16 patients with malignant lymphoma undergoing ABMT [15,35]. IL-2 was administered at a median of 51 (21 to 91) days posttransplant. Five of 16 patients underwent leukapheresis on days 6 through 8 following initial IL-2 therapy (3×10^6 RU/m^2/day for five days). Lymphocytes were incubated with IL-2 for five days in vitro to generate LAK cells. A median of 136×10^9 LAK cells were infused per patient on days 12 to 14, and low-dose IL-2 (3×10^5 RU/m^2/day) was administered on days 12 through 21. Leukapheresis was associated with severe thrombocytopenia despite aggressive platelet therapy. LAK cell infusions were generally well tolerated, with transient fever, rigors and dyspnea, which rapidly reversed. Other toxicities were similar to those occurring after IL-2 alone. Of the 16 patients treated, 11 remain in CR at 6+ to 21+ months after BMT. In another study, the Seattle group reported the feasibility of using IL-2 alone or in combination with LAK cells after autologous BMT for patients with AML in untreated first relapse or second remission [13]. The toxicities associated were comparable to previous trials [15,35]. However, collection of lymphocytes for LAK cell generation was associated with severe thrombocytopenia. Of the 14 patients treated on this trial, ten remain in continuous CR for 13+ to 48+ months.

The use of IL-2 in the transplant setting has generally been evaluated in phase I/II trials in patients who have received extensive prior therapy. Determining the efficacy of IL-2 therapy in this situation is difficult and is further compounded by the fact that most studies are uncontrolled and have a short follow-up. However, two groups have recently published results from trials using IL-2 alone or in combination with LAK cells. Hamon et al. performed ABMT in 18 patients with AML in first remission conditioned with busulfan–Cy (BU–Cy) or with Cy–TBI followed by IL-2 [40,41]. Seven patients received IL-2 after ABMT in nonrandomized fashion (determined by the availability of IL-2), and 11 patients received ABMT alone without IL-2. Otherwise, groups were comparable in respect to age, white cell count at diagnosis, interval between diagnosis and treatment, and pretransplant chemotherapy. One patient receiving IL-2 died of pulmonary edema. Of the remaining six patients, one has relapsed after a median follow up of 32 months (range 21 to 58), resulting in actuarial disease-free survival of 71%. Of the 11 patients who did not receive IL-2 following autologous BMT, the actuarial disease-free survival after a median follow-up of 29 months (range 24 to 45) was 36%.

In another study, Benyunes et al. analyzed the results of two trials using IL-2 alone or IL-2 plus LAK cells after ABMT in 14 patients with AML in first relapse or a later stage [13]. One patient died of multiple organ failure during IL-2 therapy, three patients relapsed at four, five, and ten months following BMT, and ten patients remain in CR from 13+ to 48+ months (median 34 months). The actuarial probability of relapse was 23% and the probability of survival was 71%, which was superior to the outcome of the historical controls undergoing autologous BMT without IL-2.

Allogeneic BMT. IL-2 can lead to exacerbation of GVHD by expansion and maintenance of allosensitized T cells and possibly NK cells. In experimental models, delayed institution of IL-2 treatment following allogeneic transplant potentiates GVHD [42,43]. However, early institution on the day of transplant has been associated with abrogation of GVHD [44,45]. It appears from these results that institution of IL-2 treatment after sensitization of alloreactive T cells may be associated with potentiation of GVHD, while early IL-2 may prevent or abort sensitization of unprimed alloreactive T cells. Mechanisms responsible for modulation of GVHD by IL-2 are not well understood. However, induction of veto cell activity in the host may be responsible for such an effect. Veto cells suppress the generation of cytotoxic T lymphocytes (CTL) in an MHC-specific manner, with MHC specificity determined by the antigens expressed on the surface of veto cells themselves. Preclinical studies have shown that LAK cells are capable of mediating veto activity and therefore could potentially reduce the incidence and severity of GVHD in allogeneic BMT [46]. IL-2 therapy following transplantation with T-cell-depleted allogeneic bone marrow enhances veto activity in a mouse model [47]. Interestingly, this reduction in GVHD by posttransplant IL-2 therapy is not associated with a reduction in GVT effect induced by allogeneic T cells [44,45,48]. These observations suggest a possible benefit of IL-2 therapy after allogeneic BMT. Administration of IL-2 four months after allogeneic BMT with non-T-cell-depleted bone marrow in a patient with neuroblastoma led to reactivation of GVHD. Cessation of IL-2 therapy and treatment with corticosteroids resulted in rapid resolution of GVHD [32]. More recently, Soiffer et al. administered IL-2 after allogeneic BMT with T-cell-depleted bone marrow to patients with NHL, AML, chronic myeloid leukemia (CML), or myelodysplastic syndrome (MDS) [36,49]. Low-dose IL-2 was initiated after engraftment and continued over a period of three months by continuous intravenous infusion. Toxicities were mild and consisted of fever, hypotension, nausea, vomiting, weight gain, and catheter infection. No patient developed GVHD. IL-2 induced a drop in platelet count and an increase in circulating eosinophils and lymphocytes, with a return of eosinophil count to normal approximately three months after cessation of IL-2. The increase in the lymphocyte population was predominantly due to an increase in NK cell number from 15% before therapy to 70% during therapy. These cells exhibited potent activity against both NK-sensitive and NK-resistant tumor targets. The antitumor activity of these cells rapidly fell to baseline levels after cessation of IL-2 therapy. Relapse rate and disease-free survival were determined in the 25 patients who completed at least four weeks of IL-2 treatment. The Cox proportional hazards regression model suggested that, compared with historical control patients without history of GVHD, patients treated with IL-2 had a lower risk of disease relapse (hazard ratio 0.34; range 0.14 to 0.82) and superior disease-free survival (hazard ratio 0.39; range 0.18 to 0.87) [49].

Initially, there was concern that IL-2 after BMT would delay engraftment. Early studies demonstrated suppression of progenitor cell activity of bone marrow by LAK cells in vitro [50]. Subsequently, a large number of preclinical studies both in vitro and in vivo confirmed the absence of harmful effects of IL-2 and LAK cells on bone marrow [51,52]. However, most of the clinical trials employed IL-2 therapy after the recovery of peripheral blood counts following autologous BMT. These trials were designed to avoid both hematologic and nonhematologic toxicity in patients who had received high-dose chemotherapy or chemoradiotherapy.

All the trials using IL-2 after autologous BMT have reported similar effects on hematologic parameters. In general, IL-2 treatment has been associated with a modest drop in hemoglobin levels, which could not be accounted for by blood loss from diagnostic testing [33,34]. However, since hemoglobin levels have generally been maintained above 10 gm/dl by red cell transfusions, it has been difficult to define the effect. Nonetheless, cessation of IL-2 was followed by increases in the levels of hemoglobin [35]. Administration of IL-2 is accompanied by an increase in circulating neutrophils in most patients [33,34,37]. Elevation of neutrophil counts has been related to the dose of IL-2 [35]. In all patients, neutrophil counts returned to baseline after cessation of IL-2. Administration of low doses of IL-2 for a prolonged period of time by Soiffer et al. was not accompanied by significant changes in circulating neutrophil levels but has been associated with a significant increase in eosinophil counts that has persisted for several days after cessation of IL-2 [36]. The study reported by Blaise et al. [34] showed a significant fall in neutrophil counts during the early phase of IL-2 treatment, with a subsequent rise. Nearly all studies have observed a slight initial fall in circulating lymphocytes followed by a significant rise in lymphocyte counts persisting above baseline levels for several days to weeks after discontinuation of IL-2 [33,34]. Some studies have shown an increase in both CD4$^+$ and CD8$^+$ lymphocytes, while others have observed a greater increase in CD8$^+$ than in CD4$^+$ lymphocyte populations [35]. Prolonged infusion of low-dose IL-2 has been shown to significantly increase circulating NK cells while having no significant effect on the numbers of CD3 cells [36]. Gottlieb et al. [33] and Blaise et al. [34] have reported a significant decrease in platelets during IL-2 therapy, with rapid return to normal levels after cessation of treatment.

The exact mechanisms by which IL-2 stimulates myeloid cells have not been elucidated. IL-2 may induce demargination of neutrophils into the circulation; alternatively, myeloid precursors may be stimulated directly or indirectly by the release of other cytokines. Cancer patients receiving IL-2 therapy have been reported to have an increase in the number of circulating hematopoietic precursors in their peripheral blood, attributed to the release of cytokines, which stimulate hematopoiesis [53]. Administration of IL-2 to patients undergoing autologous BMT has been reported to induce the expression of mRNA for GM-CSF, IL-3, IL-4, and IL-6 in mononuclear cells [54], which could result in induction of proliferation of myeloid precursors.

IL-2 has been shown to restore proliferative T-cell responses in vitro and to improve immunologic function by direct induction of cellular changes and indirectly by stimulating release of other cytokines in vivo [55,56]. Following BMT, endogenously generated NK cells appear 4 to 6 weeks after BMT. These cells have been shown to be highly responsive to IL-2 both in vitro and in vivo [57]. During IL-2 therapy, circulating lymphocytes exhibit increased spontaneous activity against both NK-sensitive and NK-resistant tumor targets and have been reported to inhibit the growth of autologous leukemic blasts in vitro [33]. Incubation of lymphocytes collected after IL-2 administration with IL-2 in vitro has resulted in the generation of potent antitumor effector cells [34]. These data suggest that IL-2 induces a substantial increase in both LAK effector and LAK precursor cells. During IL-2 therapy, variable effects have been observed on the phenotype of circulating cells, including an increase in activated NK cells, CD8$^+$ cytotoxic T cells, and T cells with activation markers such as IL-2 receptor and Ia [36,37,58]. In addition to inducing significant changes in the cellular compartment, IL-2 has been reported to exert an effect on the secretion of IFN and TNF, both possessing antitumor effects [59].

IL-2 also seems to alter the reactivity of the autologous lymphocytes regenerating after autologous BMT. A preliminary study has shown that the administration of IL-2 and LAK cells after autologous BMT resulted in infiltration of T cells in the skin, with the demonstration of histological changes consistent with cutaneous GVHD [60]. Since the occurrence of GVHD in allogeneic BMT has been associated with a GVL effect, it is possible that such a reaction in autologous BMT could reflect the induction of a GVL phenomenon. Whether or not the induction of autologous GVHD results in GVL remains to be determined.

Interferons after BMT

In addition to a direct cytotoxic effect on tumor cells [61], interferons act as strong immunomodulatory agents. IFN-α and IFN-γ act either alone or with IL-2 as potent inducers of cytolytic activity of NK cells and monocytes [62]. Cell surface expression of different molecules on tumor cells including integrins (involved in cell adhesion) and MHC molecules is regulated by IFN-γ [63,64]. IFN-γ upregulates MHC expression (both class I and class II) on a variety of tumor cell types [65–67]. Regulation of MHC is associated with increased immunogenicity of tumor cells, possibly mediated by improved antigen presentation by tumor cells. These properties make the interferons attractive molecules for immunotherapy. However, IFNs inhibit hematopoietic progenitor-cell proliferation [68]. Therefore, in most trials, IFN therapy has been instituted only after engraftment [69].

Several small, nonrandomized studies using IFN-α post ABMT have been performed in patients with CML, NHL, Hodgkins' disease, and multiple myeloma [70–77]. In these studies, the dose of IFN varied from 1×10^6 to 3×10^6 U/day for 3 to 7 days in a week starting at hematological reconstitution. Side effects have been limited, ranging from mild constitutional symptoms to occasional hematological toxicity in the form of thrombocytopenia. Neloni et al. reported their results with use of IFN-α in 34 patients with CML transplanted in chronic phase [78]. After a median follow-up of 13 months, 12 of 12 patients who received IFN and 19 of 22 untreated patients were in CR. In another study [75], 13 CML patients in chronic phase and two patients in accelerated phase or blast crisis were treated with IFN-α following ABMT. Five of eight patients in first chronic phase were in complete hematological remission after 8 to 19 months, while 2 of 7 patients in second chronic phase or accelerated/blastic phase were in complete hematological remission after more than 16 months. Ascensao et al. reported results of IFN-α therapy in 58 patients with NHL or Hodgkins disease [79]. After minimal follow-up of 19 months, overall survival was 83%, with event-free survival at 64%. Attal et al. [77] reported progression-free survival of 53% at 33 months post-BMT in patients with multiple myeloma treated with IFN. These results indicate that

IFN-α can be used safely following ABMT. However, in the absence of large controlled randomized trials, valid conclusions for efficacy of treatment cannot be determined.

After allogeneic BMT. IFN-α therapy has been employed in patients with CML in combination with donor leukocyte infusion as discussed below. Meyers et al. [70] evaluated IFN for patients with ALL. Treatment was instituted after engraftment and continued for 80 days after transplant. This therapy led to significant reduction in the incidence of relapse at four years.

CsA induced autologous GVHD

GVHD is a common occurrence after allogeneic BMT and simulates many features of autoimmune diseases [80,81]. GVHD contributes to the GVL effect of allogeneic BMT and reduces relapse rates as compared to ABMT [1,82–84]. Glazier et al. [85] described the development of syngeneic GVHD after syngeneic or autologous transplantation in rats after brief treatment of these animals with cyclosporine (CsA). Since then, this autologous-immune phenomenon of CsA-induced GVHD has been studied extensively.

Cytotoxic lymphocytes circulating in animals with GVHD lyse Ia^+ tumor cells [86]. Tumor cells in different neoplastic disorders, particularly lymphoid tumors, express class II MHC antigens, and in other disorders MHC expression can be induced by IFN. Tumor cells with class II MHC molecules can thus be susceptible to lysis by autoreactive lymphocytes induced by CsA therapy posttransplant [86,87]. Based on precursor clinical studies, this technique of inducing GVHD is being evaluated in clinical trials in an attempt to obtain GVHD/GVL effects following autologous transplantation [88,89]. CsA has been evaluated in phase I/II trials in patients with metastatic breast cancer, lymphoma, CML, and ANLL in dosages of 1–3.75 mg/kg/day from day 0 to day 28. Most of the patients treated with CsA developed evidence of grade I–II cutaneous GVHD. However, visceral manifestations of GVHD were not observed. Decreased relapse rate and improved disease-free survival have been reported in a study on 14 patients with NHL when compared to historical controls [90]. In other studies, due either to the small number of patients or short follow-up, it is difficult to draw conclusions about the antitumor effect of this mode of therapy.

IL-2 with IL-2-activated bone marrow or PBSC grafts

Reinfusion of clonogenic tumor cells with the marrow and lack of a GVL effect are possible factors responsible for the higher relapse rates seen with ABMT than with allogeneic BMT [4,91,92]. Several methods have been used to remove malignant cells contaminating autologous marrow [93–95]. In vitro purging of the autograft may be critical, but the overall impact in decreasing relapse rate remains to be defined [4]. Recent studies favor the view that relapse following ABMT is predominantly the result of residual disease escaping the high-dose chemotherapy or chemoradiotherapy [96]. This could be due to the fact that the autograft lacks the GVL effect that plays a critical role in eradication of MRD or in maintaining tumor dormancy in allogeneic BMT [97]. The importance of the GVL effect and the immune mechanisms involved are corroborated by the fact that in the setting of allogeneic BMT, patients who receive T-cell-depleted grafts with or without GVHD after transplant have a higher risk of relapse than recipients of unmanipulated grafts without GVHD. Those patients who have GVHD have the lowest probability of relapse [98]. These data support an antileukemic effect independent of GVHD that is altered by T-cell depletion. In addition, it is clear that recipients of syngeneic transplants have a higher probability of relapse than patients receiving allografts when conditioned with the same treatment regimen. In patients with CML, several investigators have demonstrated NK cell deficiency, which has led to attempts to induce GVL activity in vitro by generation of donor peripheral blood LAK cells that have been shown to kill recipient CML cells in ^{51}Cr release assays and to selectively inhibit growth of recipient CML CFU-GM but not normal donor CFU-GM [99,100]. Such an effect may be clinically relevant, since it has been shown that the risk of relapse after BMT for CML was significantly increased in patients who failed to generate LAK cell lytic activity against host-derived CML targets as compared to those who did [101].

Current ABMT protocols do not have the immune capabilities of allogeneic bone marrow transplant. Therefore, it may be important to explore strategies aimed at in vitro purging of the autograft and to simultaneously induce a GVL effect. Our group [31,102] has demonstrated that IL-2-activated marrow has significant antitumor activity in vitro and in vivo. This property of marrow can be exploited to purge marrow of contaminating tumor cells [52] and, in addition, to generate cytotoxic effector cells that can mediate a GVL effect in vivo. Thus, IL-2 incubation of the graft is a potential approach to therapy that might decrease relapse rates following ABMT.

Studies with both murine and human bone marrow suggest that incubation of bone marrow cells with IL-2 leads to generation of potent cytotoxic effector cells [52,102–105]. These effector cells, generated by IL-2, like LAK cells, lyse a wide variety of both NK-sensitive and NK-cell-resistant tumor cell targets in an MHC unrestricted manner. However, the cytolytic activity of these cells was found to be superior to that of LAK cells and was maintained for longer periods of time [102,106]. The in vivo antitumor effects of activated bone marrow were shown in a murine melanoma model in which transplant of IL-2 incubated bone marrow followed by IL-2 treatment led to regression of pulmonary metastases consisting of drug- and radiation-resistant B16 and MCA tumors in mice [102,106]. Subsequently, similar observations were made in murine AML models [31,103]. In these studies, it was shown that transplantation with IL-2 activated bone marrow combined with posttransplant IL-2 was associated with significant antitumor responses. These results are summarized in figure 1. As is apparent from figure 1, treatment with IL-2 following

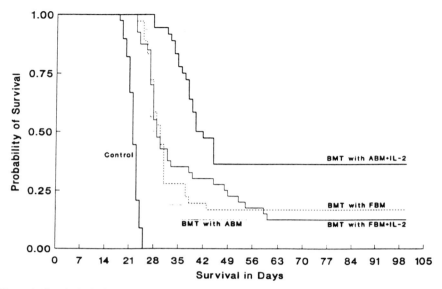

Figure 1. Survival of mice with acute myeloid leukemia (AML) given IL-2-activated bone marrow and posttransplant IL-2 therapy. AML was induced in C57B1/6 mice by injection with 2×10^5 C1498 cells. BMT was performed three days after injection of leukemic cells, and mice were reconstituted with fresh bone marrow (FBM) or IL-2-activated BM (ABM). Systemic IL-2 therapy was started immediately following transplant in the groups shown and was continued for seven days. Pooled results from ten experiments are shown. There was significant improvement in survival of mice given ABM + IL-2 as compared to those given FBM ($p < .001$).

transplantation with unmanipulated fresh bone marrow or transplantation with IL-2 activated bone marrow alone without posttransplant IL-2 led to a decrease in the cure rate. Again, in a comparable set of in vivo experiments, splenic LAK cells demonstrated far less antitumor activity than IL-2-activated bone marrow cells [106]. Further studies suggested that tumor eradication resulted when IL-2 was instituted immediately posttransplant in a state of minimal residual disease [103]. The superior antitumor effect seen with IL-2-activated marrow and posttransplant administration of IL-2 may be due to the fact that effectors primed in vitro with high doses of IL-2 can maintain their cytotoxic potential in vivo with low serum levels of IL-2, and without undue toxicity [107]. Several studies suggest that to be successful, immunotherapeutic modalities must be instituted in a state of low tumor burden [108,109]. IL-2-activated bone marrow followed by low-dose IL-2 has the advantage of mediating antitumor responses immediately following transplantation. The early institution of IL-2 may be necessary for in vivo survival and expansion of antitumor effector cells.

Similar to results with murine bone marrow, short-term (24-hour) activation with IL-2 of normal human marrow was associated with generation of potent cytotoxic effector cells. However, studies conducted with leukemic marrow show reduced cytotoxicity dependent on the degree of leukemic infiltration of the marrow [110]. Whether this finding is a quantitative phenomenon due to a decreased proportion of cytotoxic precursors in the infiltrated marrow or a qualitative defect is unclear. It is possible that both factors may be responsible. However, since most patients are transplanted in remission, the effect of leukemic infiltration may not be relevant in most clinical circumstances.

In addition to the generation of cytotoxic effector cells that mediate GVT effects in vivo, eradication of contaminating tumor cells in the graft while maintaining the capacity to reconstitute hematopoiesis is critically important for successful application of this strategy. Therefore, both these parameters were evaluated with human and murine bone marrow. Short-term culture of bone marrow with IL-2 was associated with significant clearing of contaminating leukemic cells [52]. Increasing duration of bone marrow culture, regardless of the presence or absence of IL-2, was associated with a decline in the number of clonogenic hematopoietic cells. However, at 24 hours, there was generation of potent cytotoxicity with maintenance of the intial number of hematopoietic clonogenic cells [111]. In murine models, transplantation with IL-2-activated bone marrow was associated with similar reconstitution kinetics to that of fresh bone marrow [31,111]. These studies suggested that IL-2 activation of the autograft for 24 hours can lead to in vitro purging and generation of effector cells capable of mediating a GVT effect without loss of hematopoietic precursors.

It has been shown in variety of hematological malignancies that neoplastic cells undergo preferential loss in comparison with normal hematopoietic cells during long-term culture (LTC) of the bone marrow [112,113]. These investigations, coupled with studies evaluating the mechanisms of selective loss of neoplastic cells in LTC [114,115], suggest that the culture environment in LTC could provide a selective growth disadvantage for neoplastic cells [116]. This property of LTC provides a rationale for application of in vitro purging of marrow from patients with hematological malignancies. Potent NK cells and other cells capable of killing tumor cells can be generated in LTC of marrow in the presence of IL-2 [117], providing a further strategy for purging and activation of marrow. In the presence of IL-2, long-term marrow cultures may lead to more complete eradication of tumor cells and provide sufficient time for generation of more potent cytotoxic effector cells, provided the LTC could be maintained for a long period of time without compromising the reconstituting potential of marrow.

We have shown that cytotoxic effector cells generated by IL-2 in LTC (1–3 weeks) lyse a variety of tumor cell lines in vitro [118]. Prolonging the duration of IL-2 exposure in culture leads to a progressive increase in cytotoxicity. However, the number of hematopoietic precursors declines after peaking at day 7. At day 7, the number of normal hematopoietic clonogenic cells was higher than in the starting marrow inoculum [118]. These results indicated that marrow cultured for seven days with IL-2 can be successfully used for transplantation. In a model of in vitro purging, it was observed that IL-2 incubation in LTC could successfully purge marrow with 10% contaminating tumor cells [118]. Studies performed with marrows from patients with CML indicate that LTC with IL-2 leads to eradication of Ph^1 metaphases [118]. The feasibility of LTC of bone marrow autografts with IL-2 with the aim of purging and generating cytotoxic effectors has also been demonstrated by Klingemann et al. [119,120]. Earlier, several groups demonstrated that LAK cells preferentially lyse contaminating neoplastic cells present in bone marrow and that these LAK cells can be used for in vitro purging [51,121]. IL-2 activation of marrow provides a possible advantage over LAK cell purging because it is a single-step procedure that also leads to generation of effector cells that can mediate in vivo reactivity against tumor in the presence of low-dose IL-2.

Peripheral blood stem cell (PBSC) transplantation is associated with faster immunohematopoietic recovery and possibly less risk of contamination by tumor cells as compared to marrow [112,123]. PBSCs are mobilized by cytotoxic chemotherapy and/or myeloid growth factors (GM-CSF or G-CSF) [124,125]. There may be both qualitative and quantitative effects on IL-2 responsive cells under these conditions [126]. We have examined the capacity of chemotherapy- and growth-factor-mobilized PBSCs to generate antitumor

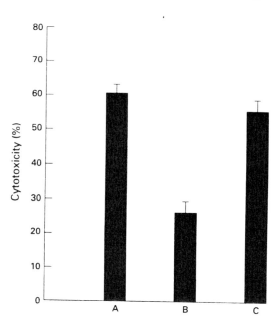

Figure 2A. Cytotoxicity of IL-2-activated PBSCs and the effect of cryopreservation. Fresh PBSCs were activated with 6000 IU/ml of IL-2, and cytotoxicity was assessed as such (fresh, activated; A) or after freezing and thawing (activated, frozen; B). Frozen PBSCs from the same harvests were activated and cytotoxicity was tested (C) along with the activated frozen and thawed sample. Data are percentage cytolysis (mean + SEM) of A375 at an E:T ratio of 50:1 from a representative experiment.

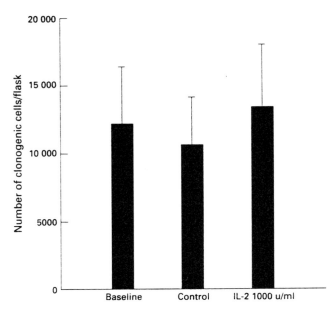

Figure 2B. Effect of IL-2 activation of PBSCs on the number of clonogenic cells. The number of clonogenic cells was assayed at baseline and after 24 hours of culture, with and without IL-2. Shown are total number of day-14 colonies (CFU-GM, BFU-E, CFU-GEMM) per flask (input: 1×10^7 cells). Data represent mean + SEM from 12 experiments with PBSCs from different patients. The number of colonies per flask was derived by the number of colonies per 1×10^5 plated cells in semisolid medium and cellular output from the flask after 24 hours of activation.

cytotoxic effector cells in vitro [127]. IL-2 activation of chemotherapy and growth factor mobilized PBSCs from patients with different neoplastic disorders leads to generation of potent cytotoxic effector cells without loss of hematopoietic progenitors. Results obtained with PBSC from breast cancer patients are shown in figure 2A and 2B. As shown in figure 2A, a decrease in cytotoxicity was seen after freezing IL-2-activated PBSC; however, cytotoxicity comparable to fresh IL-2-activated PBSC was obtained by IL-2 activation of cryopreserved PBSC. These results suggested feasibility of performing IL-2 activation of cryopreserved PBSC. Further experiments showed that the cytotoxicity achieved from growth-factor-mobilized PBSCs was equal to or higher than that achieved from bone marrow. These studies suggested that it should be possible to use PBSCs from patients with different neoplastic disorders for generation of cytotoxic effector cells by IL-2 activation.

Based on our preliminary studies discussed above, phase I/II clinical trials are in progress at our center in patients with different neoplastic disorders to evaluate the feasibility of administering IL-2-activated autografts following high-dose chemoradiotherapy. Systemic IL-2 is administered to patients after transplantation. Sixty-one patients with breast cancer have been transplanted with PBSCs mobilized with rhG-CSF and chemotherapy (either Cy (5 gms/m²)

Table 1. Clinical characteristics of breast cancer patients treated with IL-2-activated PBSC and systemic IL-2

Groups	No. of patients	IL-2 schedule Dose (IU/m²/day)	Duration	Median (age) (range in years)	Reconstitution (days) ANC	Platelets	Toxicity (level)[a] I	II	III	IV	V
1	5	No IL-2		44 (38–51)	11 ± 1.9	12.2 ± 6.4	5	4	2	1	0
2	5	6×10^5	1 week	49 (37–54)	11 ± 0.6	12.8 ± 4.6	5	4	4	0	0
3	3	6×10^5	2 weeks	44 (39–54)	12 ± 1.6	8.6 ± 0.5	3	2	0	0	0
4	6	6×10^5	4 weeks	37.5 (24–59)	13.3 ± 2.1	11.5 ± 2.5	6	5	0	0	0
5	11	1.8×10^6	4 weeks	42 (31–51)	12.6 ± 3.0	10.9 ± 7.2	11	10	4	1	0
6	8	6.0×10^6	4 weeks	46 (32–59)	12.2 ± 2.4	13.5 ± 3.9	8	7	6	0	0
7	23	1.8×10^6	4 weeks	48 (33–58)	10.4 ± 2.6^b	11.6 ± 4.5^b	23	21	11	2	1

[a] Denotes number of patients in each group developing toxicities involving any organ system.
[b] One of 23 patients died on day 11 after transplant before WBC or platelet reconstitution was achieved.

41

or paclitaxel (200–300 mg/m^2 over 24 hours)). The patient population consisted of patients with high-risk stage II ($n = 21$), stage III ($n = 15$), and stage IV disease ($n = 25$). Salient clinical features, treatment, schedule, hematopoietic reconstitution, and toxicity data are summarized in table 1. Of the 61 patients, 10 patients had resistant disease at the time of transplantation, with the remaining patients demonstrating either partial or complete response. After high-dose chemotherapy with carboplatin and Cy, PBSCs incubated for 24 hours with IL-2 were reinfused. IL-2 administration was initiated on the day of transplantation (day 0). The initial five patients received only IL-2-activated PBSC, while subsequent patients received IL-2 initially at a dose of 6×10^5 IU/m^2/day by continuous infusion starting on day 0 and continuing for five days. As shown in table 1, subsequent groups of patients received increasing doses and durations of IL-2. The maximal tolerated dose was 1.8×10^6 IU/m^2/day administered over four weeks.

Rapid hematopoietic reconstitution was achieved in all patients. The average number of days required both for the absolute neutrophil count to reach 0.5×10^9/l for three days and for the platelet count to be maintained at 20,000 $\times 10^9$/l for three days is given in table 1.

IL-2-activated PBSC transplantation followed by systemic IL-2 therapy was associated with frequent but tolerable side effects. Not all the toxicities could be attributed to IL-2 alone; some may be the result of the combination of chemotherapy and IL-2. Systemic toxicities seen in this group of patients involving any organ system are given in table 1. The most prominent toxicities included a mild elevation of liver function tests (60 of 61 patients), diarrhea (58 of 61 patients), nausea/vomiting (59 of 61 patients), and the development of a skin rash (29 of 61 patients). Seventeen patients developed pulmonary complications. Fourteen patients experienced a mild decrease in arterial oxygenation. Three patients required ventilatory assistance, with two subsequently discharged form the hospital. The remaining patient died during hospitalization due to a nontraumatic subdural hematoma. Fifteen patients experienced transient cardiac symptoms generally manifesting as rhythm disturbances. Eighteen patients developed renal abnormalities with mild elevation of blood urea nitrogen or creatinine.

A unique and interesting phenomenon was the development of autologous GVHD. All patients underwent weekly skin biopsies while hospitalized. Liver and/or gastrointestinal biopsies were performed when clinically indicated to evaluate the incidence of autologous GVHD. Although these data are presently being evaluated, we have observed autologous GVHD of the skin manifested as a diffuse erythematous rash developing initially on the trunk and back and then extending to involve all four extremities. GVHD was documented pathologically, and the rash improved within days of discontinuing the IL-2. No patient received corticosteroid for management of GVHD.

Follow-up is too short to determine the possible impact of IL-2-activated PBSC transplantation on relapse and survival in these patients. However, the development of autologous GVHD, successful hematopoietic reconstitution, and lack of undue toxicities suggest that we may have been successful in altering the immune status of autologous marrow and PBSCs. It remains to be determined if these immunological effects will translate into clinical benefit due to a possible associated autologous graft-vs.-tumor effect. However, these initial results with IL-2-activated PBSCs clearly demonstrate the feasibility of such an approach in patients with poor-prognosis solid tumors.

Donor leukocyte infusions (DLI)

The GVL effect of allogeneic BMT seems to be critically dependent on mature T cells contained in allogeneic grafts. In an effort to induce GVHD and thus augment the GVL effect posttransplant in relapsed patients, peripheral blood mononuclear cells (PBMNCs) from the original bone marrow donors have been infused into these patients [128]. This approach seems to be promising mainly for patients with CML. Helg et al. [129] reported successful reinduction of complete hematological, cytogenetic, and molecular remission in two relapsed patients who were in chronic stable phase at initiation of leukocyte infusions and IFN-α therapy. The third patient, treated in accelerated phase, died with bone marrow aplasia 39 days following PBMNC infusion. Similar results were reported by Drobyski et al. [130] and Porter et al. [3]. In a limited number of small trials, results with DLI have not been as impressive in other hematological malignancies. These results have been further confirmed in a large multicenter trial reported recently [128]. In this study, patients with CML, AML, polycythemia vera (PV), MDS, and ALL were treated with DLI. Again, the best results were seen in CML patients in whom therapy was started early, when the patients were in cytogenetic relapse or stable hematological relapse.

Considerable toxicity is associated with DLI, the most common being GVHD and bone marrow aplasia. In the study by Kolb et al. [128] mentioned above, 79 of 133 patients (59%) developed GVHD. In 55 patients (41%), the GVHD was grade II or higher, and myelosuppression was a common side effect; 50% of CML patients who were in hematological relapse with a mixed chimerism developed myelosuppression. On the contrary, patients with cytogenetic relapses or with chemotherapy-induced remission were less prone to this effect, and only 4 of 34 patients developed myelosuppression. These findings suggest that myelosuppression in these patients is the result of suppression of recipient-derived hematopoiesis. It remains to be seen whether the infusion of donor cells and the resultant immune response selectively suppress the neoplastic clone or if the recipient-derived type of hematopoietic cells are indiscriminately eliminated. Six deaths were attributable to myelosuppression, and four additional patients died of combined myelosuppression and GVHD. In most of the other patients, myelosuppression reversed spontaneously or after a boost with donor marrow without immunosuppressive therapy. Similar side effects have been reported in other studies. This topic is discussed in greater detail in the chapter by Porter and Antin in this volume.

Tumor-specific immunotherapy

The development of effective cancer vaccines for treatment of established tumors or for tumor prevention remains a goal, but decades of efforts in this direction have not been very encouraging. Active, specific immunotherapy in patients with different tumors has been attempted by several investigators [131–136]. Vaccines consisting of irradiated autologous or allogeneic tumor cells, tumor cell lysates, or purified tumor antigens in combination with different immunological adjuvants have been used to immunize these patients, with encouraging results obtained in patients with melanoma, colon cancer, and lung cancer [5,137–140].

There is compelling evidence from experimental systems and anecdotal clinical reports that at least some tumors are immunogenic and that systemic antitumor immunity plays a role in eradication or control of tumor growth or metastasis. The immune repertoire of persons with cancer contains B and T cells that recognize antigens expressed by autologous cancer cells [141]. Several immunogenic molecules have been defined on cancer cells, including products of mutated oncogenes and different differentiation antigens [141]. Although most of these antigens are expressed on normal cells, aberrant expression on tumor tissues, due to either quantitative or qualitative alterations, makes these immunogenic [137]. Despite a detectable immune response against tumor cells, tumor progression can be explained by inherently weak immunogenicity of tumor antigens [137]. However, studies in experimental models suggest that even weakly immunogenic cancers can be rejected by the host's immune response after effective immunization [142,143].

Several methods have been employed to make tumor cells more immunogenic, including culturing tumor cells with IFN-γ to upregulate MHC molecules and transfecting with genes of costimulatory molecules and cytokines such as IL-2 and IFN-γ [64,134,139,143–145]. In experimental systems, all these strategies have enhanced the immunogenic potential of tumor cells. One encouraging finding has been that antitumor immunity induced by modified tumor cells extends to wild-type tumor as well [146]. Host factors may be important determinants of the outcome of immunization, especially in the context of immunotherapy. Immunosuppression in a tumor-bearing host can be the result of several known factors, such as a defective CD3 complex in T cells [147], elaboration of cytokines such as TGF-β, and other undefined factors [148]. The magnitude of immunosuppression parallels the tumor burden [149]. Therefore, chances of success with immunotherapy are improved if it is applied in a state of minimal residual disease, such as after BMT. Several other variables associated with BMT may enhance the success of immunotherapy in this setting, including elimination of suppressor cells and disruption of the architectural integrity of residual tumor by the conditioning regimen, thus making the tumor more susceptible to damage by immune effector mechanisms. However, the phenomenon of general immune suppression associated with BMT may be a potential concern. Most of the studies addressing the immunosuppression occurring post-BMT have looked only at nonspecific functions of the majority of B and T cells, which are de novo differentiating cells [150,151]. In contrast to these studies, there are reports of successful transfer of immunity to different viral and bacterial antigens by BMT, suggesting the presence of 'carry-over' memory cells [152,153]. Further, immunity can be boosted by posttransplant immunization [154]. As far as antitumor immunity is concerned, animals show a state of higher resistance to tumor uptake after transplant as compared to normal mice [155]. In addition, the occurrence of the GVL effect with GVHD suggests that, in spite of immunosuppression associated with BMT, effective antitumor mechanisms are operative. This evidence suggests that, although there is immunosuppression associated with BMT, it is not so great as to preclude antitumor immunotherapy.

Kwak et al. demonstrated the transfer of humoral anti-idiotypic response with resultant protective immunity to a murine B-cell tumor [156]. Our results in B16 murine melanoma suggest that antitumor immunity can be successfully transferred by BMT [157]. Mice transplanted with immune bone marrow reject fresh tumor, and in tumor-bearing animals this leads to a potent antitumor effect. Our preliminary results in the same model suggest that bone marrow from animals that are not fully immune to the tumor elicit more potent immunity in secondary recipients after BMT. Thus, BMT may represent an ideal situation for application of immunotherapeutic techniques. In addition, there is possibility of in vitro manipulation of bone marrow before reinfusion into the host to augment induced immune responses by procedures such as in vitro sensitization.

Despite these possible advantages associated with the application of immunotherapeutic strategies post-BMT, efforts in this direction have been limited. So far no results have been published evaluating the role of tumor-specific immunotherapy in the setting of ABMT. Recently, Kwak et al. reported the successful transfer of myeloma idiotype-specific immunity from an actively immunized bone marrow donor [158]. A normal sibling bone marrow donor was immunized with two doses of myeloma IgG (idiotype) conjugated to KLH and emulsified in an adjuvant. Tumor-specific immunity in the form of lymphoproliferative responses was noted in the recipient at days 30 and 60 posttransplant. A $CD4^+$ cell line of donor origin was developed from the recipient's peripheral blood mononuclear cells, and this proliferated in response to immunizing antigen. The patient was clinically well with a stable M component two years posttransplant. The report suggests that it may be possible to transfer tumor-specific immunity by bone marrow transplantation. These results, in conjunction with earlier work in experimental models, should provide the basis for evaluation of this strategy in larger clinical trials.

Conclusions

Immunotherapy as a treatment modality for neoplastic disorders has been attempted for several decades, with periods of enthusiasm and disillusionment. The application of this strategy in the transplant setting is relatively new. Several approaches are being evaluated, and results published thus far make it difficult to draw valid conclusions. Donor leukocyte infusions appear promising for patients with relapsed CML. In other disorders, efficacy is yet to be established. In the future, early institution of DLI for patients who are in early relapse should decrease the incidence of bone marrow aplasia and increase the likelihood of achieving complete remission. In vitro sensitization of donor lymphocytes with recipients' cells may potentiate efficacy. It is unclear whether the GVL effect observed in these patients is part of a generalized GVH allogeneic response or is selectively directed towards the recipients' hematopoietic stem cells or, more specifically, towards the neoplastic clone. Delineation of these mechanisms will raise further possibilities of selective augmentation of donor lymphocyte clones reactive with neoplastic cells from the recipient by various strategies, such as immunization of donor or in vitro sensitization of donor marrow with neoplastic cells or antigens. Cytokine modulation of autologous grafts, particularly with IL-2, is being explored by our group and others. Early results look promising in terms of feasibility of approach and induction of autologous GVHD. Planned randomized trials will answer the question about antitumor efficacy. Several other cytokines, including IL-4, IL-7, IL-12, and other stimulators of T cells and NK cells, synergize with IL-2 in some of its action. This finding raises the possibility of using a combination of different biological response modifiers and decreasing the toxicity associated with high-dose therapy with single agents.

Effective induction of tumor-specific immune responses to prevent or treat established disease is the goal of the tumor immunobiologist. Advances in understanding tumor-associated antigens, antigen processing, MHC binding and presentation, regulation of MHC expression, and further characterization of professional antigen-presenting cells such as dendritic cells should provide novel methods to induce immunity. The mechanism of tumor-induced immunosuppression and the mechanisms by which tumor cells evade immune mechanisms are still undefined. TGF-β is one of the most potent immunosuppressive factors known to be elaborated by tumor cells. Neutralization of these factors might improve the outcome of immunotherapy. Our results in a murine melanoma model indicate that a combination of IL-2 with anti-TGF-β antibody induces potent antitumor effects in conditions when neither of the agents is effective alone. Further experiments need to be conducted to determine whether neutralization of TGF-β can be used to augment the immunization potential of different whole tumor cell vaccines. Tumor-specific immunotherapy has not been explored to any significant extent in the transplant setting. Allogeneic BMT provides an ideal situation for such a technique, provided that potent, yet safe, immunogens and immunization strategies can be defined. Thus, immunization of normal allogeneic donors will overcome some of the problems associated with immunization of the patients, such as tolerance to self-tumor antigens and tumor-induced immunosuppression. Failure to reconstitute antitumor immunity in the face of posttransplant immunodeficiency and development of GVHD remains a major concern. However, techniques of mature T-cell add-back can circumvent the immune deficiency problem. In vitro manipulation of donor marrow or peripheral blood lymphocytes (PBLs) to enrich for tumor-reactive clones may enhance the GVL effect.

The majority of potential candidates for BMT do not receive allogeneic grafts for a multiplicity of reasons. Therefore, it becomes important to develop strategies for immunization of the tumor-bearing host. In this situation, it is important to develop novel ways to break tolerance to the tumor by immunization and by counterbalancing tumor-induced immunosuppressive mechanisms. Vaccination with genetically modified tumor cells (e.g., transfected with MHC, costimulatory molecules, and/or different cytokines) or with recombinant vectors expressing tumor antigens holds promise. Methods have been developed to culture and expand dendritic cells from hematopoietic stem cells. Tumor-antigen pulsed or transfected dendritic cells can be used for in vivo immunization. It would be interesting to see whether the same system can be used to sensitize autologous bone marrow grafts in vitro before reinfusion into patients.

References

1. Barrett AJ, Horowitz MM, Gale RP, et al. Marrow transplantation for acute lymphoblastic leukemia: factors affecting relapse and survival. Blood 74:862–871, 1989.
2. Champlin R. Graft-versus-leukemia without graft-versus-host disease: an elusive goal of bone marrow transplantation. Semin Hematol 29:46–52, 1992.
3. Porter DL, Roth MS, McGarigle C, Ferrara JL, Antin JH. Induction of graft-versus-host disease as immunotherapy for relapsed chronic myeloid leukemia. N Engl J Med 330:100–106, 1994.
4. Brenner MK, Rill DR, Moen RC, et al. Gene-marking to trace origin of relapse after autologous bone-marrow transplantation. Lancet 341:85–86, 1993.
5. Quan WD Jr., Mitchell MS. Immunology and immunotherapy of melanoma. Cancer Treat Res 65:257–277, 1993.
6. Morton DL. Active immunotherapy against cancer: present status. Semin Oncol 13:180–185, 1986.
7. Wang RF, Robbins PF, Kawakami Y, Kang XQ, Rosenberg SA. Identification of a gene encoding a melanoma tumor antigen recognized by HLA-A31-restricted tumor-infiltrating lymphocytes. J Exp Med 181:799–804, 1995.
8. Bernhard H, Karbach J, Wolfel T, et al. Cellular immune response to human renal-cell carcinomas: definition of a common antigen recognized by HLA-A2-restricted cytotoxic T-lymphocyte (CTL) clones. Int J Cancer 59:837–842, 1994.
9. Van der Bruggen P, Bastin J, Gajewski T, et al. A peptide encoded by human gene mage-3 and presented by HLA-A2 induces cytolytic T lymphocytes that recognize tumor cells expressing MAGE-3. Eur J Immunol 24:3038–3043, 1994.

10. Whittington R, Faulds D. Interleukin-2: a review of its pharmacological properties and therapeutic use in patients with cancer. Drugs 46:446–514, 1993.

11. Ghosh AK, Cerny T, Wagstaff J, Thatcher N, Moore M. Effect of in vivo administration of interferon gamma on expression of MHC products and tumor associated antigens in patients with metastatic melanoma. Eur J Cancer Clin Oncol 25:1637–1643, 1989.

12. Hirte HW, Clark DA, O'Connell G, Rusthoven J, Mazurka J. Reversal of suppression of lymphokine-activated killer cells by transforming growth factor-beta in ovarian carcinoma ascitic fluid requires interleukin-2 combined with anti-CD3 antibody. Cell Immunol 142:207–216, 1992.

13. Benyunes MC, Massumoto C, York A, et al. Interleukin-2 with or without lymphokine-activated killer cells as consolidative immunotherapy after autologous bone marrow transplantation for acute myelogenous leukemia. Bone Marrow Transplant 12:159–163, 1993.

14. Simpson C, Seipp CA, Rosenberg SA. The current status and future applications of interleukin-2 and adoptive immunotherapy in cancer treatment. Semin Oncol Nurs 4:132–141, 1988.

15. Fefer A, Benyunes M, Higuchi C, et al. Interleukin-2 +/– lymphocytes as consolidative immunotherapy after autologous bone marrow transplantation for hematologic malignancies. Acta Haematol 89 (Suppl 1):2–7, 1993.

16. Pavletic Z, Benyunes MC, Thompson JA, et al. Induction by interleukin-7 of lymphokine-activated killer activity in lymphocytes from autologous and syngeneic marrow transplant recipients before and after systemic interleukin-2 therapy. Exp Hematol 21:1371–1378, 1993.

17. Rosenberg SA. Immunotherapy of cancer using interleukin 2: current status and future prospects. Immunol Today 9:58–62, 1988.

18. Champlin R. T-cell depletion for allogeneic bone marrow transplantation: impact on graft-versus-host disease, engraftment, and graft-versus-leukemia. J Hematother 2:27–42, 1993.

19. Bron D. Graft-versus-host disease. Curr Opin Oncol 6:358–364, 1994.

20. Noga SJ, Hess AD. Lymphocyte depletion in bone marrow transplantation: will modulation of graft-versus-host disease prove to be superior to prevention? Semin Oncol 20:28–33, 1993.

21. Champlin R. Immunobiology of bone marrow transplantation as treatment for hematologic malignancies. Transplant Proc 23:2123–2127, 1991.

22. Boiron JM, Cony-Makhoul P, Mahon FX, Pigneux A, Puntous M, Reiffers J. Treatment of hematological malignancies relapsing after allogeneic bone marrow transplantation. Blood Rev 8:234–240, 1994.

23. Kennedy MJ, Vogelsang GB, Jones RJ, et al. Phase I trial of interferon gamma to potentiate cyclosporine-induced graft-versus-host disease in women undergoing autologous bone marrow transplantation for breast canncer. J Clin Oncol 12:249–257, 1994.

24. Smith KA. Interleukin-2: inception, impact, and implications. Science 240:1169–1176, 1988.

25. Waldmann TA, Pastan IH, Gansow OA, Junghans RP. The multichain interleukin-2 receptor: a target for immunotherapy. Ann Intern Med 116:148–160, 1992.

26. Grimm EA, Mazumder A, Zhang HZ, Rosenberg SA. Lymphokine-activated killer cell phenomenon. Lysis of natural killer-resistant fresh solid tumor cells by interleukin 2-activated autologous human peripheral blood lymphocytes. J Exp Med 155:1823–1841, 1982.

27. Lotze MT, Grimm EA, Mazumder A, Strausser JL, Rosenberg SA. Lysis of fresh and cultured autologous tumor by human lymphocytes cultured in T-cell growth factor. Cancer Res 41:4420–4425, 1981.

28. Chadwick BS, Miller RG. Heterogeneity of the lymphokine-activated killer cell phenotype. Cell Immunol 132:168–176, 1991.

29. Rosenberg SA, Lotze MT, Yang JC, et al. Experience with the use of high-dose interleukin-2 in the treatment of 652 cancer patients. Ann Surg 210:474–484, 1989.

30. Rosenberg SA. Karnofsky memorial lecture. The immunotherapy and gene therapy of cancer. J Clin Oncol 10:180–199, 1992.

31. Charak BS, Brynes RK, Groshen S, Chen SC, Mazumder A. Bone marrow transplantation with interleukin-2-activated bone marrow followed by interleukin-2 therapy for acute myeloid leukemia in mice. Blood 76:2187–2190, 1990.

48

32. Favrot MC, Floret D, Negrier S, et al. Systemic interleukin-2 therapy in children with progressive neuroblastoma after high dose chemotherapy and bone marrow transplantation. Bone Marrow Transplant 4:499–503, 1989.
33. Gottlieb DJ, Brenner MK, Heslop HE, et al. A phase I clinical trial of recombinant interleukin 2 following high dose chemo-radiotherapy for haematological malignancy: applicability to the elimination of minimal residual disease. Br J Cancer 60:610–615, 1989.
34. Blaise D, Olive D, Stoppa AM, et al. Hematologic and immunologic effects of the systemic administration of recombinant interleukin-2 after autologous bone marrow transplantation. Blood 76:1092–1097, 1990.
35. Higuchi CM, Thompson JA, Petersen FB, Buckner CD, Fefer A. Toxicity and immunomodulatory effects of interleukin-2 after autologous bone marrow transplantation for hematologic malignancies. Blood 77:2561–2568, 1991.
36. Soiffer RJ, Murray C, Cochran K, et al. Clinical and immunologic effects of prolonged infusion of low-dose recombinant interleukin-2 after autologous and T-cell-depleted allogeneic bone marrow transplantation. Blood 79:517–526, 1992.
37. Weisdorf DJ, Anderson PM, Blazar BR, Uckun FM, Kersey JH, Ramsay NK. Interleukin 2 immediately after autologous bone marrow transplantation for acute lymphoblastic leukemia — a phase I study. Transplantation 55:61–66, 1993.
38. Papa MZ, Mule JJ, Rosenberg SA. Antitumor efficacy of lymphokine-activated killer cells and recombinant interleukin 2 in vivo: successful immunotherapy of established pulmonary metastases from weakly immunogenic and nonimmunogenic murine tumors of three district histological types. Cancer Res 46:4973–4978, 1986.
39. Peace DJ, Cheever MA. Toxicity and therapeutic efficacy of high-dose interleukin 2. In vivo infusion of antibody to NK-1.1 attenuates toxicity without compromising efficacy against murine leukemia. J Exp Med 169:161–173, 1989.
40. Gottlieb DJ, Prentice HG, Heslop HE, et al. Effects of recombinant interleukin-2 administration on cytotoxic function following high-dose chemo-radiotherapy for hematological malignancy. Blood 74:2335–2342, 1989.
41. Hamon MD, Prentice HG, Gottlieb DJ, et al. Immunotherapy with interleukin 2 after ABMT in AML. Bone Marrow Transplant 11:399–401, 1993.
42. Sprent J, Schaefer M, Gao EK, Korngold R. Role of T cell subsets in lethal graft-versus-host disease (GVHD) directed to class I versus class II H-2 differences. I. L3T4+ cells can either augment or retard GVHD elicited by Lyt-2+ cells in class I different hosts. J Exp Med 167:556–569, 1988.
43. Malkovsky M, Brenner MK, Hunt R, et al. T-cell depletion of allogeneic bone marrow prevents acceleration of graft-versus-host disease induced by exogenous interleukin 2. Cell Immunol 103:476–480, 1986.
44. Sykes M, Abraham BS, Harty MW, Pearson DA. IL-2 reduces graft-versus-host disease and preserves a graft-versus-leukemia effect by selectively inhibiting CD4+ T cell activity. J Immunol 150:197–205, 1993.
45. Sykes M, Harty MW, Szot GL, Pearson DA. Interleukin-2 inhibits graft versus host disease promoting activity of CD4+ cells while preserving CD4− and CD8− mediated graft versus leukemia effects. Blood 83:2560–2569, 1994.
46. Azuma E, Kaplan J. Role of lymphokine-activated killer cells as mediators of veto and natural suppression. J Immunol 141:2601–2606, 1988.
47. Nakamura H, Gress RE. Interleukin-2 enhancement of veto suppressor cell function in T-cell-depleted bone marrow in vitro and in vivo. Transplantation 49:931–937, 1990.
48. Sykes M, Romick ML, Sachs DH. Interleukin-2 prevents graft-versus-host disease while preserving the graft-versus-leukemia effect of allogeneic T cells. Proc Natl Acad Sci USA 87:5633–5637, 1990.
49. Soiffer RJ, Murray C, Gonin R, Ritz J. Effect of low-dose interleukin-2 on disease relapse after T-cell-depleted allogeneic bone marrow transplantation. Blood 84:964–971, 1994.
50. Fujimori Y, Hara H, Nagai K. Effect of lymphokine activated killer cell fraction on the development of human hematopoietic progenitor cells. Cancer Res 48:534–538, 1987.

51. van den Brink MRM, Voogt PJ, Marijt WAF, van Luxemburg-Heys SAP, Van Rood JJ, Brand AA. Lymphokine activated killer cells selectively kill tumor cells in bone marrow without compromising bone marrow stem cell function in vitro. Blood 74:354–560, 1989.

52. Charak BS, Malloy B, Agah R, Mazumder A. A novel approach to purging of leukemia by activation of bone marrow with interleukin-2. Bone Marrow Transplant 6:193–198, 1990.

53. Schaafsma MR, Fibbe WE, van der Harst D, et al. Increased numbers of circulating hematopoietic progenitor cells after treatment with high dose interleukin-2 in cancer patients. Br J Haematol 76:180–185, 1990.

54. Heslop HE, Bello-Fernandez C, Reittie JE, et al. Interleukin 2 infusion after autologous bone marrow transplantation or chemotherapy enhances hematopoietic regeneration (abstract). Blood 76 (Suppl 1):544a, 1990.

55. Bosly AE, Staquet PJ, Doyen CM, Chatelain BJ, Humblet YP, Symann ML. Recombinant human interleukin-2 restores in vitro T-cell colony formation by peripheral blood mononuclear cells after autologous bone marrow transplantation. Exp Hematol 15:1048–1054, 1987.

56. Borradori L, Hirt A, Baumgartner C, Morell A. Influence of exogenous interleukin-2 on the proliferation of lymphocytes from normal donors and from patients after autologous bone marrow transplantation. Acta Haematol 77:129–134, 1987.

57. Reittie JE, Gottlieb D, Heslop HE, et al. Endogenously generated killer cells circulate after autologous and allogeneic bone marrow transplantation but not after chemotherapy. Blood 73:1341–1358, 1989.

58. Bosly A, Guillame T, Brice P, et al. Effects of escalating doses of recombinant human interleukin-2 in correcting functional T-cell defects following autologous bone marrow transplantation for lymphomas and solid tumors. Exp Hematol 20:962–968, 1992.

59. Heslop HE, Gottlieb DJ, Bianchi ACM, et al. In vivo induction of γ interferon and tumor necrosis factor by interleukin-2 infusion following intensive chemotherapy or autologous bone marrow transplantation. Blood 74:1374–1380, 1989.

60. Massumoto C, Sale G, Benyunes M, et al. Cutaneous GVHD associated with IL-2 + LAK therapy after autologous bone marrow transplantation (ABMT) for hematologic malignancies (abstract). Proc Am Soc Clin Oncol 11:825a, 1992.

61. Price G, Brenner MK, Prentice HG, Hoffbrand AV, Newland AC. Cytotoxic effects of tumor necrosis factor and gamma interferon on acute myeloid leukemia blast cells. Br J Cancer 55:287–290, 1987.

62. Herberman RB, Ortaldo JR, Montovani A, Hobbs DS, Kung HF, Pestka S. Effect of human recombinant interferon on cytotoxic activity of natural killer (NK) cells and monocytes. Cell Immunol 67:160–167, 1982.

63. Guadagni F, Schlom J, Johnston WW, et al. Selective interferon-induced enhancement of tumor-associated antigens on a spectrum of freshly isolated human adenocarcinoma cells. J Natl Cancer Inst 81:502–512, 1989.

64. Jabrane-Ferrat N, Faille A, Loiseau P, Poirier O, Charron D, Calvo F. Effect of gamma interferon on HLA class-I and II transcription and protein expression in human breast adenocarcinoma cell lines. Int J Cancer 45:1169–1176, 1990.

65. Giacomini P, Fisher PB, Duigou GJ, Gambari R, Natali PG. Regulation of class II MHC gene expression by interferons: insights into the mechanism of action of interferon (review). Anticancer Res 8:1153–1161, 1988.

66. Boyer CM, Dawson DV, Neal SE, et al. Differential induction by interferons of major histocompatibility complex-encoded and non-major histocompatibility complex-encoded antigens in human breast and ovarian carcinoma cell lines. Cancer Res 49:2928–2934, 1989.

67. Nouri AM, Hussain RF, Dos Santos AV, Gillott DJ, Oliver RT. Induction of MHC antigens by tumour cell lines in response to interferons. Eur J Cancer 28A:1110–1115, 1992.

68. Carlo Stella C, Cazzola M. Interferons as biologic modulators of hematopoietic cell proliferation and differentiation. Haematologica 73:225–237, 1988.

69. Bilgrami S, Silva M, Cardoso A, Miller KB, Ascensao JL. Immunotherapy with autologous bone-marrow transplantation: rationale and results. Exp Hematol 22:1039–1050, 1994.
70. Meyers JD, Flournoy N, Sanders JE, et al. Prophylactic use of human leukocyte interferon after allogeneic marrow transplantation. Ann Intern Med 107:809–816, 1987.
71. Winston DJ, Ho WG, Schroff RW, Champlin RE, Gale RP. Safety and tolerance of recombinant leukocyte a interferon in bone marrow transplant recipients. Antimicrob Agents Chemother 23:846–851, 1983.
72. McGlave PB, Arthur D, Miller WJ, Lasky L, Kersey J. Autologous transplantation for CML using marrow treated ex vivo with recombinant human interferon gamma. Bone Marrow Transplant 6:115–120, 1990.
73. Lo Coco F, Mandelli F, Diverio D, et al. Therapy-induced Ph1 suppression in chronic myeloid leukemia: molecular and cytogenetic studies in patients treated with alpha-2b IFN, high-dose chemotherapy and autologous stem cell infusion. Bone Marrow Transplant 6:253–258, 1990.
74. Higuchi W, Moriyama Y, Kishi K, et al. Hematopoietic recovery in a patient with acute lymphoblastic leukemia after an autologous marrow graft purged by combined hyperthermia and interferon in vitro. Bone Marrow Transplant 7:163–166, 1991.
75. Kantarjian HM, Talpaz M, Le Maistre CF, et al. Intensive combination chemotherapy and autologous bone marrow transplantation leads to the reappearance of Philadelphia chromosome-negative cells in chronic myelogenous leukemia. Cancer 67:2959–2965, 1991.
76. Klingemann HG, Grigg AP, Wilkie-Boyd K, et al. Treatment with recombinant interferon (alpha-2b) early after bone marrow transplantation in patients at high risk for relapse. Blood 78:3306–3311, 1991.
77. Attal M, Huguet F, Schlaifer D, et al. Intensive combined therapy for previously untreated aggressive myeloma. Blood 79:1130–1136, 1992.
78. Neloni G, De Fabritiis P, Alimena G, et al. Autologous bone marrow or peripheral blood stem cell transplantation for patients with chronic myeloid leukemia in chronic phase. Bone Marrow Transplant 4 (Suppl 4):92, 1989.
79. Ascensao JL, Miller KB, Tuck D, et al. Immunotherapy with interferon-alpha-2b (IFN) following autologous bone marrow transplantation (ABMT) for lymphomas: an update (abstract). Proc Am Soc Clin Oncol 12:380, 1993.
80. Graze PR, Gale RP. Chronic graft versus host disease: a syndrome of disordered immunity. Am J Med 66:611–620, 1979.
81. Deeg HJ, Storb R. Acute and chronic graft versus host disease: clinical manifestations, prophylaxis, and treatment. J Natl Cancer Inst 76:1325–1328, 1986.
82. Weiden PL, Sullivan KM, Fluornoy N, Storb R, Thomas ED. Antileukemic effect of graft-versus-host disease in human recipients of allogeneic-marrow grafts. N Eng J Med 300:1068–1073, 1979.
83. Butturini A, Bortin MM, Gale RP. Graft-versus-leukemia following bone marrow transplantation. Bone Marrow Transplant 2:233–242, 1987.
84. Chopra R, Goldstone AH, Pearce R, et al. Autologous versus allogeneic bone marrow transplantation for non-Hodgkin's lymphoma: a case controlled analysis of the European Bone Marrow Transplant Group registry data. J Clin Oncol 10:1690–1695, 1992.
85. Glazier AD, Tutschka PJ, Farmer ER, Santos GW. Graft-versus-host disease in cyclosporine A treated rats following syngeneic and autologous bone marrow reconstitution. J Exp Med 158:1–8, 1983.
86. Hess AD, Horwitz L, Beschorner WE, Santos GW. Development of graft-versus-host disease-like syndrome in cyclosporine-treated rats after syngeneic bone marrow transplantation. I. Development of cytotoxic T lymphocytes with apparent polyclonal anti-Ia specificity, including autoreactivity. J Exp Med 161:718–730, 1985.
87. Hess AD, Jones RC, Santos GW. Autologous graft-versus-host disease: mechanism and potential therapeutic effect. Bone Marrow Transplant 12 (Suppl 3):S65, 1993.

88. Jones RJ, Vogelsang GB, Hess AD, Farmer ER, Mann R, Geller PB, Piantadosi S, Santos GW. Induction of graft versus host disease after autologous bone marrow transplantation. Lancet 1:754–757, 1989.

89. Yeager AM, Vogelsang GB, Jones RJ, Farmer ER, Altomonte V, Hess AD, Santos GW. Induction of cutaneous graft-versus-host reaction by administration of cyclosporine to patients undergoing autologous bone marrow transplantation for acute myeloid leukemia. Blood 79:3031–3035, 1992.

90. Santos GW. Autologous graft vs host disease (abstract). Exp Hematol 19:463, 1991.

91. Gribben JG, Freedman AS, Neuberg D, et al. Immunological purging of marrow assessed by PCR before autologous bone marrow transplantation for B cell lymphoma. N Engl J Med 325:1525–1533, 1991.

92. Ringden O, Horowitz MM. Graft-versus-leukemia reactions in humans. The Advisory Committee of the International Bone Marrow Transplant Registry. Transplant Proc 21:2989–2992, 1989.

93. Rosenfeld C, Shadduck RK, Przepiorka D, Mangan KF, Colvin M. Autologous bone marrow transplantation with 4-hydroperoxycyclophosphamide purged marrows for acute nonlymphocytic leukemia in late remission or early relapse. Blood 74:1159–1164, 1989.

94. Pole JG, Gee A, Jansen W, Lee C, Gross S. Immunomagnetic purging of bone marrow: a model for negative cell selection. Am J Pediatr Hematol Oncol 12:257–261, 1990.

95. Vogler WR, Berdel WE, Olson AC, Winton EF, Heffner LT, Gordon DS. Autologous bone marrow transplantation in acute leukemia with marrow purged with alkylysophospholipids. Blood 80:1423–1429, 1992.

96. Uckun FM, Kersey JH, Vallera DA, et al. Autologous bone marrow transplantation in high risk remission T-lineage acute lymphoblastic leukemia using immunotoxins plus 4-hydroperoxycyclophosphamide for marrow purging. Blood 76:1723–1733, 1990.

97. Truitt RL, Horowitz MM, Atasoylu AA, Drobyski WR, Johnson BD, LeFever AV. Graft-versus-leukemia effect of allogeneic bone marrow transplantation: clinical and experimental aspects of late leukemia relapse. In Stewart THM, Wheelock EF (eds), Cellular Immune Mechanisms and Tumor Dormancy. Boca Raton: CRC Press, 1992, pp. 111–128.

98. Horowitz MM, Gale RP, Sondel PM, et al. Graft-versus-leukemia reactions after bone marrow transplantation. Blood 75:555–562, 1990.

99. Chang WC, Hsiao MH, Pattengale PK. Natural killer cell immunodeficiency in patients with chronic myelogenous leukemia. IV. Interleukin-1 deficiency, gamma-interferon deficiency and the restorative effects of short term culture in the presence of interleukin-2 on natural killer cytotoxicity, natural killer-target binding and production of natural killer cytotoxic factor. Nat Immunol Cell Growth Regul 10:57–70, 1991.

100. Mackinnon S, Hows JM, Goldman JM. Induction of in vitro graft-versus-leukemia activity following bone marrow transplantation for chronic myelogenous leukemia. Blood 76:2037–2045, 1990.

101. Hauch M, Gazzold MV, Small T, et al. Anti-leukemia potential of interleukin-2 activated natural killer cells after bone marrow transplantation for chronic myelogenous leukemia. Blood 75:2250–2262, 1990.

102. Agah R, Malloy B, Kerner M, Mazumder A. Generation and characterization of IL-2 activated bone marrow cells as a potent graft versus tumor effector in transplantation. J Immunol 143:3039–3099, 1989.

103. Charak BS, Brynes RK, Katsuda S, Groshen S, Chen S-C, Mazumder A. Induction of graft versus leukemia effect in bone marrow transplantation: dosage and time schedule dependency of interleukin 2 therapy. Cancer Res 51:2015–2020, 1991.

104. Charak BS, Agah R, Gray D, Mazumder A. Interaction of various cytokines with interleukin-2 in the generation of killer cells from human bone marrow: application in purging of leukemia. Leuk Res 15:801–810, 1991.

105. Keever CA, Pekle K, Gazzola MV, Collins NH, Gillio A. NK and LAK activities from human bone marrow progenitors. I. The effects of interleukin-2 and interleukin-1. Cell Immunol 126:211–226, 1990.

106. Agah R, Malloy B, Kerner M, Girgis E, Bean P, Twomey P, Mazumder A. Potent graft antitumor effect in natural killer-resistant disseminated tumors by transplantation of interleukin-2-activated syngeneic bone marrow in mice. Cancer Res 49:5959–5963, 1989.

107. Lotze MT, Matory YL, Ettinghausen SE, et al. In vivo administration of purified human interleukin-2: half life, immunologic effects, and expansion of peripheral lymphoid cells in vivo with recombinant IL-2. J Immunol 135:2865–2875, 1985.

108. Kedar E, Klein E. Cancer immunotherapy: are the results discouraging? can they be improved? Adv Cancer Res 59:245–322, 1992.

109. Mitchell MS. Combining chemotherapy with biological response modifiers in the treatment of cancer. J Natl Cancer Inst 80:1445–1450, 1988.

110. Charak BS, Brynes RK, Chogyoji M, Kortes V, Tefft M, Mazumder A. Graft versus leukemia effect of interleukin-2-activated bone marrow: correlation with eradication of residual disease. Transplantation 56:31–37, 1993.

111. Charak BS, Agah R, Brynes RK, Chogyoji M, Groshen S, Chen S-C, Mazumder A. Interleukin-2 (IL-2) and IL-2-activated bone marrow in transplantation: evaluation from a clinical perspective. Bone Marrow Transplant 9:479–486, 1992.

112. Coulombel L, Kalousek D, Eaves CJ, Gupta CM, Eaves A. Long-term marrow culture reveals chromosomally normal hematopoietic progenitor cells in patients with Philadelphia chromosome-positive chronic myelogenous leukemia. N Engl J Med 308:1493–1498, 1983.

113. Hogge DE, Coulombel L, Kalousek DK, Eaves CJ, Eaves AC. Nonclonal hemopoietic progenitors in a G6PD heterozygote with chronic myelogenous leukemia revealed after long-term marrow culture. Am J Hematol 24:389–394, 1987.

114. Coulombel L, Eaves CJ, Kalousek DK, Gupta C, Eaves Ac. Long term marrow culture of cells from patients with acute myelogenous leukemia. J Clin Invest 75:961–969, 1985.

115. Firkin FC, Birner R, Farag S. Differential action of diffusible molecules in long term culture on proliferation of leukemic and normal hematopoietic cells. Br J Hematol 84:8–15, 1993.

116. Udomsakdi C, Eaves CJ, Swolin B, Reid DS, Barnett MJ, Eaves AC. Rapid decline of chronic myeloid leukemic cells in long term culture due to a defect at the leukemic stem cell level. Proc Natl Acad Sci 89:6192–6196, 1992.

117. Lotzova E, Savary CA. Generation of NK cell activity from human bone marrow. J Immunol 139:279–284, 1987.

118. Verma UN, Bagg A, Brown E, Mazumder A. Interleukin-2 activation of human bone marrow in long term cultures: an effective strategy for purging and generation of anti-tumor cytotoxic effectors. Bone Marrow Transplant 13:115–123, 1994.

119. Klingemann HG, Deal H, Reid D, Eaves CJ. Pre-clinical evaluation of a bone marrow autograft culture procedure for generating lymphokine-activated killer cells in vitro. Can J Infect Dis 3:123B–127B, 1992.

120. Klingemann HG, Deal H, Reid D, Eaves CJ. Design and validation of a clinically applicable culture procedure for the generation of interleukin-2 activated natural killer cells in human bone marrow autografts. Exp Hematol 21:1263–1270, 1993.

121. Long GS, Cramer DV, Harnaha JB, Hiserodt JC. Lymphokine-activated killer (LAK) cell purging of leukemic bone marrow: range of activity against different hematopoietic neoplasms. Bone Marrow Transplant 6:169–177, 1990.

122. Chao N, Schriber J, Grimes K, et al. Granulocyte colony-stimulating factor 'mobilized' peripheral blood progenitor cells accelerate granulocyte and platelet recovery after high dose chemotherapy. Blood 81:2031–2035, 1993.

123. To LB, Roberts MM, Haylock DN, et al. Comparison of hematological recovery times and supportive care requirements of autologous recovery phase peripheral blood stem cell transplants, autologous bone marrow transplants and allogeneic bone marrow transplants. Bone Marrow Transplant 9:277–284, 1992.

124. Kessinger A, Armitage JO. The evolving role of autologous peripheral stem cell transplantation following high-dose therapy for malignancies. Blood 77:211–213, 1991.

125. Kessinger A, Bierman P, Vose J, Armitage JO. High-dose cyclophosphamide, carmustine, and etopside followed by autologous peripheral stem cell transplantation for patients with relapsed Hodgkin's disease. Blood 77:2322–2325, 1991.

126. Liu K-Y, Akashi K, Harada M, Takamatsu Y, Niho Y. Kinetics of circulating hematopoietic progenitors during chemotherapy-induced mobilization with or without granulocyte colony-stimulating factor. Br J Haematol 84:31–38, 1993.

127. Verma UN, Areman E, Dickerson SA, Kotula PL, Sacher R, Mazumder A. Interleukin-2 activation of chemotherapy and growth factor mobilized peripheral blood stem cells for generation of cytotoxic effectors. Bone Marrow Transplant 15:199–206, 1995.

128. Kolb KJ, Schattenberg A, Goldman JM, et al. Graft-versus-leukemia effect of donor lymphocyte transfusions in marrow grafted patients. Blood 86:2041–2050, 1995.

129. Helg C, Roux E, Beris P, et al. Adoptive immunotherapy for recurrent CML after BMT. Bone Marrow Transplant 12:125–129, 1993.

130. Drobyski WR, Keever CA, Roth MS, et al. Salvage immunotherapy using donor leukocyte infusions as treatment for relapsed chronic myelogenous leukemia after allogeneic bone marrow transplantation: efficacy and toxicity of a defined T-cell dose. Blood 82:2310–2318, 1993.

131. Mitchell MS, Harel W, Kan-Mitchell J, et al. Active specific immunotherapy of melanoma with allogeneic cell lysates. Rationale, results, and possible mechanisms of action. Ann N Y Acad Sci 690:153–166, 1993.

132. Berd D, Maguire HC Jr., McCue P, Mastrangelo MJ. Treatment of metastatic melanoma with an autologous tumor-cell vaccine: clinical and immunologic results in 64 patients. J Clin Oncol 8:1858–1867, 1990.

133. Hanna MG Jr., Ransom JH, Pomato N, et al. Active specific immunotherapy of human colorectal carcinoma with an autologous tumor cell/Bacillus Calmette-Guerin vaccine. Ann N Y Acad Sci 690:135–146, 1993.

134. Gilboa E, Lyerly HK, Vieweg J, Saito S. Immunotherapy of cancer using cytokine gene-modified tumor vaccines. Semin Cancer Biol 5:409–417, 1994.

135. Barth A, Hoon DS, Foshag LJ, et al. Polyvalent melanoma cell vaccine induces delayed-type hypersensitivity and in vitro cellular immune response. Cancer Res 54:3342–3345, 1994.

136. Plaksin D, Porgador A, Vadai E, Feldman M, Schirrmacher V, Eisenbach L. Effective anti-metastatic melanoma vaccination with tumor cells transfected with MHC genes and/or infected with newcastle disease virus (NDV). Int J Cancer 59:796–801, 1994.

137. Finn OJ. Tumor-specific immune responses and opportunities for tumor vaccines. Clin Immunol Immunopathol 71:260–262, 1994.

138. Mastrangelo MJ, Schultz S, Kane M, Berd D. Newer immunologic approaches to the treatment of patients with melanoma. Semin Oncol 15:589–594, 1988.

139. Pardoll DM. Cancer vaccines. Trends Pharmacol Sci 14:202–208, 1993.

140. Golumbek P, Levitsky H, Jaffee L, Pardoll DM. The antitumor immune response as a problem of self–nonself discrimination: implications for immunotherapy. Immunol Res 12:183–192, 1993.

141. Houghton AN. Cancer antigens: immune recognition of self and altered self. J Exp Med 180:1–4, 1994.

142. Johnston D, Bystryn JC. Immunogenicity and tumor protective activity of B16 melanoma vaccines. Mol Biother 1:218–222, 1989.

143. Sainouchi R, Terata N, Kodama M. The induction of enhanced antitumor effect against a nonimmunogenic tumor by highly immunogenic variants obtained by mutagen treatment. Jpn J Cancer Res 79:1247–1253, 1988.

144. Guadagni F, Roselli M, Schlom J, Greiner JW. In vitro and in vivo regulation of human tumor antigen expression by human recombinant interferons: a review. Int J Biol Markers 9:53–60, 1994.

145. Pardoll DM. New strategies for enhancing the immunogenicity of tumors. Curr Opin Immunol 5:719–725, 1993.

54

146. Vanky F, Stuber G, Rotstein S, Klein E. Auto-tumor recognition following in vitro induction of MHC antigen expression on solid human tumors: stimulation of lymphocytes and generation of cytotoxicity against the original MHC-antigen-negative tumor cells. Cancer Immunol Immunother 28:17–21, 1989.
147. Mizoguchi H, O'Shea JJ, Longo DL, Loeffler CM, McVicar DW, Ochoa AC. Alterations in signal transduction molecules in T lymphocytes from tumor-bearing mice. Science 258:1795–1798, 1992.
148. Sulitzeanu D. Immunosuppressive factors in human cancer. Ady Cancer Res 60:247–267, 1993.
149. Deckers PJ, Davis RC, Parker GA, Mannick JA. The effect of tumor size on concomitant immunity. Cancer Response 33:33–39, 1973.
150. Verma UN, Mazumder A. Immune reconstitution following bone marrow transplantation. Cancer Immunol Immunother 37:351–360, 1993.
151. Roberts MM, To LB, Gillis D, et al. Immune reconstitution following peripheral blood stem cell transplantation, autologous bone marrow transplantation and allogeneic bone marrow transplantation. Bone Marrow Transplant 12:469–475, 1993.
152. Ilan Y, Nagler A, Shouval D, et al. Development of antibodies to hepatitis B virus surface antigen in bone marrow transplant recipient following treatment with peripheral blood lymphocytes from immunized donors. Clin Exp Immunol 97:299–302, 1994.
153. Ljungman P, Lewensohn-Fuchs I, Hammarstrom V, et al. Long-term immunity to measles, mumps, and rubella after allogeneic bone marrow transplantation. Blood 84:657–663, 1994.
154. Hammarstrom V, Pauksen K, Azinge J, Oberg G, Ljungman P. Pneumococcal immunity and response to immunization with pneumococcal vaccine in bone marrow transplant patients: the influence of graft versus host reaction. Support Care Cancer 1:195–199, 1993.
155. Kwak LW, Grand LC, Williams RM. Radiation-induced augmentation of host resistance to histocompatible tumor in mice. Detection of a graft antitumor effect of syngeneic bone marrow transplantation. Transplantation 51:1244–1248, 1991.
156. Kwak LW, Campbell M, Levy R. Idiotype vaccination post-bone marrow transplantation for B-cell lymphoma: initial studies in a murine model. Cancer Detect Prev 15:323–325, 1991.
157. Verma UN, Hodgson J, Brown E, Mazumder A. Anti-tumor immunity to B16 murine melanoma: induction, transfer, and generation of a graft versus tumor effect by syngeneic bone marrow transplantation with an immune graft. (Submitted.)
158. Kwak LW, Campbell MJ, Czerwinski DK, Hart S, Miller RA, Levy R. Induction of immune responses in patients with B-cell lymphoma against the surface-immunoglobulin idiotype expressed by their tumors. N Engl J Med 327:1209–1215, 1992.

3. Graft-versus-leukemia effect of allogeneic bone marrow transplantation and donor mononuclear cell infusions

David L. Porter and Joseph H. Antin

Allogeneic bone marrow transplantation (BMT) has proven to be curative for many patients with hematologic malignancies. Myeloablative doses of chemotherapy, with or without radiotherapy, are administered to patients, and normal hematopoiesis is restored with the infusion of normal donor bone marrow. Yet despite intensive conditioning therapy, many patients have residual disease that can result in recurrent leukemia. The prevalence of these residual leukemic cells is most evident after syngeneic BMT, when there is a high relapse rate. However, allogeneic bone marrow transfers not only normal hematopoietic elements but also mature alloreactive immune cells that may be capable of reacting against a host's residual leukemia. Increasing evidence suggests that this is an important immunologic mechanism that contributes to the success of transplantation by eradicating residual disease. This phenomenon is referred to as the *graft-vs.-leukemia* (GVL) effect. Hence, as suggested by Mathe, allogeneic BMT can be considered a successful form of 'adoptive immunotherapy' [1].

As supportive care after BMT has become more sophisticated and successful, relapse has become a major cause of treatment failure. The conditioning regimens currently in use in most allogeneic transplant protocols are already administered at near maximal tolerated doses, and it is unlikely that further dose intensification will have a significant impact on relapse rates.Until recently, the only curative option for patients who relapse after allogeneic transplant has been a second BMT, but this option is successful for only a minority of patients. There is a clear need to develop more effective and safer strategies to deal with minimal residual disease and relapse. This need has led to extensive efforts designed to enhance the GVL effects of allogeneic donor cells to prevent, as well as to treat, relapsed leukemia after allogeneic BMT.

Defining the GVL reaction in animal models

The first description of a GVL reaction in mice was provided by Barnes and colleagues [2,3]. In their experiments, leukemic mice received a subablative dose of radiation followed by transplantation with either syngeneic or alloge-

Jane N. Winter (ed.) BLOOD STEM CELL TRANSPLANTATION. 1997. Kluwer Academic Publishers. ISBN 0-7923-4260-7. All rights reserved.

neic bone marrow. Only the recipients of syngeneic marrow died from recurrent leukemia. Barnes et al. postulated that the antileukemic effect was due to 'a process of immunity' provided by the allogeneic marrow, now referred to as the 'GVL' effect. Interestingly, the allogeneic marrow recipients tended to die of a 'wasting syndrome' now recognized as graft-vs.-host disease (GVHD); this was the first report to highlight the intimate relationship between GVL and GVHD.

Since these early experiments, the GVL reaction has been studied in detail in murine models of transplantation, and has been reviewed elsewhere [4,5]. While these experiments are extremely useful in modeling GVL, the results must be interpreted with caution. Conclusions about the magnitude of GVL and about the effector cells responsible for GVL or GVHD may depend on the leukemia model studied, specific experimental conditions, and the degree of major histocompatability complex (MHC) variation between donor and host. In addition, many murine leukemias are virally induced, and it can be difficult to distinguish specific antiviral immunity from GVL. Ultimately, most murine experiments are performed under conditions that are unlikely to have direct clinical application. Nevertheless, these important models form the basis for many subsequent clinical trials and will be reviewed briefly.

It is generally accepted that donor T cells mediate not only acute GVHD [6] but also GVL reactivity in murine models [5,7,8]. For instance, depletion of T cells from the donor graft results in loss of both GVHD and GVL [9–11]. It is also clear that under appropriate experimental conditions in mice, GVL activity can be separated from undesirable GVHD toxicity. Bortin and colleagues first showed it was possible to dissociate GVL and GVHD in an MHC-matched, but minor-antigen-mismatched, donor–host combination (CBA into AKR, H-2^k compatible) [12]. In this model, GVL activity is enhanced without an increase in GVHD if the donor (CBA) is preimmunized with allogeneic (AKR) leukemic or nonleukemic cells, followed by adoptive transfer of donor cells to leukemic AKR mice. Preimmunization with H-2-incompatible cells induced GVL but also enhanced GVHD toxicity.

These preliminary findings have led to extensive experiments by Truitt and colleagues designed to separate and identify specific GVL and GVHD effector mechanisms; much of this work has been reviewed [4]. GVL reactivity in this system can be reliably induced only when the donor is preimmunized against minor-mismatched (non-H-2-encoded) antigens. When different strain combinations are analyzed, quantitative differences in GVL reactivity are seen, implying that specific minor antigenic differences, or the number of mismatched antigens, may influence GVL [4]. Furthermore, in this alloimmunization model, CD4+ cells are primarily responsible for GVHD, while CD8+ T cells possess the majority of cytolytic, GVL activity [4]. Subsequent experiments demonstrate that CD4+ cells are required for maximal GVL reactivity induced by the CD8+ T-cell population [11]. The finding that both CD4+ and CD8+ lymphocytes contribute to GVL is consistent with other murine models of transplantation [10,13].

In a fully mismatched model of BMT (A/J into B10 across major histocompatibility barriers), Sykes and colleagues have shown that GVHD and GVL are also separable and induced by different lymphocyte populations [8]. Similar to the findings described above, the CD4+ subset of donor T cells primarily mediate GVHD, while the CD8+ T cells are necessary for the GVL effects [14]. In a different strain combination (A/J into BALB/c), both CD4+ and CD8+ contribute to GVL reactivity [15].

To further dissociate GVL and GVHD, Sykes et al. have shown that a short course of IL-2 administration can minimize GVHD while preserving GVL, largely through selective inhibition of the CD4+ T cells [8,14]. IL-2 is a potent inducer of NK-cell activity and has been used in other model systems to augment GVL reactivity [16,17]. While there are few data definitively implicating NK cells as direct effectors of GVL in mice, it seems likely that MHC-unrestricted mechanisms would contribute to GVL. Notably, in one study, depletion of NK cells from the allogeneic graft did not influence GVL reactivity [18]. While IL-2 may induce other effector mechanisms [14], NK-cell activation is likely to be an important component of the observed GVL effect.

These models emphasize the complexity of the GVL reaction. It is most likely that more than one cell population or effector mechanism is responsible for GVL, and different effectors may be of varying importance depending on the model system under investigation. It is true that murine models may not always be directly applicable to clinical use, but they will continue to serve as a guide in designing future clinical trials.

GVL in clinical transplantation

Until recently, the evidence for a significant GVL reaction in clinical BMT has been largely circumstantial and based on several important, but indirect observations (table 1). These observations also begin to identify potential mechanisms underlying GVL reactivity, and form the basis for developing innovative approaches to immunotherapy designed to enhance and manipulate the GVL reaction for clinical benefit.

Table 1. Indirect evidence for a GVL reaction in clinical BMT

- Abrupt withdrawal of immunosuppression, or a flare of graft-vs.-host disease, may induce complete remissions in some patients with relapsed leukemia after BMT (anecdotal).
- Syngeneic BMT is associated with a higher risk of relapse than allogeneic BMT.
- Graft-vs.-host disease after BMT is associated with a lower risk of relapse.
- T-cell depletion of the donor bone marrow results in an increased risk of relapse, especially for patients with CML.

Remission after relapse can be induced by a flare of GVHD or withdrawal of immune suppression

Anecdotal reports describe patients with relapsed leukemia after allogeneic BMT that reenter at least transient remission after a flare of GVHD [19]. For patients who relapse while receiving immunosuppressive therapy, withdrawal of immunosuppression may induce a flare of GVHD and also induce complete remissions [20–22]. While abrupt discontinuation of immunosuppressive therapy is a simple maneuver as a first attempt at restoring GVL reactivity, unfortunately, it is anticipated that only occasional patients will respond.

Syngeneic marrow grafts are associated with increased relapse rates

Leukemia relapse rates are increased after syngeneic BMT when compared to matched sibling transplantation [23]. A recent update of the Seattle experience analyzed over 800 patients transplanted with advanced leukemia (ALL or ANLL in second or greater complete remission or relapse) and noted that the relapse rate was 62% for 785 recipients of allogeneic grafts compared to 75% for 53 recipients of syngeneic grafts ($p < 0.0001$) [24]. A more dramatic difference in relapse rates was noted in a multicenter analysis of patients

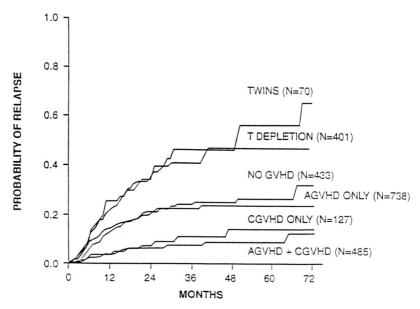

Figure 1. Probability of relapse after allogeneic bone marrow transplantation. Data are presented for 2254 patients reported to the International Bone Marrow Transplant Registry. Reprinted with permission from Horowitz et al. [27].

transplanted for AML in first remission [25]; the relapse rate for 31 recipients of syngeneic marrow grafts was increased almost threefold when compared with 339 recipients of allogeneic grafts (actuarial probability of relapse: 59 ± 20% vs 18 ± 4%).

These finding are consistent with the large retrospective analyses from the International Bone Marrow Transplant Registry (IBMTR) [26,27] (figure 1). This analysis demonstrated that the relapse rate after syngeneic BMT was higher than the relapse rate for similar patients receiving matched sibling grafts who experienced no GVHD [27]. Since recipients of syngeneic marrow experience no GVHD, the allogeneic graft may provide an important GVL effect independent of GVHD [26,27].

This high relapse rate associated with syngeneic marrow grafting is noted both in standard-risk and high-risk patients [24,25,27]. However, analysis of syngeneic BMT also suggests that the magnitude of the GVL effect may be disease specific and may be dependent on both the diagnosis and disease activity at the time of BMT. For instance, while syngeneic transplantation results in higher relapse rates for patients with CML and AML, no increase in the relapse rate for patients with ALL in first remission has been observed [26].

It has been suggested that the higher relapse rate after syngeneic BMT may be in part related to other GVL-independent factors. For instance, although the conditioning regimens for syngeneic and allogeneic BMT tend to be similar, recipients of matched sibling marrow grafts typically receive GVHD prophylaxis that typically includes methotrexate, while recipients of syngeneic grafts receive no GVHD prophylaxis. However, the relatively low total dose of methotrexate makes it unlikely that this therapy contributes to the antileukemic effect of allogeneic BMT. Another improbable concern is that the high relapse rate is actually due to de novo donor-derived leukemia; this might be impossible to distinguish from the recipients' original leukemia in syngeneic twins.

GVHD is protective against relapse

Patients who develop GVHD after allogeneic BMT have a lower risk of relapse when compared to similar patients who do not experience GVHD. This finding suggests that GVHD and GVL are similar or at least overlapping processes. This association was first noted in patients transplanted with advanced leukemia (AML or ALL in relapse, CML in accelerated phase or blast crisis, or patients in remission but at high risk of relapse) [23,28,29], and is found for patients transplanted earlier in the disease course [27,30]. Both acute and chronic GVHD appear to be protective against relapse [27,28]. Results from the IBMTR analysis for 2254 patients transplanted with 'early leukemia' (AML or ALL in first remission or CML in chronic phase) are shown in figure 1 and demonstrate that the risk of relapse after BMT is lowest in patients experiencing acute and chronic GVHD, and that patients with either acute or chronic GVHD have a lower relapse rate than patients without GVHD [27].

There also appears to be disease and stage specificity for the magnitude of the GVL effect associated with GVHD. The Seattle data demonstrated a significant GVL effect associated with GVHD for patients with ALL or AML transplanted in relapse, while no protection against relapse was noted for patients transplanted in remission [31]. For patients with CML, acute or chronic GVHD was associated with a GVL effect and protection from relapse only when BMT was performed for advanced-phase CML, but not for chronic-phase disease [28]. The IBMTR analysis also demonstrated disease specificity for GVL associated with GVHD; for recipients of unmanipulated donor marrow grafts, acute GVHD protected against relapse for patients with ALL, while the combination of acute and chronic GVHD was protective against relapse for patients with ALL, AML, and CML [27].

Depletion of donor T cells results in increased relapse rates

It has been well established that the donor T cells included in the bone marrow graft are in large part responsible for acute GVHD. This finding has led to numerous trials confirming that depletion of T cells from the donor graft is one of the most successful means of limiting the incidence and severity of GVHD after allogeneic BMT [32–38]. Unfortunately, while T-cell depletion is associated with lower transplant-related morbidity and mortality, improved survival rates have not been reliably demonstrated [30,37,39–41]. This has been due, in large part, to a reciprocal increase in the subsequent relapse rate, as well as graft failure and other complications in these patients. These findings are strong, though indirect , evidence that implicate donor T cells as important effectors for the GVL effect associated with allogeneic marrow transplantation.

The GVL effect provided by donor T cells also exhibits disease specificity; the increase in relapse rate after T-cell depletion has been most dramatic in patients with CML where the incidence of relapse is as high as 50%, compared to 10%–20% when unmanipulated donor marrow is transplanted [27,30,41]. the IBMTR analysis reported that patients with CML receiving T-cell-depleted marrow grafts have a relative risk of relapse of 6.91 when compared to a reference group of patients receiving unmanipulated marrow who develop no GVHD [27].

Treatment of relapsed leukemia after allogeneic BMT

Relapse after allogeneic BMT remains a significant cause of treatment failure. Previously, the only definitive and curative option for patients who relapsed after allogeneic BMT was second marrow transplantation. Although second transplants may be curative for a minority of patients, they are associated with very high morbidity, relapse, and mortality rates [42–44]. As described above, abrupt withdrawal of immunosuppression may induce remission for a small number of patients [20,21]. Some patients with relapsed CML have achieved complete remissions with the use of IFN-α alone, although, with relatively short follow-up, many of these patients have exhibited recurrent disease [45,46]. The inadequacies of these therapeutic approaches for relapse highlight the need for safer, more effective therapy for this group of patients.

Donor MNC infusions for relapsed CML

Given the evidence that donor lymphocytes are important mediators of GVL, it was logical to test whether the infusion of donor mononuclear cells (MNCs) could directly induce a GVL reaction without the need for second BMT. Kolb et al. first showed that complete cytogenetic remissions (in three patients with relapsed CML after allogeneic BMT) occurred by treatment with IFN-α and the infusion of MNC collected by leukapheresis of the original transplant donor [47]. This was the first reported demonstration of a direct GVL reaction in the clinical setting. Since this initial report, these results have been confirmed and expanded on by several investigators, and adoptive immunotherapy with donor MNC infusions has been used to treat over 100 patients worldwide for relapsed CML. At Brigham and Women's Hospital, 19 patients with relapsed CML have been treated with a combination of IFN-α and donor MNC infusions as diagrammed in figure 2. Patients receive up to 5 million units/M^2 of IFN-α for 6 to 12 weeks prior to donor MNC infusions. As would be anticipated, this short course of IFN-α did not result in a significant cytogenetic response in any patient [48]. Donor MNCs are collected by leukapheresis and immediately infused unmanipulated once weekly for four weeks without the use of GVHD prophylaxis. Patients who develop acute GVHD prior to subsequent infusions would not receive additional donor MNC, although in our series, GVHD did not limit the number of infusions received by any

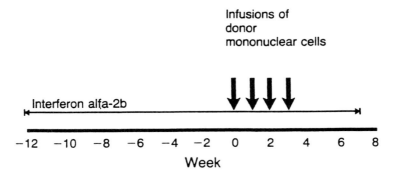

Figure 2. Treatment protocol for adoptive immunotherapy to treat relapsed chronic myelogenous leukemia used at Brigham and Women's Hospital. Reprinted with permission from Porter et al. [48].

patient. A median MNC dose of 4.2×10^8 MNC/kg (range 0.8–8.4) was administered; 10 of 14 patients treated with chronic phase relapse (12 patients), cytogenetic relapse (1 patient) or molecular relapse (1 patient) had a complete response. The magnitude of the response is highlighted by the fact that all patients with a complete cytogenetic response had no detectable cells containing the bcr/abl mRNA transcript as assayed by reverse transcription and polymerase chain reaction (RT-PCR). this technique is capable of detecting one CML cell in 10^6 normal cells [49]. Therefore, assuming that clinical relapse of CML represents a minimum leukemia cell burden of

Table 2. Adoptive immunotherapy for relapsed CML

Author [ref]	N	Disease status		IFN-α	MNC dose (10^8/kg)	Complete cytogenetic response	Complete molecular response
Kolb [47]	3	CP:	3	3	4.4–7.4	3/3	ND
Bar [51]	6	CP:	6[a]	4	0.34–5.2	5/6	4/6
Drobyski [52]	8	CP:	6[b]	3	2.6–4.0[e]	6/6	5/6
		AP/BC:	2	1		1/2	0/2
Helg [53]	3	CP:	3[c]	3	3.8–12.3	3/3	2/2
Hertenstein [54]	8	CP:	6	0	3.0–5.5	3/6	3/6
		AP/BC:	2			0/2	0/2
van Rhee [57]	14	CP:	12[d]	0	0.6–10.0	10/12[f]	8/12
		AP/BC:	2			0/2	0/2
Porter [48]	18[g]	CP:	13	14	0.9–8.4	9/13	9/13
		AP/BC:	5			0/5	0/3
Collins [56]	6	CP	4	ns	1.2–16.4	3/4	3/4
		AP/BC	2			0/2	0/2
Mackinnon [58]	22	CP[h]	18	1[i]	0.16–16.2	15/16	14/17
		AP	4		0.25–17.9	1/3	1/3
TOTAL	88	CP:	71	29/88	0.16–16.4	57/69 (82%)	48/66 (73%)
		AP/BC:	17		0.25–17.9	2/16 (12.5%)	1/14 (7%)

[a] One patients had a cytogenetic relapse only.

[b] These patients were clinically in chronic phase, although the authors classified them as 'accelerated phase' due to complex chromosomal abnormalities. Because the majority of patients who relapse after allogeneic BMT have complex chromosomal abnormalities (personal observation), we have classified these patients as chronic phase unless other criteria are present.

[c] One patient had a cytogenetic relapse only.

[d] Seven patients had hematologic relapse, 5 had cytogenetic relapse only, and two had a molecular relapse only.

[e] This number refers to number of T lymphocytes infused.

[f] Seven of ten CRs occurred in patients with cytogenetic or molecular relapse only. Three of seven patients in hematologic relapse achieved cytogenetic remission.

[g] Seventeen of these patients have been reported in abstract form as referenced. One patient is previously unreported.

[h] Ten of these patients had hematologic relapse in chronic phase, six had cytogenetic relapse only, and two had molecular relapse only.

[i] One patient was pretreated with IFN. Three other patients received IFN after donor MNC infusions had failed to induce a response alone.

Abbreviations: AP, accelerated phase; BC, blast crisis; CP, chronic phase; MNC, mononuclear cell; IFN, interferon; nd, not done; ns, not stated.

approximately 10^{12} cells, this GVL reaction is responsible for at least a six-log cell kill [50]. No responses occurred in our series in patients with more advanced CML.

Similar results have been achieved by several groups [47,48,51–59], and the results of therapy for 88 patients reported in the literature are summarized in table 2. Although the treatment protocols vary slightly among institutions, there is a consistent complete cytogenetic and molecular response rate of 70% to 80% for patients treated with either early (cytogenetic or molecular) or chronic-phase relapse. Patients with more advanced disease (accelerated phase or blast crisis) are unlikely to respond. A similar summary of 84 patients treated with relapsed CML reported to the European Group for Blood and Marrow Transplantation (EBMT) includes some, but not all, of these patients, and overall results are similar [60].

The remissions induced by donor MNC infusions for patients with CML are durable. At Brigham and Women's Hospital, one of the ten patients who had achieved a complete molecular remission had a subsequent relapse of CML. The median follow-up for these ten patients is 169 weeks. Recently, Kolb et al. reported that 3 of 54 patients treated for cytogenetic or hematologic relapse of CML developed recurrent leukemia, while 3 of 5 patients responding with advanced phases of CML subsequently relapsed [60]. These findings are significant given that relapse rates after second BMT for relapsed CML may be as high as 43% to 58% [43,44]. It is unknown why the GVL reaction after donor MNC infusions should be more sustained than that after second BMT, but these results are intriguing and lend strong support for the role of donor MNC infusions to treat relapsed CML.

Toxicity of adoptive immunotherapy for patients with relapsed CML (table 3)

Pancytopenia and bone marrow aplasia. Pancytopenia with marrow aplasia is a major complication of donor MNC infusions. Many patients experience at least transient absolute neutropenia and thrombocytopenia, and may be dependent on platelet and blood transfusions; aplasia and cytopenias have con-

Table 3. Toxicity after donor MNC infusions

- GVHD
Acute
Chronic
- Infections
Bacterial, fungal, viral
    Related to neutropenia and marrow aplasia
    Related to immunosuppression used to treat GVHD
- Pancytopenia
Bleeding (thrombocytopenia)
Infections
Transfusion requirements

tributed significantly to morbidity and have resulted in the death of several patients.

Marrow aplasia presumably results from destruction of the host leukemia cells prior to recovery of normal donor hematopoiesis. This hypothesis is supported by the observation that patients treated with donor MNC infusions for cytogenetic or molecular relapse rarely experience pancytopenia (unpublished observation and [60]. In addition, although the clinical findings are reminiscent of transfusion-associated GVHD (TA-GVHD) [61], unlike TA-GVHD, marrow aplasia is usually transient. Patients relapsing after allogeneic BMT, unlike patients who develop GVHD after a transfusion, presumably have an adequate number of donor stem cells, either persisting from the transplant or infused with the donor MNC fraction, that restore hematopoiesis after aplasia.

Occasionally marrow aplasia has been persistent [48,52,62], although this condition has been successfully reversed with the infusion of additional donor bone marrow in some patients [48,52] (figure 3). It is unknown why some patients spontaneously recover hematopoiesis and others do not, although it is not related simply to an absolute lack of normal donor stem cells. Figure 3 diagrams the response of a patient who had detectable normal donor hematopoiesis prior to donor cell infusions but was not protected against aplasia; following the GVL response, all detectable hematopoiesis was of donor origin, yet marrow hypoplasia and pancytopenia persisted. Marrow recovery did not

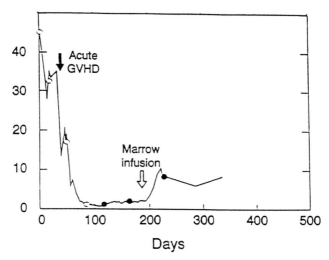

Days

Figure 3. Response to adoptive immunotherapy for a patient with relapsed chronic myelogenous leukemia. Acute GVHD was associated with cytoreduction and a drop in the WBC (solid arrow), followed by complete remission (closed circles). Additional donor bone marrow was infused on day 186 to correct persistent marrow aplasia (open arrow) and was followed by prompt hematopoietic recovery. 'O' represents a positive test for the presence of bcr/abl mRNA by reverse transcription and polymerase chain reaction (RT-PCR). '●' represents a negative RT-PCR test and complete molecular remission. Reprinted with permission from Porter et al. [48].

occur until the infusion of additional donor bone marrow, suggesting that the number of donor stem cells may have been insufficient to sustain normal hematopoietic function. Furthermore, the stem cells contained in the peripheral blood leukapheresis product were necessarily inadequate to sustain hematopoiesis. Recent reports suggest that similar donor MNC products collected by leukapheresis are a sufficient source of stem cells for allogeneic BMT [63–65], but these studies use G-CSF mobilized peripheral blood MNC. Future studies using G-CSF mobilized donor MNC for adoptive immunotherapy might therefore be appropriate in an attempt to limit the complication of marrow aplasia.

Graft-vs.-host disease. Most studies have identified an association of acute and chronic GVHD with response to donor MNC infusions [66–68] (table 4). However, despite the relatively high number of T cells administered without the use of GVHD prophylaxis, the severity of GVHD has generally been mild to moderate. Approximately 36% to 40% of patients develop no acute GVHD, and another 15% to 30% have grade I acute GVHD (table 5). Twenty percent to 50% of patients may have grade II–IV acute GVHD, but in our experience, this disease is typically responsive to immunosuppressive therapy. A recent analysis of 141 patients from 26 North American centers treated with donor MNC infusions for relapse of a variety of diseases found a 96% incidence of acute GVHD and 78% incidence of chronic GVHD in 49 complete responders. Only 35% and 13% of 92 patients who did not achieve complete remission had acute and chronic GVHD, respectively [66].

In contrast to most published series, a recent study from Memorial Sloan Kettering shows no relationship between response and acute GVHD, although the development of chronic GVHD correlated with complete remission [58]. Potential explanations for these findings include 1) a relatively low dose of donor MNC was administered to many of their patients, which might limit GVHD; 2) half of their complete responders were treated with low tumor

Table 4. Association of GVHD with clinical response to adoptive immunotherapy for patients with relapsed CML[a]

$N = 83$	Response (66/83)	No response (17/83)
GVHD	51/66 (77%)	3/17[b] (18%)
No GVHD	15/66 (23%)	13/17 (76%)

[a] Data are compiled from nine reports in which the association of GVHD and response could be determined [47,48,51–54,57–59].

Seven patients are included from our unpublished data. The majority of patients responding had complete cytogenetic and/or molecular remissions after donor mononuclear cell infusions, although several patients classified as responders for the purpose of this analysis died before remission could be documented.

[b] One patient was not evaluable.

Table 5. GVHD occurring after donor mononuclear cell infusions

Disease	N	Acute GVHD grade 0	Acute GVHD grade 1	Acute GVHD grade II–IV	Chronic GVHD limited/extensive
CML	90	38 (42%)	26 (29%)	26 (29%)	Limited: 17/65 (26%) Extensive: 12/65 (18%)
Acute Leukemia, MDS, MM, NHL, HD	50	18 (36%)	7 (14%)	25 (51%)	Most not reported
Total	140	56 (40%)	33 (24%)	51 (36%)	

Data for CML patients is compiled from eight reports in which details on GVHD were available [47,51–55,57–59,62]. Data for patients with diseases other than CML are compiled from eight reports in which details on GVHD were available [56,92–97,126]. Abbreviations: CML, chronic myelogenous leukemia; GVHD, graft-vs.-host disease; HD, Hodgkin's disease; MDS, myelodysplasia; MM, multiple myeloma; NHL, non-Hodgkin's lymphoma.

Table 6. Mortality associated with adoptive immunotherapy for relapsed CML[a]

Deaths	16/60	(27%)
• Therapy Related:	10/60	(17%)
GVHD	5/60	(8%)
CML CP:	3/48	
Advanced CML[b]	2/12	
Marrow aplasia	4/60	(7%)
and/or infection:		
CML CP:	3/48	
Advanced CML:	1/12	
Other	1/60	(2%)
CML CP	1/48	
• Disease Progression	6/60	(10%)
CML CP:	0/44	
Advanced CML:	6/12	

[a] These data represent a compilation of patients from seven centers that have reported outcome and cause of death in patients receiving donor MNC infusions for relapsed CML [47,48,51–53,57,127], and includes several previously unpublished cases treated at our institution.
[b] Advanced CML refers to patients with accelerated phase or blast crisis CML [48,52] or greater than second chronic phase [54].
Abbreviations: CML, chronic myelogenous leukemia; CP, chronic phase.

burdens (cytogenetic or molecular relapse), which may influence subsequent GVHD; or 3) the treatment protocol included sequential escalation of donor MNC infusions over time, which may also influence subsequent development of acute GVHD.

GVHD after donor MNC infusions has generally been responsive to immunosuppressive therapy, and the mortality rate from GVHD has been low (table 6). Although 5% to 8% of patients may die from direct complications of GVHD, another 7% to 12% may die from infectious complications, either related to marrow aplasia or immune suppression as therapy for treatment of GVHD; the overall treatment-related mortality after MNC infusions may be as high as 20% (table 6). This result is still favorable compared to the anticipated 40% or higher treatment-related mortality associated with second BMT [43]. In the future, the early administration of donor bone marrow to rescue patients from marrow aplasia [48,52], and the development of strategies to limit GVHD without sacrificing GVL as highlighted below, should result in even lower morbidity and mortality from donor MNC infusions.

The role of interferon for GVL induction

The contribution of IFN-α to successful adoptive immunotherapy has generated discussion in the literature [58,68,69]. The use of IFN-α alone results in complete cytogenetic remission for patients with untreated CML [70–72] and relapsed CML after allogeneic BMT [42,45,46]. However, it is unlikely that the short course of IFN-α used in most adoptive immunotherapy trials results in significant cytogenetic remissions, and molecular remissions from the use of IFN-α are rare [46,73]. Clearly, the use of IFN-α is not an absolute requirement for remission induction, since many patients have achieved complete responses after donor MNC infusions without the simultaneous use of IFN-α [52,54,57,58,60,68] (see table 2). However, it is notable that some patients failing to respond to donor MNC infusion entered complete remission only after the addition of IFN-α [58]. It is possible that IFN-α may influence the tempo of the GVL reaction and shorten the interval required for complete remission [69], although this hypothesis is not supported by all studies [58]. Ultimately, the importance of IFN-α to the GVL reaction, remission duration, and survival will have to be determined by further trials and longer follow-up.

While it is unknown how IFN-α may influence the GVL reaction, there are several biological properties of this cytokine that make it a logical adjunct to adoptive immunotherapy. It has known antiproliferative effects and causes cytoreduction prior to cellular therapy. In addition, IFN-α may increase the expression of several important cell surface antigens, such as HLA class I and II molecules [74,75] and the adhesion molecule LFA-3 [76] on leukemic cells; these changes could make leukemia cells better targets for cellular immunotherapy. IFN-α may also influence production of other important cytokines [77] and effector cells to further influence the GVL reaction.

Is there a dose–response relationship for donor MNC and GVL?

No correlation between MNC dose and GVHD or GVL has yet been noted, and the cell dose used to induce a GVL response has varied greatly among published reports (table 2). It is possible that most patients already receive MNC doses above a theoretical 'threshold' and that a dose–response relationship would be identified at lower MNC doses. For instance, one recent report suggests that a low MNC dose (as low as 10^7 cells/kg) may retain antileukemic effects while limiting clinically evident GVHD, particularly for patients with only minimal residual disease (cytogenetic or molecular relapse [58]). This finding may suggest an important relationship between the number of effector and target cells; patients with only minimal disease may achieve remission with fewer donor cells than patients with larger leukemia cell burdens. Fewer numbers of effector cells in these patients may not induce clinically apparent GVHD. However, it is also likely that differences in minor histocompatibility antigens, in addition to the leukemia cell burden, will have a significant influence on the number of MNCs required to induce both GVL and GVHD.

Is GVL separable from GVHD?

The majority of patients who respond to donor MNC infusions also develop acute or chronic GVHD (tables 4, 5), suggesting that GVL and GVHD are overlapping processes. For patients with relapsed CML, approximately 77% of responding patients develop clinical evidence of GVHD, while 23% of responders have no evidence of GVHD (table 4). It is of interest that some patients enter remission without clinical evidence of acute GVHD, suggesting that, at least in some cases, clinical GVHD and GVL may be distinct processes [54,57,58,60]. However, other factors may be involved in limiting GVHD in this setting. In a recent report from Memorial Sloan Kettering, only 1 of 22 patients treated with donor MNC infusions experienced acute GVHD [58]. These patients were treated with sequential escalating doses of donor MNCs until remission was achieved, and seven of these patients received less than 10^8 MNC/kg. As discussed, it is possible that a quantitative threshold exists below which clinical GVHD is not evident, while the GVL reaction still occurs. It is notable that 8 of 16 patients entering molecular remission were treated at a time of low leukemia cell burden (cytogenetic or molecular relapse), and received the lowest cell doses in this study (1 or 2 infusions of 1.5 $\times 10^7$ to 1.4×10^8 MNC/kg). If an important effector–target ratio exists, fewer numbers of donor MNC would be needed to eradicate fewer leukemia cells while limiting generalized alloreactivity. Hence clinical GVHD may be separable from clinical GVL. This does not explain why the majority of the other patients in this study, who received cell doses comparable to other reported patients, had a very low incidence of acute GVHD. Hypothetically, the strategy of sequential escalation of donor MNC doses could induce allogeneic tolerance without effecting the GVL response. It is also possible that for some responding patients who have no GVHD, donor MNC are targeting only leukemia-specific antigens or minor histocompatibility antigens that are present only on host hematopoietic or leukemia cells; a more generaliged GVHD reaction would therefore be absent. It can be hoped that these intriguing data may lead to experiments that will provide a better understanding of the GVL reaction, and ultimately lead to the more effective and safer use of allogeneic immunotherapy.

Future approaches to posttransplantation immunotherapy

The potent GVL effect induced by unmanipulated donor MNC infusions has been conclusively demonstrated. Newer approaches to adoptive immuno-therapy that are currently under investigation may preserve GVL reactivity while limiting toxicity. One such strategy is the administration of donor MNCs depleted of effectors suspected of causing GVHD. In bone marrow transplan-tation, donor grafts depleted of CD8+ cells may be associated with less GVHD than unmanipulated marrow grafts and yet retain GVL properties when com-pared to pan-T-cell-depleted marrow [78]. Studies of CD8+ depleted donor MNC infusions are currently under way and suggest that GHVD can be minimized; conclusions regarding the GVL effects will await further follow-up [79].

Another approach that may enhance the efficacy of and limit toxicity from donor MNC infusions is to administer donor cells prior to clinical relapse. Patients with minimal residual disease treated with lower doses of donor MNC may be at less risk for marrow aplasia or GVHD as described above [58]. Since patients with minimal residual disease who are at high risk for clinical relapse can be reliably identified by sequential positive PCR tests for bcr/abl mRNA transcripts [80], a logical strategy would be to administer donor MNC at the time of PCR positivity for bcr/abl mRNA but before hematologic relapse.

Ultimately, the best approach to relapse is prevention, and it may be pos-sible to design transplant strategies that augment GVL at the time of BMT to reduce subsequent relapse rates.The Seattle group attempted to augment GVL at the time of BMT for a group of high-risk patients with acute leukemia by withholding GVHD prophylaxis [81,82]. While they found that the inci-dence of significant acute GVHD was increased, no decrease in relapse rate was identified. A similar trial withholding GVHD prophylaxis did show an improvement in relapse rate and survival [83], although follow-up was short; it remains possible that this approach will benefit a small group of patients, although toxicity is expected to be significant.

An analogous study reported by the Seattle group attempted to enhance GVL by manipulating GVHD rater than by just withholding prophylactic therapy [84]. Patients with advanced leukemia undergoing allogeneic BMT received one of three regimens: standard GVHD prophylaxis with a long course of methotrexate (control arm), a short course of methotrexate, or the short course of methotrexate plus the addition of donor buffy-coat cells given at the time of BMT. The two arms that resulted in enhanced GVHD (short MTX or donor buffy-coat infusions) failed to show an improvement in either relapse or overall survival, in part due to the increase in non-relapse-related mortality seen in these patients. This finding does not exclude the possibility that manipulation of GVL and GVHD at the time of BMT is effective. For instance, the patient population and the timing of the immune manipulation may be critical; patients with advanced leukemia at high risk for relapse may not be the appropriate group to study. Regardless, any strategy anticipated to enhance toxicity from GVHD at the time of BMT should be approached with extreme caution.

The timing of GVHD and GVL induction in relation to BMT may be critical. For instance, while the studies described above failed to demonstrate lower relapse rates or improved survival, this was in part due to the increased toxicity of GVHD induction. Recent data suggest that the toxicity from GVHD may be minimized if dissociated from the other acute toxicities of transplantation (e.g., toxicity related to the conditioning regimen, tissue damage, and infections) [85]. In dogs, allogeneic lymphocytes can be administered safely after chimerism has been established [86]. In mice, the administration of donor lymphocytes at the time of BMT results in severe GVHD; when donor lymphocytes are given 21 days after the conditioning therapy, they retain significant GVL effects without inducing severe GVHD [87]. Similar findings have been noted in other murine models [88], and it has been postulated that this limited toxicity may be due to the separation of the cytokine phases that occur after BMT [85,89].

The use of delayed GVL induction with donor MNC infusions to prevent relapse after BMT is now being tested clinically, and results show that this approach can be taken without excessive toxicity. Slavin and colleagues have developed a protocol of incremental T-cell repletion after T-cell-depleted allogeneic BMT [89,90]. Escalating doses of donor T cells are given to patients beginning on day +1 (recipients of Campath-1M-treated grafts) or day +28 (recipients of Campath-1G-treated grafts) and repeated weekly or monthly. T-cell reinfusions resulted in an increase in the risk of GVHD, but no effect on event-free survival could be demonstrated. Donor T-cell reinfusions resulted in a nonstatistically significant trend toward lower relapse rates only in recipients of Campath-1M-treated marrow. A similar study has recently been initiated at the NIH with incremental doses of donor T cells administered beginning 30 days after BMT [91]. Significant acute GVHD has not occurred in five patients reported to date, and longer follow-up will determine the ultimate effect on GVL and relapse. Taken together, the experimental and clinical data suggest that posttransplantation cellular immunotherapy can be performed safely and effectively, but optimization of patient selection, cell dose, and timing of administration may all serve to enhance the potential GVL effects.

Adoptive immunotherapy for relapse of diseases other than CML

Donor MNC infusions appear to be less effective for patients who relapse after allogeneic BMT with diseases other than CML, although for some patients, a

Table 7. Adoptive immunotherapy for relapse of diseases other than CML

Disease	North America [66]	EBMT [60]	Total
AML	6/40 (15%)	5/17 (29%)	11/57 (19%)
ALL	3/15 (20%)	0/12 (0%)	3/27 (11%)
MDS	3/6 (50%)	1/4 (20%)	4/10 (40%)
NHL	0/8 (0%)	NR	0/8 (0%)
Multiple myeloma	2/5 (40%)	NR	2/5 (40%)

definitive GVL effect can be induced and sustained remissions will be achieved [92–98]. Data compiled from 26 North American transplant centers, or from the EBMT, suggest that the approximately 15%–30% of patients treated for relapsed AML and 0%–20% of patients treated for relapsed ALL will reenter remission [60,66] (table 7). In addition, several patients with relapsed myelodysplasia and multiple myeloma have responded, although the small number of patients treated precludes definitive conclusions regarding the efficacy for these diseases. No lasting responses have yet been reported for relapsed lymphoma or CLL. The toxicity of donor MNC in this group of patients is similar to that seen in patients treated with CML. Given the poor outcome anticipated for relapsed patients undergoing a second BMT [42–44], an initial trial of adoptive immunotherapy is a reasonable alternative for these patients.

The lower response rate to donor MNC infusions in these patients compared to patients with CML is consistent with a large retrospective analysis of BMT that demonstrates that donor lymphocytes are most important for the GVL effects against CML [27]. This finding further implies that the immunologic properties of the tumor cells strongly influence GVL. For instance, it is possible that leukemia-specific antigens effect the GVL reaction. The bcr/abl protein would be a likely candidate antigen. In mice, T-cell-specific immunity to the bcr/abl peptide can be demonstrated [99], although the clinical significance of this finding is uncertain. It is also possible that disease specificity is determined by minor histocompatibility antigens expressed on some leukemia cells and not others. It should be noted, however, that the median time to response for patients with CML is approximately 8 to 14 weeks after donor MNC infusions [48,58], and some patients with relapsed acute leukemia will not survive long enough to benefit from GVL induction.

What are the effector cells responsible for GVL reactivity?

The identity of the effector mechanisms responsible for GVL induction remains an enigma, and it is likely that several mechanisms are involved. As discussed above, the majority of evidence implicates donor T cells as vital effectors of GVL, and both MHC-restricted and MHC-unrestricted cell-mediated immune responses have been implicated in GVL reactivity. In murine models, donor T cells are important for GVL [7,10], and several model systems implicate CD8+ T cells as important mediators of GVL in mice [4,8,14]. Other models using different strain combinations demonstrate that both CD4+ and CD8+ cells contribute to GVL induction [10,11,13,15]. MHC-unrestricted mechanisms may also be important mediators of GVL, and the GVL effect of allogeneic BMT is dependent on NK/LAK cell activity in certain systems [100].

As in murine models, most evidence from clinical BMT suggests that both donor-derived T cells and NK cells may be important mediators of the GVL reaction. T-cell depletion of the donor graft, when used as GVHD prophylaxis, results in a significant increase in relapse rates, especially for patients with CML [27,30,40,41,101]. The fact that most strategies for T-cell purging leave other potential effector cells intact (i.e., NK cells) [32,33,40] further supports the role of T cells as mediators of GVL. It is not yet known which specific T-cell subset is required for GVL induction, although CD4+ cells are likely candidates. Selective CD8+ depletion of the donor graft for patients with CML has resulted in a low incidence of GVHD and a low incidence of relapse, indicating that at least for CML, CD8+ T cells may not be necessary for GVL induction. After allogeneic BMT, it has been reported that higher numbers of circulating cytotoxic T-cell precursors directed against the patient's leukemia may correlate with relapse-free survival, and some patients will have CD4+ cells circulating after BMT that specifically lyse cryopreserved leukemic cells in vitro [102,103]. Furthermore, donor T-cell populations have been identified with specific cytolytic activity against allogeneic leukemia cells [104,105]. Sosman et al. have further isolated and characterized these cells as phenotypically CD3+, CD4+, and α/β T-cell receptor-positive and have demonstrated cytolytic activity specifically against allogeneic leukemic but not nonleukemic targets [105].

There is significant evidence suggesting that NK cells are active participants in the GVL reaction in clinical BMT. Since NK cells generally have the capacity to lyse the CML-derived cell line K562 in vitro, it is logical to suspect that they may play an important role in GVL induction. After BMT, the number and activity of NK cells is typically increased in the peripheral blood [106,107], and NK-cell isolates can be identified that will lyse cryopreserved host leukemia cells [106,108,109]. Nk cells isolated after BMT have also been shown to inhibit leukemic progenitor colony growth [110]. In addition, the use of IL-2 after BMT, which stimulates NK-cell number and activity, may result in lower relapse rates, presumably due to enhanced GVL activity [88,111,112] (see below).

It is presumed that similar effector cells are responsible for the potent GVL reaction that occurs when donor mononuclear cells are administered to treat patients who relapse after allogeneic BMT, although no formal proof exists for this assumption. Most groups administer unfractionated donor mononuclear

74

cell preparations that contain all lymphocytes, NK cells, and other MNC populations. Similar to data after BMT, there is evidence that the T-cell fraction is important for GVL after MNC infusions. Bunjes et al. detected an increase in host-reactive T-helper precursor cells in five patients who responded to donor MNC infusions for relapsed CML [113]. The one patient who failed to respond had no detectable increase in the frequency of T-helper precursor cells. This group noted no consistent increase in host-reactive cytotoxic T-cell precursors in the responding five patients. Lymphocyte profiles for two patients treated with donor MNC infusions for relapsed CML were analyzed by Jiang et al.; an increase in cytotoxic T-cell precursor frequency against cryopreserved host leukemia cells relative to host lymphocytes was noted in both patients following donor cell infusions [109]. In this analysis, NK-cell activity initially decreased but recovered to levels higher than preinfusion values, and this change preceded evidence of GVL. The significance of these phenotypic changes is unclear, but future analysis may help determine which MNC subsets are important for GVL induction.

One approach that will help identify important effector cells for GVL induction will be the selective infusion or depletion of donor MNC populations used to treat relapse. Trials are already underway using CD8+ depleted donor MNC infusions to treat relapse of CML; initial results suggest that CD8+ depleted MNC infusions will minimize GVHD and still retain GVL activity [79]. The effect of CD8+ depletion on the magnitude and duration of the GVL potential of donor MNC infusions will have to await further follow-up.

Cytokine-mediated immunotherapy

It is becoming increasing clear that GVHD results from a complex interaction of effector cells and cytokines [85]; it is also likely that qualitative and quantitative changes in cytokine production will influence the GVL reaction. Interleukin-2 (IL-2) has been studied in some detail due to the ability of this molecule to augment the immune system [114] and enhance NK-cell number and function. Initial studies provide substantial indirect evidence to suggest that IL-2-activated NK cells may be important determinants for GVL reactivity. NK cells will lyse tumor cells in vitro, and this activity is augmented by in vitro incubation with IL-2 [106,110]. Early after autologous or allogeneic BMT, activated lymphocytes can be isolated from patients that will lyse NK-resistant targets [107,115]. In addition, NK-cell number and activity is increased in the peripheral blood of patients after BMT [106,107], and for patients with CML transplanted with T-cell-depleted marrow grafts, the ability of IL-2-stimulated peripheral blood MNCs to lyse leukemic targets may correlate with protection from relapse [106].

Reports of clinical trials now demonstrate that varying doses of IL-2 can be safely administered to patients after autologous BMT, and initial results have been encouraging [33,88,116,117]. After T-cell-depleted allogeneic BMT, the administration of low-dose IL-2 (200,000–500,000 units/M^2) has been safe and can reliably result in up to a tenfold increase in the number of circulating NK cells [111]. These data suggest that relapse rates may be lower in the patients receiving low-dose IL-2 when compared to similar patients not treated with post-BMT immunotherapy, suggesting that IL-2 may be capable of restoring GVL reactivity. It is notable that IL-2 in this setting has not resulted in an exacerbation of GVHD, perhaps because at these doses, NK cells may be selectively activated without additional T-cell stimulation [111]. The optimal timing and dose of IL-2 will need to be further defined, and ultimately, the results of randomized trials will be useful to elucidate the impact of post-BMT IL-2-mediated immunotherapy.

Adoptive immunotherapy for nonrelapse complications after allogeneic BMT

Defective-cell-mediated immunity after allogeneic BMT, particularly when the marrow graft has been depleted of donor T cells, may limit the success of BMT due to complications other than leukemic relapse. T-cell-depleted marrow grafts have been associated with an increase in Epstein–Barr-virus-associated B-cell lymphoproliferative disorders (BLPD) [32,118]. These aggressive lymphomas are typically of donor origin and presumably arise due to uncontrolled proliferation of EBV-infected B cells in the absence of appropriate virus-specific cytotoxic T lymphocytes. They are characteristically unresponsive to standard therapy and are most often fatal in the setting of allogeneic BMT [119]. Donor MNCs have been used to successfully induce complete remissions in several patients with BLPD, presumably due to restoration of cell-mediated immunity [120,121]. Unfortunately, several of these patients experienced severe complications from the infusion of unselected donor lymphocytes. An elegant strategy to limit toxicity from GVHD in this setting has been described that uses donor lymphocytes transfected with the herpes virus thymidine kinase (HSV-TK) gene. Expression of HSV-TK confers sensitivity of these cells to gancyclovir. These cells have induced remissions of BLPD, and subsequent administration of gancyclovir has resulted in the resolution of complicating GVHD [122,123]. Recently, Rooney et al. described the generation of EBV-specific T cells from allogeneic marrow donors and showed that administration of up to 1×10^8 cells is safe and may be effective therapy for controlling proliferation of EBV-infected B cells [124].

Undoubtedly, the use of donor lymphocytes to restore defective-cell-mediated immunity will undergo further evaluation for a variety of posttransplantation complications. For instance, donor MNC infusions have been used effectively to reverse a life-threatening adenoviral infection after allogeneic BMT [125]. The ability to modify cells with appropriate 'suicide' genes and to generate and transfer antigen-specific donor lymphocytes may ultimately broaden the application of adoptive immunotherapy for use in a variety of infectious and malignant complications.

Summary

The significance and potency of GVL can no longer be argued. It is very clear that an allogeneic bone marrow graft provides an important GVL component critical to the success of BMT for many patients. The extraordinary success of donor MNC infusions to treat relapse after BMT shows that it is now possible to manipulate the GVL reaction to treat leukemia. The identity of the effector cells and target antigens remains unclear, but no doubt future experiments will begin to dissect out the complex cellular and cytokine interactions that mediate GVL reactivity. It also remains unclear whether GVL is distinct from GVHD; ultimately, the ability to harness GVL without excessive toxicity from GVHD will be a central challenge in BMT and cellular immunotherapy. There is now an excellent opportunity to understand the detailed mechanisms of GVL and to begin to design clinical strategies to harness the potent GVL effects of allogeneic donor cells for greater therapeutic benefit.

Acknowledgments

This work was supported in part by NIH grant CA58661 (JHA). DLP is a Fellow of the Leukemia Society of America.

References

1. Mathe G, Amiel J, Schwarzenberg L, Cattan A, Schneider M. Adoptive immunotherapy of acute leukemia: Experimental and clinical results. Cancer Res 25:1525–1531, 1965.
2. Barnes D, Corp M, Loutit J, Neal F. Treatment of murine leukaemia with X rays and homologous bone marrow. Preliminary communication. Br Med J 2:626–630, 1956.
3. Barnes D, Loutit J. Treatment of murine leukaemia with X-rays and homologous bone marrow. Br J Haematol 3:241–252, 1957.
4. Truitt R, LeFever A, Shih C-Y, Jeske J, Martin T. Graft-vs-leukemia effect. In Burakoff S, Deeg H, Ferrara J, Atkinson K (eds), Graft-vs.-Host Disease: Immunology, Pathophysiology, and Treatment, vol. 12. New York: Marcel Dekker, 1990, pp. 177–204.
5. Truitt R, LeFever A, Shih C-Y. Graft-versus-leukemia reactions: experimental models and clinical trails. In Gale R, Champlin R (eds), Progress in Bone Marrow Transplantation. New York: Alan R. Liss, 1987, pp. 219–232.
6. Korngold R, Sprent J. T cell subsets and graft-versus-host disease. Transplant 44:335–339, 1987.
7. Truitt R, Shih C, Lefever A, Tempelis L, Andreani M, Bortin M. Characterization of alloimmunization-induced T lymphocytes reactive against AKR leukemia in vitro and correlation with graft-vs-leukemia activity in vivo. J Immunol 131:2105–2058, 1983.
8. Sykes M, Romick M, Sachs D. Interleukin 2 prevents graft-versus-host disease while preserving the graft-versus-leukemia effect of allogeneic T cells. Proc Natl Acad Sci 87:5633–5637, 1990.

9. Okunewick J, Kochiban D, Machen L, Buffo M. Comparison of the effects of CD3 and CD5 donor T cell depletion on graft-versus-leukemia in a murine model for MHC-matched unrelated donor-transplantation. Bone Marrow Transplant 13:11–18, 1994.

10. Weiss L, Weigensberg M, Morecki S, Bar S, Cobbold S, Waldmann H, Slavin S. Characterization of effector cells of graft-vs-leukemia following allogeneic bone marrow transplantation in mice inoculated with murine B-cell leukemia. Cancer Immunol Immunother 31:236–242, 1990.

11. Truitt R, Atasoylu A. Contribution of CD4+ and CD8+ T cells to graft-versus-host disease and graft-versus-leukemia reactivity after transplantation of MHC-compatible bone marrow. Bone Marrow Transplant 8:51–58, 1991.

12. Bortin M, Truitt R, Rimm A, Bach F. Graft-versus-leukemia reactivity induced by alloimmunization without augmentation of graft-versus-host reactivity. Nature 281:490–491, 1979.

13. Okunewick J, Kochiban D, Machen L, Buffo M. The role of CD4 and CD8 T-cells in the graft-versus-leukemia response in Rauscher murine leukemia. Bone Marrow Transplant 8:445–452, 1991.

14. Sykes M, Abraham V, Harty M, Pearson D. IL-2 reduces graft-versus-host disease and preserves a graft-versus-leukemia effect by selectively inhibiting CD4+ T cell activity. J Immunol 150:197–205, 1993.

15. Sykes M, Harty M, Szot G, Pearson D. Interleukin-2 inhibits graft-versus-host disease-promoting activity of CD4+ cells while preserving CD4- and CD8-mediated graft-versus-leukemia effects. Blood 83:2560–2569, 1994.

16. Weiss L, Reich S, Slavin S. Use of recombinant human interleukin-2 in conjunction with bone marrow transplantation as a model for control of minimal residual disease in malignant hematological disorders. Treatment of murine leukemia in conjunction with allogenic bone marrow transplantation and IL2-activated cell-mediated immunotherapy. Cancer Invest 10:19–26, 1992.

17. Slavin S, Eckerstein A, Weiss L. Adoptive immunotherapy in conjunction with bone marrow transplantation-amplification of natural host defense mechanisms against cancer by recombinant IL2. Nat Immun Cell Growth Reg 7:180–184, 1988.

18. Johnson B, Truitt R. A decrease in graft-vs-host disease without loss of graft-vs-leukemia reactivity after MHC matched bone marrow transplantation by selective depletion of donor NK cells in vivo. Transplantation 54:104–112, 1992.

19. Odom L, August C, Githens J, Humbert J, Morse H, Peakman D, Sharma B, Rusnak S, Johnson F. Remission of relapsed leukaemia during a graft-versus-host reaction. A 'graft-versus-leukaemia reaction' in man? Lancet 2:537–540, 1978.

20. Collins R, Rogers Z, Bennett M, Kumar V, Nikein A, Fay J. Hematologic relapse of chronic myelogenous leukemia following allogeneic bone marrow transplantation: apparent graft-versus-leukemia effect following abrupt discontinuation of immunosuppression. Bone Marrow Transplant 10:391–395, 1992.

21. Higano C, Brixey M, Bryant E, Durnam D, Doney K, Sullivan K, Singer J. Durable complete remission of acute nonlymphocytic leukemia associated with discontinuation of immunosuppression following relapse after allogeneic bone marrow transplantation. A case report of a probable graft-versus-leukemia effect. Transplantation 50:175–177, 1990.

22. Sullivan K, Shulman H. Chronic graft-versus-host disease, obliterative bronchiolitis, and graft-versus-leukemia effect: case histories. Transplant Proc 21:51–62, 1989.

23. Weiden P, Flournoy N, Donnall Thomas E, Prentice R, Fefer A, Buckner C, Storb R. Antileukemic effect of graft-versus-host disease in human recipients of allogeneic-marrow grafts. N Engl J Med 300:1068–1073, 1979.

24. Fefer A, Sullivan K, Weiden P, Buckner C, Schoch G, Storb R, Thomas E. Graft versus leukemia effect in man: the relapse rate of acute leukemia is lower after allogeneic than after syngeneic marrow transplantation. In Truitt R, Gale R, Bortin M (eds), Cellular Immunotherapy of Cancer. New York: AR Liss, 1987, pp. 401–408.

25. Gale R, Champlin R. How does bone-marrow transplantation cure leukaemia? Lancet 2:28–30, 1984.
26. Gale R, Horowitz M, Ash R, Champlin R, Goldman J, Rimm A, Ringden O, Veum Stone J, Bortin M. Identical-twin bone marrow transplants for leukemia. Ann Intern Med 120:646–652, 1994.
27. Horowitz M, Gale R, Sondel P, Goldman J, Dersey J, Kolb H, Rimm A, Ringden O, Rozman C, Speck B, Truitt R, Zwaan F, Bortin M. Graft-versus-leukemia reactions after bone marrow transplantation. Blood 75:555–562, 1990.
28. Sullivan K, Weiden P, Storb R, Witherspoon R, Fefer A, Fisher L, buckner C, Anasetti C, Appelbaum F, Badger C, Beatty P, Bensinger W, Berenson R, Bigelow C, Cheever M, Clift R, Deeg H, Doney K, Greenberg P, Hansen J, Hill R, Loughran T, Martin P, Neiman P, Peterson F, Sanders J, Singer J, Stewart P, Thomas E. Influence of acute and chronic graft-versus-host disease on relapse and survival after bone marrow transplantation from HLA-identical siblings as treatment of acute and chronic leukemia. Blood 73:1720–1728, 1989.
29. Weiden P, Sullivan K, Flournoy N, Storb R, Thomas E. Antileukemic effect of chronic graft-versus-host disease. Contribution to improved survival after allogeneic marrow transplantation. N Engl J Med 304:1529–1533, 1981.
30. Goldman J, Gale R, Horowitz M, Biggs J, Champlin R, Gluckman E, Hoffmann R, Jacobsen S, Marmont A, McGlave P, Messner H, Rimm A, Rozman C, Speck B, Tura S, Weiner R, Bortin M. Bone marrow transplantation for chronic myelogenous leukemia in chronic phase. Ann Intern Med 108:806–814, 1988.
31. Sullivan K, Fefer A, Witherspoon R, Storb R, Buckner C, Weiden P, Schoch G, Thomas E. Graft-versus-leukemia in man: relationship of acute and chronic graft-versus-host disease to relapse of acute leukemia following allogenic bone marrow transplantation. In Truitt R, Gale R, Bortin M (eds), Cellular Immunotherapy of Cancer. New York: A.R. Liss, 1987, pp. 391–399.
32. Antin J, Bierer B, Smith B, Ferrara J, Guinan E, Sieff C, Golan D, Macklis R, Tarbell N, Lynch E, Reichert T, Blythman H, Bouloux C, Rappeport J, Burakoff S, Weinstein H. Selective depletion of bone marrow T lymphocytes with anti-CD5 monoclonal antibodies: effective prophylaxis for graft-versus-host disease in patients with hematologic malignancies. Blood 78:2139–2149, 1991.
33. Soiffer R, Murray C, Mauch P, Anderson K, Freedman A, Rabinowe S, Takvorian T, Robertson M, Spector N, Gonin R, Miller K, Rudders R, Freeman A, Blake K, Coral F, Nadler L, Ritz J. Prevention of graft-versus-host disease by selective depletion of CD6-positive T lymphocytes from donor bone marrow. J Clin Oncol 10:1191–1200, 1992.
34. Wagner J, Santos G, Noga S, Rowley S, Davis J, Vogelsang G, Farmer E, Zehnbauer B, Saral R, Donnenberg A. Bone marrow graft engineering by counterflow centrifugal elutriation: results of a phase I–II clinical trial. Blood 75:1370–1377, 1990.
35. Waldmann H, Polliak A, Hale G, et al. Elimination of GVHD by in-vitro depletion of alloreactive lymphocytes with a monoclonal rat anti-human lymphocyte antibody (Campath-1). Lancet ii:483–486, 1984.
36. Martin P, Hansen J, Buckner C, Sanders J, Deeg H, Stewart P, Appelbaum F, Clift R, Fefer A, Witherspoon R, Kennedy M, Sullivan K, Flournoy N, Storb R, Thomas E. Effects of in vitro depletion of T cells in HLA-identical allogeneic marrow grafts. Blood 66:664–672, 1985.
37. Mitsuyasu R, Champlin R, Gale R, Ho W, Lenarsky C, Winston D, Selch M, Elashoff R, Giorgi J, Wells J, Terasaki P, Billing R, Feig S. Treatment of donor bone marrow with monoclonal anti-T-cell antibody and complement for the prevention of graft-versus-host disease. Ann Intern Med 105:20–26, 1986.
38. Young J, Papadopoulos E, Cunningham I, Castro-Malaspina H, Flomenberg N, Carabasi M, Gulati S, Brochstein J, Heller G, Balck P, Collins N, Shank B, Kernan N, O'Reilly R. T-cell depleted allogeneic bone marrow transplantation in adults with acute nonlymphocytic leukemia in first remission. Blood 79:3380–3387, 1992.

39. Goldman J, Apperley J, Jones L, Marcus R, Gollden A, Batchelor R, Hale G, Waldmann H, Reid C, Hows J, Gordon-Smith E, Catovsky D, Galton D. Bone marrow transplantation for patients with chronic myeloid leukemia. N Engl J Med 314:202–207, 1986.

40. Marmont A, Horowitz M, Gale R, Sobocinski K, Ash R, van Bekkum D, Champlin R, Dicke K, Goldman J, Good R, Herzig R, Hong R, Masaoka T, Rimm A, Ringden O, Speck B, Weiner R, Bortin M. T-cell depletion of HLA-identical transplants in leukemia. Blood 78:2120–2130, 1991.

41. Apperley J, Mauro F, Goldman J, Gregory W, Arthur C, Hows J, Arcese W, Papa G, Mandelli F, Wardle D, Gravett P, Franklin I, Bandini G, Ricci P, Tura S, Iacone A, Torlontano G, Heit W, Champlin R, Gale R. Bone marrow transplantation for chronic myeloid leukaemia in first chronic phase: importance of a graft-versus-leukaemia effect. Br J Haematol 69:239–245, 1988.

42. Arcese W, Goldman J, D'Arcangelo E, Schattenberg A, Nardi A, Apperley J, Frassoni F, Aversa F, Prentice H, Ljungman P, Ferrant A, Marosi C, Sayer H, Niederwieser D, Arnold R, Bandini G, Carreras E, Parker A, Frappaz D, Mandelli F, Gratwohl A. Outcome for patients who relapse after allogeneic bone marrow transplantation for chronic myeloid leukemia. Blood 82:3211–3219, 1993.

43. Mrsic M, Horowitz M, Atkinson K, Biggs J, Champlin R, Ehninger G, Gajewski J, Gale R, Herzig R, Prentice H, Rozman C, Sobocinski K, Speck B, Bortin M. Second HA-identical sibling transplants for leukemia recurrence. Bone Marrow Transplant 9:269–275, 1992.

44. Radich J, Sanders J, Buckner C, Martin P, Petersen F, Bensinger W, McDonald G, Mori M, Schoch G, Hansen J. Second allogeneic marrow transplantation for patients with recurrent leukemia after initial transplant with total-body irradiation-containing regimens. J Clin Oncol 11:304–313, 1993.

45. Higano C, Raskind W, Flowers M. Alpha interferon (IFN) results in high complete cytogenetic response rate in patients with cytogenetic-only relapse of chronic myelogenous leukemia (CML) after marrow transplantation (BMT). Blood 82 (Supplt): 661a, 1993.

46. Higano C, Raskind W, Singer J. Use of alpha interferon for the treatment of relapse of chronic myelogenous leukemia in chronic phase after allogeneic bone marrow transplantation. Blood 80:1437–1442, 1992.

47. Kolb H, Mittermuller J, Clemm C, Holler E, Ledderose G, Brehm G, Heim M, Wilmanns W. Donor leukocyte transfusions for treatment of recurrent chronic myelogenous leukemia in marrow transplant patients. Blood 76:2462–2465, 1990.

48. Porter D, Roth M, McGarigle C, Ferrara J, Antin J. Induction of graft-versus-host disease as immunotherapy for relapsed chronic myeloid leukemia. N Engl J Med 330:100–106, 1994.

49. Roth M, Antin J, Bingham E, Ginsberg D. Detection of Philadelphia chromosome-positive cells by the polymerase chain reaction following bone marrow transpant for chronic myelogenous leukemia. Blood 74:882–885, 1989.

50. Antin J. Graft-versus-leukemia: no longer an epiphenomenon. Blood 82:2273–2277, 1993.

51. Bar B, Schattenberg A, Mensink E, Geurts Van Kessel A, Smetsers T, Knops G, Linders E, De Witte T. Donor leukocyte infusions for chronic myeloid leukemia relapsed after allogeneic bone marrow transplantation. J Clin Oncol 11:513–519, 1993.

52. Drobyski W, Keever C, Roth M, Koethe S, Hanson G, McFadden P, Gottschall J, Ash R, van Tuinen P, Horowitz M, Flomenberg N. Salvage immunotherapy using donor leukocyte infusions as treatment for relapsed chronic myelogenous leukemia after allogeneic bone marrow transplantation: efficacy and toxicity of a defined T-cell dose. Blood 82:2310–2318, 1993.

53. Helg C, Roux E, Beris P, Cabrol C, Wacker P, Darbellay R, Wyss M, Jeannet M, Chapuis B, Roosnek E. Adoptive immunotherapy for recurrent CML after BMT. Bone Marrow Transplant 12:125–129, 1993.

54. Hertenstein B, Wiesneth M, Novotny J, Bunjes D, Stefanic M, Heinze B, Hubner G, Heimpel H, Arnold R. Interferon-α and donor buffy coat transfusions for treatment of relapsed chronic myeloid leukemia after allogeneic bone marrow transplantation. Transplant 56:1114–1118, 1993.

55. Porter D, Roth M, McGarigle C, Ferrara J, Antin J. Induction of graft-vs-leukemia (GVL) reaction as therapy for relapsed leukemia after allogeneic bone marrow transplantation (BMT). J Cell Biochem 18B:94a, 1994.
56. Collins R, Wolff S, List A, Christiansen N, Pineiro L, Greer J, Goodman S, Dalton W, Gonzalez G, Herzig G, Phillips G, Fay J. Prospective multicenter trial of donor buffy coat infusion for relapsed hematologic malignancy post-allogeneic bone marrow transplantation (BMT). Blood 84:333a, 1994.
57. van Rhee F, Lin F, Cullis J, Spencer A, Cross N, Chase A, Garicochea B, Bungey J, Barrett J, Goldman J. Relapse of chronic myeloid leukemia after allogeneic bone marrow transplant: the case for giving donor leukocyte transfusions before the onset of hematologic relapse. Blood 83:3377–3383, 1994.
58. Mackinnon S, Papadopoulos E, Carabasi M, Reich L, Collins N, Boulad F, Castro-Malaspina H, Childs B, Gillio A, Kernan N, Small T, Young J, O'Reilly R. Adoptive immunotherapy evaluating escalating doses of donor leukocytes for relapse of chronic myeloid leukemia after bone marrow transplantation: separation of graft-versus-leukemia responses from graft-versus-host disease. Blood 86:1261–1268, 1995.
59. Leber B, Walker I, Rodriguez A, McBride J, Carter R, Brain M. Reinduction of remission of chronic myeloid leukemia by donor leukocyte transfusion following relapse after bone marrow transplantation: recovery complicated by initial pancytopenia and late hematomyositis. Bone Marrow Transplant 12:405–407, 1993.
60. Kolb H, Schattenberg A, Goldman J, Hertenstein B, Jacobsen N, Arcese W, Ljungman P, Ferrant A, Verdonck L, Niederwieser D, van Rhee F, Mittermueller J, de Witte T, Holler E, Ansari H. Graft-versus-leukemia effect of donor lymphocyte transfusions in marrow grafted patients. Blood 86:2041–2050, 1995.
61. Anderson K, Weinstein H. Transfusion-associated graft-versus-host disease. N Engl J Med 323:315–321, 1990.
62. Frassoni F, Fagioli F, Sessarego M, Gualandi F, van Lint M, Lamparelli T, Occhini D, Figari O, Valbonesi M, Bacigalupo A. The effect of donor leucocyte infusion in patients with leukemia following allogeneic bone marrow transplantation. Exp Hematol 20:712, 1992.
63. Korbling M, Przepiorka D, Huh Y, Engel H, van Besien K, Giralt S, Anderson B, Kleine H, Seong D, Deisseroth A, Andreeff M, Champlin R. Allogeneic blood stem cell transplantation for refractory leukemia and lymphoma: potential advantage of blood over marrow allografts. Blood 85:1659–1665, 1995.
64. Bensinger W, Weaver C, Appelbaum F, Rowley S, Demirer T, Sanders T, Sanders J, Storb R, Buckner C: Transplantation of allogeneic peripheral blood stem cells mobilized by recombinant human granulocyte colony-stimulating factor. Blood 85:1655–1658, 1995.
65. Schmitz N, Dreger P, Suttorp M, Rohwedder E, Haferlach T, Loffler H, Hunter A, Russell N. Primary transplantation of allogneic peripheral blood progenitor cells mobilized by filgrastim (granulocyte colony-stimulating factor). Blood 85:1666–1672, 1995.
66. Collins R, Shpilberg O, Drobyski W, Porter D, Antin J, Wolfe S, Giralt S, Chetrit A, Ognoskie N, Prine S, Nemunaitis J. Donor leukocyte infusion (DLI) for post-bone marrow transplant (BMT) relapse-retrospective cohort analysis of 141 cases (abstract). Blood, 86:563a, 1995.
67. Porter D, Antin J. Adoptive immunotherapy in bone marrow transplantation. In Burakoff S, Deeg H, Ferrara J (eds), Graft-versus-Host-Disease. New York: Marcel Dekker, 733–754, 1996.
68. Kolb H, Mittermuller J, Hertenstein H, Schumm M, Holler E, de Witte T, Gunther W, Ljungman P, Goldman J. Adoptive immunotherapy in human and canine chimeras — the role of Interferon alfa. Semin Hematol 30:37–39, 1993.
69. Porter D, Antin J. Adoptive immunotherapy for relapsed leukemia following allogeneic bone marrow transplantation. Leukemia Lymphoma 17:191–197, 1995.
70. Ozer H, George S, Schiffer C, Rao K, Rao N, Wurster-Hill D, Arthur D, Powell B, Gottlieb A, Peterson B, Rai K, Testa J, LeBeau M, Tantravahi R, Bloomfield C. Prolonged subcutaneous administration of recombinant a2b Interferon in patients with previously untreated

81

Philadelphia chromosome-positive chronic-phase chronic myelogenous leukemia: effect on remission duration and survival: Cancer and Leukemia Group B study 8583. Blood 82:2975–2984, 1993.

71. Leukemia. ICSGoCM: Interferon alfa-2a as compared with conventional chemotherapy for the treatment of chronic myeloid leukemia. New Engl J Med 330:820–825, 1994.

72. Talpaz M, Kantarjian H, Kurzrock R, Trujillo J, Gutterman J. Interferon-alpha produces sustained cytogenetic responses in chronic myelogenous leukemia: Philadelphia chromosome-positive patients. Ann Intern Med 114:532–538, 1991.

73. Lee M, Kantarjian H, Talpaz M, Freireich E, Deisseroth A, Trujillo J, Stass S. Detection of minimal residual disease by polymerase chain reaction in Philadelphia chromosome positive chronic myelogenous leukemia following interferon therapy. British J Haematol 82:708–714, 1992.

74. Gressler V, Weinkauff R, Franklin W, Golomb H. Moldulation of the expression of major histocompatibility antigens on splenic hairy cells — differential effect upon in vitro treatment with alpha-2b-interferon, gamma-interferon, and interleukin-2. Blood 72:1048–1053, 1988.

75. Balkwill F. Interferons. New York: Oxford University Press, 1989.

76. Upadhyaya G, Gupta S, Sih S, Feinberg A, Talpaz M, Kantarjian H, Deisseroth A, Emerson S. Interferon-alpha restores the deficient expression of the cytoadhesion molecule lymphocyte function antigen-3 by chronic myelogenous leukemia progenitor cells. J Clin Invest 88:2131, 1991.

77. Peschel C, Aman M, Rudolf G, Aulitzky W, Huber C. Regulation of the cytokine network by interferon: a potential mechanism of interferon in chronic myelogenous leukemia. Semin Hematol 30:28–31, 1993.

78. Nimer S, Giorgi J, Gajewski J, Ku N, Schiller G, Lee K, Territo m, Ho W, Feig S, Selch M, Isacescu V, Reichert T, Champlin R. Selective depletion of CD8+ cells for prevention of graft-versus-host disease after bone marrow transplantation. Transplant 57:82–87, 1994.

79. Giralt S, Hester J, Huh Y, Hirsch-Ginsberg C, Rondon G, Guo J, Lee M, Gajewski J, Talpaz M, Kantarjian H, Fischer H, Deisseroth A, Champlin R. CD8+ depleted donor lymphocyte infusions as treatment for relapsed chronic myelogenous leukemia (CML) after allogeneic bone marrow transplantation (BMT): graft vs leukemia without graft vs host disease (GVHD). Blood 84:538a, 1994.

80. Roth M, Antin J, Ash R, Terry V, Gotlieb M, Silver S, Ginsburg D. Prognostic significance of Philadelphia chromosome-positive cells detected by the polymerase chain reaction after allogeneic bone marrow transplant for chronic myelogenous leukemia. Blood 79:276–282, 1992.

81. Sullivan K, Deeg H, Sanders J, Losterman A, Amis D, Shulman H, Sale G, Martin P, Witherspoon R, Appelbaum F, Doney K, Stewart P, Meyers J, McDonald G, Weiden P, Fefer A, Buckner C, Storb R, Thomas E. Hyperacute graft-v-host disease in patients not given immunosuppression after allogeneic marrow transplantation. Blood 67:1172–1175, 1986.

82. Sullivan K, Storb R, Witherspoon R, Weiden P, Anasetti C, Appelbaum F, Beatty P, Buckner C, Deeg H, Doney K, Fisher L, Loughran T, Martin P, Meyers J, McDonald G, Sanders J, Shulman H, Steewart P, Thomas E. Deletion of immunosuppressive prophylaxis after marrow transplantation increased hyperacute graft-versus-host disease but does not influence chronic graft-versus-host disease or relapse in patients with advanced leukemia. Clin Transplant 3:5–11, 1989.

83. Elfenbein G, Graham-Pole J, Weiner R, Goedert T, Gross S. Consequences of no prophylaxis for acute graft-versus-host disease after HLA-identical bone marrow transplantation (abstract). Blood 70 (Suppl 1):305a, 1987.

84. Sullivan K, Storb R, Buckner D, Fefer A, Fisher L, Weiden P, Witherspoon R, Appelbaum F, Banaji M, Hansen J, Martin P, Sanders J, Singer J, Thomas ED. Graft-versus-host disease as adoptive immunotherapy in patients with advanced hematologic neoplasms. N Engl J Med 320:828–834, 1989.

85. Antin J, Ferrara J. Cytokine dysregulation and acute graft-versus-host disease. Blood 80:2964–2968, 1992.
86. Weiden P, Storb R, Tsoi M, Graham T, Lerner K, Thomas E. Infusion of donor lymphocytes into stable canine radiation chimeras: implications for mechanism of transplantation tolerance. J Immunol 116:1212–1219, 1978.
87. Johnson B, Drobyski W, Truitt R. Delayed infusion of normal donor cells after MHC-matched bone marrow transplantation provides an antileukemia reaction without graft-versus-host disease. Bone Marrow Transplant 11:329–336, 1993.
88. Slavin S, Ackerstein A, Weiss L, Nagler A, Or R, Naparstek E. Immunotherapy of minimal residual disease by immunocompetent lymphocytes and their activation by cytokines. Cancer Invest 10:221–227, 1992.
89. Naparsteck E, Or R, Nagler A, Cividalli G, Engelhard D, Aker M, Gimon Z, Manny N, Sacks T, Tochner Z, Weiss L, Samuel S, Brautbar C, Hale G, Waldmann H, Steinberg S, Slavin S. T-cell-depleted allogeneic bone marrow transplantation for acute leukaemia using Campath-1 antibodies and posttransplant administration of donor's peripheral blood lymphocytes for prevention of relapse. Br J Haematol 89:506–515, 1995.
90. Slavin S, Naparstek E, Nagler A, Ackerstein A, Kapelushnik Y, Drakos P, Or R. Graft vs leukemia (GVL) effects with controlled GVHD by cell mediated immunotherapy (CMI) following allogeneic bone marrow transplantation (BMT). Blood 82:423a, 1993.
91. Couriel D, Cottler-Fox M, Burt R, Dunbar C, Hensel N, Young N, Barrett A. T-cell depleted marrow transplants with delayed lymphocyte add-back to prevent relapse in patients with leukemia and MDS. Blood 84:334a, 1994.
92. Porter D, Roth M, McGarigle C, Lee S, Ferrara J, Antin J. The graft-vs-leukemia (GVL) effect of donor mononuclear cell (MNC) infusions for patients with relapsed acute leukemia and myelodysplasia (MDS) after allogeneic bone marrow transplantation. Blood 84:338a, 1994.
93. Pati A, Godder K, Lamb L, Gee A, Henslee-Downey P. Donor leukocyte infusions (DLI) to treat relapsed acute myeloid leukemia (AML) following partially mismatched related donor (PMRD) bone marrow transplantation (BMT). Blood 84:339a, 1994.
94. Szer J, Grigg A, Phillipos G, Sheridan W. Donor leucocyte infusions after chemotherapy for patients relapsing with acute leukaemia following allogeneic BMT. Bone Marrow Transplant 11:109–111, 1993.
95. Vesole D, Tricot G, Jagannath S, Barlogie B. Induction of graft-versus-myeloma (GVM) effect following allogeneic bone marrow transplantation. Blood 84:331a, 1994.
96. Ferster A, Bujan W, Mouraux T, Devalck C, Heimann P, Sariban E. Compalete remission following donor leukocyte infusion in ALL relapsing after haploidentical bone marrow transplantation. Bone Marrow Transplant 14:331–332, 1994.
97. Verfaillie C, Weisdorf D, McGlave P, Vercellotti G, Enright H, Burns L, Miller J. High dose donor mononuclear cell infusion in post-transplant relapsed AML/MDS. Blood 84:333a, 1994.
98. Mehta J, Powles R, Singhal S, Tait D, Swansbury J, Treleaven J. Cytokine-mediated immunotherapy with or without donor leukocytes for poor-risk acute myeloid leukemia relapsing after allogeneic bone marrow transplantation. Bone Marrow Transplant 16:133–137, 1995.
99. Chen W, Peace D, Rovira D, You S, Cheever M. T-cell immunity to the joining region of p210 BCR-ABL protein. Proc Natl Acad Sci USA 89:1468–1472, 1992.
100. Uharek L, Glass B, Gaska T, Zeiss M, Gassmann W, Loffler H, Muller-Ruchholtz W. Natural killer cells as effector cells of graft-versus-leukemia activity in a murine transplantation model. Bone Marrow Transplant 12:S57–60, 1993.
101. Maraninchi D, Blaise D, Rio B, Leblond V, Dreyfus F, Gluckman E, Guyotat D, Pico J, Michallet M, Ifrah N, Bordigoni A. Impact of T-cell depletion on outcome of allogeneic bone-marrow transplantation for standard-risk leukaemias. Lancet 2:175–178, 1987.
102. Faber L, van Luxemburg-Heijs A, Veenhof W, willemze R, Falkenburg J. Generation of CD4+ cytotoxic T-lymphocyte clones from a patient with severe graft-versus-host disease

after allogeneic bone marrow transplantation: implications for graft-versus-leukemia reactivity. Blood 86:2821–2828, 1995.

103. Jiang Y, Kanfer E, MacDonald D, Cullis J, Goldman J, Barrett A. Graft versus leukaemia following allogeneic bone marrow transplantation: emergence of cytotoxic T lymphocytes reacting to host leukaemia cells. Bone Marrow Transplant 8:253–258, 1991.

104. Datta A, Barret A, Jiang Y, Guimaraes A, Mavroudis D, van Rhee F, Gordon A, Madrigal A. Distinct T cell populations distinguish chronic myeloid leukaemia cells from lymphocytes in the same individual: a model for separating GVHD from GVL reactions. Bone Marrow Transplant 14:577–524, 1994.

105. Sosman J, Oettel K, Smith S, Hank J, Fisch P, Sondel P. Specific recognition of human leukemic cells by allogeneic T cells: II. Evidence for HLA-D restricted determinants on leukemic cells that are crossreactive with determinants present on unrelated nonleukemic cells. Blood 75:2005–2016, 1990.

106. Hauch M, Gazzola M, Small T, Bordignon C, Barnett L, Cunningham I, Castro-Malaspinia H, O'Reilly R, Keever C. Anti-leukemia potential of interleukin-2 activated natural killer cells after bone marrow tranplantation for chronic myelogenous leukemia. Blood 75:2250–2262, 1990.

107. Reittie J, Gottlieb D, Heslop H, Leger O, Drexler H, Hazlehurst G, Hoffbrand A, Brenner M. Endogenously generated activated killer cells circulate after autologous and allogeneic marrow transplantation but not after chemotherapy. Blood 73:1351–1358, 1989.

108. Hercend T, Takvorian T, Nowill A, Tantravahi R, Moingeon P, Anderson K, Murray C, Bohuon C, Ythier A, Ritz J. Characterization of natural killer cells with antileukemia activity following allogeneic bone marrow transplantation. Blood 67:722–728, 1986.

109. Jiang Y, Cullis J, Kanfer E, Goldman J, Barrett A. T cell and NK cell mediated graft-versus-leukaemia reactivity following donor buffy coat transfusion to treat relapse after marrow transplantation for chronic myeloid leukaemia. Bone Marrow Transplant 11:133–138, 1993.

110. Mackinnon S, Hows J, Goldman J. Induction of in vitro graft-versus-leukemia activity following bone marrow transplantation for chronic myeloid leukemia. Blood 76:2037–2045, 1990.

111. Soiffer R, Murray C, Gonin R, Ritz J. Effect of low-dose interleukin-2 on disease relapse after T-cell-depleted allogeneic bone marrow transplantation. Blood 84:964–971, 1994.

112. Verdonck L, van Heugten H, Giltay J, Franks C. Amplification of the graft-versus-leukemia effect in man by interleukin-2. Transplantation 51:1120–1124, 1991.

113. Bunjes D, Theobald M, Hertenstein B, Wiesneth M, Novotny J, Arnold R, Heimpel H. Successful therapy with donor buffy coat transfusions in patients with relapsed chronic myeloid leukemia after bone marrow transplantation is associated with high frequencies of host-reactive interleukin 2-secreting T helper cells. Bone Marrow Transplant 15:713–719, 1995.

114. Smith K. Lowest dose interleukin-2 immunotherapy. Blood 81:1414–1423, 1993.

115. Ikinciogullari A, Oblakowski P, Hamon M, et al. Activation marker expression on the peripheral blood lymphocytes of normal volunteers, recipients of interleukin 2 and patients undergoing bone marrow transplantation. Exp Hematol 20:819, 1992.

116. Benyunes M, Massumoto C, York A, Higuchi C, Buchner C, Thompson J, Petersen F, Fefer A. Interleukin-2 with or without lymphokine-activated killer cells as consolidative immunotherapy after autologous bone marrow transplantation for acute myelogenous leukemia. Bone Marrow Transplant 12:159–163, 1993.

117. Hamon M, Prentice H, Gottlieb D, Macdonald I, Cunningham J, Smith O, Gilmore M, Gandhi L, Collis C. Immunotherapy with interleukin 2 after ABMT in AML. Bone Marrow Transplant 11:399–401, 1993.

118. Zutter M, Maretin P, Sale G, Shulman H, Fisher L, Thomas E, Durnam D. Epstein–Barr virus lymphoproliferation after bone marrow transplantation. Blood 72:520–529, 1988.

119. Shapiro R, McClain K, Frizzera G, Gajl-Peczalska K, Kersey J, Blazar B, Arthur D, Patton D, Greenberg J, Burke B, Ramsay N, McGlave P, Filipovich A. Epstein–Barr virus associ-

ated B cell lymphoproliferative disorders following bone marrow transplantation. Blood 71:1234–1243, 1988.

120. Papadopoulos E, Ladanyi M, Emanuel D, Mackinnon S, Boulad F, Carabasi M, Castro-Malaspina J, Childs B, Gillio A, Small T, Young J, Kernan N, O'Reilly R. Infusions of donor leukocytes to treat Epstein–Barr virus-associated lymphoproliferative disorders after allogeneic bone marrow transplantation. N Engl J Med 330:1185–1191, 1994.

121. Porter D, Orloff G, Antin J. Donor mononuclear cell infusions as therapy for B-cell lymphoproliferative disorder following allogeneic bone marrow transplant. Transplant Science 4:11–15, 1994.

122. Servida P, Rossini S, Traversari C, Ferrari G, Bonini C, Nobili N, Vago L, Faravelli A, Vanzulli A, Mavillio F, Bordignon C. Gene transfer into peripheral blood lymphocytes for in vivo immunomodulation of donor anti-tumor immunity in a patient affected by EBV-induced lymphoma. Blood 82:214a, 1993.

123. Bonini C, Verzeletti S, Servida P, Rossini S, Traversari C, Ferrari G, Nobili N, Mavillo F, Bordignon C. Transfer of the HSV-TK gene into donor peripheral blood lymphocytes for in vivo immunomodulation of donor anti-tumor immunity after allo-BMT. Blood 84:110a, 1994.

124. Rooney C, Smnith C, Ng C, Loftin S, Li C, Krance R, Brenner M. Use of gene-modified virus-specific T lymphocytes to control Epstein–Barr-virus-related lymphoproliferation. Lancet 345:9–13, 1995.

125. Hroma R, Cornetta K, Srour E. Donor leukocyte infusion as therapy of life-threatening adenoviral infections after T-cell-depleted bone marrow transplantation (letter). Blood 84:1690–1691, 1994.

126. Takahashi S, Nagayama H, Nagamura F, Inoue T, Okamoto S, Tani K, Ikebuchi K, Sato N, Ozawa K, Hirano T, Oshimi K, Asano S. Graft versus leukemia (GVL) effect with fatal graft versus host disease (GVHD) by donor leukocyte transfusion (DLT) in post-transplantation acute leukemia relapse: reports of two cases. Blood 84:338a, 1994.

127. Heberman R, Ortaldo J, Rjubinstein M, Pestka S. Augmentation of natural and antibody-dependent cell-mediated cytotoxicity by pure human leukocyte interferon. J Clin Immunol 1:149–153, 1981.

4. Graft-versus-host disease: implications from basic immunology for prophylaxis and treatment

Georgia B. Vogelsang

Graft-vs.-host disease (GVHD) continues to be a major complication after allogeneic bone marrow transplantation, especially with the increasing use of unrelated and mismatched donors. To understand how best to prevent GVHD and to treat GVHD should prophylaxis fail, it is necessary to have a good understanding of the underlying immunology of GVHD. There has been recent progress in understanding two basic aspects of the immune response in GVHD — the immunologic target and the effector mechanisms. First, the target of the immune response in GVHD has been identified as histocompatibility antigens possessed by the host but not the donor. Recognition of self antigens in GVHD has been documented, showing that GVHD is more than simple alloreactivity. Second, the effector mechanism in GVHD was initially thought to be direct cytotoxicity by alloreactive T cells. Cytokines are now known to play a central role in mediating many of the clinical and experimental manifestations of GVHD.

Immunologic background

Graft-vs.-host disease was originally called 'secondary disease' to differentiate it from the radiation sickness and aplasia occurring after total body irradiation [1]. Mice receiving syngeneic transplants recovered normally. Animals receiving allogeneic transplants developed erythroderma, wasting, diarrhea, and jaundice, and ultimately died of 'secondary disease.' Skin biopsies of these animals showed vacuolar alteration of the basilar epidermis and dyskeratotic epithelial cells in the epidermis or hair follicle. As the disease advanced, the vacuoles at the basement membrane progressed to cleft and frank subepidermal bulla formation. In the liver, lymphocytic infiltration and necrosis of the small bile ducts were seen. Crypt necrosis leading to eventual mucosal denudation was seen in the intestinal tracts of animals with GVHD [1]. Further experimental work showed that F1 hybrid recipients given parental haploidentical marrow developed secondary disease, but parental strain recipients given F1 hybrid marrow did not [2]. These observations led to the conclusion that secondary disease was due to recognition of host histocompat-

Jane N. Winter (ed.) BLOOD STEM CELL TRANSPLANTATION. 1997. Kluwer Academic Publishers. ISBN 0-7923-4260-7. All rights reserved.

ibility antigens by donor (graft) lymphocytes — hence the name graft-versus-host disease [3]. Billingham summarized these observations by defining the classical requirements for GVHD [3]. These requirements were the following:

1. The graft must contain immunologically competent cells.
2. The host must possess important transplantation alloantigens that are lacking in the donor graft, so that the host appears foreign to the graft and is therefore capable of stimulating it antigenically.
3. The host itself must be incapable of mounting an effective immunological reaction against the graft, at least for sufficient time for the latter to manifest its immunological capabilities: that is, it must have the security of tenure.

The immunologic recognition and response seen in GVHD were felt to be due to histocompatibility differences between the donor and recipient. This classic concept of GVHD as delineated by Billingham accounted for the GVHD seen both after marrow transplantation and in immunoincompetent individuals receiving unirradiated blood products. The manifestations of GVHD in the animals were duplicated in the initial human transplants. This construct also accounted for the therapeutic approaches used for GVHD. The original agents used for prophylaxis and treatment of GVHD were lymphocytotoxic agents (i.e., steroids, methotrexate, cyclophosphamide, and antithymocyte globulin) used to destroy cytotoxic T cells.

There were several cases reported of patients who received syngeneic or autologous transplants and developed clinical GVHD [4–6]. In most cases, the GVHD involved the skin only. In a few cases, multiorgan disease with involvement of the liver and/or gut was observed [5]. These cases were at first attributed to unirradiated blood products or severe infections such as CMV-mimicking GVHD. Over time, however, a more subtle explanation was appreciated. GVHD in these patients arose from recognition of self antigens. The development of an animal model of autologous GVHD allowed new insights into the complexity of GVHD.

Autologous GVHD

Glazier et al. initially described an animal model of autologous GVHD [7]. Rats given total body irradiation followed by syngeneic transplants and cyclosporine would develop a syndrome that clinically and histologically resembles allogeneic GVHD. The possibility of strain drift accounting for this observation was discounted by performing autologous transplants in which the animals were allowed to reconstitute from a single shielded limb [8]. In both cases (animals receiving syngeneic marrow or animals undergoing autologous reconstitution), the animals developed autologous GVHD, as shown by erythroderma and histology consistent with GVHD. Further laboratory work has shown that autologous GVHD is directed against an apparent public determinant of the MHC class II [9,10]. Monoclonal antibodies against class II antigens blocked this recognition (in vitro and in vivo), whereas monoclonal antibodies to class I antigens were ineffective. Paradoxically, the cells initially involved in this reaction were CD8 positive, whereas class-II-restricted T cells belong to the CD4 subset. As the disease progressed, both CD4 and CD8 positive cells were involved in the reaction.

The concept of autoreactive T cells was not new. However, this study was the first demonstration of an auto-aggression syndrome due to the failure to recognize autologous MHC antigens. The requirements for induction of this syndrome have been elucidated elsewhere [11–14]. Thymic damage was critical for its development. Animals who were thymectomized or in whom the thymuses were shielded during total body irradiation failed to develop this syndrome. Second, total body irradiation was very important, primarily because of the thymic damage induced and the elimination of a peripheral host resistance mechanism (see below). Third, cyclosporine was also needed to induce this syndrome in the majority of animals.

Cyclosporine has many complicated effects on the thymus. Cyclosporine ablates the thymic medulla and depletes reticuloepithelial cells within the cortex [15–17]. Class II expression is markedly reduced within the medulla [18]. T-cell differentiation is significantly affected by cyclosporine [18–22]. Thymocytes expressing the α/β T-cell receptor and single positive CD4 and CD8 cells are reduced. Immature CD4 CD8 double-negative and CD4 CD8 double-positive thymocytes are increased, implying a maturational arrest. These immature cells have been detected in the peripheral circulation. The normal mechanism of clonal deletion of self-reactive T cells is inhibited by CsA, again resulting in release of autoreactive cells into the peripheral immune system [18,21].

This disorder is not as simple as production of an autoreactive cell. For the disease to be expressed, autoreactive cells need to be present and the normal peripheral autoregulatory mechanisms need to be interrupted. Autologous GVHD can be adoptively transferred from animals receiving posttransplant cyclosporine into fresh irradiated recipients. If normal splenocytes are added, the secondary recipients do not develop autologous GVHD [9,10]. Animals receiving cyclosporine alone, without a transplant, can be shown to develop autocytotoxic T cells in increased numbers, which can cause autologous GVHD if the animals remain on cyclosporine for prolonged periods of time more than six months [23]. Thus, there is both the need for an autocytotoxic cell and disruption of normal regulatory mechanisms for autologous GVHD to develop clinically.

Recent work has centered on the thymic repertoire involved in autologous GVHD. The same limited repertoire of Vβ 8.5 and Vβ 10 cells that has been implicated in spontaneously occurring or in genetically determined autoimmune disorders in the rat has also been implicated in autologous GVHD [24]. Cells bearing these markers are expressed in much higher frequencies in animals with autologous GVHD, suggesting that much of this disorder is clonally regulated [25,26]. Depletion of these cells from effector splenocytes inhibits the ability to adoptively transfer this syndrome.

Autologous GVHD may play a role in both acute and chronic GVHD occurring after an allogeneic transplant [27–29]. The intrathymic and peripheral conditions that result in autologous recognition occur after both autologous and allogeneic BMT. Animals receiving allogeneic major histocompatibility complex (MHC) mismatched transplants do not develop GVHD while maintained on cyclosporine. Upon cyclosporine withdrawal, the majority of animals will develop the clinical manifestation and histological manifestations of acute GVHD. Could the GVHD seen in the allogeneic recipient include an autologous GVHD component? To answer this question, cells from animals developing GVHD were adoptively transferred into irradiated recipients of the host and donor strain. If the GVHD seen after withdrawal of cyclosporine was purely allogeneic, donor strain animals should not develop GVHD. However, if there was an autologous component, animals of both the donor and host strain would be expected to develop GVHD. The results were indeed surprising: both donor and host strains developed GVHD, implicating an autologous component to the GVHD after immunosuppression with cyclosporine [27]. Finally, there is intriguing data to suggest that the chronic GVHD seen after allogeneic transplant may be related to poor/dysfunctional immunologic recovery akin to autologous GVHD. The same Vβ repertoire is expressed in experimental chronic GVHD (without cyclosporine therapy) as in autologous GVHD, suggesting that chronic GVHD includes an autoimmune component [28]. This hypothesis is supported by the recent demonstration of class-II-specific donor antidonor autoreactive T cells in humans and in mice with chronic GVHD [29]. Should this finding of a restricted T-cell repertoire be confirmed in human GVHD (either acute or chronic), one exciting application would be the use of monoclonal antibodies with binding restricted to certain V regions to treat GVHD. This should provide more specific therapy with less global immunosuppression.

Autologous GVHD is currently being investigated clinically for its potential antitumor effects. Animal models of autologous GVHD have shown that the effector cells of autologous GVHD are capable of recognizing tumor cells with MHC class II antigens [30]. Uncontrolled clinical trials have shown promising results, with lower relapse rates in patients developing autologous GVHD [31–35]. Randomized trials are just starting to verify that there is indeed a benefit to autologous GVHD.

Cytokines and GVHD — Overview

GVHD was first conceived of as a T-cell-mediated disease. The cellular injury in GVHD was thought to be due to infiltration of target tissues by effector cells with resultant destruction. This explanation for the destruction seen in GVHD was based on the frequent observation of lymphocytes accompanying dying cells (satellitosis) in the skin of patients or animals with GVHD. Consequently, it was concluded that the target cell was being destroyed by the effector cell. However, immunohistochemical analysis has shown that many, but not all, of these cells are phenotypically natural killer cells rather than mature T cells [36]. These observations have been confirmed by electron microscopy. Many investigators have rethought GVHD based on these findings. A new model of the effector phase of GVHD has been proposed [37]. GVHD is seen as a 'cytokine storm.' Cytokines are initially released during the preparative regimen, and then this process is perpetuated by T-cell recognition of histocompatibility antigens. The cytokines released start a positive feedback loop that results in the actual disease/destruction in GVHD.

The cytokine model of the effector phase of GVHD accounts for many of the observations that have been made about this process and has already led to new lines of therapy. This model proposes that damage to host tissues occurring during chemotherapy, radiotherapy, and infection results in release of inflammatory cytokines such as tumor necrosis factor-α (TNF-α) and IL-1. These cytokines cause increased MHC expression and upregulate other adhesion molecules. The recognition of recipient/donor differences by alloreactive T cells in the donor graft is increased because of the increased recipient expression of MHC and adhesion molecules. The reactive donor T cells then proliferate and secrete cytokines, most particularly IL-2. The cytokines then activate additional donor T cells and mononuclear cells. Macrophages are induced to secrete IL-1 and TNF-α. The cytokines will stimulate both autoreactive and alloreactive T cells. Patients developing either spontaneous or cyclosporine-induced autologous GVHD do so during lymphocyte recovery, again adding substantial credibility to the existence of this cascade. Thus, an inflammatory response involving multiple cytokines is established, recruiting additional cells into the response and damaging more tissue. The resulting cytokine cascade eventually produces the clinical manifestations of the syndrome called graft-versus-host disease. Several factors, including gut decontamination, the use of a sterile environment, and the administration of IV immunoglobulin, all of which have been found to decrease the incidence of GVHD, interrupt this cascade [38,39]. In part, lymphocyte depletion of a marrow graft may decrease GVHD by temporarily removing the lymphocytes necessary to maintain the cytokine cascade. These observations raise the question of whether delaying the infusion of alloreactive T cells until after the initial cytokine wave (arising from damage from the preparative regimen) is over would prevent GVHD while maintaining a graft-versus-leukemia effect. Increased relapse rates observed after lymphocyte depletion of marrow grafts have largely negated the anti-GVHD benefit of these manipulated marrow grafts. Maintaining the graft-versus-leukemia effect while eliminating or reducing GVHD has remained an elusive goal. Animal experiments suggest that delayed infusion of lymphocytes may achieve this goal by interrupting the cytokine cascade [40]. Delayed infusion of normal donor cells after MHC-matched bone marrow transplantation provides an antileukemic reaction without GVHD.

IL-2 was considered to be critical in the development of GVHD even before the concept of a cytokine cascade had been proposed to explain the clinical manifestations of GVHD. IL-2 was one of the first cytokines to be identified and was found to be critical in T-cell activation. Cyclosporine, an agent that inhibits IL-2 secretion, inhibits experimental GVHD and has been shown to be useful in multiple studies of clinical prophylaxis of GVHD, especially when combined with methotrexate and/or steroids [41–44]. Much of the early work on the importance in cytokines concentrated on the influence of IL-2. Recent studies have emphasized the importance of IL-2 as an initiating agent in GVHD. Several groups have shown that the precursor frequency of antihost-specific IL-2-producing cells predicts for GVHD in HLA identical sibling transplants [45–47]. The prominence of IL-2 as the presumed (but now disputed, as discussed below) pivotal cytokine in GVHD also meant that some of the first trials using anticytokine therapy were directed against IL-2. Herve et al. used an anti-IL-2 receptor monoclonal antibody to treat steroid-resistant, severe GVHD. Although frequently not sustained, responses were seen in over 80% of patients [48]. Recent work has concentrated on the use of humanized anti-IL-2-receptor monoclonal antibodies [49]. Media reports have suggested that these trials are not going to show the desired benefits; however, lessons learned from studies using humanized monoclonal antibodies should have significant implications for other monoclonal antibody trials.

Another line of evidence for the involvement of IL-2 in GVHD is the effectiveness of cyclosporine in the treatment of experimental and clinical GVHD [41–44]. Cyclosporine inhibits IL-2 production and, at higher concentrations, expression of the IL-2 receptor [22].

The important role of TNF-α in GVHD has become apparent from two lines of evidence. In experimental animal models, TNF-α was found to be an important mediator of the disease, and its production was increased [50]. When infused into animals, TNF has many effects that mimic the effects of GVHD. These include cachexia, runting, hematopoietic failure, erythroderma, diarrhea, alveolar damage, and ultimately, death. Treatment of animals with anti-TNF antibodies can blunt or prevent many of the findings found in GVHD. Clinical studies have confirmed these results and again emphasized the interactive nature of the multiple events occurring during marrow transplantation with GVHD [51]. Investigators found that TNF-α levels were increased in patients with GVHD and in patients with hepatic toxicity (veno-occlusive disease of the liver) from the preparative regimen. One clincial study has examined the use of anti-TNF-α monoclonal antibodies in severe steroid-resistant GVHD [52]. As predicted by the cytokine cascade model, responses in these heavily pretreated patients were short-lived. Blocking a mediator with a monoclonal antibody would be expected to affect the disease only during exposure to the reagent. Since multiple cytokines would be released, a multiprong approach using multiple anticytokine reagents would be expected to have a more profound influence and potentially induce complete responses. Similarly, for these agents to be maximally effective, they would have to be used early in GVHD, before wholesale activation of the immune system occurs.

Recognition that TNF plays an important role in GVHD has led to the study of several agents that may decrease TNF production. The best known is pentoxifylline, a xanthine derivative, that downregulates TNF-α production in vitro. Unfortunately, the initial pilot data supporting the use of this agent in preventing toxicity, both from preparative regimens and GVHD, have not been reproduced in a large randomized study [53,54]. Recent studies have shown that thalidomide may also be exerting its influences in treatment and prevention of GVHD, partially through inhibition of TNF-α production by stimulated monocytes [55].

Another cytokine to achieve considerable attention is IL-1. IL-1 is a cytokine produced by monocytes. Studies with a transplant model that uses mice of different strains with minor histocompatibility antigen differences have shown that IL-1 may be the critical effector molecule in GVHD [56].

IL-2 mRNA was upregulated only during the first week posttransplant in this model. IL-1 and, to a lesser degree, TNF were found to be increased during GVHD. Inhibition of IL-1 by an IL-1 receptor antagonist prevented severe GVHD in this animal model. Because of these observations, phase I/II trials using an IL-1 receptor antagonist for patients with steroid-resistant GVHD have been undertaken and show very encouraging early results.

Although the role of interferon in the cytokine cascade has not clearly been elucidated, the interferon most likely to be involved in GVHD is gamma interferon. Gamma interferon may be induced during the initial injury caused by chemotherapy and/or infection. Interferon has been found to be increased in patients and in animal models of GVHD [57,58]. Gamma interferon may function by upregulating histocompatibility antigens and inducing release of TNF [59]. Gamma interferon primes macrophages to release TNF after exposure to lipopolysaccharide (LPS). LPS is a potent trigger for induction of experimental GVHD, and endogenous LPS has been detected in the serum of animals with lethal GVHD [59]. Thus, LPS represents another component in the cascade that results in GVHD.

Certainly, many other cytokines may be important in GVHD. However, other cytokines such as IL-6, IL-4, IL-8, and IL-10 have not been thoroughly studied in GVHD. The potential role of other cytokines, as well as the interaction among cytokines and different T-cell subsets (especially Th1 and Th2), needs further delineation. Experimental animal data suggest that the Th2 subpopulation of CD4+ lymphocytes (which produces IL-4 and IL-10) prevents LPS-induced, TNF-mediated lethal GVHD [60]. In these animals, there was suppression of gamma interferon mRNA, reduction of TNF levels in the serum, increased IL-4 mRNA, and decreased CD8+ lymphoid engraftment. In certain experimental animal models in which GVHD is mediated by CD4+ cells, it has been observed that administration of IL-2 actually reduced mortality from GVHD; this effect may be due to generation of Th2 cells [61]. These data suggest that Th2 cells may play a major role in establishing tolerance after marrow transplant.

Thus, a model can be constructed showing the interactive nature of cytokines that have been implicated in GVHD. Many of the effects of GVHD are caused directly by the cytokines themselves (TNF being the primary example) or by secondary activation of bystander cells such as NK cells, which may cause much of the cytotoxic damage seen in GVHD.

The view of GVHD has changed significantly over the last few years. The targets of immune recognition and the effector mechanisms are much more complex than previously appreciated. However, this very complexity has shown many new ways of preventing and treating GVHD. These more specific maneuvers are not only likely to lead to better control of GVHD but to less global immunosupression. These therapies should result in improved survival and should facilitate the increasing use of mismatched/unrelated donors.

References

1. Barnes DWH, Loutit JF. Spleen protection: the cellular hypothesis. In Bacq ZM (ed), Radiobiology Symposium Liegè. London: Butterworths, 1955, p. 134.
2. Trentin JJ. Mortality and skin transplantability in irradiated mice receiving isologous or heterologous bone marrow. Proc Soc Exp Biol Med 92:688, 1956.
3. Billingham RE. The biology of graft-versus-host reactions. Harvey Lectures (1966–67) 62:21, 1967.
4. Gluckman E, Devergie A, Sohier J, Sauret SH. Graft versus host disease in recipients of syngeneic bone marrow. Lancet i:253, 1980.
5. Thien SW, Goldman JM, Galton DG. Acute 'graft versus host disease' after autologous grafting for chronic granulocytic leukemia in transplantation. Ann Intern Med 94:210, 1981.
6. Hood AF, Vogelsang GB, Black C, Farmer ER, Santos GW. Acute graft versus host disease: development following autologous and syngeneic bone marrow transplantation. Arch Dermatol 123:745, 1987.
7. Glazier A, Tutschka PJ, Farmer ER, Santos GW. Graft-versus-host disease in cyclosporin A treated rats after syngeneic and autologous bone marrow reconstitution. J Exp Med 158:1, 1983.
8. Glazier A, Tutschka PJ, Farmer ER. Studies on the immunobiology of syngeneic and autologous graft-versus-host disease in cyclosporine treated rats. Transplant Proc 15:3035, 1983.
9. Hess AD, Horwitz L, Beschorner WE, Santos GW. Development of graft-versus-host disease-like syndrome in cyclosporine-treated rats after syngeneic bone marrow transplantation. I. Development of cytotoxic T-lymphocytes with apparent polyclonal anti-Ia specificity, including autoreactivity. J Exp Med 161:718, 1985.
10. Hess AD, Horwitz LR, Laulis MK. Cyclosporine induced syngeneic graft-vs-host disease: recognition of self MHC class II antigens in vivo. Transplant Proc 25:1218, 1993.
11. Cheney RT, Sprent J. Capacity of cyclosporine to induce autograft-versus-host disease and impair intrathymic T-cell differentiation. Transplant Proc 17:528, 1985.
12. Beschorner WE, Shinn CA, Hess AD, Suresch DL, Santos GW. Immune related injury to endothelium associated with acute graft-vs-host disease in the rat. Transplant Proc 21:3025, 1989.
13. Shinozawa T, Beschorner WE, Hess AD. Prolonged administration of cyclosporine and the thymus: irreversible immunopathologic changes associated with autologous pseudo-graft-vs-host disease. Transplant 50:106, 1990.

14. Beschorner WE, Ren H, Phillip J, Pulido HB, Hiaban RH, Hess AD. Recovery of thymic microenvironment after cyclosporine prevents syngeneic graft-vs-host disease. Transplant 52:668, 1991.
15. Ryffel B, Deyssenroth H, Borel JH. Cyclosporin A: effects on the mouse thymus. Agents Actions 11:373, 1981.
16. Beschorner WE, Nammorim JF, Hess AD, Shinn CA, Santos GW. Cyclosporine A and the thymus: immunopathology. Am J Pathol 126:487, 1987.
17. Fabien NH, Auger C, Moreira A, Monier JC. Effects of cyclosporin A on mouse thymus: immunochemical and ultrastructural studies. Thymus 20:153, 1992.
18. Beschorner WE, Suresch DL, Shinozawa T, Santos GW, Hess AD. Influence of irradiation and age on the CsA induced thymic immunopathology. Transplant Proc 20:1072, 1988.
19. Beschorner WE, Ren H, Phillip J, Pulido HB, Hruban RH, Hess AD. Recovery of thymic microenvironment after cyclosporine prevents syngeneic graft-vs-host disease. Transplant 52:668, 1991.
20. Fischer AC, Laulis MK, Horwitz L, Hess AD. Effect of cyclosporine on T lymphocyte development: relationship to syngeneic graft-versus-host disease. Transplant 51:252, 1991.
21. Zhang H, Horwitz LR, Fischer AC, Colombani PM, Hess AD. Adoptive transfer of cyclosprine-induced MHC class II autoreactive cells prolong heart allograft survival. Transplant Sci 3:17, 1993.
22. Hess AD, Vogelsang GB, Heyd J, Beschorner WE. Cyclosporine induced syngeneic graft-vs-host disease, assessment of T-cell differentiation. Transplant Proc 19:2683, 1987
23. Shinozawa T, Beschorner WE, Hess AD. Prolonged administration of cyclosporine irreversible immunopathologic changes associated with autologous pseudo-graft-vs-host disease. Transplant 50:106, 1990.
24. Herber-Katz E, Acha-Orbea H. The v-region hypothesis: evidence from autoimmune encephalomyelitis. Immunol Today 10:64, 1989.
25. Severino ME, Laulis MK, Horwitz LR, Hess AD. Cyclosporine preferentially inhibits clonal deletion of CD8 positive T-cells with an MHC class II restricted autoreactive T-cell receptor. Transplant 25:520, 1993.
26. Hess AD, Fischer AC, Ruvolo PP, Fuchs EJ. A failure of central and peripheral tolerance mechanisms. In Ildstad S (ed), Chimerism and Tolerance. Austin, TX: Landes, in press.
27. Hess AD, Vogelsang GB, Silankis M, Friedman KA, Beschorner WE, Santos GW. Syngeneic graft-vs-host disease (GVHD) after allogeneic bone marrow transplantation and cyclosporine treatment. Transplant Proc 20:487, 1988.
28. Severino ME, Laulis MK, Horwitz LR, Hess AD. Cyclosporine preferentially inhibits clonal deletion of CD8 positive T cells with an MHC class II restricted autoreactive T cell receptor. Transplant Proc 25:520, 1993.
29. Parkman R. Clonal analysis of graft-vs-host disease. In Burkoff, Deeg HJ, Ferrara J (eds), Graft-vs-Host Disease. New York: Marcal Dekker, 1990, p. 51.
30. Geller R, Esa A, Benhomer W, Frondoza C, Santos GW, Hess AD. Successful in vitro graft-versus-tumor effect against an Ia-bearing tumor using cyclosporine induced syngeneic graft-versus-host disease in the rat. Blood 74:1165, 1989.
31. Kennedy MJ, Vogelsang GB, Beveridge RA, Farmer ER, Altomonte V, Huelskamp AM, Davidson NE. Phase I trial of intravenous cyclosporine A to induce graft-versus-host disease in women undergoing autologous bone marrow transplantation for breast cancer. J Clin Oncol 11:478, 1993.
32. Jones RJ, Vogelsang GB, Hess AD, Farmer ER, Mann RB, Geller RB, Piantadosi S, Santos GW. Induction of graft versus host disease after autologous bone marrow transplantation. Lancet i:754, 1989.
33. Kennedy MJ, Vogelsang GB, Jones RJ, Farmer ER, Hess AD, Altomonte V, Huelskamp AM, Davidson NE. Phase I trial of interferon-gamma to potentiate cyclosporine A induced graft-versus-host disease in women undergoing autologous bone marrow transplantation for breast cancer. J Clin Oncol, in press.
34. Yeager AM, Vogelsang GB, Jones RJ, Farmer ER, Hess AD, Santos GW. Cyclosporine-

induced graft-versus-host disease after autologous bone marrow transplantation for acute myeloid leukemia. Leukemia Lymphoma 11:215, 1993.

35. Jones RJ, Vogelsang GB, Ambinder RF, Santos GW, Hess AD. Autologous marrow transplant with cyclosporine induced autologous graft-versus-host disease for relapsed aggressive non-Hodgkin's lymphoma. Blood 78:287a, 1991.

36. Guillen FJ, Ferrara J, Hancock WW, Messadi D, Fonferko E, Burakoff SJ, Murphy GF. Acute cutaneous graft-versus-host disease to minor histo-compatibility antigens in a murine model: evidence that large granular lymphocytes are effector cells in the immune response. Lab Invest 55:35, 1986.

37. Ferrara J, Burakoff S. The pathophysiology of acute graft-versus-host disease in a murine bone marrow transplant model. In Burakoff S, Deeg HJ, Ferrara J, Atkinson K (eds), Graft-versus-Host Disease: Immunology, Pathophysiology and Treatment. New York: Marcel Dekker, 1990, p. 9.

38. Vossen JM, Heidt PJ. Gnotobiotic measure for the prevention of acute graft-versus-host disease. In Burakoff S, Deeg HJ, Ferrara J, Atkinson K (eds), Graft-versus-Host Disease: Immunology, Pathophysiology and Treatment. New York: Marcel Dekker, 1990, p. 403.

39. Sullivan KM, Kopecky KS, Jocom J, Fisher L, Buckner CD, Meyers J, Counts G, Bowden R, Petersen F, Witherspoon R, Budninger M, Schwartz R, Appelbaum F, Clift R, Hansen J, Sanders J, Thomas ED, Storb R. Immunomodulatory and antimicrobial efficacy of intravenous immunoglobulin in bone marrow transplantation. N Engl J Med 323:705, 1990.

40. Johnson BD, Drobyski WR, Truitt RL. Delayed infusion of normal donor cells after MHC-matched bone marrow transplantation provides an antileukemia reaction without graft-vs-host disease. Bone Marrow Transplant 11:329, 1993.

41. Tutschka PJ, Beschorner WE, Allison AC, Burns WH, Santos GW. Use of cyclosporine A in allogeneic bone marrow transplant in the rat. Nature 280:148, 1979.

42. Storb R, Deeg HJ, Whithead J, Appelbaum FR, Beatty P, Bensinger W, Buckner CD, Clift R, Doney K, Farewell V, Hansen J, Hill R, Lum L, Martin P, McGuffin R, Sandors J, Stewart P, Sullivan K, Witherspoon R, Yee G, Thomas ED. Methotrexate and cyclosporine compared with cyclosporine alone for prophylaxis of acute graft versus host disease after marrow transplantation for leukemia. N Engl J Med 314:729, 1986.

43. Santos GW, Tutschka PJ, Brookmyer R, Beschorner WF, Bias WB, Braine HG, Burns WH, Famer ER, Hess AD, Kaizer H, Mellitis D, Sensenbrenner L, Stuart R, Yeager AM. Cyclosporine plus methylprednisolone versus cyclophosphamide plus methylprednisolone as prophylaxis for graft-versus-host disease. A randomized double-blind study in patients undergoing allogeneic marrow transplantation. Clin Transplant 1:21, 1987.

44. Chao NS, Schmidt G, Niland J, Amylon M, Dagio A, Long G, Nademanee A, Negrin R, O'Donnell M, Parker P, Smith E, Snyder D, Stein A, Wong R, Blume K, Forman S. Cyclosporine, methotrexate and prednisone compared with cyclosporine and prednisone for prophylaxis of acute graft-versus-host disease. N Engl J Med 329:1225, 1993.

45. Theobald M, Nierle T, Bunjes D, Arnold R, Heimpel H. Host-specific interleukin-2-secreting donor T-cell precursors as predictors of acute graft-versus-host disease in bone marrow transplantation between HLA-identical siblings. N Engl J Med 327:1613, 1992.

46. Schwarer A, Jiang Y, Brookes P, Barrett AJ, Batchelor JR, Goldman JM, Lechler RI. Frequency of antirecipient alloreactive helper T-cell precursors in donor blood in graft-vs-host disease after HLA identical siblings bone marrow transplantation. Lancet i:203, 1993.

47. Nierle T, Bunjes D, Arnold R, Heimpel H, Theobald M. Quantitative assessment of post transplant host-specific interleukin-2-secreting T-helper cell precursors in patients with and without graft-vs-host after allogeneic HLA-identical sibling bone marrow transplants. Blood 81:841, 1993.

48. Herve P, Wijdenes J, Bergerat JP, Bordigioni P, Milpied N, Cahn JY, Clement C, Beliard R, Morel-Fourrier B, Racadot E. Treatment of corticosteroid resistant acute graft-versus-host disease by in vivo administration of anti-interleukin-2 receptor monoclonal antibodies (B-B10). Blood 75:1017, 1990.

49. Anasetti C, Hansen JA, Waldmann T, Diagi MH, Mould D, Satoh H, Appelbaum FR, Deeg

HJ, Doney K, Martin PS, Nack R, Sullivan KM, Witherspoon R, Storb R. Treatment of acute graft-versus-host disease with a humanized monoclonal antibody specific for the IL-2 receptor. Blood 80:1484, 1992.

50. Piguet PF. Tumor necrosis factor and graft-versus-host disease. In Burakoff SJ, Deeg HJ, Ferrara J, Atkinson K (eds), Graft-versus-Host Disease: Immunology, Pathophysiology, and Treatment. New York: Marcel Dekker, 1990, p. 255.

51. Holler E, Kolb HJ, Hintermeier-Knabe R, Mittermuller J, Thierfelder S, Kaul M, Wilmanns W. Role of tumor necrosis factor alpha in acute graft-versus-host disease and complications following allogeneic bone marrow transplantation. Transplant Proc 25:1234, 1993.

52. Herve P, Flesch M, Tiberghien P, Wijdenes J, Racadot E, Bordigoni P, Plouvier E, Stephan JL, Bourdeau H, Holler E. Phase I-II trial of monoclonal anti-tumor necrosis alpha antibody for the treatment of refractory severe acute graft-versus-host disease. Blood 79:3362, 1992.

53. Bianco JA, Appelbaum FR, Nemunaitis J, Almgren J, Andrews F, Kettner P, Shields A, Singer JW. Phase I–II trial of pentoxifylline for prevention of transplant-related toxicities following bone marrow transplantation. Blood 78:1205, 1991.

54. Clift RA, Bianco JA, Appelbaum FR, Buckner CD, Singer JW, Bakke L, Bensinger W, Bowden R, McDonald G, Schubert M, Shields A, Slattery W, Storb R, Fisher L, Mori M, Thomas ED, Hansen JA. A randomized controlled trial of pertoxicylline for the prevention of regimen-related toxicities in patients undergoing allogeneic transplantation. Blood 82:2025, 1993.

55. Sampaio EP, Sarno EN, Galilly R, Cohn ZA, Kaplan G. Thalidomide selectively inhibits tumor necrosis factor alpha production by stimulated human monocytes. J Exp Med 173:699, 1991.

56. Abhyankar S, Gilliand D, Ferar A. Interleukin 1 is a critical effector molecule during cytokine dysregulation and graft-vs-host disease to minor histocompatibility antigens. Transplantation 56:1518, 1994.

57. Niederwieser D, Herold M, Woloszczuk W, Aulitzky W, Meister B, Tilg H, Gastl G, Bowden R, Huber C. Endogenous INF-gamma during human bone marrow transplantation. Analysis of serum levels of interferon and interferon-dependent secondary messages. Transplantation 50:620, 1990.

58. Allen RD, Staley TA, Sidman CL. Differential cytokine expression in acute and chronic murine graft-versus-host disease. Eur J Immunol 23:333, 1993.

59. Nestel FP, Price KS, Seemayer TA, Lapp WS. Macrophage priming and lipopolysaccharide-triggered release of tumor necrosis factor alpha during graft-versus-host disease. J Exp Med 175:405, 1992.

60. Fowler DH, Kurasawa K, Husebekk A, Cohen P, Gress R. Cells of Th2 cytokine phenotype prevent LPS-induced lethality during murine graft-versus-host reaction. J Immunol 152:1004, 1994.

61. Sykes M, Abraham VS, Harty M, Pearson D. IL-2 reduces graft-versus-host disease and preserves a graft-versus-leukemia effect by selectively inhibiting CD4+ T cell activity. J Immunol 150:197, 1993.

5. The detection of minimal residual disease: implications for bone marrow transplantation

John G. Gribben and Joachim L. Schultze

The source of relapse in patients who achieve complete clinical remission is residual cancer cells that number below the limits of detection using standard diagnostic techniques. Therefore, considerable effort has been made over the past decade to develop new techniques that have greatly increased the sensitivity of detection of small numbers of residual neoplastic cells. In particular, the identification of specific gene rearrangements and chromosomal translocations in neoplastic cells has permitted the development of sensitive molecular techniques that are capable of detecting minimal residual disease. With the development of these more sensitive techniques, especially by the application of PCR technology, the presence of residual neoplastic cells in patients in complete clinical remission, commonly called *minimal residual disease* (MRD), has been demonstrated clearly. It seems obvious to patients that if residual cancer cells can still be detected, then additional therapy is necessary for cure; nevertheless, the data demonstrating that detection of MRD using PCR-based techniques is associated with increased risk of relapse has been difficult to establish. In certain disease states, such as chronic myelogenous leukemia, there are now sufficient data demonstrating that detection of MRD is associated with a poor enough prognosis to merit experimental treatment approaches on the basis of detection of disease by PCR techniques alone. If this can be established in other malignancies, then molecular biologic techniques will become an essential part of staging and follow-up of patients and will redefine our concept of complete remission.

Assays for the detection of minimal residual disease

A variety of techniques have been used to detect MRD in different clinical settings. The tissue sites most often used to assess MRD are peripheral blood and bone marrow. Of course, other factors are also important in assessing the likelihood of successfully detecting residual cancer cells in these tissue sources. Neoplastic infiltration of bone marrow or peripheral blood is rare in some tumors, such as testicular or ovarian cancers; more common in non-Hodgkin's lymphoma and in solid tumors such as small cell lung cancer, neuroblastoma,

Jane N. Winter (ed.) BLOOD STEM CELL TRANSPLANTATION. 1997. Kluwer Academic Publishers. ISBN 0-7923-4260-7. All rights reserved.

Table 1. Sensitivity of tumor cell detection in bone marrow

Method of detection	Sensitivity	Number of tumor cells required to be detected in 10^{10} total marrow cells
Morphologic analysis		
Aspirate	5%	5×10^8
Biopsy	5%	5×10^8
Flow cytometric analysis	1–5%	$1–5 \times 10^8$
Southern blot analysis	1%	1×10^8
Fluorescence in situ hybridization	1%	1×10^8
Immunohistochemistry of cytospins	0.01%	1×10^6
Clonogenic assay	0.001%	1×10^5
Polymerase chain reaction	0.0001%	1×10^4

and breast cancer; and invariable in the leukemias. Histological assessment of bone marrow aspirates and biopsies is used to determine whether patients with leukemia have achieved complete remission and whether patients with other malignancies have evidence of bone marrow infiltration. The limit of detection of marrow infiltration by histologic examination is 5%. The techniques most widely used to detect MRD in patients in complete clinical remission are shown in table 1.

Clonogenic assays

Sensitive culture techniques were the first assays to demonstrate clearly that malignant cells could be grown from bone marrow that had no morphologic evidence of infiltration. Lymphoma cell lines could be established from the morphologically normal marrows of 17% of patients with undifferentiated lymphoma [1]. Using a sensitive liquid culture technique, 50% of patients with Burkitt's lymphoma and morphologically normal marrows had occult marrow involvement [2]. Similarly, residual acute lymphoblastic leukemia cells were detected by culture techniques from the bone marrows of children in complete clinical remission [3]. Up to one third of patients with intermediate and high-grade non-Hodgkin's lymphoma have clonogenic lymphoma cells in morphologically normal marrow at the time of autologous bone marrow harvest [4]. Culture assays are capable of detecting a malignant cell in up to 10^5 normal cells. These assays should be used in collaboration with assays that indicate the clonal population is indeed the malignant population, since there may be growth of clonal populations of nonmalignant cells, including Epstein–Barr-virus-transformed lymphoblastoid cells [4]. The major disadvantage of these assays is their low plating efficiency. In addition, we know little regarding the optimal requirements for clonogenic tumor cell growth. Once more is known about the biology of the stromal cell/tumor cell interactions, clonogenic culture systems should become applicable to a wider variety of tumor types.

In disease settings such as breast cancer, immunohistochemistry is a useful adjunct to detect the presence of infiltrating breast cancer cells. Fluorescent activated flow analysis has the potential to greatly increase the level of detection of marrow contamination and, in specialized hands, has been reported to be a very sensitive technique to detect tumor contamination. However, this technique is handicapped by the lack of true tumor-specific monoclonal antibodies and relies on the detection of an increase in the percentage of cells expressing antigens that occur on tumor cells but only rarely on normal cells.

Molecular biologic techniques to assess minimal residual disease

The underlying principle for the application of molecular biologic techniques to the diagnosis and detection of cancers is the detection of a clonal population of cells. Tumor-specific DNA sequences occur at the sites of nonrandom chromosomal translocations and are candidates for detection by PCR amplification if the sequences at the sites of the chromosomal breakpoints are known. Because of the specific nature of gene rearrangements occurring at the antigen receptors, the lymphoid malignancies have been studied most extensively. Since B- and T-cell malignancies undergo antigen-receptor gene rearrangements, their clonal progeny have the identical antigen-receptor rearrangement [5]. Initially, the most widely used molecular biologic technique was DNA restriction fragment analysis with Southern blot hybridization. This technique is capable of detecting neoplastic cell infiltration [5]. DNA hybridization techniques have confirmed that residual cancer cells could indeed be detected in the peripheral blood of patients who were judged to be in complete clinical remission by established diagnostic criteria [6]. DNA restriction fragment analysis with Southern blot hybridization with Ig and T-cell receptor (TCR) probes has demonstrated the presence of clonal lymphoid populations in the majority of lymphoid neoplasms, including acute and chronic leukemias, myeloma, non-Hodgkin's lymphoma, angioimmunoblastic lymphadenopathy, and some cases of Hodgkin's disease [7–9]. Although these techniques represented a major advance in minimal disease detection, they only increased the level of detection of minimal disease to the 1% level and were labor intensive to perform.

Polymerase chain reaction

More recently, the sensitivity of detection of minimal residual disease has been greatly increased with the development of the polymerase chain reaction (PCR) [10,11]. This technique specifically amplifies DNA and involves repeated cycles of denaturation of DNA, annealing of oligonucleotide primers, and extension of the primers using heat-stable bacterial DNA polymerase. The specificity of the procedure can be increased by the re-amplification of an aliquot of the amplified product using internal oligonucleotide primers. This

Table 2. Chromosomal translocations and gene rearrangements

Myeloid leukemia	Non-Hodgkin's lymphomas	Lymphoid leukemia	CLL myeloma
t(19;22)	t(14;18)	t(9;22)	CDR III
t(8;11)	t(8;14)	t(8;21)	FR1
t(15;17)	t(8;21)	t(1;19)	
t(6;9)	t(11;14)	t(1;14)	
	CDR III	t(10;14)	
	FR1	t(17;19)	
		TAL-deletion	
		TCR γ/δ	
		CDR III	
		FR1	

Abbreviations: CDR, complementarity determining region; FR, framework region; TCR, T-cell receptor.

procedure is known as *nested PCR*. A major disadvantage to the use of PCR is that DNA polymerase can only add nucleotides to the 3′ end of a preexisting single-stranded DNA oligonucleotide sequence. This means that for sensitive detection of MRD by PCR amplification, sequence information is required on both sides of the gene sequence to be amplified. Tumor-specific DNA sequences occur at the sites of nonrandom chromosomal translocations and are candidates for detection by PCR amplification if the sequences at the breakpoints are known. A number of chromosomal translocations and gene rearrangements have been identified and the breakpoints sequenced. The translocations given in table 2 are therefore applicable for PCR detection of tumor cells, and this list is growing as more chromosomal translocation sites are sequenced. The application of PCR has greatly increased the sensitivity of detection of disease, such that one malignant cell can be detected in up to 10^6 normal cells. By far the most widely studied specific gene re-arrangements detected using PCR amplification are associated with chronic myelogenous leukemia and t(14;18), associated with non-Hodgkin's lymphoma.

Detection of chimeric bcr/abl by PCR amplification. The t(9;22) is formed by the fusion of the bcr gene on chromosome 22 with the abl proto-oncogene on chromosome 9 and occurs in the vast majority of patients with chronic myeloid leukemia (CML) and in up to 20% of adult patients with acute lymphoblastic leukemia (ALL). The chronic myeloid leukemic cells transcribe an 8.5-kbp chimeric mRNA that is translated into a 210-kDa protein with tyrosine kinase activity. The breakpoints at the abl gene can occur at any point up to 200 kbp upstream in the intron and therefore cannot easily be amplified by PCR using genomic DNA. In contrast, the chimeric mRNA will usually be of two possible types (figure 1). It is therefore possible to amplify the chimeric mRNA by first reverse transcribing to cDNA. Using this technique, it is possible to detect one leukemic cell in up to 10^6 normal cells.

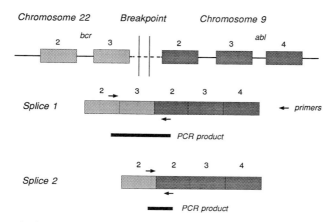

Figure 1. Organization of the t(9;22) translocation. The gene locus of the bcr gene on chromosome 22 is translocated to the abl gene locus on chromosome 9. Genomic DNA cannot be used for PCR amplification, since the breakpoint region is several kilobases in length. Therefore, mRNA is reverse transcribed and cDNA analyzed by PCR. Two splice variants of the fusion mRNA exist: one variant includes exon 3 of the bcr gene, and the other is characterized by fusion of exon 2 of the bcr gene to exon 2 of abl. Primers chosen as indicated in this figure detect both splice variants of the fusion RNA.

PCR analysis of t(14;18). The t(14;18) occurs in up to half of all patients with non-Hodgkin's lymphoma, including 85% of patients with follicular lymphoma and 30% of patients with diffuse lymphoma [14–16]. In the t(14;18), the bcl-2 proto-oncogene on chromosome 18 is juxtaposed with the immunoglobulin (Ig) heavy chain locus on chromosome 14 (figure 2). The breakpoints have been cloned and sequenced [17–19] and have been shown to cluster at two main regions 3' to the bcl-2 coding region. The major breakpoint region (MBR) occurs within the 3' untranslated region of the bcl-2 gene [17–19], and the minor cluster region (mcr) is located some 20kb downstream [20]. The clustering of the breakpoints at these two main regions at the bcl-2 gene and the availability of consensus regions of the Ig heavy chain (IgH) J regions [21] make this an ideal candidate for PCR amplification to detect lymphoma cells containing this translocation [22]. This extremely sensitive technique is capable of detecting one lymphoma cell in 10^6 normal cells. Since there is variability in the site of the breakpoint at the bcl-2 gene, and since the translocation occurs into the IgH variable region, the PCR products are of different sizes and have unique sequences. The size of the PCR product can be assessed by gel electrophoresis. A major advantage in the detection of lymphoma cells bearing the bcl-2/IgH translocation is that DNA can be used to detect the translocation and there is no need for reverse transcription before performing PCR amplification.

PCR detection of antigen receptor gene rearrangements. Although most follicular lymphomas exhibit t(14;18), the majority of patients with lymphoid

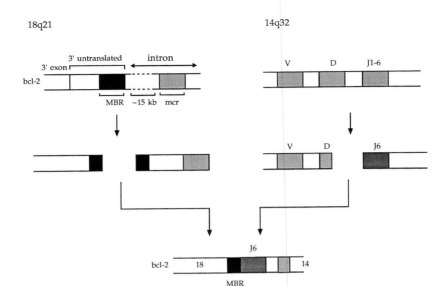

18q21   14q32

Figure 2. Organization of the t(14;18) translocation. On chromosome 18, the major breakpoint region (MBR) is within the 3' untranslated region, and the minor cluster region (mcr) is located downstream within the intron. In this figure, the derived t(14;18) has a breakpoint at the MBR and translocates to J6 in the immunoglobulin heavy chain region on chromosome 14. Primers at the MBR region on chromosome 18 and the consensus Jh region will therefore amplify in a PCR reaction.

malignancies do not demonstrate nonrandom chromosomal translocations. Lymphoid neoplasms usually demonstrate a rearrangement of either TCR or Ig genes or both, and their clonal progeny have the identical antigen-receptor rearrangement [5,7–9,23,24]. B-cell neoplasms, including ALL, non-Hodgkin's lymphoma, myeloma, and chronic lymphocytic leukemia (CLL), undergo somatic rearrangement of the IgH locus, providing a useful marker of clonality and stage of differentiation in these tumors [25–29].

The third complementarity-determining region (CDR III) of the IgH gene is generated early in B-cell development and is the result of rearrangement of germline variable (V), diversity (D), and joining (J) region elements. In a similar mechanism in both Ig and TCR genes, the enzyme terminal deoxynucleotidyl transferase (TdT) inserts random nucleotides at two sites: the V–D and D–J junctions. At the same time, random deoxynucleotides are removed by exonucleases [30]. Antibody diversity is increased further by somatic mutation. The final V–N–D–N–J sequence (CDR III) is unique to that cell, and if the cell expands to form a clone, then this region may act as a unique marker for that leukemic clone. PCR amplification of the CDR III sequence is possible due to the presence of conserved sequences within the V and J regions that are specific to the rearranged allele and serve as useful

104

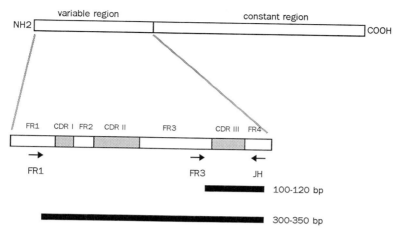

Figure 3. Structure of the immunoglobulin heavy chain (IgH). The IgH consists of the variable region and the constant region. As depicted, the variable region is divided into four framework regions (FR 1–4) and three complementary determining regions (CDR I–III). Due to highly conserved regions in the FR regions, primers can be designed that can amplify the clone-specific CDR III region. If no product is obtained using FR3- and FR4-region primers, Vh family-specific primers in the FR1 region with a consensus primer in the FR4 region can be used to amplify tumor-cell-specific clonal DNA of the IgH.

clonal markers for MRD detection (figure 3). Although these techniques have the advantage of being applicable to a greater number of patients, they are much less sensitive than the detection of chromosomal translocations. More highly sensitive tumor detection can be achieved by using primers directed against the unique junctional region sequences within the rearranged antigen-receptor genes [31]. These sequences can be cloned and sequenced from diagnostic tissue by first using primers for the conserved regions within the V and J regions for PCR amplification. Clone-specific oligonucleotides can then be constructed and used as primers for PCR amplification in that patient.

In B-lineage ALL, it would appear that IgH would be an ideal candidate gene for amplification. However, because of the large number of V regions, construction of clinically useful oligonucleotide primers is difficult. Whereas Ig genes undergo high rates of spontaneous mutation, such clonal markers change over time and may result in false-negative results using PCR amplification in at least 25% of cases [32]. IgH genes are known to show a high degree of somatic hypermutation in immature lymphoid malignancies such as B-lineage ALL so that around 25% of relapses will not be detected using CDR III sequence analysis alone [33]. Also, from previous analyses of precursor B-ALL using Southern blot analysis of the IgH gene, it is known that up to 40% of cases have multiple gene rearrangements [34]. From sequence data, it is known that the most common cause of bi- and oligoclonality is secondary gene rearrangement, e.g., V_H–V_H. Over time, there may be the appearance of secondary leukemic clones. To date, no study has demonstrated clearly that

105

eradication of PCR-detectable cells bearing clonal Ig rearrangements is necessary for cure after bone marrow transplantation.

Problems using PCR amplification. A major concern with PCR will always be the fear of false-positive results because of the ability of the technique to amplify even minute amounts of contaminating DNA. Great precautions must be taken in the laboratory to ensure that false-positive results do not occur, and every assay must be accompanied by the appropriate negative controls [35]. Amplified material must never be taken to the areas where DNA extraction is performed. It has been our experience that standard precautions and good laboratory practice make cross-contamination less of a problem than might be anticipated unless cloning and sequencing of genes have occurred within the same laboratory as the DNA extraction process. Although a number of quantitative methods have been developed [36,37], a major drawback of PCR is that it has been extremely difficult to quantitate the tumor cells in the original sample. Traditional methods for detection of minimal residual disease by PCR give a binary read-out: the presence or absence of a PCR band. The semiquantitative nature of PCR is due to minor differences in efficiency of amplification from tube to tube (e.g., due to variation in temperature based on the thermal cycling block position) that are accentuated during the logarithmic amplification of DNA samples. However, these variables can be precisely controlled by using an internal standard that controls for amplification efficiency. Since variation in amplification efficiency can also be attributed to primer annealing efficiency, rate of template denaturation, or length of template, among other variables, the best internal standard is primed by the same primers as the target DNA, but can be distinguished from the starting template either by minor size differences or by the presence of a single-base-pair change adding or ablating a restriction endonuclease site. These quantitation strategies have been termed *competitive* or *quantitative* PCR (figure 4) [37].

Unlike cell culture assays, it is not possible to determine whether cells detected by PCR are clonogenic. Cells bearing this translocation might be committed progenitors incapable of further proliferation, or they might have been sufficiently damaged by previous exposure to chemotherapy or radiotherapy to be already dead or in the process of dying but still detectable by PCR analysis. It must also be remembered that not all patients with lymphoma have a PCR-detectable translocation or gene rearrangement that can be used to monitor minimal residual disease.

A potential problem with the use of PCR of the bcl-2/IgH translocation to detect lymphoma cells is that this translocation may not be specific for lymphoma cells. Cells bearing the translocation have been detected in hyperplastic tonsil tissue from children with no evidence of lymphoma [38], and more recently have been shown to occur rarely in normal B cells. However, in our own laboratories we have not detected cells with this translocation in bone marrow or nonfractionated peripheral blood samples from a large number of individuals who have lymphoma that does not carry this transloca-

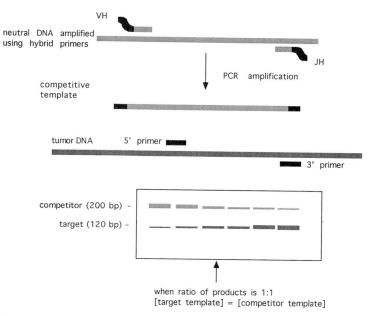

Figure 4. Competitive/quantitative PCR. To obtain a competitive template, hybrid primers are designed consisting of a sequence hybridizing to a neutral DNA and the sequence of the primers hybridizing to the tumor DNA. To obtain the competitive template, PCR amplification of the neutral DNA with the hybrid primers is performed. The amount of tumor DNA in the DNA sample is determined using serial dilutions of competitive-template DNA and equal amounts of tumor DNA in each individual PCR sample. Equal amounts of competitor template and target template are amplified at a ratio of products of 1:1.

tion. This suggests that these cells may be sufficiently rare that they will not interfere with the use of PCR at this translocation in the clinical management of patients who are being monitored for residual disease.

Clinical utility of minimal residual disease detection

Detection of MRD after BMT in chronic myeloid leukemia

CML is incurable using standard chemotherapy, and at the present time the only possibility of cure lies in allogeneic BMT. However, 20% of patients transplanted in chronic phase and more than 50% of patients transplanted in accelerated phase or blast crisis will relapse. If experimental treatment approaches are to be effective, then they should be utilized in the setting of MRD. Therefore, it is of importance to detect patients at high risk of subsequent relapse early after BMT. Considerable effort has therefore been made to establish whether persistence of MRD after allogeneic BMT is predictive of subsequent relapse of disease. Early studies utilized RT-PCR for the unique bcr-abl fusion mRNA transcript to detect MRD after BMT [39–54]. Although these studies demonstrated that PCR amplification can be used to detect minimal residual CML cells after allogeneic bone marrow transplantation, they yielded conflicting results as to the clinical implications of these results. A number of studies detected residual leukemia cells in most samples analyzed [40,55,56]. Other studies reported that there was persistence of cells with the chimeric mRNA in the early posttransplant period and that this did not adversely affect prognosis [41]. However, two studies demonstrated that the detection of residual leukemic cells after BMT was associated with subsequent relapse [43,48]. The reasons for the differences among these studies are not clear. Differences in the preparation of the patient for transplantation and in the treatment given to prevent graft-versus-host disease might affect the survival of these lymphocytes. The influence of T-cell depletion of the donor marrow is also not clearly understood. There were, in addition, different methodologies used to prepare the samples and to carry out the PCR procedure. However, a recent study from Seattle including analysis from 346 patients showed a clear association between relapse and PCR positivity [57]. Detection of MRD early after BMT does not necessarily suggest poor prognosis, and a PCR-positive sample at three months post-BMT was not informative for clinical outcome. In contrast, a PCR-positive bone marrow or peripheral blood sample at or after six months post-BMT was closely associated with subsequent relapse. Statistical analysis of the data revealed that the PCR assay for the bcr-abl fusion transcript 6 to 12 months post-BMT is an independent predictor of subsequent relapse. In contrast, no clear prediction of clinical outcome could be made in patients who tested PCR positive more than three years after BMT. This study [57] and others [58] have clearly demonstrated that most patients are PCR positive at three months after BMT, indicating that BMT preparative regimens alone do not eradicate CML cells effectively. Nevertheless, since this treatment leads to cure in more than 50% of patients, other mechanisms, e.g., immunological mechanisms, must be responsible for tumor eradication. The comparison of two patient groups treated with either T-cell-depleted bone marrow or untreated marrow underlines this presumption [58]. A defect of this study is that the two patient populations studied were treated at different institutions and used different preparative regimens. However, samples obtained 7 to 12 months after BMT were PCR positive in 88% of patients treated with T-cell-depleted marrow, whereas only 30% of recipients of untreated bone marrow were PCR-positive. When patients were grouped by PCR results, most of the patients with persistently PCR positive samples were recipients of T-cell-depleted allografts (24 of 29). Moreover, in this study there was also a strong association with clinical outcome, since patients with persistently PCR-positive samples relapsed, whereas patients with persistently PCR-negative samples were in complete remission. When PCR patterns were associated with GVHD, a clear correlation was observed: 95% of patients with GVHD were either intermittently or persistently PCR negative. These findings indicate that in addition to BMT, immunological mechanisms are responsible for the eradication of minimal residual disease and that the monitoring of MRD by RT-PCR is a very important indicator for clinical outcome in those patients.

Assessment of MRD by RT-PCR may prove useful as a surrogate endpoint to measure the effect of novel therapeutic strategies to eradicate remaining CML cells after BMT. Recent studies utilizing adoptive transfer of donor lymphocytes after BMT to eradicate CML cells showed the importance of MRD detection in these patients [59–62]. In a more recent study of patients treated with low doses of donor T cells, 15 to 17 patients became bcr-abl negative by PCR, indicating that this therapy achieved either eradication of the entire malignant clone or suppression below the limit of detection by PCR [62]. This question is not yet answered, since long-term follow-up is necessary to decide whether donor T-cell infusions can eradicate remaining CML cells. To date, monitoring MRD by PCR over long time periods seems to be the only method sensitive enough to answer this question. Based on these findings, future strategies could change our approach to curing CML with BMT. T-cell-depleted bone marrow would be used instead of untreated bone marrow to reduce the acute morbidity and mortality associated with GVHD. Detection of patients who have a high probability of relapse, based on persistence of detectable MRD or rise in leukemic burden as assessed by quantitative PCR, would allow targeting of adoptive immunotherapy (for example, donor lymphocyte infusions) to these high-risk patients. The success of this part of the therapeutic strategy would be monitored by assessment of MRD during the period of adoptive transfer. Detection of MRD will therefore likely have an important place in future curative therapies for this disease.

Detection of MRD after ABMT in non-Hodgkin's lymphoma

In non-Hodgkin's lymphoma patients, the disease-free survival after ABMT was adversely influenced by the persistence or reappearance of residual detectable lymphoma cells after high-dose therapy [63]. In 134 patients with B-cell non-Hodgkin's lymphoma with a documented PCR-detectable bcl-2 translocation, the failure to achieve or maintain a complete remission as assessed by PCR analysis of bone marrow was predictive of which patients will relapse. In contrast to the findings that all patients had bone marrow infiltration following conventional dose therapy, no PCR-detectable lymphoma cells could be detected in the most recent bone marrow sample obtained from 77 patients (57%) patients following high-dose chemoradiotherapy and autologous BMT. All 33 patients who relapsed had PCR-detectable lymphoma cells in the bone marrow prior to relapse, irrespective of the site of relapse. In contrast, of the 77 patients who had no PCR-detectable lymphoma cells in their most recent marrow sample, none had relapsed. Therefore, the detection of MRD by PCR following autologous BMT in patients with lymphoma would appear to identify those patients who require additional treatment for cure and suggests that our therapeutic goal should be to eradicate all PCR-detectable lymphoma cells.

In the remaining 41 patients, three distinct patient subgroups could be identified. In 14 patients, lymphoma cells could not be detected early after transplantation but reappeared at a later time. In these patients, lymphoma cells either remained in the marrow below the limit of detection by PCR or reseeded the bone marrow from extramedullary sites. Six patients in this group have relapsed to date, and lymphoma cells were detected by PCR in the marrow of all six patients before clinical relapse. Therefore, the reappearance of lymphoma cells in the marrow appears to be associated with a poor prognosis. In eight patients, residual lymphoma cells were detected in some but not all samples obtained at the time of each follow-up visit. In the final group of 19 patients, residual lymphoma cells in the bone marrow were detected early following transplantation and then were consistently absent. Two explanations are possible. First, residual lymphoma cells may already have been irreversibly damaged by the high dose therapy and were destined to die. Alternatively, an endogenous immune mechanism may be capable of eliminating residual lymphoma cells in some patients. Irrespective of the mechanism, once these patients had complete disappearance of residual lymphoma cells in their bone marrow, they had excellent prognoses, since none have relapsed.

In this study, 24 patients were identified who had detectable lymphoma cells in their marrow for varying lengths of time and who have not relapsed to date. A major question is whether all such patients with PCR-detectable disease will ultimately relapse. However, only one patient was identified in this study who was a long-term disease-free survivor despite the presence of PCR-detectable lymphoma cells in the marrow. These results have recently been confirmed by analysis of the results of detection of minimal residual disease after ABMT in patients treated in first remission (Gribben, unpublished results).

PCR assessment of the efficacy of purging autologous bone marrow

Autologous stem cell support from either bone marrow or peripheral blood stem cells (PBSCs) has permitted the use of chemotherapy dose escalation for a large number of patients with a number of hematologic and solid tumors [64–70]. The major obstacle to the use of autologous stem cells is that contaminating tumor cells will also be infused back to the patient and contribute to subsequent relapse. To minimize this risk, most centers obtain autologous bone marrow either when the patient is in complete remission or when there is no history of bone marrow infiltration. Others believe that PBSCs may provide a source that is less likely to be contaminated with malignant cells and use this as a rationale to move from autologous bone marrow to PBSC transplants. However, it is now clear that a number of patients with no morphological evidence of disease in the bone marrow or peripheral blood have contaminating malignant cells when assessed by more sensitive techniques. Therefore, an increasing effort has been made to attempt to determine the relative contribution of reinfusion of minimal numbers of malignant cells to subsequent relapse of disease. An alternative approach to decrease tumor contamination of stem cells is to 'purge' malignant cells. The aim of purging is to eliminate any contaminating malignant cells yet leave intact hematopoietic stem cells necessary for engraftment. The development of purging techniques has led subsequently to a number of studies of autologous BMT in patients with either a previous history of bone marrow infiltration or even overt marrow infiltration at the time of bone marrow harvest [66,67,70,71]. These clinical studies have demonstrated that purging can deplete malignant cells in vitro without significantly impairing hematologic engraftment.

Whereas the rationale for removing any contaminating tumor cells from the autologous marrow appears to be compelling, the issue of purging remains highly controversial. To date, there have been no clinical trials testing the efficacy of purging by comparison of infusion of purged versus unpurged autologous bone marrow, due primarily to the large number of patients that would be required for such studies. Intense argument therefore persists as to whether attempts to remove residual tumor cells from the harvested bone marrow have contributed to improving disease-free survival in these patients. In addition, the finding that the majority of patients who relapse after ABMT do so at sites of prior disease has led to the widespread view that purging of autologous marrow could contribute little to subsequent outcome after ABMT.

Assessment of the efficacy of purging

In tumor cell line model systems set up to optimize purging, clonogenic assays have been used to demonstrate the efficacy of multiple monoclonal antibodies (mAbs) and complement mediated lysis [72]. Multiple sequential treatments were shown to be more efficient than single treatments, and the combination of two or more antibodies was also more efficient than a single mAb to eliminate tumor cells [73]. Clonogenic lymphoma cell assays also demonstrated that different anti-B-cell mAbs differ in their efficiency in depleting lymphoma cells [74]. Similar assay systems were used to examine the efficacy of different complement sources [75] and to demonstrate synergy between chemotherapeutic agents and mAb-mediated purging [76]. A cocktail of two mAbs was used to assess the relative efficiency of purging of two different immunomagnetic particles [77]. Using a single cycle of treatment with multiple mAbs and beads, approximately 2.5 logs of small cell lung cancer lines could be depleted, although there was variability in the efficiency of purging different cell lines [78]. In parallel studies, there was no significant toxicity noted to myeloid progenitors. Anti-CD15 mAb, expressed on a variety of human cancer cell lines, was capable of depleting up to 3 logs of breast cancer cells from normal marrow using immunomagnetic bead depletion but minimally affected normal hematopoietic progenitors [79]. Using two small cell lung cancer lines, immunomagnetic bead depletion was shown to result in a 4- to 5-log reduction of cancer cells and did not adversely affect bone marrow colony growth [80]. The combination of 4-hydroperoxycyclophosphamide and immunomagnetic bead depletion removed 4 to 5 logs of clonogenic breast cancer cells [81]. Evaluation of the purging efficiency of an immunotoxin prepared by conjugating anti-CD7 with pokeweed anti-viral protein revealed that approximately 3 logs of clonogenic T cells could be eliminated; however, the addition of 2'-deoxycoformycin and deoxyadenosine to the immunotoxin resulted in the elimination of up to 6 logs of the T-cell line, but also resulted in decreased myeloid progenitor colony assay growth [82].

PCR analysis has been used recently to assess the efficacy of immunologic purging both in cell line models [83] and in patient samples [84,85]. Treatment of harvested bone marrow samples from lymphoma patients with either a three- or a four-mAb cocktail followed by immunomagnetic bead depletion resulted in the loss of all PCR-detectable cells after three cycles of treatment in all patients studied [85]. This study suggests that immunomagnetic bead depletion is significantly more efficient than complement-mediated lysis in depleting lymphoma cells. In addition, the ability of immunomagnetic beads to deplete residual lymphoma cells that survived complement-mediated cytolysis with the identical mAb cocktail suggests that the mechanism whereby lymphoma cells survive complement-mediated purging is not by failure to express the targeted antigen.

Contribution of infused tumor cells to relapse

Three independent lines of evidence have suggested that the reinfusion of tumor cells in autologous bone marrow may indeed contribute to relapse. Firstly, gene-marking studies performed at St. Jude Children's Hospital have demonstrated that at the time of relapse, 'marked' autologous marrow cells are detected, suggesting that the reinfused tumor cells contribute to relapse [86]. Second, studies at the University of Nebraska have demonstrated that those patients who are reinfused with morphologically normal bone marrow containing clonogenic lymphoma cells have an increased incidence of relapse after ABMT [4]. Thirdly, patients whose marrows contain PCR-detectable lymphoma cells after immunological purging had an increased incidence of relapse after ABMT [84].

If a marker gene were transfected into clonogenic malignant cells and the majority of cells at the site of relapse expressed the marker gene, this would provide compelling evidence that infused malignant cells contribute to relapse. Since the efficiency of transfection is low using existing technology, a negative result would still not be definitive. However, results published to date have demonstrated that when relapse occurs there is evidence of malignant cells, with the marker gene suggesting strongly that the reinfused malignant cells contributed to relapse [86,87].

Recent studies from Nebraska have confirmed the earlier finding [4] that detection of clonogenic cells in the autologous bone marrow or peripheral blood predicts for subsequent relapse. The actuarial relapse-free survival at five years for patients who received stem cells that were free of tumor contamination was 64% for those receiving PBSCs and 57% for those receiving autologous bone marrow. In contrast, those patients who received a histologically negative bone marrow that contained minimally detectable lymphoma cells had a relapse-free survival at five years of only 17% [88].

In studies at the Dana-Farber Cancer Institute, PCR amplification of the t(14;18) was used to detect residual lymphoma cells in the bone marrow before and after purging to assess whether efficient purging had any impact on disease-free survival [84]. In this study, 114 patients with B-cell non-Hodgkin's lymphoma and the bcl-2 translocation were studied. Residual lymphoma cells were detected in all patients in the harvested autologous bone marrow. Following three cycles of immunologic purging using the anti-B-cell mAbs J5 (anti-CD10), B1 (anti-CD20), and B5 and complement-mediated lysis, PCR amplification detected residual lymphoma cells in 57 of these patients. The incidence of relapse was significantly increased in patients who had residual detectable lymphoma cells compared to those in whom no lymphoma cells were detectable after purging. The elimination of PCR-detectable lymphoma cells was independent of the histology of the lymphoma, the degree of bone marrow infiltration, or remission status at the time of autologous BMT. These findings suggest that the infusion of detectable lymphoma cells is indeed associated with subsequent relapse.

The majority of patients who relapse do so at sites of previous disease, suggesting that the major contribution to subsequent relapse came from endogenous disease. However, in 60 consecutive patients with a PCR-detectable bcl-2 translocation who had undergone immunologic purging and autologous BMT, there was also an association between the presence of residual lymphoma cells after purging and the presence of circulating lymphoma cells that could be detected as early as two hours after infusion of bone marrow [89]. It is possible that these circulating lymphoma cells are capable of homing back to the sites of previous disease and that these sites provide the microenviromental conditions conducive for cell growth.

A randomized trial using purged versus unpurged autologous marrow would likely provide a definitive answer. This would require a multicenter study of several hundred patients. However, several ethical questions would have to be addressed in the design of such a study. Although purging appears to have no significant toxicity, it is expensive and there are no definitive data showing that unpurged marrow contributes to relapse. Although studies do not prove that purging is essential, they are consistent with the interpretation that MRD in the marrow may contribute to relapse. If patients with 5% marrow infiltration were randomized to receive unpurged marrows, then malignant cells would be infused. On the other hand, patients with minimal marrow infiltration should not necessarily be prevented from receiving autologous BMT, since those patients with histologic marrow involvement whose marrows purged to PCR negativity had excellent disease-free survival.

Therefore, there is again increasing interest in methods of obtaining autologous bone marrow that is free of tumor contamination. An alternative and highly attractive strategy is positive selection of hematopoietic stem cells. There are a number of mAbs that recognize the human hematopoietic progenitor cell antigen CD34, which may be used to positively select CD34+ cells. Precursors of all human hematopoietic lineages, including B and T lymphocytes, express CD34, and studies in primates and humans have shown that isolated CD34+ cells are capable of reestablishing hematopoietic engraftment [90,91]. Endothelial cells appear to be the only other cell type that expresses CD34. The CD34+ population represents less than 2% of the low-density human mononuclear marrow cells, and increasing interest is now being placed on the use of PBSCs rather than bone marrow as a source of hematopoietic progenitors. Peripheral blood is less frequently involved than bone marrow at presentation, but is a more frequent finding as disease progresses [92,93]. Two recent studies of patients at the time of presentation have suggested a high level of concordance between the detection of lymphoma cells in the peripheral blood and bone marrow when assessed by PCR [94,95]. However, other studies have found that the bone marrow is more likely than peripheral blood to contain infiltrating lymphoma cells in previously untreated patients [96]. The positive selection of CD34+ cells from autologous marrow with or without negative selection to purge any more mature contaminating neoplastic cells is likely to become increasingly important as a source of stem cells.

Conclusions

Over the past decade, a number of methodologies capable of detecting minimal residual disease have been developed. These techniques have clearly illustrated that patients in clinical complete remission often harbor malignant cells in low numbers. The clinical significance of the detection of such MRD is still being evaluated and remains unclear in many diseases and at different stages of disease. After BMT, detection of minimal residual tumor cells early after transplantation does not appear to affect prognosis adversely.

The prognostic significance of the achievement of a 'molecular complete remission' has remained elusive, and few studies to date have been able to demonstrate the importance of eradicating MRD in the patient to achieve cure. However, the largest studies that have been performed to date suggest that in CML and in NHL, eradication of MRD is necessary for cure. The results of additional studies will be necessary to determine whether minimal disease detection will have a major clinical impact on experimental therapeutic strategies utilized at the time patients have only MRD. Therefore, we are rapidly approaching the time when molecular detection of residual cancer cells will become as much a routine staging procedure as morphologic assessment of the bone marrow is today.

References

1. Benjamin D, Magrath IT, Douglass EC, Corash LM. Derivation of lymphoma cell lines from microscopically normal bone marrow in patients with undifferentiated lymphoma: evidence of occult bone marrow involvement. Blood 61:1017–1019, 1983.
2. Favrot MC, Herve P. Detection of minimal malignant cell infiltration in the bone marrow of patients with solid tumors, non-Hodgkin's lymphomas and leukemias. Bone Marrow Transplant 2:117–122, 1987.
3. Estrov Z, Grunberger T, Dube ID. Detection of residual acute lymphoblastic leukemia cells in cultures of bone marrow obtained during remission. N Engl J Med 315(9):538–542, 1986.
4. Sharp JG, Joshi SS, Armitage JO, et al. Significance of detection of occult non-Hodgkin's lymphoma in histologically uninvolved bone marrow by culture technique. Blood 79:1074–1080, 1992.
5. Cleary ML, Chao J, Wanke R, Sklar J. Immunoglobulin gene rearrangement as a diagnostic criterion of B cell lymphoma. Proc Natl Acad Sci U S A 81:593–597, 1984.
6. Hu E, Trela M, Thompson J, et al. Detection of B cell lymphoma in peripheral blood by DNA hybridization. Lancet ii:1092–1095, 1985.
7. Arnold A, Cossman J, Bakhshi A, Jaffe ES, Waldmann TA, Korsmeyer SJ. Immunoglobulin gene rearrangements as unique clonal markers in human lymphoid neoplasms. N Engl J Med 309:1593–1599, 1983.
8. Toyonaga B, Mak TW. Genes of the T-cell antigen receptor in normal and malignant T cells. Annu Rev Immunol 5:585–620, 1987.
9. Griesser H, Tkachuk D, Reis MD, Mak TW. Gene rearrangements and translocations in lymphoproliferative diseases. Blood 73:1402–1415, 1989.
10. Saiki RK, Gelfand DH, Stoffel S, et al. Primer-directed enzymatic amplification of DNA with a thermostable DNA polymerase. Science 239:487–491, 1988.
11. Saiki RK, Scharf F, Faloona F, et al. Enzymatic amplification of betaglobin genomic sequences and restriction site analysis for diagnosis of sickle cell anemia. Science 230:1350–1352, 1985.
12. Dubrovic A, Trainor KJ, Morley AA. Detection of the molecular abnormality in chronic myeloid leukemia by use of the polymerase chain reaction. Blood 72:2063–2965, 1988.
13. Lee MS, LeMaistre A, Kantarjian HM, et al. Detection of two alternative bcr/abl mRNA junctions and minimal residual disease in Philadelphia chromosome positive chronic myelogenous leukemia by polymerase chain reaction. Blood 73:2165–2170, 1989.
14. Yunis JJ, Oken MM, Kaplan ME, Theologides RR, Howe A. Distinctive chromosomal abnormalities in histological subtypes of non-Hodgkin's lymphoma. N Engl J Med 307:1231–1236, 1982.
15. Weiss LM, Warnke RA, Sklar J, Cleary ML. Molecular analysis of the t(14;18) chromosomal translocation in malignant lymphomas. N Engl J Med 317:1185–1189, 1987.
16. Aisenberg AC, Wilkes BM, Jacobson JO. The bcl-2 gene is rearranged in many diffuse B-cell lymphomas. Blood 71(4):969–972, 1988.
17. Cleary ML, Sklar J. Nucleotide sequence of a t(14;18) chromosomal breakpoint in follicular lymphoma and demonstration of a breakpoint cluster region near a transcriptionally active locus on chromosome 18. Proc Natl Acad Sci U S A 82:7439–43, 1985.

18. Tsujimoto Y, Finger LR, Yunis J, Norwell PC, Croce CM. Cloning of the chromosome breakpoint of neoplastic B cells with the t(14;18) chromosome translocation. Science 226:1097–1099, 1984.
19. Bakshi A, Jensen JP, Goldman P, et al. Cloning the chromosomal breakpoint of t(14;18) human lymophomas: clustering around J_H on chromosome 14 and near a transcriptional unit on 18. Cell 41:899–906, 1985.
20. Cleary ML, Galili N, Sklar J. Detection of a second t(14;18) breakpoint cluster region in human follicular lymphomas. J Exp Med 164:315–320, 1986.
21. Ravetch JV, Siebenlist U, Korsmeyer S, Waldman T, Leder P. Structure of the human immunoglobulin μ locus: characterization of embryonic and rearranged J and D genes. Cell 27:583–591, 1981.
22. Crescenzi M, Seto M, Herzig GP, Weiss PD, Griffith RC, Korsmeyer SJ. Thermostable DNA polymerase chain amplification of t(14;18) chromosome breakpoints and detection of minimal residual disease. Proc Natl Acad Sci U S A 85(13):4869–4873, 1988.
23. Berliner N, Ault K, Martin P, Weisberg DS. Detection of clonal excess in lymphoproliferative disease by kappa/lambda analysis: correlation with immunoglobulin gene DNA arrangements. Blood 67:80–85, 1986.
24. Aisenberg AC. Utility of gene rearrangements in lymphoid malignancies. Annu Rev Med (44):75–84, 1993.
25. Steward CG, Potter MN, Oakhill A. Third complementarity determining region (CDR III) sequence analysis in childhood B-lineage acute lymphoblastic leukaemia: implications for the design of oligonucleotide probes for use in monitoring minimal residual disease. Leukemia 6(11):1213–1219, 1992.
26. Yamada M, Hudson S, Tourney O, et al. Detection of minimal disease in hematopoietic malignancies of the B-cell lineage by using third complementarity-determining region probes. Proc Natl Acad Sci U S A 86:5123–5127, 1989.
27. Yamada M, Wasserman R, Lange B, Reichard BA, Womer RB, Rovera G. Minimal residual disease in childhood B-lineage lymphoblastic leukemia. N Engl J Med 323:448–455, 1990.
28. Bakkus MH, Heirman C, Van RI, Van CB, Thielemans K. Evidence that multiple myeloma Ig heavy chain VDJ genes contain somatic mutations but show no intraclonal variation. Blood 80(9):2326–2335, 1992.
29. Billadeau D, Quam L, Thomas W, et al. Detection and quantitation of malignant cells in the peripheral blood of multiple myeloma patients. Blood 80(7):1818–1824, 1992.
30. Tonegawa S. Somatic generation of antibody diversity. Nature 302:575–581, 1983.
31. Billadeau D, Blackstadt M, Greipp P, et al. Analysis of B-lymphoid malignancies using allele-specific polymerase chain reaction: a technique for sequential quantitation of residual disease. Blood 78(11):3021–3029, 1991.
32. Wasserman R, Yamada M, Ito Y, et al. VH gene rearrangement events can modify the immunoglobulin heavy chain during progression of B-lineage acute lymphoblastic leukemia. Blood 79(1):223–228, 1992.
33. Steward CG, Goulden NJ, Potter MN, Oakhill A. The use of the polymerase chain raction to detect minimal residual disease in childhood acute lymphoblastic leukaemia. Eur J Cancer 8:1192–1198, 1993.
34. Osada H, Seto M, Ueda R, et al. bcl-2 gene rearrangement analysis in Japanese B cell lymphoma; novel bcl-2 recombination with immunoglobulin kappa chain gene. Jpn J Cancer Res 80(8):711–715, 1989.
35. Kwok S, Higuchi R. Avoiding false positives with PCR. Nature 339:237–238, 1989.
36. Wang AM, Doyle MV, Mark DF. Quantitation of mRNA by the polymerase chain reaction. Proc Natl Acad Sci U S A 86(24):9717–9721, 1989.
37. Gilliland G, Perrin S, Balnchard K, Bunn HF. Analysis of cytokine mRNA and DNA: detection and quantitation by competitive polymerase chain reaction. Proc Natl Acad Sci U S A 87:2725–2729, 1990.
38. Limpens J, de Jong D, Voetdijk AMH, et al. Translocation t(14;18) in benign B lymphocytes. Blood 76 (Suppl 1):237a, 1990.

116

39. Morgan GJ, Janssen JWG, Guo AP, et al. Polymerase chain reaction for detection of residual leukaemia. Lancet i:928–929, 1989.
40. Gabert J, Lafage M, Maraninchi D, Thuret I, Carcasonne Y, Mannoni P. Detection of residual bcr/abl translocation by polymerase chain reaction in chronic myeloid leukemia patients after bone marrow transplantation. Lancet ii:1125–1128, 1989.
41. Martiat P, Maisin D, Philippe M, et al. Detection of residual bcr/abl transcripts in chronic myeloid leukaemia patients in complete remission using the polymerase chain reaction and nested primers. Br J Haematol 75:355–358, 1990.
42. Kohler S, Galili N, Sklar JL, Donlon TA, Blume KG, Cleary ML. Expression of bcr-abl fusion transcripts following bone marrow transplantation for Philadelphia chromosome-positive leukemia. Leukemia 4:541–547, 1990.
43. Sawyers CL, Timson L, Kawasaki ES, Clark SS, Witte ON, Champlin R. Molecular relapse in chronic myelogenous leukemia patients after bone marrow transplantation detected by polymerase chain reaction. Proc Natl Acad Sci U S A 87:563–567, 1990.
44. Delfau MH, Kerckaert JP, Collyn d'Hooghe M, et al. Detection of minimal residual disease in chronic myeloid leukemia patients after bone marrow trasplantation by polymerase chain reaction. Leukemia 4:1–5, 1990.
45. Delage R, Soiffer RJ, Dear K, Ritz J. Clinical significance of bcr-abl gene rearrangement detected by polymerase chain reaction after allogeneic bone marrow transplantation in chronic myelogenous leukemia. Blood 78(10):2759–2767, 1991.
46. Hughes TP, Morgan GJ, Martiat P, Goldman JM. Detection of residual leukemia after bone marrow transplant for chronic myeloid leukemia: role of polymerase chain reaction in predicting relapse. Blood 77:874–878, 1991.
47. Guerrasio A, Martinelli G, Saglio G, et al. Minimal residual disease status in transplanted chronic myelogenous leukemia patients: low incidence of polymerase chain reaction positive cases among 48 long disease-free subjects who received unmanipulated allogeneic bone marrow transplants. Leukemia 6(6):507–512, 1992.
48. Roth MS, Antin JH, Ash R, et al. Prognostic significance of Philadelphia chromosome-positive cells detected by the polymerase chain reaction after allogeneic bone marrow transplant for chronic myelogenous leukemia. Blood 79:276–282, 1991.
49. Thompson JD, Brodsky I, Yunis JJ. Molecular quantification of residual disease in chronic myelogenous leukemia after bone marrow transplantation. Blood 79(6):1629–1635, 1992.
50. Lee M, Khouri I, Champlin R, et al. Detection of minimal residual disease by poylmerase chain reaction of bcr/abl transcripts in chronic myelogenous leukaemia following allogeneic bone marrow transplantation. Br J Haematol 82(4):708–714, 1992.
51. Cross NC, Feng L, Bungey J, Goldman JM. Minimal residual disease after bone marrow transplant for chronic myeloid leukaemia detected by the polymerase chain reaction. Leuk Lymphoma 1:39–43, 1993.
52. Cross NC, Feng L, Chase A, Bungey J, Hughes TP, Goldman JM. Competitive polymerase chain reaction to estimate the number of BCR-ABL transcripts in chronic myeloid leukemia patients after bone marrow transplantation. Blood 82(6):1929–1936, 1993.
53. Arnold R, Janssen JW, Heinze B, et al. Influence of graft-versus-host disease on the eradication of minimal residual leukemia detected by polymerase chain reaction in chronic myeloid leukemia patients after bone marrow transplantation. Leukemia 7(5):747–751, 1993.
54. Miyamura K, Tahara T, Tanimoto M, et al. Long persistent bcr-abl positive transcript detected by polymerase chain reaction after marrow transplant for chronic myelogenous leukemia without clinical relapse: a study of 64 patients. Blood 81:1089–1093, 1993.
55. Lange W, Snyder DS, Castro R, Rossi JJ, Blume KG. Detection by enzymatic amplification of bcr/abl mRNA in peripheral blood and bone marrow cells of patients with chronic myelogenous leukemia. Blood 73:1735–1741, 1989.
56. Pignon JM, Henni T, Amselem S, et al. Frequent detection of minimal residual disease by use of polymerase chain reaction in long-term survivors after bone marrow transplantation for chronic myeloid leukemia. Leukemia 4:83–86, 1990.

117

57. Radich JP, Gehly G, Gooley T, et al. Polymerase chain reaction detection of the BCR-ABL fusion transcript after allogeneic marrow transplantation for chronic myeloid leukemia: results and implications in 346 patients. Blood 85(9):2632–2638, 1995.

58. Pichert G, Roy DC, Gonin R, et al. Distinct patterns of minimal residual disease associated with graft-versus-host disease after allogeneic bone marrow transplantation for chronic myelogenous leukemia. J Clin Oncol 13(7):1704–1713, 1995.

59. Kolb HJ, Mittermuller J, Clemm C, et al. Donor leukocyte transfusions for treatment of recurrent chronic myelogenous leukemia in marrow transplant patients. Blood 76:2462–2465, 1990.

60. Drobyski WR, Keever CA, Roth MS, et al. Salvage immunotherapy using donor leukocyte infusions as treatment for relapsed chronic myelogenous leukemia after allogeneic bone marrow transplantation: efficacy and toxicity of a defined T-cell dose. Blood 82:2310–2318, 1993.

61. Porter DL, Roth MS, McGarigle C, Ferrara JLM, Antin JH. Induction of graft-vs-host disease as immunotherapy for relapsed chronic myelogenous leukemia. N Engl J Med 330:100–105, 1994.

62. Mackinnon S, Papadopoulos EB, Carabasi MH, et al. Adoptive immunotherapy evaluating escalating doses of donor leukocytes for relapse of chronic myeloid leukemia after bone marrow transplantation: separation of graft-versus-leukemia responses from graft-versus-host disease. Blood 86(4):1261–1268, 1995.

63. Gribben JG, Neuberg D, Freedman AS, et al. Detection by polymerase chain reaction of residual cells with the bcl-2 translocation is asocied with increased risk of relapse after autologous bone marrow transplantation for B-cell lymphoma. Blood 81(12):3449–3457, 1993.

64. Armitage JO. Bone marrow transplantation in the treatment of patients with lymphoma. Blood 73:1749–1758, 1989.

65. Ball ED, Mills LE, Cornwell GG, et al. Autologous bone marrow transplantation for acute myeloid leukemia using monoclonal antibody-purged bone marrow. Blood 75:1199–1206, 1990.

66. Freedman AS, Nadler LM. Developments in purging in autotransplantation. Hematol Oncol Clin North Am 7(3):687–715, 1993.

67. Freedman AS, Takvorian T, Anderson KC, et al. Autologous bone marrow transplantation in B-cell non-Hodgkin's lymphoma: very low treatment-related mortality in 100 patients in sensitive relapse. J Clin Oncol 8(5):784–791, 1990.

68. Gribben JG, Goldstone AH, Linch DC, et al. Effectiveness of high-dose combination chemotherapy and autologous bone marrow transplantation for patients with non-Hodgkin's lymphomas who are still responsive to conventional dose therapy. J Clin Oncol 7:1621–1629, 1989.

69. Peters WP, Shpall EJ, Jones RB. High dose combination combination alkylating agents with bone marrow support as initial treatment for metastatic breast cancer. J Clin Oncol 6:1501–1515, 1988.

70. Hurd DD, LeBien TW, Lasky LC, et al. Autologous bone marrow transplantation in non-Hodgkin's lymphoma: monoclonal antibodies plus complement for ex vivo marrow treatment. Am J Med 85:829–834, 1988.

71. Takvorian T, Canellos GP, Ritz J, et al. Prolonged disease-free survival after autologous bone marrow transplantation in patients with non-Hodgkin's lymphoma with a poor prognosis. N Engl J Med 316:1499–1505, 1987.

72. Bast RC, De Fabritiis P, Lipton J, et al. Elimination of malignant clonogenic cells from human bone marrows using multiple monoclonal antibodies and complement. Cancer Res 45:499–503, 1985.

73. LeBien TW, Stepan DE, Bartholomew RM, Strong RC, Anderson JM. Utilization of a colony assay to assess the variables influencing elimination of leukemic cells from human bone marrow with monoclonal antibodies and complement. Blood 65:945–950, 1985.

74. Kvalheim G, Sorensen O, Fodstad O, et al. Immunomagnetic removal of B-lymphoma cells

118

from human bone marrow: a procedure for clinical use. Bone Marrow Transplant 3:31–41, 1988.

75. Roy DC, Felix M, Cannady WG, Cannistra S, Ritz J. Comparative activities of rabbit complements of different ages using an in-vitro marrow purging model. Leuk Res 14:407–416, 1990.

76. De Fabritiis P, Bregni M, Lipton J, et al. Elimination of clonogenic Burkitt's lymphoma cells from human bone marrow using 4-hydroperoxycyclophosphamide in combination with monoclonal antibodies and complement. Blood 65:1064–1070, 1985.

77. Trickett AE, Ford DJ, Lam-Po-Tang PRL, Vowels MR. Immunomagnetic bone marrow purging of common acute lymphoblastic leukemia cells: suitability of BioMag particles. Bone Marrow Transplant 7:199–203, 1991.

78. Elias AD, Pap SA, Bernal SD. Purging of small cell lung cancer-contaminated bone marrow by monoclonal antibodies and magnetic beads. Prog Clin Biol Res 333(1):263–275, 1990.

79. Vrendenburgh J, Simpson W, Memoli VA, Ball ED. Reactivity of anti-CD15 monoclonal antibody PM-81 with breast cancer and elimination of breast cancer cell lines from human bone marrow by PM-81 and immunomagnetic beads. Cancer Res 51:2451–2455, 1991.

80. Vrendenburgh JJ, Ball ED. Elimination of small cell carcinoma of the lung from human bone marrow by monoclonal antibodies and immunomagnetic beads. Cancer Res 50:7216–7120, 1990.

81. Schpall EJ, Bast RC, Joines WT, et al. Immunomagnetic purging of breast cancer from bone marrow for autologous transplantation. Bone Marrow Transplant 7:145–151, 1991.

82. Montgomery RB, Kurtzberg J, Rhinehardt-Clark A, et al. Elimination of malignant clonogenic T cells from human bone marrow using chemoimmunoseparation with 2'-deoxycoformycin, deoxyadenosine and an immunotoxin. Bone Marrow Transplant 5:395–402, 1990.

83. Negrin RS, Kiem HP, Schmidt WI, Blume KG, Cleary ML. Use of the polymerase chain reaction to monitor the effectiveness of ex vivo tumor cell purging. Blood 77(3):654–660, 1991.

84. Gribben JG, Freedman AS, Neuberg D, et al. Immunologic purging of marrow assessed by PCR before autologous bone marrow transplantation for B-cell lymphoma. N Engl J Med 325(22):1525–1533, 1991.

85. Gribben JG, Saporito L, Barber M, et al. Bone marrows of non-Hodgkin's lymphoma patients with a bcl-2 translocation can be purged of polmerase chain reaction-detectable lymphoma cells using monoclonal antibodies and immunomagnetic bead depletion. Blood 80(4):1083–1089, 1992.

86. Brenner MK, Rill DR, Moen RC, et al. Gene-marking to trace origin of relapse after autologous bone-marrow transplantation. Lancet 341:85–86, 1993.

87. Rill DR, Santana VM, Roberts WM, et al. Direct demonstration that autologous bone marrow transplantation for solid tumors can return a multiplicity of tumorigenic cells. Blood 84:380–383, 1994.

88. Sharp JG, Kessinger A, Mann S, et al. Outcome of high dose therapy and autologous transplantation in non-Hodgkin's lymphoma based on the presence of tumor in the marrow or infused hematopoietic harvest. J Clin Oncol 14:214–219, 1996.

89. Gribben JG, Nadler LM. Detection of minimal residual disease in patients with lymphomas using the polymerase chain reaction. Important Adv Oncol:117–129, 1994.

90. Berenson RJ, Andrews RG, Bensinger WI. Antigen CD34+ marrow cells engraft lethally irradiated baboons. J Clin Invest 81:951–955, 1988.

91. Berenson RJ, Bensinger WI, Hill RS. Engraftment after infusion of CD34+ marrow cells in patients with breast cancer or neuroblastoma. Blood 77:1717–1722, 1991.

92. Ault KA. Detection of small numbers of monoclonal B lymphocytes in the blood of patients with B cell lymphoma. N Engl J Med 300:1401–1405, 1979.

93. Horning SJ, Galila N, Cleary M, Sklar J. Detection of non-Hodgkin's lymphoma in the peripheral blood by analysis of the antigen receptor gene rearrangements: results of a prospective trial. Blood 75:1139–1145, 1990.

94. Berinstein NL, Reis MD, Ngan BY, Sawka CA, Jamal HH, Kuzniar B. Detection of occult

lymphoma in the peripheral blood and bone marrow of patients with untreated early stage and advanced stage follicular lymphoma. J Clin Oncol 11:1344–1352, 1993.

95. Yuan R, Dowling P, Zucca E, Diggelmann H, Cavalli F. Detection of bcl-2/JH rearrangement in follicular and diffuse lymphoma: concordant results of peripheral blood and bone marrow analysis at diagnosis. Br J Cancer 67(5):922–925, 1993.

96. Berinstein NL, Jamal HH, Kuzniar B, Klock RJ, Reis MD. Sensitive and reproducible detection of occult disease in patients with follicular lymphoma by PCR amplification of t(14;18) both pre- and post-treatment. Leukemia 7(1):113–119, 1993.

120

6. The use of radiolabeled antibodies in bone marrow transplantation for hematologic malignancies

Dana C. Matthews, Frederick R. Appelbaum, Oliver W. Press, Janet F. Eary, and Irwin D. Bernstein

Blood stem cell transplantation has been widely used in the treatment of leukemia and lymphoma for more than two decades. The majority of bone marrow transplant preparative regimens have incorporated total body irradiation (TBI) because lymphohematopoietic cells and their malignant derivatives are relatively radiosensitive. Such preparative regimens have cured a substantial proportion of patients with both acute and chronic leukemia as well as lymphoma. However, despite the radiation sensitivity of hematologic malignancies, relapse remains a major cause of failure.

While a higher radiation dose would be predicted to decrease the risk of relapse, escalation of the dose of radiation delivered as TBI is limited by normal organ toxicity, principally to the liver, lung, and gastrointestinal tract. For example, in two randomized studies comparing the efficacy of 12 Gray (Gy) vs. 15.75 Gy TBI combined with cyclophosphamide (CY) in patients receiving HLA-matched related marrow transplants for acute myeloid leukemia (AML) in first remission [1] and chronic myelogenous leukemia (CML) in chronic phase [2], the higher dose of TBI was associated with a significantly lower relapse rate (12% vs. 35% for AML, 0% vs. 25% for CML). However, in both studies mortality rates not related to relapse were higher for patients receiving the higher radiation dose, resulting in no difference in long-term, disease-free survival with the two TBI doses.

The lower relapse rates with higher radiation doses confirm that leukemias are radiosensitive, with a relatively steep dose–response curve. We and others have hypothesized that if supplemental radiation could be delivered to the lymphohematopoietic tissues where leukemia and lymphoma cells arise and reside, while sparing to a great degree critical normal organs such as liver, lung, and mucosa, an increased cure rate might result without significantly increased toxicity.

Radionuclide conjugates of monoclonal antibodies reactive with lymphohematopoietic antigens have been demonstrated in both preclinical [3–13] and clinical [14–30] studies to deliver greater doses of radiation to target tissues (including bone marrow, spleen, and lymphomatous masses) than to normal, nontarget organs. Below, we discuss the factors to be considered when designing a radioimmunotherapy trial. The results of clinical studies using

Jane N. Winter (ed.) BLOOD STEM CELL TRANSPLANTATION. 1997. Kluwer Academic Publishers. ISBN 0-7923-4260-7. All rights reserved.

targeted therapy in high-dose, marrow-ablative preparative regimens for patients undergoing transplantation for hematologic malignancies are reviewed, with a focus on the principles of radioimmunotherapy elucidated by these first-generation studies. Finally, potential means of improving upon current approaches are discussed.

Designing a radioimmunotherapy trial

The radiation absorbed dose delivered to a tissue by a radioimmunoconjugate is a result of the concentration of the isotope in the organ over time as well as 'cross-fire' from neighboring organs. The 'therapeutic ratio' of radiation doses delivered to target as compared to nontarget tissues thus depends upon the relative concentrations and residence times of the isotope in each tissue. The biodistribution of a radioimmunoconjugate can be measured in patients by serial quantitative gamma camera scanning following the administration of a dose of antibody labeled with a trace amount of isotope. Such biodistribution studies result in estimates of radiation absorbed doses (per millicurie of isotope) delivered to target and nontarget tissues with any given antibody–isotope conjugate. Studies both in animals and man have shown that the biodistribution, and therefore the radiation absorbed doses, of a given antibody-isotope conjugate dose can vary widely between two subjects. Thus, biodistribution studies are useful in determining the appropriate dose of isotope to be administered, particularly in clinical trials employing radiation doses near those that are the maximum tolerated. These biodistribution studies have also served to define some of the variables (table 1) that affect the uptake and retention of various radioimmunoconjugates by both tumor and normal, nontarget tissues.

The target antigen has a major effect in determining the relative biodistribution of radiolabeled antibodies. Ideally, the antigen should be expressed in high copy numbers by the majority of the malignant cells, and should be of restricted specificity to minimize the delivery of radiation to nontarget tissues. Antigens that remain stable on the cell surface after antibody binding allow for continued accumulation of antibody by unbound antigenic sites as long as appreciable levels of immunoreactive antibody persist in circulation, and result in minimal metabolism of the radioimmunoconjugate by the target cell. In contrast, the binding of antibody to a 'modulating' antigen results in the internalization of the antibody–antigen complex into the cell, which may result in metabolism and dehalogenation of iodinated antibodies and rapid excretion of ^{131}I from the cell. Thus, for conventionally iodinated antibodies, modulating antigens may present a relative disadvantage by limiting the retention of ^{131}I at the target site, and by causing the transient loss of surface expression of target antigen after modulation. However, when using an antibody–radiometal chelate that is retained intracellularly after metabolism, of alternative labeling methods for ^{131}I that are not susceptible to

122

Table 1. Factors influencing the biodistribution of radioimmunoconjugates

Factor	Attribute
Target antigen	Copy number per target cell Expression by nontarget tissues Internalizing or 'surface stable' after antibody binding
Radioisotope	Energy/path length Half-life Stability of labeling method and retention in cells
Antibody	Dose Dose schedule Size (whole Ig vs. F(ab')$_2$ vs. F(ab') or single chain Fv)
Tumor	Bulk Vascularity

Table 2. Potential radioisotopes for radiolabeled antibody therapy

Radionuclide	Mean range (mm)[a]	Particulate energy (MeV)	Half-life	Comments
β-emitters				
Iodine-131	0.4	0.6	8.1 days	High-energy gamma component delivers 'TBI' and requires treatment in radiation isolation
Yttrium-90	2.8	2.3	2.7 days	No gamma component; must use Indium-111 for imaging
Rhenium-186	0.9	1.1	3.7 days	Gamma component suitable for imaging
Lutetium-177	0.3	0.5	6.7 days	Gamma component suitable for imaging
Copper-67	0.3	0.6	2.6 days	Gamma component suitable for imaging
α-emitters				
Bismuth-212	0.06	6.1	1 hour	Short half-life limits treatment options
Astatine-211	0.06	5.9	7.2 hours	
Electron capture				
Iodine-125	0.001–0.02	7.5	60.1 days	Very short path length limits cell kill to cells directly binding antibody

[a] Mean range is the distance in which 60% of decay energy is deposited.

deiodination, internalizing antigens may improve the accumulation of isotope at the target site, since the isotope–antibody cannot 'fall off' the cell surface once internalized.

Several isotopes are available for radioimmunotherapy, each with advantages and disadvantages resulting from its specific energy, half-life, and radiolabeling characteristics (table 2). Iodine-131 has been used medically for decades, and simple radiolabeling methods are well established. Its significant component of gamma energy allows direct quantitative imaging and provides an element of 'TBI' that may have therapeutic benefit for hematologic malignancies. However, the TBI component of ^{131}I also increases the nonspecific organ toxicity of radioiodinated antibody, and the long-range gamma energy presents a short-term radiation hazard to staff and to the family of the patient, which necessitates treatment in radiation isolation, increasing the cost of therapy.

Yttrium-90 has a longer-ranged beta particle than ^{131}I, which should decrease the heterogeneity of radiation delivery in target tissue. It has no significant gamma component and thus is safer for both staff and family, allowing patients to be treated in the outpatient setting. The absence of a gamma component with ^{90}Y necessitates that imaging/biodistribution studies be performed with a different isotope, usually Indium-111. However, many radioimmunoconjugates of these radiometals have not been stable in vivo, and thus the biodistribution of ^{111}In-labeled antibodies have not always predicted the localization of ^{90}Y, especially given the propensity of free ^{90}Y to bind to bone and liver. Newer chelation methods appear to result in more stable radiometal immunoconjugates. As noted, radiometals such as ^{90}Y may have superior intracellular retention when internalizing antigens are targeted. As yet, there are no studies that have adequately compared the use of conventionally iodinated antibodies reactive with noninternalizing antigens to radiometal-labeled antibodies reactive with internalizing antigens. Other potential radioisotopes such as ^{186}Rhenium, ^{67}Copper, and ^{177}Lutetium are under study. There is also great interest in alpha emitters because their short range and high energy may result in more specific and effective cell kill. However, their short half-life may limit their utility for large tumor masses where diffusion of antibody into tumor occurs over days rather than hours, and there are many difficulties associated with radiolabeling antibodies with these isotopes.

Finally, the optimum antibody dose and dose schedule must be determined. High doses of antibody result in high serum levels and prolonged circulation, which may improve the penetration of antibody into larger tumor masses. However, the longer circulation time increases the radiation dose delivered to nontarget organs, and the use of large amounts of monoclonal antibodies is costly. Smaller doses of antibody may be used when targeting well-vascularized sites such as marrow, or when targeting antigens of limited expression where higher antibody doses would lead to saturation of antigen and circulation of excess antibody. The use of very low doses of antibody may also limit the amount of radioisotope that can be delivered at a single treatment, because labeling the antibody to a very high specific activity (i.e., mCi/mg antibody) may adversely affect immunoreactivity.

The total radiation dose to be delivered can be administered as a single or divided dose. Divided doses delivered at short intervals without allowing marrow recovery may prolong the period of neutropenia, yet separating such doses by an interval that allows marrow recovery may also allow tumor regrowth and thus may be less effective than a single, higher-dose treatment. Repetitive antibody doses may be limited by the development of human antimouse antibody (HAMA), which might be prevented by the use of 'humanized' antibody.

In summary, many characteristics of a radioimmunoconjugate, including the target antigen, radioisotope, and antibody dose and schedule, may affect the distribution and retention of the radionuclide at target and nontarget tissues as well as the antitumor effect. Further, initial clinical studies have defined patient factors, including tumor burden, affecting antibody localization. The relative roles of some of these variables in the treatment of lymphoma and leukemia are illustrated by the studies detailed below, while others remain to be tested.

Radioimmunotherapy trials in non-Hodgkin's lymphoma

The initial experience using radioimmunoconjugates for the treatment of non-Hodgkin's lymphoma in Seattle was obtained in a phase 1 dose-escalation trial using ^{131}I-labeled anti-CD20 and anti-CD37 antibodies in patients with B-cell lymphoma in relapse [16,26]. Because we wished to deliver maximum doses of radiation to lymphoma to optimize the therapeutic effect, this study required that patients had stored autologous marrow available in order that radiation doses likely to be marrow ablative could be delivered. The objectives of this study were to determine the biodistribution of ^{131}I-labeled anti-B-cell antibodies in patients with relapsed lymphoma, to determine the toxicity and efficacy of radiolabeled antibodies, and to estimate the maximum tolerated dose of radiation that could be delivered with autologous marrow rescue.

Patients first underwent biodistribution studies in which, during successive weeks, trace ^{131}I-labeled antibodies (antibody doses of 0.5, 2.5, and 10 mg/kg) were administered. Patients were followed with serial quantitative gamma camera images, blood samples, and when possible, tumor biopsies for determination of the concentration of antibody in tumor and in normal tissues (lung, liver, and kidney) over time. The curves of radionuclide concentration over time were used to calculate estimated radiation absorbed doses for each tissue using standard dosimetry methods [31–33].

Those patients in whom the estimated radiation absorbed dose to each evaluable tumor site was greater than that to any normal organ were considered to have 'favorable biodistribution' and were eligible to receive a therapeutic infusion of ^{131}I-labeled anti-B-cell antibody. The antibody dose resulting in the best tumor-to-normal-organ ratio was labeled with the amount of ^{131}I calculated to deliver a predetermined estimated radiation absorbed dose to the normal organ receiving the highest dose. The predetermined dose was escalated in groups of three patients. The therapeutic dose was delivered in special lead-lined rooms on the oncology ward, where patients remained in radiation isolation until their total body activity was less than 30 mCi, as estimated by a dose rate of less than 5 mR/hour at one meter from the patient. Patients whose absolute neutrophil count fell below 200/mm^3 for two consecutive days received their autologous purged marrow when their total body activity had dropped below 2 mR/hr at one meter.

Forty-three patients were entered in the study, the majority of whom had lymphomas of low-grade histology. They were a heavily pretreated group, having received an average of more than three previous chemotherapy treatment regimens.

Eighty-four percent of patients had positive tumor imaging, and favorable biodistribution was achieved in 56% of patients. Several factors influencing the biodistribution of antibody and the chance of achieving favorable biodistribution were defined. Very few patients with splenomegaly (2 of 15) had favorable biodistribution, while the majority of those with normal spleen size (17 of 23) or those who had previously undergone splenectomy (5 of 5) had favorable biodistribution. A large tumor burden similarly was associated with poor antibody biodistribution, with only 1 of 12 patients with greater than 500 ml of tumor burden achieving favorable biodistribution, compared with 23 of 31 patients with less than 500 ml of tumor ($p < 0.001$). We interpret the poor biodistribution of ^{131}I-anti-B-cell antibody in patients with splenomegaly and/or large tumor burden to reflect uptake of antibody by the large number of tumor cells and normal B cells in the spleen, which then resulted in limited penetration of the radionuclide conjugate into large tumor masses. The antibody dose also influenced biodistrbution, and for each antibody a different dose seemed preferable. For the MB-1 (anti-CD37) antibody, the highest dose tested (10 mg/kg) more often achieved favorable biodistribution than lower doses, while the majority of patients receiving 2.5 mg/kg of B1 (anti-CD20) antibody had favorable biodistribution, and this percent was not increased by giving a higher antibody dose.

Nineteen of the 24 patients with favorable biodistribution received a therapeutic dose of ^{131}I-labeled anti-B-cell antibody. Three eligible patients developed human anti-mouse antibodies (HAMA) prior to potential therapy and were not treated with a therapeutic dose. The lung was the normal organ with the highest estimated radiation absorbed dose in most patients. The maximum estimated radiation absorbed dose to normal organs ranged from 10.0 Gy to 30.75 Gy, with estimated doses to tumor ranging from 10.1 Gy to 91.5 Gy (table 3). Fifteen of 19 treated patients received their autologous marrow (13 to 31 days after therapy), with engraftment occuring at the expected interval after transplantation for recipients of autologous marrow. Toxicities included three serious and six minor infections, with fever, nausea, alopecia, elevated thyrotropin, and transient, mild elevations in bilirubin and transaminases occurring in some, but not all, patients. Life-threatening (i.e., grade III) cardiopulmonary toxicities occurred in two patients in whom the estimated radiation absorbed doses to lung were 27 and 31 Gy, respectively. Thus, the maximum

Table 3. Estimated radiation absorbed doses with ^{131}I-anti-B-cell antibodies

Site	Absorbed radiation dose	Tumor/tissue absorbed dose ratio (Mean ± SE)
Tumor	10.0–91.5	—
Lungs	6.5–31.0	1.8 ± 0.2
Liver	3.8–19.3	3.0 ± 0.3
Kidneys	5.4–21.6	3.4 ± 0.3
Marrow	1.0–6.4	10.2 ± 1.1
Total body	1.0–5.7	10.4 ± 1.0

tolerated dose was estimated to be approximately 25 Gy. While the severity of the toxicities seen correlated with the estimated radiation absorbed doses delivered, even the patients treated at the higher doses appeared less ill than the typical patient receiving a conventional autologous marrow transplant.

The clinical responses in this phase I trial were impressive. Complete remissions were seen in 16 of 19 patients, with two having a partial response and one a minor response. These responses were durable, and 8 of 16 patients remain in CR 3 to $7\frac{1}{2}$ years after therapy.

Based on the encouraging results of this phase I trial, a phase II trial of ^{131}I-B1 antibody in patients with relapsed non-Hodgkin's lymphoma was conducted [29]. Twenty-five patients underwent a biodistribution dose of 2.5 mg/kg trace ^{131}I-labeled B1 antibody, with 22 of 25 patients eventually achieving favorable biodistribution. The higher rate of favorable biodistribution in this study as compared to the phase I study reflected the overall lower tumor burden in this group and the use of B-1 as the sole anti-B-cell antibody. Three patients initially having unfavorable biodistribution when studies with a large tumor burden (1259 to 3610 ml) subsequently achieved favorable biodistribution after receiving chemotherapy to debulk tumor (posttreatment tumor burdens of 400 to 659 ml).

Twenty-one of the 22 patients with favorable biodistribution received a therapeutic dose of ^{131}I-labeled B-1 antibody, the remaining patient having developed HAMA. Estimated radiation absorbed doses to the normal organ receiving the highest dose (the lung in 20 of 21 treated patients) ranged from 25 to 27 Gy, requiring 345 to 785 mCi [131]I. All patients received either autologous marrow (19) or peripheral blood stem cell (2) infusions 12 to 18 days after therapy, followed by granulocyte colony stimulating factor. The toxicities were similar to those seen in the latter half of the phase I trial. Serious infections occurred in three patients, with one death. By design, this trial included four patients treated at the 27 Gy dose level in the phase I trial. Two patients of the first eight treated at this dose level developed grade III toxicity, establishing this as the maximum tolerated dose.

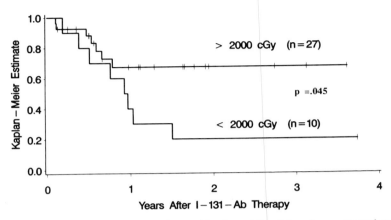

Progression – Free Survival
on Phase I & II Studies

Figure 1. Progression-free survival of patients with relapsed B-cell lymphomas treated on phase I and II trials using ^{131}I-anti B-cell antibodies and autologous stem cell rescue. The delivery of estimated radiation absorbed doses of more than 20 Gy to the normal organ receiving the highest dose was associated with improved progression-free survival. From *Lancet* 346:336, 1995, with permission.

Complete remissions were seen in 16 of 21 patients, with a partial response in two and a minor response in one. One patient had progression of a high-grade immunoblastic diffuse large cell lymphoma and died 1.5 months after therapy. When the data from both the phase I and II studies are combined, there is an apparent correlation between patients receiving a higher estimated radiation dose (>20 Gy) to normal organs, and improved progression-free survival (figure 1).

In summary, the vast majority of studied patients with relapsed non-Hodgkin's lymphoma without bulky disease were able to receive a greater dose of radiation to tumor as compared to normal organs using ^{131}I-anti-B-cell antibodies. Using the B1 antibody reactive with the noninternalizing CD20 antigen at relatively high antibody doses (2.5 mg/kg), the ^{131}I was retained at tumor sites, with tumor-to-normal-organ ratios as high as 3 to 1. A single, high-dose treatment of ^{131}I-B1 antibody was well tolerated in these patients and resulted in encouraging clinical responses, which were often durable. In an effort to combine this promising form of radioimmunotherapy with the potential benefits of high-dose chemotherapy, the current study in Seattle is a phase I/II study in which high-dose ^{131}I-B1 antibody is combined with cyclophosphamide and etoposide. Ultimately, the goal will be to see if the substitution of targeted radiotherapy in a transplant preparative regimen offers an advance over the use of nonspecific TBI.

Radiolabeled antibody studies for Hodgkin's lymphoma

Vriesendorp et al. have used ^{90}Y-labeled polyclonal antiferritin immunoglobulin to treat patients with advanced, end-stage Hodgkin's disease [20,30]. Forty of 45 patients receiving biodistribution doses of ^{111}In-labeled rabbit, pig, or baboon polyclonal antiferritin (2–5 mg) showed uptake of radiolabel in tumor. Thirty-nine of these patients then received a therapeutic dose of polyclonal immunoglobulin labeled with 20 to 50 mCi ^{90}Y, delivering estimated radiation absorbed doses to tumor of between 3 and 30 Gy, and a maximum dose to liver of 7 Gy. Nineteen patients received an infusion of autologous marrow 18 days after therapy, which accelerated recovery of hematopoiesis after 30 or 40 mCi, but not after 20 mCi doses of ^{90}Y-antiferritin. Patients received up to five cycles of therapy. The MTD was defined as 40 mCi ^{90}Y, in that higher activities led to a degree of marrow aplasia that required hospitalization.

Complete responses were seen in ten (36%) patients, with partial responses in another 10 patients. Response and response duration were not correlated with the dose of ^{90}Y administered, but responses were more frequent in patients with higher whole blood activity after antibody infusion. Fifty percent of patients survived longer than six months, but overall survival was less than 20% by two years, and of the survivors, 4 of 5 have active Hodgkin's disease. The relative safety of ^{90}Y allowed this therapy to be administered in the outpatient setting. Positive tumor imaging was achieved in most patients, despite the use of a much smaller dose of antibody than used in the anti-B-cell studies described above for non-Hodgkin's lymphoma. However, since three different polyclonal reagents were used, and since higher antibody doses were not studied, it is difficult to draw particular conclusions from these reports about the potential effect of antibody dose on biodistribution.

Bierman et al. have combined ^{90}Y-labeled antiferritin with high-dose chemotherapy in patients with poor prognosis Hodgkin's [27]. All 12 patients entered had imaging of tumor after a biodistribution dose of ^{111}In-antiferritin, and were treated with ^{90}Y-antiferritin (18 to 33 mCi) on days −13, −12, or −11. Estimated radiation absorbed doses of 5 to 10 Gy to tumor (with 0.18 Gy/mCi to marrow and 0.3 Gy/mCi to liver) were delivered over the first week after therapeutic antibody infusion. This was followed by cyclophosphamide (total dose 6 gm/m^2), carmustine (total dose 300 mg/m^2), and etoposide (total dose 750 mg/m^2) on days −6 to −3, with autologous marrow reinfusion on day 0. Four patients died early from transplant-related causes. Successful engraftment occurred in the eight evaluable patients. Three patients were free of disease progression 24 to 28 months posttransplant at the time of their report. The estimated progression-free survival rate at one year was 21%. While the early death rate was high in this study, this group of patients was heavily pretreated and all patients who died early after treatment had received prior chest irradiation. This combined preparative regimen may have less toxicity and improved efficacy in patients treated earlier in their disease course.

Radiolabeled antibody trials in acute leukemia

Studies with anti-CD33 antibody

The first trials of radiolabeled antibody in the treatment of acute myelogenous leukemia (AML) utilized ^{131}I-anti-CD33 antibody because the CD33 antigen is expressed on more than 90% of AML samples and has limited expression beyond immature myeloid cells in the marrow [23,34,35]. In a phase I dose-escalation trial conducted in Seattle [23], ^{131}I-p67 (anti-CD33) antibody was combined with cyclophosphamide 120 mg/kg and 12 Gy TBI followed by autologous or matched related allogeneic marrow transplantation. As in our trials of anti-B-cell antibodies in lymphoma patients, patients first underwent biodistribution doses of trace ^{131}I-labeled p67 antibody followed by serial quantitative gamma camera imaging, blood sampling, and bone marrow biopsies. Patients in whom the marrow and spleen had a higher estimated radiation absorbed dose than any normal organ were eligible to receive a therapeutic dose of ^{131}I-p67 antibody, followed by CY/TBI. We elected to combine radiolabeled antibody with a conventional marrow-transplant preparative regimen because we wished to be certain that the preparative regimen would deliver enough immunosuppression to prevent rejection of allogeneic marrow, and that at least a minimum dose of therapy would be delivered to sanctuary sites where leukemic cells might not be accessible to antibody.

Nine patients with AML in second remission ($n = 5$) or in relapse ($n = 4$) underwent biodistribution studies at antibody doses ranging from 0.05 to 0.5 mg/kg. While ^{131}I-labeled p67 antibody could deliver greater radiation to the marrow compared to normal organs in some patients, the differences were modest. Only 4 of 9 patients achieved 'favorable biodistribution,' with an average ratio of estimated radiation dose delivered to marrow as compared to the normal organ receiving the highest dose of only 1.2. Since the CD33 antigen modulates upon binding of antibody, internalization of the antibody–antigen complex led to rapid deiodination and release of ^{131}I from target tissues (average marrow $T\frac{1}{2}$ of 21.4 hours). In addition, low antigen expression limited both the initial uptake of antibody in some patients and the total dose of antibody that could be delivered without saturation of antigen (0.05 mg/kg).

Four patients were treated with p67 antibody labeled with the amount of ^{131}I estimated to deliver 1.8 Gy to the normal organ (liver or lung) receiving the highest dose (dose level 1), followed by CY/TBI. There were no grade III–IV toxicities in this group of patients. The planned escalation to dose level 2 (3.5 Gy) was not possible, however, because of the limited amount of ^{131}I with which 0.05 mg/kg of p67 antibody could be labeled without adversely affecting its immunoreactivity. Thus, the study was halted. Three of the four treated patients went on to relapse after transplant, and one patient survives more than five years after transplant.

Scheinberg et al. studied the biodistribution of a different anti-CD33 antibody, ^{131}I-M195, in ten patients with relapsed or refractory AML ($n = 9$) or untreated chronic myelomonocytic leukemia ($n = 1$) [22]. The reported concentrations of ^{131}I in marrow biopsies at one hour and 2 to 4 days after antibody infusion suggested longer retention time in some patients than was observed with p67 antibody. Reasons for a difference between these two antibodies, which appear to detect the same or close-by epitopes, are not clear, but in both studies marrow retention was relatively short. Like the study of p67, this study also demonstrated that antigen saturation occurred at relatively low (>3 mg/m^2) antibody doses. A humanized version of this antibody had similar biodistribution [36].

In a dose-escalation trial of ^{131}I-M195 alone in 24 patients (16 refractory, relapsed, or secondary AML; five blastic myelodysplastic syndromes; and one chronic myelogenous leukemia (in blast crisis)), patients were treated with 50 to 210 mCi/m^2 of ^{131}I administered in 2 to 4 divided doses at least 48 hours apart, to allow reexpression of antigen after modulation from the previous dose [34]. Antibody doses were adjusted for leukemic burden by adding 0.1 mg/m^2 of M195 for every 10,000 peripheral WBCs/μL to a starting dose of 3 mg/m^2. Because of concerns that higher ^{131}I doses would be marrow ablative, delivery of 160 mCi/m^2 or more was allowed only in patients with a suitable source of marrow rescue (allogeneic or previously stored autologous marrow). Fourteen patients required treatment with antibiotics, and there were nine documented infections. Eight patients required infusion of marrow. Substantial cytoreduction was seen in patients above the first two dose levels, and three of the patients requiring marrow transplantation achieved a CR (one fo nine months, and one of more than six months).

This group has also combined ^{131}I-M195 antibody with a basic preparative regimen of busulfan 16 mg/kg and cyclophosphamide 120 mg/kg (BU/CY) in recipients of allogeneic marrow transplants [35]. Nine patients with advanced/refractory AML received total doses of 120–160 mCi/m^2 ^{131}I in 2 to 3 divided doses over 5 to 7 days, followed by BU/CY, with cyclosporine and methotrexate as graft-vs.-host-disease prophylaxis. Toxicity was acceptable, although three patients died of infections. In the initial report, four patients were surviving disease-free 5 to 16 months after transplantation, and there were two relapses.

In summary, the use of an internalizing antigen expressed in low copy number as a target for conventionally iodinated antibody has limited the ratio of radiation delivered to marrow as compared to normal organs in many patients, particularly those in remission. The total radiation dose deliverable has also been restricted by the amount of ^{131}I with which small doses of antibody can be radiolabeled.

Studies with anti-CD45 antibody

To overcome the limitations of anti-CD33 antibody for AML and to expand this approach to include the treatment of patients with acute lymphoblastic leukemia (ALL), we have studied the biodistribution of an ^{131}I-labeled antibody reactive with an alternative hematopoietic antigen, CD45, which is expressed at high copy numbers and which does not internalize upon binding with antibody [28]. A phase I dose escalation study combining ^{131}I-BC8 (anti-CD45) antibody with CY/TBI was initiated in patients with AML or ALL beyond first remission and advanced myelodysplastic syndromes. Patients first underwent a biodistribution dose of trace ^{131}I-labeled BC8 antibody, and those with favorable biodistibution were treated with the amount of ^{131}I determined by a dose escalation scheme to deliver a given estimated radiation absorbed dose (starting at 3.5 Gy) to the normal organ receiving the highest dose. The therapeutic dose of ^{131}I-BC8 antibody was administered on day −14, followed by CY 60 mg/kg × 2, TBI 2 Gy × 6, and infusion of HLA-matched related allogeneic or previously stored autologous marrow on day 0. GVHD prophylaxis for allogeneic recipients consisted of conventional methotrexate and cyclosporine.

Twenty-four patients underwent biodistribution infusions of 0.5 mg/kg trace ^{131}I-labeled BC8 antibody (figure 2). Fifteen had AML (first relapse, 4; second remission, 7; third remission, 1; refractory disease, 3), seven had ALL (second remission, 4; refractory disease, 3), and two had myelodysplastic syndromes

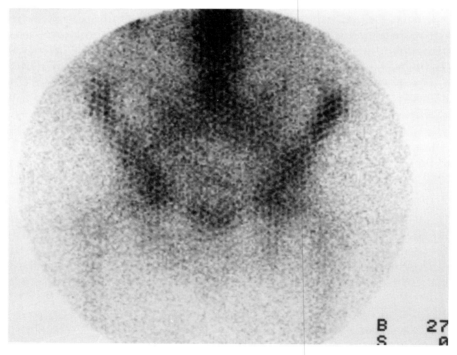

Figure 2. ^{131}I-anti-CD45 antibody localization in patient 7378 immediately following infusion of trace-labeled BC8 antibody. This anterior gamma camera image shows accumulation of ^{131}I in marrow in the lower lumbar vertebral bodies and the pelvic axial skeleton.

(refractory anemia with excess blasts, $n = 1$; refractory anemia with excess with blasts in transformation, $n = 1$). Favorable biodistribution of ^{131}I-BC8 antibody was seen in 21 of 24 patients. The ^{131}I-BC8 antibody was cleared relatively rapidly from blood, presumably because the CD45 antigen was present in vast excess on hematopoietic tissue despite the administration of up to 50 mg of antibody. The retention of ^{131}I in marrow was much longer targeting this noninternalizing antigen (43.2 hours) than with anti-CD33 antibody (21.4 hours, $p < 0.001$). This longer retention and the higher average initial marrow uptake of ^{131}I-BC8 antibody led to a higher average radiation absorbed dose to marrow (7.2 cGy/mCi ^{131}I) than was seen with ^{131}I-p67 antibody (1.6 cGy/mCi, $p < 0.001$). The liver was the organ that took up the most ^{131}I-BC8 antibody after marrow, presumably due to the binding of antibody to CD45-expressing resident macrophages as well as sequestration of antibody-coated circulating leukocytes. An attempt to prevent uptake of cells coated with radiolabeled antibody by administering the first 7.5 mg of BC8 antibody as unlabeled antibody failed to decrease the hepatic localization of the subsequent ^{131}I-BC8 antibody, despite preclinical models suggesting the efficacy of such an approach [37]. Nevertheless, the improved marrow uptake and retention of ^{131}I-BC8 antibody resulted in an average 'therapeutic ratio' of radiation dose delivered to the marrow as compared to the liver of 2.7, compared to a ratio of 1.2 when using ^{131}I-p67 antibody. Patients with AML in relapse had higher estimated marrow radiation absorbed doses compared to patients with ALL in remission or relapse and AML in remission, due to both higher initial uptake and prolonged retention of ^{131}I in marrow (table 4). Patients with AML in relapse had a higher 'therapeutic ratio' (3.7) of radiation to marrow as compared to liver than other patients (2.1).

Twenty-one patients received a therapeutic dose of ^{131}I-BC8 antibody, labeled with the amount of ^{131}I estimated to deliver a radiation absorbed dose of from 3.5 Gy (level 1) to 7.0 Gy (level 3) to the liver. This was followed by a

Table 4. Estimated radiation absorbed doses per mCi I-131 administered (mean ± SE) using ^{131}I-anti-CD45 antibodies

Patient group	Tissue (cGy/mCi)					
	Marrow	Spleen	Liver	Lungs	Kidney	Total body
All patients	7.2 ± 0.8	10.8 ± 1.3	2.7 ± 0.2	2.1 ± 0.1	0.6 ± 0.1	0.4 ± 0.03
AML remission	5.2 ± 0.7	8.1 ± 1.1	2.4 ± 0.2	1.8 ± 0.2	0.6 ± 0.03	0.4 ± 0.02
AML/MDS Relapse	11.3 ± 1.3	12.2 ± 2.5	2.8 ± 0.4	2.5 ± 0.2	0.6 ± 0.1	0.6 ± 0.07
ALL Remission	5.5 ± 0.3	13.8 ± 3.3	2.6 ± 0.1	2.0 ± 0.3	0.9 ± 0.5	0.4 ± 0.04
ALL Relapse	4.9 ± 0.5	11.4 ± 6.3	3.0 ± 0.9	2.2 ± 0.4	0.8 ± 0.2	0.4 ± 0.08

Abbreviations: AML, acute myeloid leukemia; ALL, acute lymphoblastic leukemia; MDS, myelodysplastic syndrome.

standard preparative regimen of CY and 12 Gy TBI. The ^{131}I-BC8 antibody delivered radiation doses of 4 to 31 Gy to marrow and 8 to 60 Gy to spleen. Toxicities of this combined preparative regimen have not been appreciably greater than that expected from CY/TBI alone, and the maximum tolerated dose had not yet been defined. Four patients died of infection within the first 40 days. Of 11 patients with AML or myelodysplastic syndrome evaluable for relapse (i.e., surviving the first 100 days posttransplant), one relapsed seven months posttransplant, and ten are surviving disease free a median of 28 months posttransplant. Four of six evaluable patients with ALL have relapsed between two weeks and 12 months after transplant, while two survive disease-free 32 and 20 months after transplant.

Thus, ^{131}I-anti-CD45 antibody can deliver greater radiation doses to the target organs of marrow and spleen than to normal, nontarget organs in most patients with acute leukemia, with the greatest specificity in patients with AML in relapse. Appreciable supplemental doses have been delivered to marrow and spleen via radiolabeled antibody without excessive toxicity. Although this phase I study was not designed to determine the efficacy of this treatment, the low relapse rate in patients transplanted for recurrent or refractory AML is encouraging.

Based on the demonstration of the hematopoietic specificity of ^{131}I-anti-CD45 antibody and the low toxicity associated with the delivery of a dose of targeted radiation when combined with CY/TBI, we initiated a phase I/II study combining ^{131}I-BC8 with BU/CY for patients with AML in first remission, untreated first relapse, and second remission receiving HLA-matched related transplants. Since there is evidence that BU/CY is better tolerated than CY/TBI [38], more supplemental radiation delivered via ^{131}I-labeled antibody could possibly be combined with BU/CY. Thus, the goal of this study is to gain experience with the efficacy and toxicity of ^{131}I-BC8 antibody when combined with BU/CY. The initial experience with this preparative regimen is promising, with all eight patients treated thus far in first remission alive and disease-free 2 to 20 months after transplant. Should the efficacy and toxicity of this combination of targeted therapy with BU/CY compare favorably with historical experience using conventional transplant preparative regimens, we envision an ultimate comparison to BU/CY alone in a phase III trial.

Future directions

The success of the first-generation studies using targeted radiotherapy as part or all of the preparative regimen for patients undergoing marrow transplantation for hematologic malignancies supports the promise of this approach. Although the studies reported above suggest that appreciable doses of radiation can be delivered to target tissues using radiolabeled antibodies without unacceptable toxicities, their ultimate efficacy in terms of enhancing disease-free survival remains to be tested in phase III studies. Although preliminary results are encouraging, the ratios of radiation delivered to target as compared to nontarget tissues have often been modest, with few patients achieving ratios in excess of 3:1. To be maximally effective and minimally toxic, better specificity of radiation delivery is needed, and approaches that may improve targeting deserve further study.

For example, although the best targeting to date has been achieved using anti-CD20 for non-Hodgkin's lymphoma and anti-CD45 antibody for leukemia, other antigens may result in superior uptake of radioimmunoconjugate in target tissues. The enhanced localization of ^{131}I-anti-CD45 antibody in patients with AML in relapse as compared to remission suggests that maximizing the potential number of antibody binding sites may improve antibody uptake. Thus, an antigen expressed in high copy numbers per cell may result in better uptake than one present in lower numbers. Alternatively, increasing in a target site the number of cells that express antigen, whether by selecting an antigen of broader specificity or by expanding a cell population and increasing overall cellularity using hematopoietic growth factors, may improve antibody uptake. A short course of G-CSF prior to the administration of an ^{131}I-antimyeloid antibody in the canine model improved marrow uptake of antibody, and this approach is being tested with ^{131}I-anti-CD45 antibodies in a macaque preclinical model.

An alternative approach to improving the ratio of radiation delivery to target as compared to nontarget tissues is to alter the immunoconjugate to hasten its clearance from the blood in order to minimize the nonspecific radiation delivery from circulating radioisotope. Although smaller molecules such as $F(ab')_2$ or $F(ab')$ fragments and single-chain Fv molecules are cleared more quickly from blood, they are also often cleared more rapidly from tumor [10,39]. Furthermore, their shortened time in circulation leads to a decreased concentration gradient between the circulation and tumor, which may limit the localization and diffusion of antibody into large tumor masses. Thus, these smaller molecules have not been definitively shown to result in improved ratios of radiation delivery to tumor as compared to normal organs.

A novel approach to decreasing the time during which radionuclide circulates non-specifically involves 'pretargeting' tumor with a streptavidin conjugate of *non-radiolabeled* monoclonal antibody. This is followed 24 to 48 hours later by a biotin-clearing agent compound that binds circulating streptavidin-antibody with extremely high avidity and results in clearance of this complex by the liver. The final step is the administration of a radioisotope-biotin moiety, which is of low molecular weight and thus diffuses rapidly into tumor, where it binds to the streptavidin-antibody conjugate. Non-bound isotope-biotin is cleared promptly through the kidneys. Animal studies have demonstrated a tenfold improvement in target-to-normal-organ ratios [40], and impressive responses to therapy with ^{90}Y-DOTA-biotin have been seen, without apparent marrow toxicity, in a murine subcutaneous tumor xenograft model [41]. Trials of this approach in humans with solid tumors are under way.

Most studies reported to date have used ^{131}I as the therapeutic radioisotope, conjugated to antibody using the chloramine T method. However, as noted, a disadvantage of conventionally radioiodinated antibody was its rapid degradation and clearance from target cells seen when targeting an internalizing antigen such as CD33. We have demonstrated that the use of a non-metabolizable carbohydrate linker tyramine cellobiose (TCB) to conjugate ^{131}I to antibody led to improved retention of ^{131}I in cells in a subcutaneous xenograft murine model of myeloid leukemia [42], and in a single patient receiving ^{131}I-p67 antibody labeled via the TCB method. Similarly, radiometal isotopes such as ^{90}Y and ^{111}In have been demonstrated to have improved intracellular retention, compared to conventionally labeled ^{131}I, when delivered by antibody binding to internalizing antigens [11]. The theoretical advantages and disadvantages of alternative isotopes have been discussed, but few have been put to test in clinical settings.

The production of HAMA has not been a major limitation in the treatment of patients with radiolabeled antibodies in the setting of bone marrow transplantation, where often only a single therapeutic infusion is administered. However, a minority of patients made HAMA in response to their biodistribution infusion, and HAMA may limit the delivery of repetitive therapeutic doses in some patients. Humanized or human monoclonal antibodies reactive with many relevant hematopoietic antigens have been produced and should minimize this problem. Some of these reagents have been cleared more slowly from blood than their murine counterparts, which may increase nonspecific radiation.

Conclusion

The studies conducted to date incorporating radioimmunotherapy as part or all of the preparative regimen for patients undergoing marrow transplantation for non-Hodgkin's lymphoma and acute leukemia have demonstrated that large doses of radiation can be delivered to target tissues with this approach. The delivery of the highest possible radiation doses to target tissues, possible in the setting of hematopoietic stem cell rescue, is likely to result in the best cure rate for these radiosensitive diseases. The clinical response rates seen in these phase I and II studies have been encouraging, and toxicities have been acceptable. Planned phase III studies should provide further information about the efficacy of targeted therapy and should better define its role in the therapy of hematologic malignancies. Ultimately, new radioimmunoconjugates may improve the specificity of radiation delivery and result in improved clinical outcomes for these patients.

Acknowledgments

The authors gratefully acknowledge the scientific collaboration of Drs. Paul Martin, Darrell Fisher, Edmond Hui, David Mitchell, Stephan Glenn, and Wil

Nelp, the nursing care of Sherri Bush, R.N., and Donna Kelly, R.N., and the technical support of Larry Durack, Minna Zheng, Carol Dean, Caroline Thostenson, Karen Richter, and Linda Risler. Antibodies were provided by Coulter Corporation (B1) and Idec Pharmaceutical Corporation (MB-1). This work was supported by NIH Grants No. CA44991, CA18029, CA47748, CA18221, and HL36444.

References

1. Clift RA, Buckner CD, Appelbaum FR, Bearman SI, Petersen FB, Fisher LD, Anasetti C, Beatty P, Bensinger WI, Doney K, Hill R, McDonald G, Martin P, Sanders J, Singer J, Stewart P, Sullivan KM, Witherspoon R, Storb R, Hansen J, Thomas ED. Allogeneic marrow transplantation in patients with acute myeloid leukemia in first remission. A randomized trial of two irradiation regimens. Blood 76:1867–1871, 1990.
2. Clift RA, Buckner CD, Appelbaum FR, Bryant E, Bearman SI, Petersen FB, Fisher LD, Anasetti C, Beatty P, Bensinger WI, Doney K, Hill RS, McDonald GB, Martin P, Meyers J, Sanders J, Singer J, Stewart P, Sullivan KM, Witherspoon R, Storb R, Hansen JA, Thomas ED. Allogeneic marrow transplantation in patients with chronic myeloid leukemia in the chronic phase: a randomized trial of two irradiation regimens. Blood 77:1660–1665, 1991.
3. Redwood WR, Tom TD, Strand M. Specificity, efficacy and toxicity of radioimmunotherapy in erythroleukemic mice. Cancer Res 44:5681–5687, 1984.
4. Badger CC, Krohn KA, Shulman H, Flournoy N, Bernstein ID. Experimental radio-immunotherapy of lymphoma with ^{131}I-labeled anti-T-cell antibodies. Cancer Res 46:6223–6228, 1986.
5. Macklis RM, Kaplan WD, Ferrara JL, Kinsey BM, Kassis AI, Burakoff SJ. Biodistribution studies of anti-Thy 1.2 IgM immunoconjugates: implications for radioimmunotherapy. Int J Radiat Oncol Biol Phys 15:383–389, 1988.
6. Knox SJ, Levy R, Miller Ra, Uhland W, Schiele J, Ruehl W, Finston R, Day-Lollini P, Goris ML. Determinants of the antitumor effect of radiolabeled monoclonal antibodies. Cancer Res 50:4935–4940, 1990.
7. Nourigat CL, Badger CC, Bernstein ID. Treatment of lymphoma with radiolabeled antibody: elimination of tumor cells lacking target antigen. J Natl Cancer Inst 82:47–50, 1990.
8. Schmidberger H, Buchsbaum DJ, Blazar BR, Everson P, Vallera DA. Radiotherapy in mice with yttrium-90-labeled anti-Ly1 monoclonal antibody: therapy of the T cell lymphoma EL4. Cancer Res 51:1883–1890, 1991.
9. Matthews DC, Appelbaum FR, Eary JF, Hui TE, Fisher DR, Martin PJ, Durack LD, Nelp WB, Press OW, Badger CC, Bernstein ID. Radiolabeled anti-CD45 monoclonal antibodies target lymphohematopoietic tissue in the macaque. Blood 78:1864–1874, 1991.
10. Matthews DC, Badger CC, Fisher DR, Hui TE, Nourigat C, Appelbaum FR, Martin PJ, Bernstein ID. Selective radiation of hematolymphoid tissue delivered by anti-CD45 antibody. Cancer Res 52:1228–1234, 1992.
11. van der Jagt RH, Badger CC, Appelbaum FR, Press OW, Matthews DC, Eary JF, Krohn KA, Bernstein ID. Localization of radiolabeled antimyeloid antibodies in a human acute leukemia xenograft tumor model. Cancer Res 52:89–94, 1992.
12 Buchsbaum DJ, Wahl RL, Normolle DP, Kaminski MS. Therapy with unlabeled and ^{131}I-labeled pan-B-cell monoclonal antibodies in nude mice bearing Raji Burkitt's lymphoma xenografts. Cancer Res 52:6476–6481, 1992.
13. Huneke RB, Pippin CG, Squire RA, Brechbiel MW, Gansow OA, Strand M. Effective alpha-particle radioimmunotherapy of murine leukemia. Cancer Res 52:5818–5820, 1992.
14. Lenhard RE Jr., Order SE, Spunberg JJ, Asbell SO, Leibel SA. Isotopic immunoglobulin: a new systemic therapy for advanced Hodgkin's disease. J Clin Oncol 3:1296–1300, 1985.

137

15. Rosen ST, Zimmer AM, Goldman-Leiken R, Gordon LI, Kazikiewicz JM, Kaplan EH, Variakojis D, Marder RJ, Dykewicz MS, Piergies A, Silverstein EA, Roenigk HH Jr., Spies SM. Radioimmunodetection and radioimmunotherapy of cutaneous T-cell lymphomas using an ^{131}I-labeled monoclonal antibody: an Illinois Cancer Council Study. J Clin Oncol 5:562–573, 1987.
16. Press OW, Eary JF, Badger CC, Martin PJ, Appelbaum FR, Levy R, Miller R, Brown S, Nelp WB, Krohn KA, Fisher D, DeSantes K, Porter B, Kidd P, Thomas ED, Bernstein ID. Treatment of refractory non-Hodgkin's lymphoma with radiolabeled MB-1 (anti-CD37) antibody. J Clin Oncol 7:1027–1038, 1989.
17. DeNardo GL, DeNardo SJ, O'Grady LF, Levy NB, Adams GP, Mills SL. Fractionated radioimmunotherapy of B-cell malignancies with [131]I Lym-1. Cancer Res 50:1014s–1016s, 1990.
18. Scheinberg DA, Straus DJ, Yeh SD, Divgi C, Garin-Chesa P, Graham M, Pentlow K, Coit D, Oettgen HF, Old LJ. A phase I toxicity, pharmacology, and dosimetry trial of monoclonal antibody OKB7 in patients with non-Hodgkin's lymphoma: effects of tumor burden and antigen expression. J Clin Oncol 8:792–803, 1990.
19. Parker BA, Vassos AB, Halpern SE, Miller Ra, Hupf H, Amox DG, Simoni JL, Starr RJ, Green MR, Royston I. Radioimmunotherapy of human B-cell lymphoma with 90Y-conjugated antiidiotype monoclonal antibody. Cancer Res 50:1022s, 1990.
20. Vriesendorp HM, Herpst JM, Germack MA, Klein JL, Leichner PK, Loudenslager DM, Order SE. Phase I–II studies of yttrium-labeled antiferritin treatment for end-stage Hodgkin's disease. J Clin Oncol 9:918–928, 1991.
21. Goldenberg DM, Horowitz JA, Sharkey RM, Hall TC, Murthy S, Goldenberg H, Lee RE, Stein R, Siegel JA, Izon DO, Burger K, Swayne LC, Belisle E, Hansen HJ, Pinsky CM. Targeting, dosimetry, and radioimmunotherapy of B-cell lymphomas with iodine-131-labeled LL2 monoclonal antibody. J Clin Oncol 9:548–564, 1991.
22. Scheinberg DA, Lovett D, Divgi CR, Graham MC, Berman E, Pentlow K, Feirt N, Finn RD, Clarkson BD, Gee TS, Larson SM, Oettgen HF, Old LJ. A phase I trial of monoclonal antibody M195 in acute myelogenous leukemia: specific bone morrow targeting and internalization of radionuclide. J Clin Oncol 9:478–490, 1991.
23. Appelbaum FR, Matthews DC, Eary JF, Badger CC, Kellogg M, Press OW, Martin PJ, Fisher DR, Nelp WB, Thomas ED, Bernstein ID. The use of radiolabeled anti-CD33 antibody to augment marrow irradiation prior to marrow transplantation for acute myelogenous leukemia. Transplantation 54:829–833, 1992.
24. Waldmann TA, Pastan IH, Gansow OA, Junghans RP. The multichain interleukin-2 receptor: a target for immunotherapy. Ann Intern Med 116:148–160, 1992.
25. Kaminski MS, Zasadny KR, Francis IR, Milik AW, Ross CW, Moon SD, Crawford SM, Brugess JM, Petry NA, Butchko GM, Glenn SD, Wahl RL. Radioimmunotherapy of B-cell lymphoma with ^{131}I] anti-B1 (anti-CD20) antibody. N Engl J Med 329:459–465, 1993.
26. Press OW, Eary JF, Appelbaum FR, Martin PJ, Badger CC, Nelp WB, Glenn S, Butchko G, Fisher D, Porter B, Matthews DC, Fisher LD, Bernstein ID. Radiolabeled antibody therapy of B cell lymphomas with autologous bone marrow support. N Engl J Med 329:1219–1224, 1993.
27. Bierman PJ, Vose JM, Leichner PK, Quadri SM, Armitage JO, Klein JL, Abrams RA, Dicke KA, Vriesendorp HM. Yttrium 90-labeled antiferritin followed by high-dose chemotherapy and autologous bone marrow transplantation for poor-prognosis Hodgkin's disease. J Clin Oncol 11:698–703, 1993.
28. Matthews DC, Appelbaum FR, Eary JF, Fisher DR, Durack LD, Bush SA, Hui TE, Martin PJ, Mitchell D, Press. OW, Badger CC, Storb R, Nelp WB, Bernstein ID. Development of a marrow transplant regimen for acute leukemia using targeted hematopoietic irradiation delivered by ^{131}I-labeled anti-CD45 antibody, combined with cyclophosphamide and total body irradiation. Blood 85:1122–1131, 1995.
29. Press OW, Eary JF, Appelbaum FR, Martin PJ. Nelp WB, Glenn S, Fisher DR, Porter B, Matthews DC, Gooley T, Bernstein ID. Phase II trial of ^{131}I-B1 (anti-CD20) antibody therapy

with autologous stem cell transplantation for relapsed B cell lymphomas. Lancet 346:336–340, 1995.

30. Herpst JM, Klein JL, Leichner PK, Quadri SM, Vriesendorp HM. Survival of patients with resistant Hodgkin's disease after polyclonal yttrium 90-labeled antiferritin treatment. J Clin Oncol 13:2394–2400, 1995.

31. Society of Nuclear Medicine. MIRD Primer for Absorbed Dose Calculations. Washington, D.C.: Society of Nuclear Medicine, 1988.

32. Christy M, Eckerman KF. Specific Absorbed Fractions of Energy at Various Ages from Internal Photon Sources. ORNL/TM-8381, vols. 1–7. Oak Ridge, TN: Oak Ridge National Laboratory, 1987.

33. Fisher DR, Badger CC, Breitz H, Eary JF, Durham JS, Hui TE, Hill RL, Nelp WB. Internal radiation dosimetry for clinical testing of radiolabeled monoclonal antibodies. Antib Immunoconj Radiopharm 4:655–664, 1991.

34. Schwartz MA, Lovett DR, Redner A, Finn RD, Graham MC, Divgi CR, Dantis L, Gee TS, Andreeff M, Old LJ, Larson SM, Scheinberg DA. Dose-escalation trial of M195 labeled with Iodine 131 for cytoreduction and marrow ablation in relapsed or refractory myeloid leukemias. J Clin Oncol 11:294–303, 1993.

35. Papadopoulos EB, Caron P, Castor-Malaspina H, Childs B, Mackinnon S, Young JW, Jurcic, J, Finn R, Larson S, O'Reilly RJ, Scheinberg DA. Results of allogeneic bone marrow transplant following ^{131}I-M195/busulfan/cyclophosphamide (BU/CY) in patients with advanced/refractory myeloid malignancies. Blood 82:80a, 1993.

36. Caron PC, Jurcic JG, Scott AM, Finn RD, Divgi CR, Graham MC, Jureidini IM, Sgouros G, Tyson D, Old LJ, Larson SM, Scheinberg DA. A phase 1B trial of humanized monoclonal antibody M195 (Anti-CD33) in myeloid leukemia: specific targeting without immunogenicity. Blood 83:1760–1768, 1994.

37. Bianco JA, Sandmaier B, Brown PA, Badger C, Bernstein I, Eary J, Durack L, Schuening F, Storb R, Appelbaum F. Specific marrow localization of an ^{131}I-labeled anti-myeloid antibody in normal dogs: effects of a 'cold' antibody pretreatment dose of marrow localization. Exp Hematol 17:929–934, 1989.

38. Clift RA, Buckner CD, Thomas ED, Bensinger WI, Bowden R, Bryant E, Deeg HJ, Doney KC, Fisher LD, Hansen JA, Martin P, McDonald GB, Sanders JE, Schoch G, Singer J, Storb R, Sullivan KM, Witherspoon RP, Appelbaum FR. Marrow transplantation for chronic myeloid leukemia. A randomized study comparing cyclophosphamide and total body irradiation with busulfan and cyclophosphamide. Blood 84:2036–2043, 1994.

39. Yokota T, Milenic DE, Whitlow M, Schlom J. Rapid tumor penetration of single-chain Fv and comparison with other immunoglobulin forms. Cancer Res 52:3402–3408, 1992.

40. Axworthy DB, Fritzberg AR, Hylarides MD, Mallett RW, Theodore LJ, Gustavson LM, Su F, Beaumier PL, Reno JM. Preclinical evaluation of an anti-tumor monoclonal antibody/streptavidin conjugate for pretargeted ^{90}Y radioimmunotherapy in a mouse xenograft model. J Immunother 16:158, 1995.

41. Axworthy DB, Fritzberg AR, Hylarides MD, Mallett R, Theodore LJ, Gustavson L, Su F-M, Beaumier PL, Reno JM. Durable complete regressions of breast, lung and colon tumor xenografts with a single dose of pretargeted Y-90 in a mouse model. J Nucl Med 56:217P, 1995.

42. Ali S, Warren S, Richter K, Badger C, Eary J, Press O, Krohn K, Bernstein I, Nelp W. Improving the tumor retention of radiolabeled antibody: Aryl carbohydrate adducts. Cancer Res 50:783s–788s, 1990.

II

Sources of Hematopoietic Stem Cells and Their Ex Vivo Expansion

7. Peripheral blood stem cell harvesting and CD34-positive cell selection

Elizabeth J. Shpall, Pablo J. Cagnoni, Scott I. Bearman, Maureen Ross, Yago Nieto and Roy B. Jones

High-dose chemotherapy is effective treatment for patients with a variety of high-risk malignancies who have little chance of long-term survival with standard-dose regimens [1–3]. Such therapy produces profound myelosuppression that may be ameliorated by transplantation of allogeneic or autologous hematopoietic progenitor cells (AHPCs). The most conventional source of cells for repopulating the hematopoietic compartment has been bone marrow that is aspirated from the patient's iliac crests while under general anesthesia. Recently, peripheral blood progenitor cells (PBPCs) have replaced marrow as the major source of hematopoietic support. This shift from marrow to PBPCs occurred because many of the PBPC-supported studies have shown significantly faster engraftment rates, particularly for platelets, when compared to similar studies of conventional bone marrow transplants [1–5]. Additionally, the leukapheresis procedure is considered to be less morbid than a marrow harvest by most patients. Several studies with multiyear follow-up have now confirmed the durability of hematopoietic reconstitution produced with PBPCs as sole hematopoietic support, leading to the increased use of this technology [1,6–8].

The collection of peripheral blood progenitor cells

An outpatient leukapheresis procedure is performed for the collection of PBPCs. The procedure is typically performed over 3 to 6 hours on 1 to 5 consecutive days, using a continuous-flow blood cell separator. The COBE-Spectra and the Fenwall CS-3000 are the two most commonly employed leukapheresis machines. Approximately 9 to 20 liters of patient blood are processed with each procedure. The vast majority of the blood is returned to the patient. A final PBPC volume of approximately 80 to 200 mls is collected and in most cases cryopreserved. Patients then receive high-dose chemotherapy and/or radiotherapy followed by infusion of the thawed PBPC support. Within days of high-dose therapy administration, the patients develop profound myelosuppression, which is ameliorated by the hematopoietic cell transplant. The time to hematopoietic reconstitution or engraftment, which is

Jane N. Winter (ed.) BLOOD STEM CELL TRANSPLANTATION. 1997. Kluwer Academic Publishers. ISBN 0-7923-4260-7. All rights reserved.

commonly defined as a granulocyte count of 500 cells $\times$ 10^9/L and a platelet count of 20×10^9/L, reflects the quality of the infused progenitors.

Evaluation of a leukapheresis product

There is currently no universally accepted definition of the optimal leukapheresis product. Several different parameters considered to be surrogate markers of human hematopoietic-cell repopulating potential are used, including the total number of mononuclear cells, CD34-positive (+) cells [9], and myeloid progenitors measured as colony-forming units granulocyte-macrophage (CFU-GM) [8].

Studies have been published showing a correlation between engraftment rates and the PBPC graft content of mononuclear cells [10], CD34+ cells [9], and CFU-GM [8]. Other studies report no such correlation [11]. Given the lack of standardization among laboratories of the CD34 or CFU-GM assays, the total mononuclear cell count is probably the most consistent (although not necessarily the most predictive) parameter to discuss. Generally, transplant centers attempt to collect, per kilogram of patient weight, a total of $4.0-6.0 \times 10^8$ mononuclear cells, $1.5-5.0 \times 10^6$ CD34+ cells, and $0.5-30.0 \times 10^4$ CFU-GM. The number of leukaphereses performed to reach these target parameters depends upon whether the cells are collected from patients in a *steady state*, or following chemotherapy and/or growth factor treatment, which mobilizes the hematopoietic progenitors from the bone marrow to the peripheral blood. Whether tumor cells are also mobilized with chemotherapy and/or growth factors is unknown and under investigation.

Collection of PBPCs in the steady state

Steady state refers to the clinical situation in which patients have *not* received chemotherapy or growth factor treatment within several weeks of the leukapheresis procedure. In the steady state, six or more leukapheresis procedures may be required to reach one or more of the target parameters described above. This approach was employed initially, before the development of PBPC mobilization techniques. Kessinger et al. showed that patients who received nonmobilized PBPCs had a median recovery of granulocytes in eight days and platelets in 23 days [1]. This result was comparable to that of their patients who received autologous marrow support [10]. Williams et al. reported median time to granulocyte and platelet recovery of 15 and 42 days, respectively, with nonmobilized PBPCs [12]. In the latter study, delayed platelet recovery was noted in 22% of patients, which stimulated interest in the development of mobilization techniques to improve platelet recovery. Steady-state collections are now generally reserved for patients who are mobilization failures due to extensive prior therapy or substantial tumor cell contamination of the marrow [13].

Mobilization of PBPCs with chemotherapy

Mobilization refers to a treatment designed to stimulate the exodus of hematopoietic progenitors cells from the marrow cavity to the peripheral blood, where they can be collected via leukapheresis. Chemotherapy-induced mobilization occurs following administration of nonmyeloablative high-dose chemotherapy. The most commonly used mobilization regimen is cyclophosphamide in a single dose of 4 to 7 grams/m^2 [14]. As shown in figure 1, the patient's white blood count will decrease rapidly following the cyclophosphamide administration, with the lowest level or nadir occurring approximately 14 days later followed by a rapid rise back to the normal range. The patient is leukapheresed as the peripheral leukocyte count is recovering, generally beginning with the first day that the leukocyte count reaches $1-2 \times 10^9$/L, with collections continuing daily for 3 to 4 consecutive days.

Chemotherapy-mobilized PBPCs have been shown to contain a significantly higher CFU-GM content than those collected in the steady state [6]. To

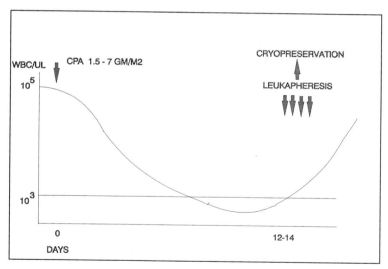

Figure 1. Chemotherapy-induced mobilization of peripheral blood progenitor cells. Cyclophosphamide in a single dose of 4–7 grams/m^2 is administered on day 0. The patient's white blood count will decrease rapidly, with the lowest level (or nadir) occurring approximately 14 days later, followed by a rapid rise back to the normal range. The patient is leukapheresed as the peripheral leukocyte count is recovering, generally beginning with the first day that the leukocyte count reaches $1-2 \times 10^6$/μl, with collections continuing daily for 3 to 4 consecutive days. WBC/μl, white blood cell count per microliter; CPA, cyclophosphamide.

et al. reported that patients who received chemotherapy-mobilized PBPCs had a significantly faster recovery of both granulocytes and platelets (11 and 13.5 days, respectively) than patients who received either autologous marrow support (22 and 32 days, respectively) or allogeneic marrow support (24.5 and 33 days, respectively) [15]. Other studies reported similar data, with hematopoietic recovery occurring approximately one week earlier when chemotherapy-mobilized PBPCs are compared to marrow support [11,16]. The drawback to this technique is the lack of standardization with respect to the chemotherapy mobilization regimens employed and the optimal timing of collections. With patient to patient variability in the time to marrow recovery, it can be difficult to predict when to schedule the leukapheresis. Additionally, giving the high-doses of cyclophosphamide without growth factor support has been associated with neutropenic fevers, which have rarely resulted in toxic death [6].

Mobilization of PBPCs with recombinant growth factors

The recombinant growth factors granulocyte colony stimulating factor (G-CSF) [3,4,17], granulocyte-macrophage colony stimulating factor (GM-CSF) [4,18–20], and more recently, interleukin-3 (IL-3) [21] have been administered for PBPC mobilization. As shown in figure 2, the growth factor is typically

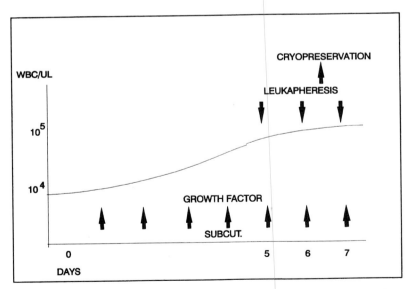

Figure 2. Growth-factor-induced mobilization of peripheral blood progenitor cells. The growth factor is typically administered for several days, with the leukophereses performed during the final consecutive days of therapy (i.e., days 5, 6, and 7 of a growth factor course). WBC/µl, white blood cell count per microliter.

146

administered for 6 to 8 days, with 3 to 6 leukaphereses performed during the final days of therapy (i.e., days 5, 6, and 7 of six-day growth factor course). As with chemotherapy-induced mobilization, the number of CFU-GM in the peripheral blood is substantially higher following treatment with G-CSF [22] and GM-CSF [23] when compared to the steady state. The reproducibility of growth factor-induced mobilization makes this approach logistically easier to arrange than mobilization with chemotherapy.

A consistent finding among studies that employed G-CSF- or GM-CSF-mobilized PBPCs is improvement in the time to platelet recovery compared to that of historical controls who received no PBPC support. An example are the studies by Sheridan et al., where the time to reach a platelet count of 50×10^9/ L was shortened significantly from 39 days in patients who received marrow support to 15 days with G-CSF-mobilized PBPCs in addition to marrow [3]. Of interest in that study were the bone marrow biopsy results at engraftment, which showed normal or increased numbers of megakaryocytes in 7 of 11 patients (64%) who received G-CSF-mobilized PBPCs, compared to 18 control patients whose biopsies showed no evidence of megakaryocyte production [3]. The reason platelet recovery is superior when mobilized PBPCs are used has not been definitively explained. It is likely that megakaryocyte precursors in the peripheral blood are elicited by the growth factor and/or chemotherapy mobilization regimens. Further study of this issue is warranted. Strategies to improve PBPC mobilization are in progress with combinations of growth factors [24–26], as well as chemotherapy plus growth factor regimens [27]. Additionally, the development of newer growth factors such as stem cell factor (SCF) may open new avenues of PBPC support [28].

In animal studies, SCF has been shown to stimulate more primitive hematopoietic cells than the other recombinant growth factors in clinical use [29]. The most impressive effects, however, have been demonstrated when SCF and G-CSF are combined. With a low dose of SCF plus G-CSF, synergistic increases in the number of PBPCs, CFU-GM, and the more primitive high proliferative potential colony-forming cells (HPP-CFC) have been demonstrated [30]. Andrews et al. reported similar data in their primate studies [31]. These preclinical data suggested that SCF plus G-CSF may produce a PBPC product that requires fewer leukaphereses and contains higher numbers of both myeloid and megakaryocytic precursors than PBPCs mobilized with the individual growth factors described above. Glaspy et al. reported the preliminary results of G-CSF with or without SCF for PBPC mobilization in patients with high-risk breast cancer prior to high-dose chemotherapy [32]. This study showed that the combination of SCF 15 ug/kg with G-CSF 10 ug/kg/d increased the number of mononuclear cells in the pheresis product when compared with either G-CSF (same dose) or SCF (5 ug/kg) alone. The use of SCF was associated with local injection site reactions, but no generalized adverse side effects occurred. These preliminary clinical results appear to confirm preclinical studies, and suggest that the use of SCF in combination with G-CSF might reduce the number of aphereses required prior to high-dose chemotherapy. A randomized phase III study of G-CSF versus SCF + G-CSF to confirm these results is currently ongoing.

Tumor-cell contamination of peripheral blood progenitor cells

Over the past few years, PBPCs have been employed as a substitute for bone marrow in patients with known marrow metastases due to the belief that peripheral blood contained fewer tumor cells than the corresponding marrow [33]. Although this may still be the case, the recent development of sensitive detection techniques, as shown in the representative studies summarized in tables 1 and 2, have revealed that contamination of peripheral blood with malignant cells is common, and much more prevalent than routine histology would suggest [17,34–38]. Brugger et al. have shown that the percentage of patients with tumor cells in PBPC collections markedly increased following mobilization with chemotherapy and growth factors [39]. Their study was not able to determine, however, whether the increase in circulating tumor cells had an impact on clinical outcome. Vredenburgh et al. recently reported that

Table 1. Detection of breast cancer cells in marrow and PBPC fractions

%Marrow+	%PBPC+	Method	Sensitivity	Reference
37	24	Immunostain	$1: 1 \times 10^6$	Shpall [38]
42	16	Culture	$1: 1 \times 10^5$	Sharp [35]
56	22/78	Immunostain	$1: 4 \times 10^5$	Brugger [39]
62	10	Immunostain	$1: 5 \times 10^5$	Ross [37]

Four different studies reported the percent of breast cancer patients with metastases documented in their bone marrow (column 1) and corresponding peripheral blood progenitor cell (column 2) fractions, using sensitive detection methods (column 3) that included immunohistochemistry or long-term culture. The sensitivity of the assay used (column 4) and the reference (column 5) are described.

Table 2. Detection of non-Hodgkin's lymphoma in marrow and PBPC fractions

%Marrow+	%PBPC+	Method	Sensitivity	Reference
36	5	Culture	$1: 1 \times 10^5$	Sharp [35]
100	50	PCR	$1: 1 \times 10^6$	Gribben [41]
100	86	PCR	$1: 1 \times 10^5$	Negrin [34]

Three different studies reported the percent of non-Hodgkins lymphoma patients with metastases documented in their bone marrow (column 1) and corresponding peripheral blood progenitor cell (column 2) fractions, using sensitive detection methods (column 3) that included polymerase chain reaction assays or long-term culture. The sensitivity of the assay used (column 4) and the reference (column 5) are described.

148

the presence of occult bone marrow micrometastases is a poor prognostic factor in patients with high-risk breast cancer that undergo high-dose chemotherapy with AHPC support [40]. Infusion of bone marrow containing residual tumor detected by polymerase chain reaction (PCR) was associated with a significantly higher relapse rate in non-Hodgkin's lymphoma patients than infusion of marrow that was normal by PCR analysis [41].

Whether the infusion of tumor in PBPC autografts will have an impact on clinical outcome remains to be determined. Results of a study conducted by Rill and collaborators suggests that it might. The investigators marked the bone marrow cells of patients with neuroblastoma and leukemia using retroviral gene-mediated transfer of a neomycin-resistant gene. The majority of patients who have relapsed have phenotypic and genotypic evidence of the marker gene in the malignant cells [42]. Many different methods have been developed to purge the bone marrow of contaminated tumor cells. Because of potential toxicity to the progenitors, chemical or immunologic purging of PBPCs has not been extensively studied. This fact stimulated the investigation of positive selection methods by which CD34+ progenitors could be isolated from the malignant cells for clinical use, thus depleting the grafts of tumor without untoward toxicity to the normal progenitors.

Positive selection of CD34+ hematopoietic progenitor cells

The CD34 antigen is expressed on both the pluripotent and committed hematopoietic progenitors, but not on NHL, myeloma and most solid tumors [43]. A number of methods are being investigated preclinically or clinically for the isolation of CD34+ hematopoietic progenitor cells. All employ one of the many monoclonal antibodies summarized in table 3 that target different epitopes on the human CD34 antigen [15,44–50]. With most of the methods, separation is effected by collection of the antibody-sensitized cells onto a solid

Table 3. Monoclonal antibodies that target the CD34 antgen

Anti-CD34 antibody	Investigator	Reference
12.8	Andrews	[43]
MY 10	Civin	[44]
B1.3C5	Katz	[45]
ICH3	Watt	[46]
QBend 10	Fina	[47]
Tuk3	Uchanska	[48]
9C5	Landsdorp	[49]

These antibodies interact with different epitopes on the human CD34 antigen, which is expressed by 1% to 4% of normal bone marrow cells, including those progenitors required for short- and long-term engraftment.

phase such as magnetic beads, plastic plates, or columns of nonmagnetic particles, while nontarget cells remain in suspension. Alternatively, high-speed flow cytometry has been employed to sort subpopulations of CD34+ cells identified by their failure to bind monoclonal antibodies directed against differentiation-associated antigens [50]. All the methods described below have been used to isolate CD34+ cells from bone marrow, peripheral blood, and umbilical cord blood.

Immunomagnetic selection

Superparamagnetic microspheres (Dynal Inc, Trondheim Norway) were initially used widely in purging regimens and more recently have been used in positive selection procedures. These polystyrene beads are 0.45 nm in diameter and contain 20% magnetite by weight dispersed throughout their volume. More recently, they have been employed in a positive selection procedure for the isolation of CD34+ cells using the Isolex device containing permanent magnets (Baxter Biotech/Dynal Inc). Hematopoietic cells are sensitized with the anti-CD34 antibody 9C5 developed by Lansdorp et al. [49], which results in rosetting between the target cells and the immunobeads. Collection of the rosetted cells is accomplished by sliding a built-in array of permanent magnets into direct contact with the chamber containing the rossetted cells; the nonadherent cells are drained from the chamber by gravity. Chymopapain is added, which will cleave the epitope where the antibody is attached, releasing the cells from the beads. The beads are then collected with the magnets, and the released CD34+ cells are drained from the chamber [51]. In a clinical study, Civin et al. used immunomagnetically isolated CD34+ bone marrow progenitors to support the high-dose therapy regimens of pediatric solid tumors patients [52]. The mean CD34 purity achieved was 60.4%, with an average recovery of 35.3%. The patients received a mean of 1.33×10^6 CD34+ cells/kg. Engraftment, defined as a white blood cell count of 1.0×10^9/L, was achieved in an average of 34 days, and a platelet count of 50.0×10^9/L was achieved in an average of 39 days. These engraftment rates were similar to those obtained historically using unmanipulated bone marrows in similarly treated patients. Williams et al. reported results from a clinical study where CD34+ PBPCs were successfully isolated using the Isolex device and then cultured ex vivo prior to transplantation [53].

More recently, a direct immunomagnetic separation method that employs microspheres precoated with anti-CD34 monoclonal antibody (Dynabeads CD34) has been studied. The beads are subsequently detached from the CD34+ cells with an anti-mouse Fab polyclonal antibody commercially available as the 'Detachabead' [54]. Clinical application of this method is being evaluated.

A newer immunomagnetic technique, developed by Miltenyi et al. (now in collaboration with Amcell Inc.), uses biodegradable paramagnetic nanoparticles, rather than larger microspheres, as the solid phase for collection of the target CD34+ cells [55]. The hematopoietic cells are incubated with the anti-CD34 monoclonal antibody Q-BEND 10, washed, and mixed with the 60 nm iron-dextran paramagnetic microspheres that recognize the monoclonal antibody. A high gradient field is then used to attract and retain the rosetted target cells. Non-CD34+ cells flow through the column, and the CD34+ cells are then collected by removing the column from the magnetic field and thus demagnetizing it. Preclinical studies demonstrate that the system can routinely produce positively selected hematopoietic fractions with more than 93% CD34+ cells. A prototype clinical-scale system has recently been developed (AmCell Inc.). Using this AmCell device, positive selection of G-CSF-mobilized leukapheresis products donated for research by University of Colorado transplant patients have contained an average of 89% CD34+ cells. Clinical studies with this device will soon be initiated.

Immunoadherent selection

The CELLector device (Applied Immune Sciences Inc.) consists of polystyrene surfaces in the form of cell culture flasks or multiple layered sheets onto which soybean agglutinin or the anti-CD34 monoclonal antibody ICH3 have been covalently bound [56]. This method involves a two-step separation with sequential negative and positive selection procedures. In the first step, the hematopoietic cells are incubated with soybean agglutinin (SBA)-coated flasks to debulk the sample of irrelevant CD34-negative cells. In the second step, flasks coated with the anti-CD34 monoclonal antibodies are loaded with the SBA-depleted cells. After incubation, the CD34-selected cells are drained and concentrated. Incubation of the cells in the SBA device results in removal of B cells, erythrocytes, fat cells, fibroblasts, endothelial cells, and certain T cells and tumor cells. The final product obtained from preclinical bone marrow studies contained 30% of the original number of CD34+ cells with a purity of 74.2% [57]. Clinical studies with this device have not yet been initiated.

Flow cytometry

Sorting of CD34+ cells by flow cytometry has been performed successfully to simultaneously isolate highly purified CD34+ subpopulations on the basis of multiple surface antigens from small hematopoietic specimens [58]. The use of flow cytometry as a single method to separate large volumes of hematopoietic cells for clinical use, however, has many inherent technologic problems that are unlikely to be overcome. Cell yields are typically insufficient for clinical use, thereby limiting the feasibility of fast, effective isolation of rare cell populations. The maximal rate at which cells can be sorted with a standard flow cytometer (approximately 5–10×10^3/second) makes the time required to perform a clinical separation technically difficult. Systemix Inc. has developed a system whereby a series of depletion steps are performed to eliminate the committed (lineage+) progenitors prior to high-speed cell sorting for CD34-positive cell enrichment, which makes the procedure feasible, with less than six hours required to complete the selection procedure [59]. There are advantages to using such a system, however, which produces a CD34+ cell product higher in purity than the selected fractions produced with any of the other methods described in this chapter. Approximately 40% to 60% of acute and chronic leukemias express the CD34 antigen [60]. The malignant cells have been shown to be eradicated, however, when highly purified CD34+/lineage-negative subpopulations are isolated. Since acute and chronic leukemia are potentially curable with hematopoietic-cell-supported high-dose therapy, the clinical development of highly purified hematopoietic cell subpopulations might increase the number of patients who could benefit from this therapeutic approach. Preliminary preclinical results with molecular detection techniques demonstrated a substantial (6–7 log) depletion of myeloma cells from patient marrow and/or blood using this high-speed method [59]. A clinical trial using this technology has recently been initiated for multiple myeloma patients receiving double transplants. The engraftment rates from the first transplant have been acceptable in three of the first four patients entered on study [59]. Further data will be forthcoming from this study.

Immunoadsorption

At the University of Colorado, CD34+ hematopoietic progenitor cells have been isolated from high-risk breast cancer patients using an immuno-adsorption technique. The hematopoietic cell fractions were incubated with the biotinylated anti-CD34 antibody 12.8. The coated cells were applied to a column of avidin coated beads (CellPro Inc, Bothell, WA), and the CD34+ cells were isolated and cryopreserved [17]. A total of 130 patients have received CD34 selected bone marrow and/or PBPCs. Engraftment rates were comparable to those obtained when unmanipulated bone marrow or PBPCs were used. Immunohistochemical staining for breast cancer was performed on all grafts before and after the CD34-selection [61]. For the initial 35 patients with evidence of breast cancer in the graft prior to positive selection, an average two-log depletion of breast cancer cells was documented (range 1 to more than 4). The disease-free survival for these patients is shown in figure 3. The disease-free survival for patients with immmunohistochemically negative hematopoietic cell grafts after CD34-selection was 45%. In contrast, for patients with hematopoietic cell grafts that remained positive despite CD34 selection, the disease-free survival is only 13%. This difference is statistically significant ($p = 0.035$). A multivariate analysis was performed [62]. The grafts that contained breast cancer before and after the CD34-selection procedure were used as reference, and several covariates, including grafts that became negative after the selection procedure, were analyzed. The purification of a graft to negativity independently predicted for a significantly better disease-free survival ($p = 0.005$). Longer follow-up will be required to assess the

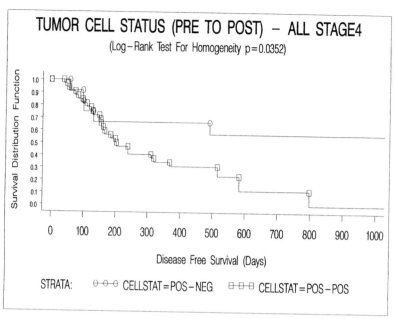

Figure 3. Breast cancer patients with tumor cells in hematopoietic fractions prior to positive selection. Immunohistochemical staining for breast cancer was performed on all grafts before and after the CD34 selection. The disease-free survival for the 47 stage-IV patients who had immuno-histochemical evidence of tumor in the marrow or blood prior to purification is shown. No breast cancer was detected in the hematopoietic grafts of 13 patients whose disease-free survival is shown in the top curve (45%). This result is significantly higher than that of the remaining 34 patients, represented in the lower curve (13%), whose grafts still contained tumor following positive selection (*p* = 0.035).

durability of engraftment produced with the CD34+ PBPCs, as well as the ultimate therapeutic effect of this approach.

The CellPro column is currently being evaluated in a wide variety of clinical settings. For autologous marrow transplantation, a randomized trial of CD34+ marrow versus buffy-coat support was completed for breast cancer patients receiving high-dose therapy [60]. A phase I–II trial with CD34+ PBPC support for patients with multiple myeloma was completed [63], and a randomized trial initiated in that disease. In the allogeneic transplant setting, the column is being evaluated as a means to T-deplete and thus reduce GVHD in patients receiving allogeneic hematopoietic cell support [64]. The column is also being used to isolate CD34+ marrow and PBPCs for gene transfer studies with the neomycin resistance gene in patients with multiple myeloma, chronic myelog-enous leukemia (CML), and breast cancer [58,65]. Similar studies are in progress using the multidrug resistance gene to transduce the CD34+ marrow cells of patients with CML [26].

In conclusion, the ongoing studies to optimize the collection and positive selection of PBPCs described in this chapter should bring many exciting advances to the field of stem cell transplantation over the next several years.

References

1. Kessinger A, Armitage JO, Landmark JD, Smith DM, Weisenburger D. Autologous peripheral hematopoietic stem cell transplantation restores hematopoietic function following marrow ablative therapy. Blood 71:723–727, 1988.
2. Juttner CA, To LB, Ho JQ, Bardy PG, Dyson PG, et al. Early lymphohematopoietic recovery after autografting using peripheral blood stem cells in acute nonlymphoblastic leukemia. Transplant Proc 20:40–42, 1988.
3. Peters WP, Davis R, Shpall EJ, Jones RB, Ross M, et al. Adjuvant chemotherapy involving high-dose combination CPA/BCNU/cDDP with bone marrow support for stage II/II breast cancer involving ten or more lymph nodes (CALGB 8782): a preliminary report. Proc Am Soc Clin Oncol 31:22, 1990.
4. Sheridan W, Begley CG, Juttner CA, Szer J, To LB, et al. Effect of peripheral blood progenitor cells mobilized by filgrastim (G-CSF) on platelet recovery after high-dose chemotherapy. Lancet 1:640–644, 1992.
5. Gianni AM, Bregni Siena S, Villa S, Sciorelli GA, et al. Rapid and complete hematopoietic reconstitution following combined transplantation of autologous blood and bone marrow cells. A changing role for high-dose chemoradiotherapy? Hematol Oncol 7:139–143, 1989.
6. Juttner CA, To LB, Roberts MM, Haylock D, Dyson PG, et al. Comparison of hematologic recovery, toxicity, and supportive care of autologous PBSC, autologous BM, and allogeneic BM transplants. Int J Cell Cloning 10:160, 1992.
7. Reiffers J, Castaigne S, Tilly H, Lepage E, Leverger G, et al. Hematopoietic reconstitution after autologous blood stem cell transplantation. A report of 46 cases. Plasma Ther Transfus Technol 8:360–364, 1987.
8. Stiff PJ, Murgo AJ, Wittes RE, et al. Quantification of peripheral blood colony forming unit-culture rise following chemotherapy: could leukocytaphereses replace bone marrow for autologous transplantation? Transfusion 23:500–503, 1983.
9. Sienna S, Bregni M, Brando B, Belli N, Ravagnani F, et al. Flow cytometry for clinical estimation of circulating hematopoietic progenitors for autologous transplantation in cancer patients. Blood 77:400–406, 1991.
10. Kessinger A, Armitage JO. The evolving role of autologous peripheral stem cell transplantation following high-dose therapy for malignancies. Blood 77:211–213, 1991.
11. Reiffers J, Faberes C, Commenges D, Marit G, Ferrer AM, et al. The CD34 assay is not of predictive value for engraftment after PBSC transplantation. Proc 2nd Int Symp Peripheral Blood Stem Cell Autografts. Mulhouse, France, 1991.
12. Williams SF, Bitran JD, Richards JM, DeChristopher PJ, Barker E, et al. Bone Marrow Transplant 5:129–133, 1990.
13. Cantin G, Marchand-Laroche D, Bouchard MM, Leblond PF. Blood-derived stem cell collection in acute nonlymphoblastic leukemia: predictive factors for a good yield. Exp Hematol 17:1991, 1989.
14. Juttner C, To LB. Peripheral blood stem cells: mobilization by myelosuppressive chemotherapy. Proc 5th Int Symp Autologous Bone Marrow Transplantation, Omaha, Nebraska. University of Nebraska Press, 1991, pp. 783–788.
15. To LB, Shepperd KM, Haylock DN, Dyson PG, Charles P, et al. Single high doses of cyclophosphamide enable the collection of high numbers of stem cells from the peripheral blood. Exp Hematol 18:442, 1990.
16. Kessinger A, Armitage JO, Smith DM, Landmark JD, Bierman PJ, Weisenburger D. High-dose therapy and autologous marrow peripheral blood stem cell transplantation for patients with lymphoma. Blood 74:1260, 1989.

154

17. Shpall EJ, Jones RB, Bearman SI, Franklin WA, Archer PG, et al. Transplantation of CD34-positive autologous marrow into breast cancer patients following high-dose chemotherapy: influence of CD34-positive peripheral-blood progenitors and growth factors on engraftment. J Clin Oncol 12:28–36, 1994.
18. Elias A, Mazanet R, Anderson K, Ayash L, Wheeler C, GM-CSF mobilized stem cell autografts. Proc 2nd Int Symp Peripheral Blood Stem Cell Autografts. Mulhouse, France, 1991.
19. Gianni AM, Siena S, Bregni M, Tarella C, Stern AC, et al. Granulocyte-macrophage colony stimulating factor to harvest circulating hematopoietic stem cells for autotransplantation. Lancet 2:580–586, 1989.
20. Haas R, Ho AD, Bredthauer U, Cayeux S, Egerer G, et al. Successful autologous transplantation of blood stem cells mobilized with recombinant human granulocyte-macrophage colony stimulating factor. Exp Hematol 18:94, 1990.
21. Vose JM, Kessinger A, Bierman P, Sharp G, Garrison L, Armitage JO. The use of rh-IL-3 for mobilization of peripheral blood stem cells in previously treated patients with lymphoid malignancies. Proc 2nd International Symposium on Peripheral Blood Stem Cell Autografts. Mulhouse, France, 1991.
22. Duhrsen U, Villeval JL, Boyd J, Kannourakis G, Morstyn G, Metcalf D. Effects of recombinant granulocyte colony stimulating factor on hematopoietic progenitor cells in cancer patients. Blood 72:2047–2081, 1988.
23. Socinski MA, Cannistra SA, Elias A, Antman KH, Schnipper L, Griffin JD. Granulocyte-macrophage colony stimulating factor expands the circulating hematopoietic progenitor cell compartment in man. Lancet 1:1194–1198, 1988.
24. McNiece I, Langley KE, Zsebo KM. Recombinant SCF synergizes with GM-CSF, G-CSF, IL-3 and Epo to stimulate human progenitor cells of the myeloid and erythroid lineages. Exp Hematol 19:226–231, 1992.
25. Hara H, Namiki M. Mechanism of synergy between GM-CSF and G-CSF in colony formation from human marrow cells in vitro. Exp Hematol 17:816–821, 1989.
26. Brucher J, Martin H, Hess U, Claude R, Ottmann G, et al. Interleukin-3 combined with rGM-CSF efficiently mobilizes circulating hematopoietic progenitor cells without prior chemotherapy. Proc 2nd Int Symp Peripheral Blood Stem Cell Autografts. Mulhouse, France, 1991.
27. Spitzer G, Huan SD, Hester J, Yau J, Dunphy F, et al. Influence of mobilized peripheral blood cells on the hematopoietic recovery from autologous marrow and recombinant granulocyte-macrophage colony stimulating factor (rhGM-CSF) following high-dose cyclophosphamide, etoposide, and cisplatin. Proc 2nd Int Symp Peripheral Blood Stem Cell Autografts. Mulhouse, France.
28. Zsebo K, Williams D, Geissler EN, Broudy VC, Martin FH, et al. Stem cell factor is encoded at the S1 locus of the mouse and is the ligand for the c-kit tyrosine kinase receptor. Cell 63:213–219, 1990.
29. Andrews RG, Bartelmez SH, Knitter GH, Myerson D, Bernstein ID, et al. A c-kit ligand, recombinant human stem cell factor mediates reversible expansion of CD34+ colony-forming cells types in blood and marrow of baboons. Blood 80:920–925, 1992.
30. Briddell RA, Hartley CA, Smith KA McNiece IK. Recombinant rat SCF synergizes with recombinant human G-CSF in vivo to mobilize PBPCs which have enhanced repopulating potential. Blood 82:1720–3, 1993.
31. Andrews RG, Appelbaum FR, Bensinger WI, McNiece IK, Bernstein ID, Zsebo K. Stem cell factor stimulates the in vivo expansion of hematopoietic progenitor cells and stimulates circulation of cells that engraft and rescue lethally irradiated recipients. Proc 6th Int Symp Autologous Bone Marrow Transplantation. Dicke K (ed), Houston, TX, 1992.
32. Glaspy J, McNiece I, LeMaistre F, Menchaca D, Briddell R, et al. Effects of stem cell factor (rhSCF) and filgrastim (rhG-CSF) on mobilization of peripheral blood progenitor cells (PBPC) and on hematological recovery posttransplant: early results from a phase I/II study. Proc Am Soc Clin Oncol 13:68, 1994.

33. Sharp JG, Armitage J, Grouse D, et al. Are occult tumor cells present in peripheral stem cell harvests of candidates for autologous transplantation? Proc 4th Int Symp Autologous Transplantation. Houston: M.D. Anderson Press, 1989, pp. 693–3.

34. Negrin RS, Pesando J, Long GD, Chao NJ, Horning SJ, Blume K. Comparison of tumor cell contamination of 'purged' bone marrow to peripheral blood mononuclear cells assessed by PCR in non-Hodgkin's lymphoma (abstract). Blood 80(Suppl 1):235a, 1992.

35. Sharp J, Kessinger A, Mann S, Crouse D, Dicke J, et al. Detection and clinical significance of minimal tumor cell contamination of peripheral blood stem cell harvests. Int J Cell Cloning 10:92–94, 1992.

36. Osborne MP, Wong GY, Gonzalez A, Potter C, Vlamis V, Cote RJ. Bone marrow micrometastases (BMM) in breast cancer: the effect of tumor cell (TC) burden on early relapse. Proc Am Soc Clin Oncol 12:75, 1993.

37. Ross AA, Cooper BW, Lazarus H, Peters WP, Vredenburgh JJ, et al. Incidence of tumor cell contamination in peripheral blood stem cell (PBSC) collections from breast cancer patients. Proc Am Soc Clin Oncol 12:68, 1993.

38. Shpall EJ, Jones RB. Release of tumor cells from bone marrow. Blood 83:623–625, 1994.

39. Brugger W, Bross KJ, Glatt M, Weber F, Mertelsman R, Kanz L. Mobilization of tumor cells and hematopoietic progenitor cells into peripheral blood of patients with solid tumors. Blood 83:636–640, 1994.

40. Vredenburgh J, Silva O, de Sombre K, Franklin W, Cirrincione C, et al. The significance of bone marrow micrometastases for patients with breast cancer and ≥10+ nodes treated with high-dose chemotherapy and hematopoietic support. Proc Am Soc Clin Oncol 14:317, 1995.

41. Gribben J, Freedman A, Neuberg D, Roy D, Blake K, et al. Immunologic purging of marrow assessed by PCR before autologous bone marrow transplantation for B-cell lymphoma. N Engl J Med 325:1525–1533, 1991.

42. Rill DR, Santana VM, Roberts WM, Nilson T, Bowman LC, et al. Direct demonstration that autologous bone marrow transplantation for solid tumors can return a multiplicity of tumorigenic cells. Blood 84:380–383, 1994.

43. Andrews RG, Singer JW, Bernstein ID. Monoclonal antibody 12–8 recognizes a 115-kd molecule present on both unipotent and multipotent hematopoietic coclony-forming cells and their precursors. Blood 67:842–845, 1986.

44. Civin CI, Strauss LC, Brovall C, Fackler MJ, Schwartz JF, Sharper JH. Antigenic analysis of hematopoiesis. III. A hematopoietic progenitor cell surface antigen defined by a monoclonal antibody raised against KG-1a cells. J Immunol 133:157–162, 1984.

45. Katz F, Tindle RW, Sutherland DR, Greaves MF. Identification of a membrane glycoprotein associated with hematopoietic progenitor cells. Leuk Res 9:191, 1985.

46. Watt SM, Karhi K, Gatter K, Furley A, Katz FE, Healy L, Atlass LJ, Bradley NJ, Sutherland DR, Levinsky R, Greaves MF. Distribution and epitope analysis of the cell membrane glycoprotein (HPCA-1) associated with human hematopoietic progenitor cells. Leukaemia 1:41, 1987.

47. Fina L, Molgaard HV, Robertson D, Bradley N, Monaghan P, Della D, Sutherland DR, Baker M, Greaves MF. Expression of the CD34 gene in vascular endothelial cells. Blood 74:2417, 1990.

48. Uchanska-Ziegler B, Petrasch S, Michel J, Ziegler A. Characterization of the CD34-specific monoclonal antibody TUK3. Tissue Antigens 33:230, 1989.

49. Lansdorp PM, Dragowska W, Mayani H. Ontogeny-related changes in proliferative potential of human hematopoietic cells. J Exp Med 178:787–791, 1993.

50. Uchida N, Combs A, Conti S, Chen S, Gianni A, Smith S, T Kholodenko, Chen B, Hoffman R, Tsukamota A. The in vivo hematopoietic population of a rhodamine 123 low population of human marrow. Exp Hematol 22:755, 1994.

51. Ishizawa L, Burgess J, Hardwick A, et al. In Wunder E, Sovalat H, Henon P, Serke S (eds), Hematopoietic Stem Cells: The Mulhouse Manual. Dayton, OH: AlphaMed, 1994, pp. 177–182.

52. Civin C, Trischmann T, Davis J, Noga S, Cohen B, Cohen K, Duffy B, Wiley J, Law P,

Hardwick A, Oldham F, Gee A. Highly purified CD34+ cells reconstitute hematopoiesis. Proc Am Soc Clin Oncol 14:437, 1995.

53. Williams SF, Lee WJ, Bender JG, Zimmerman T, Swinney P, Blake M, Carreon J, Schilling M, Smith S, Williams DE, Oldham F, Van Epps D. Selection and expansion of peripheral blood CD34+ cells in autologous stem cell transplantation for breast cancer. Blood 87:1687–91, 1996.

54. Herikstad BV, Lien E. In Wunder E, Sovalat H, Henon P, Serke S (eds), Hematopoietic Stem Cells: The Mulhouse Manual. Dayton, OH: AlphaMed, 1994, pp. 149–160.

55. Miltenyi S, Muller W, Weichel W, Radbruch A. High-gradient magnetic cell separation with MACS. Cytometry 11:231–236, 1994.

56. Lebkowski JS, Schain LR, Okrongly D, Levinsky R, Harvey MJ, Okarma TB. Rapid isolation of human CD34 hematopoietic stem cell-purging of human tumor cells. Transplantation 53:1011–1019, 1992.

57. Lebkowski J, Schain L, Harvey M, et al. In Wunder E, Sovalat H, Henon P, Serke S (eds), Hematopoietic Stem Cells: The Mulhouse Manual. Dayton OH: AlphaMed, 1994, pp. 2115–2230.

58. Uchida N, Combs A, Conti S, Chen S, Gianno A, Smith S, T Kholodenko, Chen B, Hoffman R, Tsukamoto A. The in vivo hematopoietic population of a rhodamine 123 low population of human marrow. Exp Hematol 22:755, 1994.

59. Redding C, Sasaki D, Leemhuis T, Tichenor E, Chen B, Tsao M, Gazitt Y, Trioct G, Hoffman R. Clinical scale purification of CD34 + Thy + lin-stem cells from mobilized peripheral blood by high-speed fluorescence-activated cell sorting for use as an autograft for multiple myeloma patients. Blood 84:399a, 1994.

60. Shpall EJ, Ball ED, Champlin RE, LeMaistre CF, Holland HK, Saral R, Hoffman E, Berenson RJ. A prospective randomized phase III study using the ceprate SC stem cell concentrator to isolate CD34+ hematopoietic progenitors for autologous marrow transplantation after high-dose chemotherapy. Blood 82:82a, 1993.

61. Franklin WA, Shpall EJ, Archer P, Johnston CS, Garza-Williams S, et al. Immunohistochemical detection and quantitation of metastatic breast cancer in human bone marrow and peripheral blood. Breast Cancer Res Treat, in press.

62. Cagnoni PJ, Jones RB, Franklin W, et al. Use of CD34-positive autologous hematopoietic progenitors to support patients with breast cancer after high-dose chemotherapy. Blood 86:386a, 1995.

63. Schiller G, Vescio R, Freytes C, et al. Transplantation of CD34+ peripheral blood progenitor cells after high-dose chemotherapy for patients with advanced multiple myeloma. Blood 86:390–397, 1995.

64. Link H, Arseniev L, Bahre O, Battmer K, Kadar J, Jacobs R, Lohmann D, Casper J, Kuhl J, Schubert J, Diedrich H, Poliwada H. Combined transplantation of allogeneic bone marrow and peripheral blood progenitor cells. Blood 84:713a, 1994.

65. Dunbar CE, Doren S, Sassel A, Fox M, Boine DM, O'Shaughnessy J, Sorrentino B, Donahue R, McDonagh D, Karlsson S, Liu J, Walsh C, Nienhuis AW. Gene transfer to hematopoietic stem cells. Cancer Gene Ther 1:142, 1994.

157

8. Ex vivo expansion of hematopoietic stem and progenitor cells for transplantation

Jennifer A. LaIuppa, E. Terry Papoutsakis, and William M. Miller

Over the past few years, there has been a heightened interest in the development of clinical-scale culture systems for ex vivo expansion of hematopoietic cells. Ex vivo expanded hematopoietic cells are useful for a variety of clinical applications such as transplantation, tumor purging, and gene therapy. The anticipated benefits of ex vivo expanded hematopoietic cells over bone marrow or peripheral blood for transplant patients include a shortened engraftment period following chemotherapy and reduction in the number of harvested bone marrow or peripheral blood progenitor cells required for an adequate autograft. However, several key issues need to be addressed before ex vivo expanded cells can be used clinically. The culture conditions and systems used for expansion of these cells will need to be established, since the growth factors and other culture parameters used in the expansion process greatly influence the lineage and maturation stage of the cells produced. These factors are considered below, along with regulatory and safety issues, with the goal of providing a framework for consistent and reproducible ex vivo expansion for clinical application.

Potential applications

Transplantation

Ex vivo expansion promises to improve the current methodology for blood cell progenitor transplantation following chemotherapy by increasing both the number and maturity of cells available for transplantation. One of the side effects associated with bone marrow (BM) transplantation is a period of chemotherapy-induced neutropenia and thrombocytopenia in which neutrophil counts take 26 days and platelet counts take 29 days to recover [1]. The recovery time for these cell types can be reduced by transplanting progenitors that have been mobilized into the peripheral blood (PB) with chemotherapy and/or growth factors. However, neutrophil recovery still takes approximately 8 to 9 days, and platelet recovery takes approximately 12 days [2]. Conceptually, the remaining period of cytopenia could be largely eliminated by admin-

Jane N. Winter (ed.) BLOOD STEM CELL TRANSPLANTATION. 1997. Kluwer Academic Publishers. ISBN 0-7923-4260-7. All rights reserved.

istering mature cells and late neutrophil and megakaryocyte progenitors derived from ex vivo expansion. Ex vivo expansion could also decrease the number of bone marrow or peripheral blood cells required to reconstitute hematopoiesis and/or provide the large numbers of cells needed to support multiple courses of high-dose chemotherapy. This would be a great benefit, since patients generally do not have enough cells available from a single harvest to support multiple infusions.

Tumor purging

Ex vivo expansion of hematopoietic cells also has the potential to purge tumor cells from the autograft, since in vitro culture conditions favor the maintenance of normal cells over leukemic cells [3]. Several theories have been advanced to explain the loss of leukemic cells in long-term cultures. The observation that clonogenic cells of chronic myeloid leukemia patients cannot attach to marrow stromal cells or to the extracellular matrix might indicate that their access to necessary factors is limited or that these factors are removed during feeding [4]. However, the differentiation of leukemic cells in culture might also explain their disappearance [3,5,6].

A number of clinical studies on tumor purging have been performed in which BM cells were cultured for 7 to 10 days prior to autologous transplantation [7–9]. While the results of these studies are promising, large-scale purging is not currently practical due to the large number of normal progenitor cells lost during culture and the substantial number of tissue culture flasks required for each patient. The large loss of progenitors could be overcome by ex vivo expansion using growth factors. Ex vivo expansion of cells could also be used to make up for loss of normal cells that are damaged during chemical or immunologic purging.

Gene therapy

Replacement of missing or damaged genes and introduction of new or modified genes into cellular targets are the primary goals of gene therapy. For example, if drug resistance genes could be introduced into hematopoietic stem cells to provide protection against chemotherapy, considerable dose escalation would be possible [10]. Recombinant retroviral vectors are the best characterized and only vector type currently used in clinical trials directed at the hematopoietic system [10]. However, other vector systems are under investigation. High-efficiency gene transfer and expression is routinely achieved in murine systems, but is less successful in large animal models. The rarity of stem cells makes gene transfer a difficult prospect. To complicate matters, hematopoietic stem cells are mostly quiescent and thus resistant to retroviral transduction [10]. Ex vivo expansion of hematopoietic cells would increase the percentage of primitive cells in the cell cycle. This effect, coupled with the resultant increase in primitive cell numbers, would increase the likelihood of

160

successful retroviral transduction. Improvements in retroviral transduction have already been achieved in vitro through addition of cytokines and a stromal layer [11,12]. An increased culture time has the potential to improve the process further.

Characterization of cells to measure culture performance

In vitro assays

As cells progress from stem cells to committed progenitors and then to mature cell types, they become more restricted in their developmental potential and highly proliferative. Various assays are used to evaluate the different stages of commitment. Committed progenitors are restricted to one of a few lineages such as granulocyte, monocyte, megakaryocyte, or erythrocyte. These progenitors are also known as colony-forming cells (CFCs) because of the assay commonly used for their detection. In the CFC assay, cells are plated in semisolid medium for two weeks in the presence of growth factors, after which time the plates are examined for colonies of mature blood cells. Colonies of greater than 50 cells are designated according to the mature cell types they produce: colony forming units-granulocyte, monocyte (CFU-GM), burst-forming unit-erythroid (BFU-E), and CFU-granulocyte, erythroid, monocyte, megakaryocyte (CFU-GEMM or CFU-mix).

Several assays are used for detection of earlier CFCs. The CFU-blast (CFU-Bl) assay detects an early hematopoietic cell type with high secondary recloning capacity [13]. The high proliferative potential CFU (HPP-CFU) assay detects colonies of greater than 0.5 mm diameter, containing greater than 50,000 cells per clone [14]. An assay for very primitive hematopoietic progenitors is the long-term culture-initiating cell (LTC-IC) assay [15]. LTC-IC assays are evaluated 5 to 8 weeks after initiation; more mature CFCs do not produce additional CFCs five weeks after initiation of long-term cultures, while primitive LTC-ICs sustain hematopoiesis in long-term cultures for 5 to 12 weeks.

Flow cytometry can be used to distinguish between various cell types produced in culture using fluorescently tagged antibodies against unique surface antigens. The percent of primitive (CD34$^+$) cells in a harvest or culture is commonly measured using this method. Some antigens used for detection of mature cell lineages are CD15 (granulocyte), CD11b (monocyte), glycophorin A (erythrocyte), and CD41a (megakaryocyte).

In vivo assays

In contrast with the murine system, direct evidence that human hematopoietic stem cells have the potential for self-renewal, to differentiate into multiple lineages, and to populate the marrow has been difficult to obtain due to the lack of an appropriate in vivo assay system. Nevertheless, in vivo assays for human hematopoietic stem cells have been devised using immunodeficient mice [16,17] or fetal sheep [18]. Implantation of immunodeficient mice with either human fetal liver along with thymus [16,19] or with fetal bone containing marrow [20] has resulted in maintenance of multilineage human hematopoietic activity within the graft for as long as 20 weeks. Transplantation of human adult BM cells [21], human CD34+HLA-DR− BM cells [22], or human fetal liver cells [18] in utero into preimmune fetal sheep has resulted in the establishment and maintenance of chimeric human hematopoiesis with differentiation into all blood cell lineages. While these assays show that human stem cells partially repopulate the myeloid and lymphoid compartments of the foreign host, the assays are not quantitative.

Cell sources and cell processing

Cell sources

Several sources of stem cells and progenitors are used in hematopoietic cell cultures: BM, umbilical cord blood (CB), and PB. BM harvests yield 1 to 2 liters of a mix of hematopoietic cells, stromal cells, and extracellular matrix. Unfortunately, the procedure is very invasive and must be performed under general or spinal anesthesia. CB from newborns is another rich source of hematopoietic stem cells and progenitors. The major limitation here is the small volume of CB obtained from a newborn — typically 60–150 ml — which limits the number of cells that can be obtained. PB harvests involve several hours of blood processing on apheresis machines, which collect the fraction of blood containing stem cells and progenitors. Harvest of normal PB furnishes very few hematopoietic progenitors. However, progenitors can be mobilized from the BM into the circulation through administration of growth factors. The number of progenitors in PB is also increased during the recovery period following chemotherapy. The number of progenitors mobilized into the PB varies with the mobilization regimen utilized. While 1% to 3% of cells harvested from BM or CB are CD34+ cells [23], harvests from mobilized PB show more variation in the percentage of CD34+ cells, ranging from 0.1% to 16.4% [24]. The distribution of the types of CFC (CFU-GM, BFU-E, CFU-mix) also varies depending on the cell source [25,26]. Thus, the performance of the cells expanded ex vivo would be expected to vary depending on the source from which they are derived.

Cell processing

Hematopoietic culture has been performed using samples that vary significantly in stem cell purity, ranging from unprocessed cells to highly purified primitive cells. Several different procedures are used to enrich for stem cells

162

and progenitors, since these cells are present at low levels in hematopoietic tissues. In the majority of hematopoietic cultures performed with mono-nuclear cells (MNCs), samples are density separated using Ficoll or Percoll to remove erythrocytes and mature neutrophils. The most common methods for further enrichment of primitive cells involve immunological selection for the CD34 cell surface marker. CD34+ cells can be selected in polystyrene flasks containing covalently attached antibodies to CD34 [27], with antibody-coated magnetic beads that bind anti-CD34 antibody [28], and on an avidin column using biotinylated anti-CD34 antibody [29]. The purity of the CD34+ cells obtained from these selection procedures covers a wide range.

There are several advantages to using purified progenitor (CD34+) cells in hematopoietic cultures. Selection of primitive progenitors can be used as a tumor-purging method in CD34- malignancies [30] or can be used along with additional selection steps for CD34+ malignancies [31]. Use of the CD34+ cell fraction minimizes the complicated interactions that occur between different cell types and eliminates accessory cells, which may produce inhibitory factors. The initial culture size will be reduced when using CD34+ cells, since the majority of the mature cells are eliminated. Culture size is an important factor for implementation of ex vivo expansion in clinical practice for transplantation and gene therapy, since larger cultures require more growth factors, medium, and equipment. However, the cells lost through the purification procedures may have a significant impact on culture productivity. Experiments with CB have shown that significant numbers of primitive cells are lost by density separation procedures [32], while procedures for enrichment of CD34+ cells also result in significant cell losses [29,33–35]. The CD34+ depleted fraction of cells has been found to contain approximately 37% of the CFU-GM [36] and 11% to 38% of the LTC-ICs [36–38]. The accessory cells and stromal cells eliminated in CD34+ selections are also important for expansion of primitive progenitors, since the addition of unknown factors produced by stromal cells to cultures of CD34+ cells increases the number of LTC-ICs produced [39].

Several studies performed in perfusion bioreactors have compared the effect of varying degrees of CD34+ cell purification on CFU-GM and LTC-IC expansion. Expansion of PB MNCs was compared to that of CD34+ cells by Sandstrom et al. [38], and the expansion potential of unprocessed, density-separated, and CD34+ BM cells was evaluated by Koller et al. [36]. When taking into account the number of cells lost in the separation procedures, the unprocessed or density-separated cultures gave greater production of colony-forming cells [36,38] and LTC-IC numbers [38] than a CD34+ fraction of the same sample (table 1). After 10 to 14 days, the cultures showed similar cell morphology, antigen expression (figure 1), and colony formation whether or not they were enriched for CD34+ cells [36,38]. While the additional manipulations involved in CD34+ selection may be useful for some applications, such as tumor purging, these extra processing steps are not necessary for progenitor expansion.

163

Table 1. Viable cells, CFU-GM, and LTC-ICs that would be produced from an initial sample of 10^9 PB MNCs cultured in perfusion as either MNCs or CD34+ cells

	Day	Mean MNCs[a]	Mean CD34+ cells[a]
Cells ($\times10^6$)	0	1000	38
	10	2661	1494
CFU-GM ($\times10^4$)	0	416	165
	10	7424	3039
LTC-ICs ($\times10^3$)	0	1532	649
	10	2609	547

[a] Obtained from the average of six experiments. PB cells were cultured in serum-containing medium supplemented with IL-3, IL-6, G-CSF, and SCF. A significant statistical difference ($p \leq 0.01$) between the MNCs and CD34+ cell cultures was found for all conditions using a paired student's t-test.
Adapted from [38].

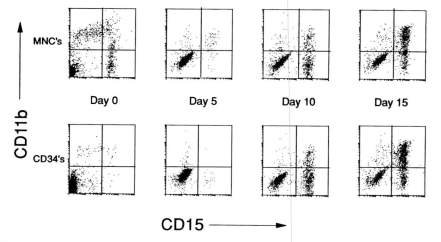

Figure 1. Two-dimensional flow cytometric analysis of MNCs and CD34+ cells from a perfusion culture (described in table 1) stained with PE-CD11b and FITC-CD15. The cells were stained before (day 0) and after 5, 10, and 15 days of perfusion culture. Reproduced from [38] with permission.

Culture conditions that affect expansion

Traditionally, growth factors were thought to have exclusive control over proliferation and differentiation in the hematopoietic system. However, cultures performed by different investigators with the same growth factor combinations often vary significantly in total cell and progenitor cell expansion. This variability is usually due to other culture variables. It is essential when comparing studies to examine not only growth factor combinations, but

164

also the presence of stroma, feeding schedule, oxygen tension, use of serum, and inoculum density. Table 2 summarizes the culture conditions used and expansions achieved in the key studies discussed throughout this chapter.

Growth factors

Colony-stimulating factors (CSFs) and interleukins (ILs) are the primary regulators of the growth and differentiation of hematopoietic cells. Although many studies have evaluated various growth factor combinations, the exact combination and amount of growth factors required for optimal expansion of hematopoietic progenitor and stem cells is still unknown. The correct combination of growth factors is especially important for those cultures performed with purified cells, due to the absence of endogenous growth factor production by stromal cells or other accessory cells.

The functions of hematopoietic growth factors fall into several categories, and hematopoietic cell cultures often contain factors from each of these categories. Most of the late-acting cytokines such as erythropoietin (EPO), thrombopoietin (TPO), and granulocyte-colony stimulating factor (G-CSF) are lineage specific and support proliferation and maturation of committed progenitors. The intermediate-acting lineage-nonspecific factors that support the proliferation of multipotential progenitors include IL-3, granulocyte macrophage-CSF (GM-CSF) [40], and PIXY321 (a fusion protein of IL-3 and GM-CSF) [41]. Other factors do not possess CSF activity on their own, but synergize with other cytokines. When combined with IL-3, factors such as IL-6, G-CSF, IL-11, stem cell factor (SCF or c-kit ligand), and flt-3 ligand have been found to bring primitive, quiescent progenitors into the cell cycle and to increase proliferation [40,42]. A number of hematopoietic growth factors such as EPO, IL-3, GM-CSF, G-CSF, and SCF are considered to be survival factors because they suppress apoptosis in cells at various stages in the hematopoietic lineage [43,44].

The most frequently used growth factors in hematopoietic cultures are IL-3 and SCF. Various other growth factors are added to this base combination to expand different lineages. When expansion of more mature cells and progenitors of the neutrophil lineage is desired, addition of one or more of the following factors is made to the base combination: IL-6, G-CSF, GM-CSF [38,45–47]. Proliferation and maturation of megakaryocytes requires TPO. Addition of TPO to cultures of human PB CD34$^+$ cells results in a culture with 20% to 100% megakaryocytes [48]. In Mk colony assays, TPO has been found to synergize with SCF, and to have an additive effect when combined with IL-3 [48]. Growth factor combinations that maximize the production of both megakaryocyte and neutrophil lineages are still under investigation.

Optimal expansion of progenitors from purified cells requires multiple growth factor combinations. Combinations of IL-3, IL-6, SCF, with IL-1, EPO, G-CSF, and/or GM-CSF [37,49–51] have been reported to give maximum expansion of progenitors. Total cell expansion of 260-fold and CFU-GM ex-

Table 2. Comparison of the effects of culture conditions on ex vivo expansion

Cell source	Cell type	Cytokines	Stroma medium oxygen	Feeding	Inoculum density (cells/ml)	Total cell expansion	Progenitor expansion	LTC-IC Expansion	Ref
BM PB	CD34+ purity 50%	• IL-3, SCF, G-CSF • IL-3, SCF, IL-6	• No stroma • Serum & SD • Ambient	Every 3-4 days	$0.5\text{-}5 \times 10^5$	• 773-fold serum (day 14) • 10–15-fold less SD	• 13-fold CFU-GM serum/G-CSF (day 17) • 2.5-fold CFU-GM serum/IL-6 (day 17)		[46]
PB	CD34+ purity 87%	• IL-3, IL-6, IL-1, EPO, SCF	• No stroma • Serum & SD + AP • Ambient	None	$0.5\text{-}15 \times 10^3$	• 260-fold serum (day 14) • 179–240-fold SD + AP (day 14)	• 190-fold CFC serum (day 14) • 130–210-fold CFC (day 14)		[49]
PB	CD34+ purity 99%	• IL-3,IL-6, IL-1, G-CSF, GM-CSF, SCF	• No stroma • Serum • Ambient	None	1×10^3	• 1320-fold (day 21)	• 66-fold CFU-GM (day 14)		[50]
BM	CD34+ purity 72%	• IL-3, IL-6, GM-CSF, SCF	• No stroma • Serum • 5% O_2	Weekly	$0.5\text{-}1.0 \times 10^5$	• 24-fold (day 10)	• 8-fold CFC (day 10)		[45]
PB	CD34+ purity 56% to 94%	• IL3,3, IL-6, G-CSF, EPO, SCF	• No stroma • Serum & SD + AP • Ambient	Weekly	4×10^4	• 501-fold serum (day 14)	• 40-fold CFC serum (day 14) • 72% of serum for SD + AP		[51]

Source	Cell/purity	Cytokines	Conditions	Feeding	Cell density	Expansion	CFU-GM	Progenitor / LTC-IC	Ref.
PB	CD34+ purity 95%	IL-3, IL-6, G-CSF, GM-CSF, SCF	• No stroma • Serum • Ambient	None	3×10^3	• 133-fold (day 7)	• 57-fold CFU-GM (day 7)		[47]
PB	CD34+ purity 61%	IL-3, IL-6, IL-1, EPO, SCF	• No stroma • SD + AP • Ambient	Weekly	3×10^4	• 70-fold (day 12)	• 50-fold CFU-GM (day 12)	• LTC-IC maintained (day 12)	[37]
BM	MNC	L-3, EPO, GM-CSF,SCF	• Stroma • Serum • Ambient	Perfusion	3×10^7 per chamber	• 10-fold (day 14)	• 21-fold CFU-GM (day 14)	• 7.5-fold (day 14)	[111]
PB	MNC	IL-3, IL-6, G-CSF,SCF	• Stroma & no stroma • Serum • Ambient	Perfusion	2×10^6 per chamber	At day 15 • stroma 5.4-fold • no stroma 9.9-fold	At day 10 CFU-GMs • stroma 17-fold • no stroma 19-fold	At day 15 • stroma 34% input • no stroma 64% input	[64]
				Every 5 days	2×10^5	At day 15 • stroma 2.4-fold • no stroma 7.4-fold	At day 10 CFU-GM • stroma 18-fold • no stroma 13-fold	At day 15 • stroma 12% input • no stroma 11% input	[64]
PB	MNC CD34+ purity 91%	IL-3, IL-6, G-CSF, SCF	• No stroma • Serum • Ambient	Perfusion	2×10^6 MNCs & 2×10^5 CD34+ per chamber	At day 15 • MNCs 9.2-fold • CD34+ 113-fold	At day 15 CFU-GM • MNCs 19-fold • CD34+ 18-fold	At day 15 • MNC 123% input • CD34+ 135% input	[38]
				Every 5 days	2×10^5 MNCs & 2×10^4 CD34+	At day 15 • MNCs 8.2-fold • CD34+ 84-fold	At day 15 CFU-GM • MNCs 19-fold • CD34+ 11-fold	At day 15 • MNC 74% input • CD34+ 72% input	[38]

AP = autologous plasma; SD = serum-depleted.
MNC = mononuclear cell.

167

pansion of 190-fold is achieved after 12 to 14 days of culture with the combination of IL-3, IL-6, SCF, IL-1, and EPO [49]. This combination also maintains the number of LTC-ICs in the culture [37]. The combination containing IL-3, IL-6, SCF, IL-1, G-CSF, and GM-CSF gives 1300-fold total cell expansion after 21 days and 66-fold expansion of CFU-GM after 14 days [50]. After 12 to 14 days, the combination of IL-3, IL-6, SCF, G-CSF, and GM-CSF gives a total cell expansion of 104-fold, and CFU-GM expansion of 14-fold [51].

Growth factor combinations for maintenance and expansion of primitive progenitors (LTC-ICs) are not as well defined. Marrow stromal cells appear to secrete some as yet undiscovered cytokines that are required for the conservation of primitive progenitors in an undifferentiated state [52]. Addition of IL-3 or multiple growth-promoting cytokines to cultures with stroma-derived factors can result in exhaustion of LTC-ICs as early as five weeks after initiation of the culture [39], which suggests that the antidifferentiation capacity of factors released by stroma can be overwhelmed by persistent stimulation with growth-promoting cytokines. Addition of IL-3 and a growth-inhibitory factor (MIP-1α) to cultures with soluble stromal factors results in maintenance of 100% of LTC-ICs for at least eight weeks in culture [53]. Total cell and CFC production in these cultures is similar to that in cultures supplemented with IL-3 alone. Thus, addition of growth-inhibitory and growth-promoting cytokines to cultures with stroma-derived factors may be necessary to prevent terminal differentiation of LTC-ICs.

Stroma

Stromal cells consist of adventitial reticular cells, endothelial cells, adipocytes, and macrophages. These cells support hematopoiesis through the production and presentation of growth factors and the synthesis of extracellular matrix [54,55]. Cultures containing a stromal layer or stroma-derived factors have greater culture longevity and progenitor cell expansion [39,56] than cultures without a stromal layer. BM stroma is also important in gene therapy, since retroviral-mediated transduction in the presence of a stromal layer increases the efficiency of the transduction [11,12] and the long-term engraftment of the transduced cells [11]. However, there are several complications and disadvantages involved in the use of a stromal layer for research and clinical applications. An additional BM cell sample would be required to establish the stromal layer for PB, CB, and CD34$^+$ cells, since these cells do not contain stromal cells. The effects and composition of stromal layers are poorly defined and variable, and the harvest of stroma-containing cultures is labor intensive and requires enzymatic treatment [57–59].

Extensive expansion of progenitor cells [49,50,60–63] and maintenance of a fraction of the LTC-ICs [37,38] can be been achieved in stroma-free cultures with addition of multiple hematopoietic growth factors. Although the maintenance and proliferation of LTC-ICs are generally not as good in stroma-free cultures as in stroma-containing static cultures [39,61], perfusion

168

cultures maintain LTC-ICs to a greater extent in stroma-free cultures than in stroma-containing cultures [64]. However, for CD34[+] cell cultures, both stroma and frequent medium exchange are important for LTC-IC expansion (figure 2c) [65]. There is reason to believe that the benefits of stromal cells can eventually be replaced by defined factors even in static cultures. LTC-ICs are actually maintained to a greater extent in cultures where progenitors are separated from stroma by a microporous membrane, which allows passage of diffusible factors [39,53,66], or supplemented daily with media conditioned by a stromal feeder layer [39]. In any event, a stromal layer is not necessary in cultures where the main goal is production of mature cells or committed progenitors.

Feeding/perfusion

The in vivo perfusion rate of plasma through the BM is approximately 0.1 ml per cc of marrow per minute [67]. Assuming a tissue cell density of 5×10^8 cells/ml, this perfusion rate corresponds to a daily replacement of medium containing 20% serum for cultures at a density of 10^6 cells/ml [68]. In contrast, the standard feeding protocol for hematopoietic cultures is a weekly exchange of 50% to 100% of the medium. In order to recreate the in vivo perfusion rate in hematopoietic cultures, culture media in flasks can be exchanged daily or cultures can be perfused continuously in a bioreactor system. Daily exchange of media improves long-term BM culture productivity and longevity [69,70], but is cumbersome to implement. Perfusion bioreactor cultures offer greater progenitor and LTC-IC expansion than static cultures [71]. Perfusion cultures also show larger and more numerous cobblestone areas of active hematopoiesis than static cultures. In addition, perfusion maintains more constant cytokine, nutrient, and by-product levels than static cultures [71]. Frequent medium exchange is not as important in BM CD34[+] cell cultures, where stromal cells are absent (figure 2) [65]. However, for maximum expansion of LTC-ICs in CD34[+] cell cultures, it may be necessary to use frequent medium exchange together with a stromal layer (figure 2c) or stromal-conditioned medium (see Stroma section above).

Oxygen tension

The oxygen tension in BM has been found to range from 10 to 50mmHg [72,73]. An environment similar to the in vivo BM microenvironment can be achieved by saturation with gas containing approximately 5% oxygen. Under reduced oxygen conditions, the size and number of hematopoietic cell colonies in semisolid medium is significantly enhanced [74–79]. In contrast, one study showed that murine myeloid colonies including HPP-CFCs were not enhanced in cultures under 7% oxygen tension [80]. Liquid cultures of CB MNCs, BM MNCs, and CB MNCs on irradiated stromal layers grown under low oxygen tension have an increased number and frequency of CFCs [56,81,82]. Progeni-

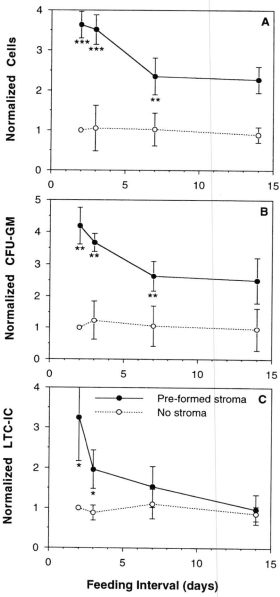

Figure 2. Effect of feeding interval and preformed stroma on BM CD34-enriched cell culture output. BM CD34-enriched cells were cultured in serum-containing medium supplemented with IL-3/GM-CSF/SCF/EPO. Data obtained in each of seven independent experiments were normalized by the values obtained from CD34-enriched cells grown in IL-3/GM-CSF/SCF/EPO without stroma and fed every other day, and then combined. Average normalized (A) total cell, (B) CFU-GM, and (C) LTC-IC numbers are shown. A normalized value of 1 corresponded to 1.23×10^6 cells (246-fold expansion), 1939 CFU-GM (4.7-fold), and 22 LTC-ICs (0.4-fold) per well. Reproduced from [65] with permission.

tors in these cultures can be maintained one to two weeks longer under 5% oxygen when fed with medium equilibrated with 5% oxygen [82]. Different types of hematopoietic progenitors display varying degrees of sensitivity to hypoxia. The most primitive progenitors show the least sensitivity to severe hypoxia [83].

Several mechanisms are involved in the enhanced colony formation in clonogenic assays and progenitor cell expansion in liquid cultures under reduced oxygen tension. The improved growth is due in part to increased responsiveness of hematopoietic cells to growth factors under 5% oxygen. Under low oxygen, CFU-E and BFU-E exhibit increased sensitivity to EPO [75] and macrophage progenitors show increased sensitivity to M-CSF [79]. Accessory cells also respond differently to varying oxygen tensions in their production of growth factors. BM-derived macrophages produce EPO and IL-3 in an oxygen-dependent manner [76]. Oxygen toxicity plays a role in the decreased colony formation at high oxygen. Addition of antioxidants such as α-thioglycerol, vitamin E, glutathione [75,76], and 2-mercaptoethanol [72,76] improve performance at high oxygen concentration, but have less of an effect at low oxygen concentrations. Studies performed in our laboratory show that in the presence of lineage-specific factors, different oxygen tensions preferentially enhance expansion of one hematopoietic cell lineage over another [84]. Greater numbers of megakaryocytes or erythrocytes are present in cultures under ambient oxygen tension supplemented with TPO or EPO, respectively. However, a greater number of granulocytes is present under reduced oxygen tension in the presence of G-CSF. Therefore, the choice of oxygen tension will help to determine the lineage and the maturity of cells present in the culture.

Serum versus serum-depleted medium

Addition of serum to a culture medium provides a source of hormones and essential nutrients and also alters the physiological and physicochemical properties of the medium such as pH, osmolarity, viscosity, and surface tension [85,86]. However, addition of serum results in a medium with an undefined composition and uncontrolled variability. The use of serum-containing medium is highly undesirable for the culture of human cells for clinical use. Medium containing animal serum could cause allergic reactions in patients [87], and while allogeneic human serum would eliminate this problem, significant concerns about the transmission of disease still remain. The potential hazards of serum use add another hurdle to the process of obtaining FDA approval for ex vivo expansion therapies [88]. However, autologous plasma (AP) may prove to be a viable alternative.

Several studies have compared the use of serum-depleted (SD) and serum-containing media for cultures performed with MNCs and CD34+ cells from PB, CB, and BM. Total cell expansion and CFU-GM expansion in serum-depleted cultures is similar to or lower than expansion in serum-containing cultures

[46,89,90]. One group examining the maturity and functionality of neutrophils produced in serum-depleted medium reports that the expanded cells are less mature and functionally less competent than cells expanded in serum-containing medium [46]. However, the addition of 1% autologous plasma increased expansion of the cells and restored their functionality almost to the level of that in serum-containing medium. Another study showed that addition of 1% autologous plasma to serum-depleted cultures retained 96% of the progenitor expansion achieved in the presence of 20% serum [51]. Several studies indicate that serum inhibits megakaryocyte production and platelet formation in culture [91–94]. Erythroid progenitors also fare better in serum-depleted cultures [89,90]. While the majority of studies performed with human plasma in the culture medium have resulted in enhanced megakaryocytopoiesis [95–97], the presence of transforming growth factor-β in the plasma can inhibit megakaryocytopoiesis and erythropoiesis [98].

Serum-depleted cultures appear to be capable of maintaining LTC-ICs. Cultures of CD34$^+$ cells in serum-depleted medium with IL-1, IL-3, IL-6, EPO, SCF, and 2% autologous plasma expanded committed progenitors while maintaining LTC-ICs [37]. Primitive BM cells (CD34$^+$45RA^{lo}71^{lo}) isolated and cultured in serum-depleted medium with IL-3, IL-6, EPO, and SCF produced large numbers of progeny without decreasing primitive cell numbers [99]. In addition, results of a study with murine cells show that serum-depleted, stroma-free cultures of primitive BM cells (Sca-1$^+$, lineage-negative, wheat-germ agglutinin-positive) maintain their in vivo reconstituting potential in the presence of IL-6, EPO, SCF, either with or without IL-3 [100]. Although serum-depleted medium is desirable for clinical applications and is able to support megakaryocytopoiesis and erythropoiesis, a component in serum appears to be necessary for greater expansion and improved functionality of the granulocyte and macrophage lineages. Addition of a small amount of autologous plasma to serum-depleted medium may be the best alternative to a completely serum-depleted system.

Seeding density effects

The effect of cell inoculum density on culture performance has been examined in cultures of BM MNCs [101] and PB MNCs and CD34$^+$ cells [102]. The cell seeding density has been found to affect total cell and progenitor expansion, as well as the percentage of progenitor cells in the culture. Lower-density cultures expand total cells preferentially over CFCs. In contrast, higher-density cultures expand CFCs to an extent comparable to that in lower-density cultures, but without the large expansion of total cells. Thus, a high-input cell density maintains progenitors and LTC-ICs better than a low inoculum density, which induces differentiation. Culture systems that can maintain high cell densities, as well as large numbers of CFU-GM, are ideal for clinical-scale applications. In this regard, a perfusion system that can maintain pH and oxygen tension in high-cell-density cultures is desirable, since studies from our

172

lab show that pH [103] and oxygen [84] strongly influence cell differentiation pattern. For example, a larger percentage of mature erythroid cells and fewer BFU-E are present at a pH of approximately 7.6 versus 7.35, suggesting that erythroid differentiation proceeds faster at higher pH.

Types and numbers of cells required for transplantation

The number and type of cells needed for transplantation depend on the aim of the procedure. Mature cells and late progenitors can be used as a graft supplement to reduce the nadir associated with myeloablative therapy or can be used alone for myelosuppressive therapy, while primitive cells are necessary for long-term engraftment. Studies of transplantation using uncultured hematopoietic cells provide the basis for most estimates of the numbers of hematopoietic cells needed for successful engraftment. For long-term repopulation of the hematopoietic system, it has been estimated (based on a murine model) that the required number of LTC-ICs is approximately 30,000 [37]. With regard to the shorter-term engraftment requirements for reducing or eliminating the period of chemotherapy-induced neutropenia and thrombocytopenia, enough cells must be administered to maintain a neutrophil count of greater than 0.5 $\times 10^9$ cells/L and a platelet count of greater than 50×10^9 cells/L. When transplanting uncultured cells, the progenitor cell dose is the most significant predictor of the rate of engraftment of neutrophils and platelets. Rapid hematopoietic engraftment occurs when 2×10^5 CFU-GM or 2×10^6 CD34$^+$ cells/ kg of body weigh are infused [104], which would be 14 million CFU-GM or 140 million CD34$^+$ cells for a 70-kg patient. However, an 8- to 12-day period of neutropenia and thrombocytopenia still occurs after this number of CFU-GM or CD34$^+$ cells is administered. Addition of mature cells and late progenitors of the neutrophil and megakaryocyte lineage has the potential to decrease this nadir. Assuming a neutrophil half-life of six hours, a blood volume of five liters, and an increased consumption of neutrophils in the neutropenic state, the approximate number of neutrophils needed to eliminate or reduce this period of neutropenia is 2×10^{11} [50]. Direct administration of this number of neutrophils from an uncultured source would be problematic. Ex vivo expansion has the potential to produce such large numbers of mature cells, as well as their precursors, on a regular basis. Since the number of clinical studies performed using cultured cells is limited at the present time, the cell doses used or estimated for uncultured cells should be used to provide initial target doses for ex vivo expanded cells. In a study by Brugger et al. [105], CD34$^+$ cells from patients were expanded ex vivo and then administered to the patients after high-dose chemotherapy. Results from this study suggest that a threshold dose of approximately 1.0×10^5 cultured CFCs/kg of body weight is needed for rapid engraftment a figure that is similar to that needed when using uncultured cells. While this finding is promising, larger studies are needed to confirm these results.

In order to efficiently obtain the target doses for long-term repopulation or short-term engraftment using ex vivo expansion, the appropriate culture conditions must be used. Successful production of a given number of cells of a desired cell type will depend on the capacity to control the generation of one cell lineage relative to another and also the capacity to control differentiation versus proliferation. Selective production of one lineage and stage of hematopoietic cell differentiation over others is controlled in large part by growth factors, but is also influenced by the other culture parameters discussed above. Serum-depleted medium containing growth factors such as TPO, G-CSF, and GM-CSF would be used to promote expansion of mature cells and late progenitors of the neutrophil and megakaryocyte lineages. To maximize expansion of more mature cells and progenitors, a low inoculum density and ambient oxygen tension would be beneficial. Stroma would be optional for this application. For long-term engraftment and gene therapy applications, culture conditions that maintain more primitive progenitors should be used. High-density perfusion cultures grown under low oxygen tension in the presence of a stromal layer may be ideal for this purpose.

Systems for expansion of hematopoietic cells

Large-scale expansion of hematopoietic stem and progenitor cells has been evaluated in many culture systems, including tissue-culture flasks [37,49,106], gas-permeable culture bags [50,51,107–110], and several types of bioreactors [38,64,71,111–115]. Tissue culture flasks are the most commonly used expansion devices for in vitro studies, but are cumbersome for large-scale applications due to the large numbers of flasks required per patient and the increased potential for contamination. While the use of culture bags is also labor and space intensive, these systems incorporate aseptic tubing technology, which decreases the probability of contamination to less than 1 in 1000 per connection [116]. These bags provide a nonadherent culture surface, which makes removal of the cells, especially BM cells, much easier and more efficient than from tissue culture flasks.

Flat-bed perfusion systems, hollow fiber reactors, and spinner cultures illustrated in figure 3 have all been evaluated for ex vivo expansion. Flat-bed perfusion bioreactor systems, employing a stromal layer to retain inoculated cells, have been very successful in expansion of stem and progenitor cells [71,111,112]. These cultures have achieved approximately a 20-fold expansion of CFU-GM, and from a twofold to sevenfold expansion of primitive LTC-ICs. A modified flat-bed bioreactor design that retains nonadherent cells with grooves instead of a stromal layer gives similar CFU-GM expansion [64]. Other bioreactor systems have been evaluated with varying degrees of success. Sardonini and Wu [114] cultured BM MNCs in suspension and microcarrier spinner flasks, airlift bioreactors, and hollow fiber bioreactors. Only the spinner flask suspension culture expanded total cells to greater extent than the

174

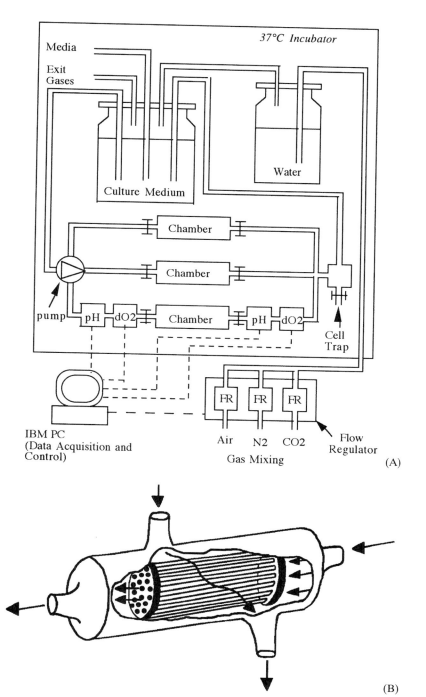

Figure 3. Bioreactor systems (A) flat-bed perfusion (reproduced from [38] with permission), (B) hollow fiber, (C) spinner (see following page).

175

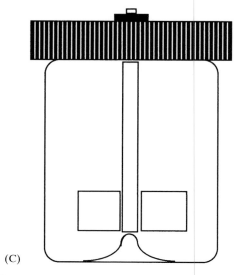

(C)

Figure 3 (continued)

static control cultures, and even for that system, progenitor expansion was minimal. The difficulty in harvesting cells from the hollow fiber reactor contributed to its poor performance. Zandstra et al. [113] have successfully cultured BM MNCs in a suspension spinner flask, showing expansion of total cells, committed progenitors, and primitive LTC-ICs. A high inoculum cell density in the suspension was reported to be a key factor in achieving these expansions. Our group has been successful in culturing PB MNCs in spinner flasks, achieving total cell and CFU-GM expansion in serum-depleted medium [102].

Bioreactor systems are advantageous because they have the potential to become automated, closed systems, thereby decreasing space and labor requirements and facilitating compliance with regulatory requirements. However, there are potential complications involved in the culture of hematopoietic cells in various bioreactor systems that deserve consideration. Of the systems discussed above, flat-bed perfusion and stirred systems show the most potential, while hollow fiber systems seem least well suited to this application. The culture environment in hollow fiber reactors is spatially inhomogeneous, which creates large concentration gradients of critical nutrients, oxygen, and pH. Gradients of pH and oxygen could result in production of different cell types in different sections of the reactor. Process monitoring could be problematic in hollow fiber reactors, since the cells cannot be easily sampled or observed during culture. In addition, limited recovery of cells from this type of reactor has been reported [114]. Flat-bed perfusion systems and stirred systems would meet regulatory requirements more easily, since these systems would allow periodic sampling for process monitoring. Flat-bed perfusion

176

systems have been studied more extensively than other types of bioreactors for ex vivo expansion of hematopoietic cells. Clinical trials have been initiated using a prototype perfusion system developed by the University of Michigan and Aastrom Biosciences [117]. A uniform culture environment and simple design are the primary advantages of stirred systems. However, if the hematopoietic cells are shear sensitive, stirred systems could be problematic, whereas flat-bed perfusion systems would provide a low-shear environment. Further studies must be done to determine the sensitivity of particular hematopoietic lineages to pH, oxygen, temperature, shear forces, and other factors to determine how tightly the culture parameters must be controlled and which bioreactor systems are best suited for a given application.

Regulatory considerations for ex vivo expansion of hematopoietic cells

Ex vivo expansion of hematopoietic cells will be regulated by the FDA as a form of somatic-cell therapy. Final products that consist of cells are complex and cannot be completely defined. Thus, testing of the final product alone cannot reliably detect or control for variability. Limits on final product testing are also imposed by the limited number of available cells and the need for timely administration of products containing living cells. Thus, quality control of the manufacturing process and facility are necessary to produce consistent products.

During development of a program to produce cells for cellular therapy, Good Manufacturing Practices (GMP) [118] and 'Points to Consider' documents on somatic-cell therapy [88] issued by the FDA should be followed in order to ensure consistency and reproducibility. The key elements of a quality control/quality assurance (QC/QA) program for cellular therapy are an extensive training program for the staff of the cell processing facility, the early establishment of specifications and standard operating procedures (SOP), and a good record-keeping system [119]. During development of cell culture procedures for somatic-cell therapy, the following issues should be addressed [88]:

- In order to ensure the reproducibility of the cell culture characteristics, the culture media should be well defined, and growth factors used in the cultures should have established measures of identity, purity, and potency.
- Those components of the culture media that have the potential to cause sensitization, such as animal sera or certain antibiotics, should be avoided.
- Laboratory procedures should be performed under conditions designed to minimize contamination of the cells with adventitious agents.
- Cultures should be monitored to determine if the cell phenotype necessary for the intended effect is present. The desired cell type should be characterized by a combination of morphology, cell surface markers, functional parameters, and biochemical features. (Compliance with this guideline could

be problematic due to the time required for the CFC and LTC-IC assays used for this purpose).

- The longevity of the cultures should be tested to determine the stability of the essential characteristics of the cultured cell population.
- The components used during the in vitro manipulation procedures such as antibodies, serum, antibiotics, and magnetic beads should be documented, along with the limits for their concentrations in the final product, methods used to remove them, the effectiveness of the methods for their removal, and the toxicity of these materials. (The biocompatibility of the materials used for culture of theses cells should also be evaluated [120].)

Compliance with GMP regulations would be easier for a closed culture system, such as culture bags or a bioreactor, that reduces the likelihood of contamination. A bioreactor system would provide a means to automatically regulate the medium flow, oxygen delivery, temperature, and pH, which would allow for a quick response to potential deviations from in-process specifications. Bioreactors would also be beneficial for validation purposes, since all culture parameters can be recorded on-line.

Clinical trials with ex vivo expanded cells

Murine

Reconstitution of lethally irradiated mice transplanted with ex vivo cultured, 5-fluorouracil (5-FU)-treated BM has been compared to that in control mice transplanted with fresh 5-FU-treated BM [121]. Those mice receiving cells cultured in the presence of IL-1 and IL-3 had a shortened period of cytopenia and required fewer transplanted BM cells for survival than did control mice. Further experiments were carried out to determine if the early hematopoietic progenitor cells were compromised by the ex vivo expansion procedure [122]. SCF was added to short-term 5-FU-treated BM cultures, and the expanded cells were administered to host mice, resulting in long-term engraftment up to 40 weeks. The engraftment and long-term rescue of mice transplanted with ex vivo expanded BM MNCs and enriched stem cell populations (Thy1+Lin−) was compared [123]. The Thy1+Lin− cells expanded significantly in cultures containing IL-3, but did not rescue lethally irradiated mice. In contrast, MNCs maintained their capacity to engraft lethally irradiated recipients, but total cell numbers did not expand in culture (final values were below input levels).

Human

Early studies evaluated the effect of culturing BM for leukemic cell purging before autologous transplantation. These studies were performed without growth factors, and as a result a large number of the normal progenitor cells

178

were lost during culture [5,7,8]. Several phase I studies have been initiated in humans to evaluate ex vivo expansion of cultured hematopoietic cells for transplantation. Aastrom Biosciences, Inc. has cultured BM MNCs in a closed perfusion bioreactor system for 9 to 14 days with IL-3, GM-CSF, EPO, and SCF in a trial done in collaboration with the University of Michigan [117] and for 12 days with PIXY321 and EPO in a trial done in collaboration with M.D. Anderson Cancer Center [115]. The cultured cells showed no evidence of toxicity in the subjects, and patients transplanted with cells expanded with PIXY321 and EPO were reported to have a median recovery of granulocytes (>500/μl) at day 11 and platelets (>25,000/μl) at day 16. Baxter Healthcare and the University of Chicago have a clinical trial underway in which PB CD34$^+$ cells are cultured for 12 days in serum-depleted medium with PIXY321 in gas-permeable culture bags [109,110]. In this study, the median times to neutrophil and platelet recovery were 9 and 10 days, respectively. Brugger et al. [105] recently published results of a clinical trial in which ex vivo expanded cells were administered to ten patients after high-dose chemotherapy. Eleven million PB CD34$^+$ cells were used to initiate the cultures, which is less than 10% of the usual number of such cells used in transplantation. PB CD34$^+$ cells were expanded in tissue culture flasks for 12 days in serum-depleted medium supplemented with 2% autologous plasma and IL-3, IL-6, IL-1, EPO, and SCF. Four patients received cultured plus uncultured cells to evaluate possible toxic effects of the cultured cells. An additional six patients received only cultured cells. Recovery of neutrophil and platelet counts in patients receiving cells generated ex vivo was similar to that in previous patients receiving unmanipulated cells. While the use of ex vivo expanded cells did not alter recovery patterns in this study, it did reduce the harvest size required for successful engraftment. A similar trial showed no difference in either platelet or neutrophil recovery between patients receiving expanded cells and historical controls [124].

The future

The field of hematopoietic stem and progenitor cell expansion has progressed rapidly since the first Dexter cultures were performed in the mid-1970s [125]. Within the last few years, progress has been especially rapid, due in part to the discovery of new growth factors and the development of improved culture conditions. The potential of ex vivo expansion is manifest, since clinicians have already begun to utilize ex vivo expanded hematopoietic cells for transplantation and gene therapy. While results of early clinical studies are promising, there are still many factors that need to be considered before the process can become a routine clinical technique. The discovery of new growth factors and the future refinement of culture conditions will undoubtedly lead to better control of the fate of stem cells cultured ex vivo and more widespread use of these cells in the clinical setting.

Acknowledgments

This work was supported by NIH grant RO1 HL 48276 (ETP and WMM).

References

1. Nemunaitis J, Rabinowe S, Singer J, et al. Recombinant granulocyte-macrophage colony-stimulating factor after autologous bone marrow transplantation for lymphoid cancer. N Engl J Med 324:1773–1778, 1991.
2. To L, Haylock D, Dyson P, Thorp D, Roberts M, Juttner C. An unusual pattern of hemopoietic reconstitution in patient with acute myeloid leukemia transplanted with autologous recovery phase peripheral blood. Bone Marrow Transplant 6:109–114, 1990.
3. Coulombel L, Eaves C, Kalousek D, Gupta C, Eaves A. Long-term bone marrow culture of cells from patients with acute myelogenous leukemia. J Clin Invest 75:961–969, 1985.
4. Gordon M, Dowding C, Riley G, Goldman J, Greaves M. Altered adhesive interactions with marrow stroma of haematopoietic progenitor cells in chronic myeloid leukemia. Nature 328(6128):342–344, 1987.
5. Saeland S, Caux C, Favre C, et al. Effects of recombinant human interleukin-3 on CD34-enriched normal hematopoietic progenitors and on myeloblastic leukemia cells. Blood 72:1580–1588, 1988.
6. Udomsakdi C, Eaves C, Swolin B, Reid D, Barnett M, Eaves A. Rapid decline of chronic myeloid leukemic cells in long-term culture due to a defect at the leukemic stem cell level. Proc Natl Acad Sci USA 89(13):6192–6196, 1992.
7. Chang J, Morgenstern G, Coutinho L, et al. The use of bone marrow cells grown in long-term culture for autologous bone marrow transplantation in acute myeloid leukemia: an update. Bone Marrow Transplant 4(1):5–9, 1989.
8. Barnett M, Eaves C, Kalousek D, et al. Successful autografting in chronic myeloid leukemia after maintenance of marrow in culture. Bone Marrow Transplant 4(4):345–351, 1989.
9. Barnett M, Eaves C, Phillips G, et al. Autografting with cultured marrow in chronic myeloid leukemia: results of a pilot study. Blood 84(3):724–732, 1994.
10. Dunbar C, Emmons R. Gene transfer into hematopoietic progenitor and stem cells: progress and problems. Stem Cells 12:563–576, 1994.
11. Nolta J, Smogorzewska E, Kohn D. Analysis of optimal conditions for retroviral-mediated transduction of primitive human hematopoietic cells. Blood 86(1):101–110, 1995.
12. Xu L, Kluepfel-Stahl S, Blanco M, Schiffmann R, Dunbar C, Karlsson S. Growth factors and stromal support generate very efficient retroviral transduction of peripheral blood CD34+ cells from Gaucher patients. Blood 86(1):141–146, 1995.
13. Nakahata T, Gross A, Ogawa M. A stochastic model of self-renewal and commitment to differentiation of the primitive hemopoietic stem cells in culture. J Cell Physiol 113:455–458, 1982.
14. Moore M. Clinical implications of positive and negative hematopoietic stem cell regulators. Blood 78:1–19, 1991.
15. Sutherland H, Eaves C, Eaves A, Dragowska W, Lansdorp P. Characterization and partial purification of human marrow cells capable of initiating long-term hematopoiesis in vitro. Blood 74:1563–1570, 1989.
16. McCune J, Namikawa R, Kaneshima H, Shultz L, Lieberman M, Weissman I. The SCID-hu mouse: murine model for the analysis of human hematolymphoid differentiation and function. Science 241:1632–1635, 1988.
17. Lapidot T, Pflumio F, Doedens M, Murdoch B, Williams D, Dick J. Cytokine stimulation of multilineage hematopoiesis for immature human cells engrafted in SCID mice. Science 255:1137–1141, 1992.

18. Zanjani E, Pallavicini M, Ascensao J, et al. Engraftment and long-term expression of human fetal hemopoietic stem cells in sheep following transplantation in utero. J Clin Invest 89:1178–1188, 1992.
19. Namikawa R, Weilbaecher K, Kaneshima H, Yee E, McCune J. Long-term human hematopoiesis in the SCID-hu mouse. J Exp Med 172(4):1055–1063, 1990.
20. Kyoizumi S, Baum C, Kaneshima H, McCune J, Yee E, Namikawa R. Implantation and maintenance of functional human bone marrow within SCID-hu mice. Blood, 79(7):1704–1711, 1992.
21. Srour E, Zanjani E, Brandt J, et al. Sustained human hematopoiesis in sheep transplanted in utero during early gestation with fractionated adult human bone marrow cells. Blood 79(6):1404–1412, 1992.
22. Srour E, Zanjani E, Cornetta K, et al. Persistence of human multilineage, self-renewing lymphohematopoietic stem cells in chimeric sheep. Blood 82(11):3333–3342, 1993.
23. Andrews R, Singer J, Bernstein I. Monoclonal antibody 12–8 recognizes a 115-kd molecule present on both unipotent and multipotent hematopoietic colony-forming cells and their precursors. Blood 67:842–845, 1986.
24. To L, Haylock D, Dowse T, et al. A comparative study of the phenotype and proliferative capacity of peripheral blood (PB) CD34+ cells mobilized by four different protocols and those of steady-phase PB and bone marrow CD34+ cells. Blood 84(9):2930–2939, 1994.
25. Richman C, Weiner R, Yankee R. Increase in circulating stem cells following chemotherapy in man. Blood 47(6):1031–1039, 1976.
26. VanEpps D, Bender J, Lee W, et al. Harvesting, characterization, and culture of CD34+ cells from human bone marrow, peripheral blood, and cord blood. Blood Cells 20:411–423, 1994.
27. Lebkowski J, Schain L, Okrongly D, Levinsky R, Harvey M, Okarma T. Rapid isolation of human CD34 hematopoietic stem cells — purging of human tumor cells. Transplant 53:1011–1019, 1992.
28. Hardwick A, Law P, Mansour V, Kulcinski D, Lshizawa L, Gee A. Development of a large-scale immunomagnetic separation system for harvesting CD34 positive cells from bone marrow. Prog Clin Biol Res 377:583–589, 1992.
29. Berenson R, Bensinger W, Hill R. Engraftment after infusion of CD34+ marrow cells in patients with breast cancer or neuroblastoma. Blood 77(8):1717–1722, 1991.
30. Fruehauf S, Haas R, Zeller W, Hunstein W. CD34 selection for purging in multiple myeloma and analysis of CD34+ cell precursors. Stem Cells 12:95–102, 1994.
31. Verfaillie C, Miller W, Boylan K, McGlave P. Selection of benign primitive hematopoietic progenitors in chronic myelogenous leukemia on the basis of HLA-DR antigen expression. Blood 79:1003–1010, 1992.
32. Broxmeyer H, Douglas G, Hangoc G. Human umbilical cord blood as a potential source of transplantable hematopoietic stem/progenitor cells. Proc Natl Acad Sci USA 86(10):3828–3832, 1989.
33. Cassel A, Cottler-Fox M, Doren S. Retroviral-mediated gene transfer into CD34-enriched human peripheral blood stem cells. Exp Hematol 21(4):585–591, 1993.
34. Traycoff C, Abboud R, Laver J. Evaluation of the in vitro behavior of phenotypically defined populations of umbilical cord blood hematopoietic progenitor cells. Exp Hematol 22(2):215–222, 1994.
35. Korbling M, Drach J, Champlin R. Large-scale preparation of highly purified, frozen/thawed CD34+ HLA-DR- hematopoietic progenitor cells by sequential immunoadsorption (CEPRATE SC) and fluorescence-activated cell sorting: implications for gene transduction and/or transplantation. Bone Marrow Transplant 13:649–654, 1994.
36. Koller M, Manchel I, Newsom B, Palsson M, Palsson B. Bioreactor expansion of human bone marrow: comparison of unprocessed, density-separated, and CD34-enriched cells. J Hematother 4:159–169, 1995.
37. Henschler R, Brugger W, Luft T, Frey R, Mertelsmann R, Kanz L. Maintenance of transplantation potential in ex vivo expanded CD34+-selected human peripheral blood progenitor cells. Blood 84(9):2898–2903, 1994.

38. Sandstrom C, Bender J, Papoutsakis E, Miller W. Effects of CD34+ cell selection and perfusion on ex vivo expansion of peripheral blood mononuclear cells. Blood, 86(3):958–970, 1995.

39. Verfaillie C. Soluble factor(s) produced by human marrow stroma increase cytokine induced proliferation and maturation of primitive hematopoietic progenitors while preventing their terminal differentiation. Blood 82:2045–2054, 1993.

40. Ogawa M. Differentiation and proliferation of hematopoietic stem cells. Blood 81(11):2844–2853, 1993.

41. Curtis B, Williams D, Broxmeyer H, et al. Enhanced hematopoietic activity of a human granulocyte/macrophage colony-stimulating factor-interleukin 3 fusion protein. Proc Natl Acad Sci USA 88:5809–5813, 1991.

42. Gabbianelli M, Pelosi E, Montesoro E, et al. Multi-level effects of flt3 ligand on human hematopoiesis: expansion of putative stem cells and proliferation of granulomonocytic progenitors/monocytic precursors. Blood 86(5):1661–1670, 1995.

43. Koury M. Programmed cell death (apoptosis) in hematopoiesis. Exp Hematol 20:391–394, 1992.

44. Brandt J, Bhalla K, Hoffman R. Effects of interleukin-3 and c-kit ligand on the survival of various classes of human hematopoietic progenitor cells. Blood 83:1507–1514, 1994.

45. Smith S, Bender J, Maples P, et al. Expansion of neutrophil precursors and progenitors in suspension cultures of CD34+ cells enriched from human bone marrow. Exp Hematol 21:870–877, 1993.

46. Lill M, Lynch M, Fraser J, et al. Production of functional myeloid cells from CD34-selected hematopoietic progenitor cells using a clinically relevant ex vivo expansion system. Stem Cells 12:626–637, 1994.

47. Sato N, Sawada K, Koizumi K, et al. In vitro expansion of human peripheral blood CD34+ cells. Blood 82(12):3600–3609, 1993.

48. Hunt P, Li Y, Nichol J, et al. Purification and biologic characterization of plasma-derived megakaryocyte growth and development factor. Blood 86(2):540–547, 1995.

49. Brugger W, Mocklin W, Heimfeld S, Berenson F, Mertelsmann R, Kanz L. Ex vivo expansion of enriched peripheral blood CD34+ progenitor cells by stem cell factor, IL-1β, IL-6, IL-3, Interferon-gamma, and erythropoietin. Blood 81(10):2579–2584, 1993.

50. Haylock D, To L, Dowse T, Juttner C, Simmons P. Ex vivo expansion and maturation of peripheral blood CD34+ cells into the myeloid lineage. Blood 80(6):1405–1412, 1992.

51. Shapiro F, Yao T, Raptis G, Reich L, Norton L, Moore M. Optimization of conditions for ex vivo expansion of CD34+ cells from patients with stage IV breast cancer. Blood 84(10):3567–3574, 1994.

52. Verfaillie C. Can human hematopoietic stem cells be cultured ex vivo? Stem Cells 12:466–476, 1994.

53. Verfaillie C, Catanzarro P, Li W. Macrophage Inflammatory Protein 1 alpha, Interleukin 3 and diffusible marrow stromal factors maintain human hematopoietic stem cells for at least eight weeks in vitro. J Exp Med 179:643–649, 1994.

54. Temeles D, McGrath H, Kittler E, et al. Cytokine expression from bone marrow derived macrophages. Exp Hematol 21:388–393, 1993.

55. Dorshkind K. Regulation of hemopoiesis by bone marrow stromal cells and their products. Annu Rev Immunol 8:111–137, 1992.

56. Koller M, Bender J, Papoutsakis E, Miller W. Effects of synergistic cytokine combination, low oxygen, and irradiated stroma on the expansion of human cord blood progenitors. Blood 80:403–411, 1992.

57. Deryugina E, Muller-Sieburg C. Stromal cells in long-term cultures: keys to the elucidation of hematopoietic development. Crit Rev Immunol 13:115–150, 1993.

58. Knospe W, Husseini S, Zipori D, Fried W. Hematopoiesis on cellulose ester membranes. XII. A combination of cloned stromal cells is needed to establish a hematopoietic microenvironment supportive of trilineage hematopoiesis. Exp Hematol 21:257–262, 1993.

182

59. Wineman J, Nishikawa S, Muller-Sieberg C. Maintenance of high levels of pluripotent hematopoietic stem cells in vitro: effect of stromal cells and c-kit. Blood 81:365–372, 1993.

60. Brandt J, Srour E, Besien K, Bridell R, Hoffman R. Cytokine-dependent long-term culture of highly enriched precursors of hematopoietic progenitor cells from human bone marrow. J Clin Invest 86(3):932–941, 1990.

61. Lansdorp P, Dragowska W, Mayani H. Ontogeny-related changes in proliferative potential of human hematopoietic cells. J Exp Med 178:787–791, 1993.

62. Brandt J, Briddell R, Srour E, Leemhuis T, Hoffman R. Role of c-kit ligand in the expansion of human hematopoietic progenitor cells. Blood 79:634–641, 1992.

63. Srour E, Brandt J, Briddell R, Grigsby S, Leemhuis T, Hoffman R. Long-term generation and expansion of human primitive hematopoietic progenitor cells in vitro. Blood 81:661–669, 1993.

64. Sandstrom C, Bender J, Miller W, Papoutsakis E. Comparison of perfused and static peripheral blood cell cultures with and wihtout stroma using a modified culture chamber for nonadherent cell retention. Biotech Bioeng 50:493–50, 1996.

65. Koller M, Palsson M, Manchel I, Palsson B. Long-term culture-initiating cell expansion is dependent on frequent medium exchange combined with stromal and other accessory cell effects. Blood 86(5):1784–1793, 1995.

66. Verfaillie C. Direct contact between human primitive hematopoietic progenitors and bone marrow stroma is not required for long-term in vitro hematopoiesis. Blood 79(11): 2821–2826, 1992.

67. Martiat P, Ferrant A, Cogneau M, et al. Assessment of bone marrow blood flow using positron emission tomography: no relationship with bone cellularity. Br J Haematol 60:307–310, 1987.

68. Caldwell J, Palsson B, Locey B, Emerson S. Culture perfusion schedules influence the metabolic activity and granulocyte-macrophage colony-stimulating factor production rates of human bone marrow stromal cells. J Cell Phys 147:344–353, 1991.

69. Schwartz R, Emerson S, Clarke M, Palsson B. In vitro myelopoiesis stimulated by rapid medium exchange and supplementation with hematopoietic growth factors. Blood 78(12):3155–3161, 1991.

70. Schwartz R, Palsson B, Emerson S. Rapid medium perfusion rate significantly increases the productivity of human bone marrow cultures. Proc Natl Acad Sci USA 88:6760–6764, 1991.

71. Koller M, Bender J, Miller W, Papoutsakis E. Expansion of primitive human hematopoietic progenitors in a perfusion bioreactor system with IL-3, IL-6, and stem cell factor. Biotechnology 11:358–363, 1993.

72. Ishikawa Y, Ito T. Kinetics of hemopoietic stem cells in a hypoxic culture. Eur J Haematol 40:126–129, 1988.

73. Lindop P, Rotblast J. Protection against acute effects of radiation by hypoxia. Nature 185:593–594, 1960.

74. Bradley T, Hodgson G, Rosendaal M. The effect of oxygen tension on hematopoietic and fibroblast cell proliferation in vitro. J Cell Physiol 97:517–522, 1978.

75. Rich I, Kubanek B. The effect of reduced oxygen tension on colony formation of erythropoietic cells in vitro. Br J Haematol 52:579–588, 1982.

76. Rich I. A role for the macrophage in normal hemopoiesis. II. Effect of varying physiological oxygen tensions on the release of hemopoietic growth factors from bone-marrow-derived macrophages in vitro. Exp Hematol 14:746–751, 1986.

77. Maeda H, Hotta T, Yamada H. Enhanced colony formation of human hemopoietic stem cells in reduced oxygen tension. Exp Hematol 14:930–934, 1986.

78. Broxmeyer H, Cooper S, Gabig T. The effects of oxidizing species derived from molecular oxygen on the proliferation in vitro of human granulocyte-macrophage progenitor cells. Ann NY Acad Sci 554:177–184, 1989.

79. Broxmeyer H, Cooper S, Lu L, Miller M, Langefeld C, Ralph P. Enhanced stimulation of

human bone marrow macrophage colony formation in vitro by recombinant human macrophage colony-stimulating factor in agarose medium and at low oxygen tension. Blood 76:323–329, 1990.

80. Muench M, Gasparetto C, Moore M. The in vitro growth of murine high proliferative potential-colony forming cells is not enhanced by growth in a low oxygen atmosphere. Cytokine 4(6):488–494, 1992.

81. Smith S, Broxmeyer H. The influence of oxygen tension on the long-term growth in vitro of haematopoietic progenitor cells from human cord blood. Br J Haematol 63:29–34, 1986.

82. Koller M, Bender J, Miller W, Papoutsakis E. Reduced oxygen tension increases hematopoiesis in long-term culture of human stem and progenitor cells from cord blood and bone marrow. Exp Hematol 20:264–270, 1992.

83. Cipolleschi M, Sbarba P, Olivotto M. The role of hypoxia in the maintenance of hematopoietic stem cells. Blood 82(7):2031–2037, 1993.

84. LaIuppa J, Miller W, Papoutsakis E. The effect of oxygen tension and cytokines on megakaryocytopoiesis and erythropoiesis. Blood 86:901a, 1995.

85. Barnes D, Sato G. Methods for growth of cultured cells in serum-free medium. Ann Biochem 102:255–270, 1980.

86. Waymouth C. Preparation and use of serum-free culture media. In Barnes D, Sirbasku D, Sato G (eds), Methods for Preparation of Media, Supplements, and Substrata for Serum-Free Animal Cell Culture. New York: Liss, 1984, pp. 23–68.

87. Cohen P, Fowler D, Kim H, et al. Propagation of mouse and human T cells with defined antigen specificity and function. Ciba Found Symp 187:179–193, 1994.

88. FDA, Points to consider in human somatic cell therapy and gene therapy. Docket No. 91N–0428, 1991.

89. Douay L, Giarratana M, Drouet X, Bardinet D. The role of recombinant haematopoietic growth factors in human long-term bone marrow culture in serum-free medium. Br J Haematol 70:27–32, 1991.

90. Sandstrom C, Collins P, Mcadams T, Bender J, Papoutsakis E, Miller W. Whole serum-deprived media for ex vivo expansion of hematopoietic progenitor cells from cord blood and peripheral blood mononuclear cells. J Hematother 5:461–473, 1996.

91. Choi E, Hokom M, Bartley T, et al. Recombinant human megakaryocyte growth and development factor (rHuMGDF), a ligand for c-Mpl, produces functional human platelets in vitro. Stem Cells 13:317–322, 1995.

92. Kimura H, Burstein S, Thorning D, et al. Human megakaryocytic progenitors (CFU-M) assayed in methylcellulose: physical characteristics and requirements for growth. J Cell Physiol 118:87–96, 1984.

93. Messner H, Jamal N, Izaguirre C. The growth of large megakaryocyte colonies from human bone marrow. J Cell Physiol Suppl 1:45–51, 1982.

94. Vainchenker W, Chapman J, Deschamps J, et al. Normal human serum contains a factor(s) capable of inhibiting megakaryocyte colony formation. Exp Hematol 10:650–660, 1982.

95. Mazur E, Basilico D, Newton J, et al. Isolation of large numbers of enriched human megakaryocytes from liquid cultures of normal peripheral blood progenitors. Blood 76(9):1771–1782, 1990.

96. Nichol J, Hornkohl A, Choi E, et al. Enrichment and characterization of peripheral blood-derived megakaryocyte progenitors that mature in short-term liquid culture. Stem Cells 12:494–505, 1994.

97. Chauvet M, Leger J, Molina L, Chabannon C, Hollard D. Study of megakaryocytic progenitors (CFU-MK) in human long-term bone marrow cultures (LTBMC): adjuvant effect of plasma from aplastic patients. Exp Hematol 18:61–64, 1990.

98. Berthier R, Valiron O, Schweitzer A, Marguerie G. Serum-free medium allows the optimal growth of human megakaryocyte progenitors compared with human plasma supplemented cultures: role of TGFβ. Stem Cells 11:120–129, 1993.

99. Lansdorp P, Dragowska W. Long-term erythropoiesis from constant numbers of CD34+ cells

184

in serum-free cultures initiated with highly purified progenitor cells from human bone marrow. J Exp Med 175:1501–1509, 1992.

100. Rebel V, Dragowska W, Eaves C, Humphries R, Lansdorp P. Amplification of Sca-1+ Lin-WGA+ cells in serum-free cultures containing steel factor, interleukin-6, and erythropoietin with maintenance of cells with long-term in vivo reconstituting potential. Blood 83(1):128–136, 1994.

101. Koller M, Manchel I, Palsson M, Maher R, Palsson B. Different measures of human hematopoietic cell culture performance are optimized under vastly different culture conditions. Biotech Bioeng 50:505–513, 1996.

102. Collins P, Miller W, Papoutsakis E. Seeding density affects proliferation, differentiation, and metabolic patterns of peripheral blood mononuclear cell cultures. Blood 86:660a, 1995.

103. McAdams T, Papoutsakis E, Miller W. Culture pH influences erythroid proliferation and differentiation. Blood 86:674a, 1995.

104. Bender J, To L, Williams S, Schwartzberg L. Defining a therapeutic dose of peripheral blood stem cells. J Hematother 1:329–341, 1992.

105. Brugger W, Heimfeld S, Berenson R, Mertelsmann R, Kantz L. Reconstitution of hematopoiesis after high-dose chemotherapy by autologous progenitor cells generated ex vivo. N Engl J Med 333(5):283–287, 1995.

106. McAlister I, Teepe M, Gillis S, Williams D. Ex vivo expansion of peripheral blood progenitor cells with recombinant cytokines. Exp Hematol 20:626–628, 1992.

107. Takaue Y, Abe T, Kawano Y, et al. Combination of recombinant cytokines fails to produce ex vivo expansion of human blood hematopoietic progenitor cells. Ann Hematol 64:217–220, 1992.

108. Lemoli R, Tafuri A, Strife A, Andreeff M, Clarkson B, Gulati S. Proliferation of human hematopoietic progenitors in long-term bone marrow cultures in gas-permeable plastic bags is enhanced by colony-stimulating factors. Exp Hematol 20:569–575, 1992.

109. Bender J, Zimmerman T, Lee W, et al. Large scale selection of CD34+ cells and expansion of neutrophil precursors in PIXY321 for clinical application. Blood 84(10):542a, 1994.

110. Zimmerman T, Bender J, Lee W, et al. Selection and expansion of CD34+ cells: feasibility and safety associated with clinical use. Blood 86(10):294a, 1995.

111. Koller M, Emerson S, Palsson B. Large-scale expansion of human stem and progenitor cells from bone marrow mononuclear cells in continuous perfusion cultures. Blood 82(2):378–384, 1993.

112. Palsson B, Paek S, Schwartz R, et al. Expansion of human bone marrow progenitor cells in a high cell density continuous perfusion system. Biotechnology 11:368–372, 1993.

113. Zandstra P, Eaves C, Piret J. Expansion of hematopoietic progenitor cell populations in stirred suspension bioreactors of normal human bone marrow cells. Biotechnology 12:909–914, 1994.

114. Sardonini C, Wu Y. Expansion and differentiation of human hematopoietic cells from static cultures through small-scale bioreactors. Biotechnol Prog 9:131–137, 1993.

115. Champlin R, Mehra R, Gajewski J, et al. Ex vivo expanded progenitor cell transplantation in patients with breast cancer. Blood 86(10):295a, 1995.

116. Armstrong R, Ogler W, Maluta J. Clinical systems for the production of human cells and tissues. Biotechnology 13:449–453, 1995.

117. Silver S, Adams P, Hutchinson R, et al. Phase I evaluation of ex vivo expanded hematopoietic cells produced by perfusion cultures in autologous bone marrow transplantation (BMT). Blood 82:297a, 1993.

118. FDA. Current Good Manufacturing Practices. Washington, DC, 1993.

119. duMoulin G, Stack J, Pitkin Z, et al. A 3-year experience of quality control and quality assurance in the multisite delivery of a lymphocyte-based cellular therapy for renal cell carcinoma. Biotech Bioeng 43:693–699, 1994.

120. LaIuppa J, McAdams T, Miller W, Papoutsakis E. Polymer and metal substrates affect the ex vivo expansion of CD34+ cells. Blood 86:231a, 1995.

121. Muench M, Moore M. Accelerated recovery of peripheral blood cell counts in mice trans-

planted with in vitro cytokine-expanded hematopoietic progenitors. Exp Hematol 20:611–618, 1992.

122. Muench M, Firpo M, Moore M. Bone marrow transplantation with interleukin-1 plus kit-ligand ex vivo expanded bone marrow accelerates hematopoietic reconstitution in mice without the loss of stem cell lineage and proliferative potential. Blood 81(12):3463–3473, 1993.

123. Knobel K, McNally M, Berson A, et al. Long-term reconstitution of mice after ex vivo expansion of bone marrow cells: differential activity of cultured bone marrow and enriched stem cell populations. Exp Hematol 22:1227–1235, 1994.

124. Holyoake T, Alcorn M, Richmond L, et al. A phase I study to evaluate the safety of re-infusing CD34 cells expanded ex vivo as part or all of a PBPC transplant procedure. Blood 86(10):294a, 1995.

125. Dexter T, Allen T, Lajitha L. Conditions controlling the proliferation of haemopoietic stem cells in vitro. J Cell Physiol 91:335–344, 1977.

9. Allogeneic umbilical cord blood transplantation

John E. Wagner

Bone marrow transplantation (BMT) from HLA-identical sibling donors has been successfully utilized in the treatment of high-risk or recurrent hematological malignancies, bone marrow failure syndromes, and selected hereditary immunodeficiency states and metabolic disorders. Use of allogeneic BMT has been limited both by the lack of suitable donors and because of the risk of life-threatening complications that arise when donor and recipient are not immunologically identical, namely, graft failure and graft-versus-host disease (GVHD).

In an attempt to increase the availability of suitable donors and reduce the morbidity and mortality associated with allogeneic BMT, clinical investigators worldwide have evaluated placental and umbilical cord blood as an alternate source of hematopoietic stem and progenitor cells for transplantation [1–14]. Early successes with the transplantation of umbilical cord blood have prompted considerable investigation into this stem cell source. Numerous laboratory investigators have subsequently confirmed the high frequency of primitive hematopoietic progenitors and have begun to describe the functional capacities of the neonatal immune system. As a result of these clinical and laboratory observations, large-scale banking of umbilical cord blood for clinical transplantation has been initiated in the U.S. and Europe.

Ontologically, hematopoiesis begins in the ventral aspect of the fetal aorta [15] and primitive yolk sac early after conception. Following a brief hepatic phase, it enters the bone marrow space at the end of the second trimester, where it remains almost exclusively throughout adulthood [16,17]. It has long been known that human placental and umbilical cord blood contains hematopoietic progenitor cells at high frequency. The frequency of granulocyte-macrophage (CFU-GM) progenitor cells equals or exceeds that of adult bone marrow and greatly surpasses that of unmobilized adult peripheral blood [18–21].

As of December 1995, umbilical cord blood from sibling and unrelated donors has been used to reconstitute hematopoiesis in more than 150 patients with malignant and nonmalignant disorders treated with myeloablative therapy. The clinical results demonstrate that transplantation of umbilical cord blood is associated with a high probability of engraftment and low risk of

Jane N. Winter (ed.) BLOOD STEM CELL TRANSPLANTATION. 1997. Kluwer Academic Publishers. ISBN 0-7923-4260-7. All rights reserved.

severe acute GVHD in children. What remains to be determined is the 'breadth of applicability' of this stem cell source: 1) are there adequate numbers of hematopoietic stem and progenitor cells to engraft adult-size recipients? and 2) is the neonatal immune system sufficiently different from that of the adult to allow greater HLA disparity between donor and recipient without concomitant increases in graft rejection or GVHD? This chapter will review the clinical results with umbilical cord blood transplantation and will introduce potential ethical issues and limitations related to this stem cell source. In addition, current information regarding hematopoietic cells circulating in placental and umbilical cord blood and the properties of the neonatal immune system will be summarized.

Historical background

The use of human umbilical cord blood as a source of transplantable hematopoietic stem cells was first suggested by Professor Edward A. Boyse in 1983. In 1984–1985, the hypothesis that umbilical cord blood contained long-term reconstituting hematopoietic stem cells was first tested in a murine model [22]. In the first of four experiments, three seven-week-old (B6 × A-T1a^b)F1 hybrid males were irradiated with 862.8 rads and then transplanted with 0.17 mL heparinized whole blood obtained from near-term (B6-T1a^a × A)F1 mouse embryos. As shown in table 1 (experiment 1), 2 of 3 recipients of fetal blood survived to day 30, in contrast to 0 of 7 controls. Thirty-day survivors were subsequently typed for the T1a markers distinguishing donor from recipient lymphohematopoietic cells. In both instances, animals demonstrated repopulation with donor cells, showing that lethally irradiated mice could be reconstituted with blood from near-term embryos.

This was followed by a second experiment in which ten animals were each injected with either blood from near-term embryos (at a smaller volume than used in experiment 1) or blood from adult donors (table 1, experiment 2). Notably, none of the 20 mice receiving either adult blood or no blood survived, while 5 of 10 recipients of 0.02 mL of near-term embryo blood survived to day 30. In all cases, 30-day survivors had evidence of the T1a^a marker, again confirming the presence of donor cells.

Together with two additional experiments evaluating the engraftment potential of neonatal blood (donors <24 hours of age) and smaller volumes of blood (table 1, experiments 3 and 4, respectively), the results showed that near-term and neonatal blood contained sufficient numbers of stem and progenitor cells to allow both early lymphohematopoietic recovery and sustained engraftment of donor cells.

These results in the murine model supported the hypothesis that small quantities of neonatal blood were sufficient for at least short-term hematopoietic recovery of donor origin. Together with previous data documenting the presence of circulating hematopoietic progenitors in human umbilical cord

Table 1. Successful lymphohematopoietic reconstitution of lethally irradiated mice transplanted with blood from near-term embryos or neonates ≤24 hours of age

Experiment 1[a]		
Treatment group	Day of death	30-day survival
0.17 mL near-term fetal blood	14	2/3
No treatment control	11, 12, 12, 13, 13, 15, 15	0/7

Experiment 2[a]		
Treatment group	Day of death	30-day survival
0.02 mL near-term fetal blood	10, 12, 12, 14, 14	5/10
0.02 mL adult blood	11, 11, 12, 12, 12, 13, 14, 14, 15, 15	0/10
No treatment control	9, 10, 10, 11, 11, 12, 12, 12, 15, 23	0/10

Experiment 3[a]		
Treatment group	Day of death	30-day survival
0.04 mL neonatal blood	12	4/5
0.02 mL neonatal blood	14, 18	3/5
0.01 mL neonatal blood	12, 12, 14, 14	1/5
No treatment control	5, 6, 9, 10, 11	0/5

Experiment 4[b]		
Treatment group	Day of death	30-day survival
0.015 mL neonatal blood	12, 12, 12, 13, 13, 13	4/10
0.01 mL neonatal blood	12, 16	3/5
No treatment control	12, 13, 14, 17, 22	0/5

[a] In experiments 1–3, seven-week-old (B6 × A-Tla[b])F1 hybrid males were first treated with 862.8 rads (107.85 rad/min) using a ^{137}Cs source (LD100/30 days) and subsequently transplanted with near-term or neonatal or adult blood from (B6-Tla[a] × A)F1 hybrid male donors within two hours of irradiation.

[b] In experiment 4, recipient mice were female. Chimerism was established by typing for the Tla marker by cytotoxicity assay of thymocytes.

blood, the next obstacle was the establishment of a practical and efficient method of collecting and storing umbilical cord blood for clinical use. With the aid of several obstetrical services, Broxmeyer et al. [20,21] evaluated the nucleated cell and progenitor content and sterility of more than 100 umbilical cord blood specimens before and after cryopreservation. The fact that umbilical cord blood remained viable at 4°C or 25°C for at least three days after collection confirmed that cell viability during transport between hospitals would not be compromised prior to cryopreservation. Studies to maximize the collection of placental and umbilical cord blood proved that the task of collection was remarkably simple, requiring only the patience of the obstetrical team. Moreover, Broxmeyer et al. demonstated that umbilical cord blood progenitors responded normally to stimulation by various recombinant human hematopoietic growth factors. Another observation of practical importance was that procedures to remove erythrocytes or granulocytes prior to cryopreservation entailed significant loss of progenitors, suggesting that such procedures might be detrimental to engraftment. In summary, these results suggested that unprocessed umbilical cord blood from a single donor could serve as a sufficient source of hematopoietic stem and progenitor cells for an autologous or allogeneic recipient.

Based on results of in vitro assays of human umbilical cord blood and the finding that fetal blood from mice could rescue lethally irradiated adult recipients, Professor Boyse and Judith Bard first considered the possibility of harvesting umbilical cord blood with therapeutic intent. An international collaboration led to the first human umbilical cord blood transplant in Paris on October 6, 1988. A year later, the results were reported [1]. The investigators had clearly demonstrated that a 19-kilogram patient with Fanconi anemia had complete hematopoietic recovery with 150/150 bone marrow metaphases being of donor origin at day 120.

Clinical results

Despite several editorials [23,24] suggesting that umbilical cord blood would have limited applicability in the clinical transplant setting, numerous investigators worldwide began to explore the potential of umbilical cord blood stem cells. Many questions were raised. Would this stem cell source engraft larger recipients (>19 kilograms) with diseases other than Fanconi anemia? Would lethal GVHD occur because of maternal lymphocyte contamination? Alternatively, would umbilical cord blood lymphocytes be less likely to cause a graft-versus-host reaction because of 'immunologic naivete'? Would there be a greater risk of leukemic relapse? While some questions have yet to be answered, we now know that the observations made in that first child with Fanconi anemia regarding engraftment and absence of GVHD were not unique.

Sibling donor umbilical cord blood transplantation

Patient population. Data on patients receiving umbilical cord blood transplants for malignant and nonmalignant disorders have previously been reported [25]. As of November 1995, 62 patients have been reported by 22 transplant teams to the International Cord Blood Transplant Registry (table 2). Patients were aged 0.5 to 16 years. Eleven patients received HLA 1–3 antigen mismatched grafts. Prophylaxis for acute GVHD consisted of cyclosporine A alone or in combination with methylprednisolone or an anti-T-cell antibody ($n = 40$), cyclosporine A with short-course methotrexate ($n = 18$), or methotrexate alone or in combination with methylprednisolone ($n = 2$); two

190

Table 2. Diseases treated by umbilical cord blood transplantation using sibling donors

Malignant diseases	Nonmalignant diseases
Acute lymphocytic leukemia	Fanconi anemia
Acute myelocytic leukemia	Idiopathic aplastic anemia
Juvenile chronic myelogeneous leukemia	Thalassemia
Chronic myelogeneous leukemia	Sickle cell anemia
Neuroblastoma	Severe combined immunodeficiency
Myelodysplastic syndrome	X-linked lymphoproliferative syndrome
	Wiskott–Aldrich syndrome
	Hurler syndrome
	Hunter syndrome
	Gunther disease

patients received no prophylaxis. Hematopoietic growth factors were used early after the infusion of umbilical cord blood in 37 patients by study design; 20 received granulocyte-macrophage colony stimulating factor (GM-CSF), 14 received granulocyte colony stimulating factor (G-CSF), and 3 received both simultaneously.

Umbilical cord blood graft characteristics. The method of umbilical cord blood collection varied significantly between institutions; however, the majority of collections were performed by obstetricians or nurse midwives without any prior experience in the large-scale collection of placental and umbilical cord blood. The median volume of umbilical cord blood collected was 98 mL (range: 42.1–282 mL). The median number of cells and colony forming unit-granulocyte macrophages (CFU-GMs) in the graft on the basis of the recipient's body weight was 4.7×10^7/kg (range: $1.0–33.0 \times 10^7$) and 1.7×10^4/kg (range $<0.1–25.6 \times 10^4$), respectively. Despite the diversity of collection systems and inexperience of collectors, the majority of samples were sterile. In 6 of 44 reported cases, the cord blood was contaminated with bacteria. Notably, bacterial contamination of the cord blood graft did not have any demonstrable impact on the posttransplant morbidity in any patient.

Hematopoietic recovery and engraftment. For recipients of HLA-matched or HLA-1 antigen mismatched umbilical cord blood grafts, the actuarial probability of hematopoietic recovery at 60 days after transplantation was 0.91 ± 0.08 (figure 1). Median time to neutrophil recovery (defined as time to achieve an absolute neutrophil count [ANC] $\geq 5 \times 10^8$/L) and platelet recovery (defined as platelet count $\geq 5 \times 10^{10}$/L untransfused for seven days) was 22.0 days (range: 9 to 46) and 51 days (range: 15 to 117) after transplantation, respectively. Four patients never had signs of hematopoietic recovery, and one patient had early recovery but cells were entirely host in origin. Of the five patients without donor cell engraftment, four had undergone umbilical cord blood transplantation for the treatment of a bone marrow failure syndrome and one for the treatment of Hunter syndrome.

191

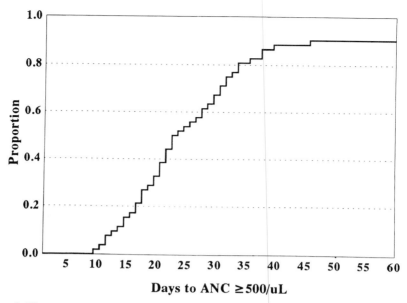

Figure 1. Time to neutrophil recovery (i.e., absolute neutrophil count ≥500/uL) in recipients transplanted with HLA-identical or HLA-1 antigen disparate sibling donor umbilical cord blood.

Correlation between nucleated cell count or hematopoietic progenitor cell content (not shown) of the graft and time to neutrophil recovery or probability of engraftment has yet to be demonstrated (figure 2). While the use of hematopoietic growth factors has not appreciably shortened the time to neutrophil recovery, the possibility of patient selection bias prevents definitive conclusion.

Graft-versus-host disease. Acute GVHD has occurred very infrequently in recipients of HLA-matched and HLA-1 antigen mismatched umbilical cord blood transplants. The actuarial probability of grade II–IV GVHD at 100 days after transplantation remains 0.02 ± 0.02. Notably, no patient has been reported to have grade III–IV acute GVHD. Of the entire cohort of patients, chronic GVHD has been reported in only three patients to date, with no patient having had extensive disease.

Interestingly, moderate to severe GVHD has infrequently been observed in eight evaluable patients with haploidentical sibling donors. Of these eight patients, three were mismatched at one antigen, one was mismatched at two antigens, and four were mismatched at three antigens. As shown in table 3, donor–recipient pairs mismatched at the maternal allele appeared to be less likely to develop grade II–IV GVHD than donor–recipient pairs mismatched at the paternal allele. This observation supports the hypothesis that partial tolerance may develop to the noninherited maternal allele during gestation.

192

Nucleated Cells/kg (x10e7)

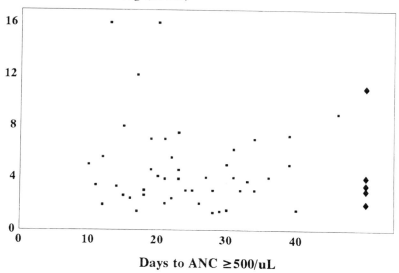

Days to ANC ≥500/uL

Figure 2. Comparison between the number of nucleated cells per kilogram recipient body weight and time to neutrophil recovery (ANC ≥500/uL) after sibling donor transplantation. Number of nucleated cells per kilogram transplanted in recipients failing to engraft are also shown (♦).

Table 3. Risk of GVHD after haploidentical sibling donor umbilical cord blood transplantation

	Disparity at the NIMA	Disparity at the NIPA
Grade 0–I GVHD	6	1
Grade II–IV GVHD	0	3

Ten patients with HLA-2 or HLA-3 antigen-disparate sibling donor grafts were evaluable for acute GVHD. Six patients received umbilical cord blood from donors disparate at the noninherited maternal allele (NIMA) and four patients received umbilical cord blood from donors disparate at the noninherited paternal allele (NIPA).

Survival. At a median follow-up of 2.0 years, the actuarial probability of survival for recipients of HLA-matched and HLA-1 antigen mismatched grafts was 0.61 ± 0.12. Causes of death were multifactorial, including graft failure, relapse, interstitial pneumonitis/adult respiratory distress syndrome, veno-occlusive disease, intracranial hemorrhage, and early bacterial sepsis. For the entire cohort, GVHD was listed as a cause of death in only one patient with an HLA-3 antigen mismatched donor graft. The actuarial probability of disease-free survival in patients transplanted for malignancy was 0.41 ± 0.11. Relapse was observed in two patients with relapsed neuroblastoma and in one patient with relapsed acute myelocytic leukemia after prior autologous BMT, in two patients with juvenile chronic myelogenous leukemia, in three patients with acute lymphocytic leukemia (one in CR1 but with the 9;22 translocation; two in CR2), and in one patient with adult-type chronic myelogeneous leukemia.

Summary. This analysis of the Registry data demonstrates that 1) the rate of neutrophil recovery is comparable to that observed after BMT, 2) use of hematopoietic growth factors does not shorten time to neutrophil recovery, 3) there is no correlation between nucleated cell count or progenitor cell content of the graft and time to neutrophil recovery or engraftment, suggesting the number of progenitor cells in umbilical cord blood exceeds the threshold needed for engraftment, 4) there is potentially a higher risk of graft failure in patients with nonmalignancy states, as compared to those with malignancy, and 5) GVHD occurs infrequently in recipients of umbilical cord blood, with results in haploidentical transplants supporting the postulate of partial tolerance to the noninherited maternal allele.

While patient age has been previously shown to be an important predictor of GVHD [26,27], it does not fully explain the extremely low incidence of grade II–IV disease observed in patients transplanted with umbilical cord blood. Properties of the neonatal immune system that might account for the relative absence of a GVH reaction are currently being explored. Recent reports, however, suggest that the frequency of helper T-lymphocyte precursors (HTLp) and cytotoxic T-lymphocyte precursors (CTLp) cells in umbilical cord blood is similar to or exceeds that in adult peripheral blood [28,29] and that activation by alloantigen is normal [28]. Other reports, however, suggest that the cytotoxic activity of umbilical cord blood does not reside with CTLs but only in the natural killer (NK) cell compartment [30]. Further, proliferative and cytotoxic responses of umbilical cord blood lymphocytes are blunted compared to those of adult peripheral blood lymphocytes [31].

Importantly, these data also suggest that maternal cell contamination of the umbilical cord blood at the time of collection may be of limited clinical importance. Kurtzberg et al. (presented by Broxmeyer et al. [2]), Wagner et al. [3] and Vilmer et al. [4] have failed to demonstrate maternal cells in the umbilical cord blood grafts by cytogenetic or DNA techniques. While maternal cell contamination is probably present in most if not all umbilical cord blood grafts [32,33], the very low incidence of GVHD observed in transplant recipients suggests that carefully collected umbilical cord blood either contains insignificant numbers of maternal T cells or that maternal T cells are not immunologically active in this context.

Unrelated donor umbilical cord blood transplantation

Since its inception in 1986, the National Marrow Donor Program (NMDP) has identified a pool of 1.92 million potential marrow donors and facilitated 3965 unrelated donor bone marrow transplants as of December 1, 1995 (personal communication, National Marrow Donor Program). While many patients have benefited from such transplants, several important obstacles prevent even greater success. These include 1) long length of the donor search process, currently a median of 3.5 months (range: one month to six years [34]), 2) limited numbers of donors in certain racial and ethnic subpopulations, 3) donor unavailability at the time of request, and 4) an increased risk of graft rejection, severe GVHD, and opportunistic infection after the transplant procedure [34]. Various strategies for ameliorating these problems are currently being investigated.

As a result of the early successes with umbilical cord blood from sibling donors, pilot programs for the banking of unrelated donor umbilical cord blood have been proposed in many countries worldwide [35,36] and initiated in New York, Milan, Dusseldorf, Paris, and London. Potential benefits of banked umbilical cord blood include 1) rapid availability (two weeks for confirmatory HLA testing), 2) absence of donor risk, 3) absence of donor attrition, and 4) very low risk of transmissible infectious diseases, such as cytomegalovirus [37] and Epstein–Barr virus [38]. Other potential advantages that remain to be determined include 1) lower risk of acute GVHD and 2) greater ability to expand the available donor pool in targeted ethnic and racial minorities currently underrepresented in all marrow donor registries.

Patient population at the University of Minnesota. Patients with high-risk leukemia, bone marrow failure syndromes, immunodeficiency states, or inborn errors of metabolism were eligible for a phase I clinical trial at the University of Minnesota, if 1) an HLA-compatible related or unrelated bone marrow donor could not be identified within four months of search request, 2) the nucleated cell count of the umbilical cord blood graft exceeded 1×10^7 per kilogram recipient body weight, and 3) patient and/or guardian consented to the transplant procedure. Algorithm for patient selection is detailed in figure 3. Thirteen patients received unrelated donor umbilical cord blood transplants for malignant and nonmalignant disorders between July 1994 and December 1995 at the University of Minnesota. The median age and weight of patients was 2.5 years (range: 0.1 to 21.3) and 12.1 kilograms (range: 3.3 to 78.8), respectively. The diagnosis and disease status of patients at the time of transplantation are shown in table 4. Five patients received grafts that were matched at HLA-A, B, and DRß1, and eight received grafts that were disparate at one to three HLA loci.

Pretransplant conditioning varied according to the patient's disease. At the University of Minnesota, all patients with acute lymphocytic leukemia (ALL) were treated with hyperfractionated total body irradiation (TBI) 1375 cGy, cyclophosphamide 120 mg/kg, and antithymocyte globulin (ATGAM, Upjohn) 60 mg/kg; all patients with acute myelogenous leukemia (AML) and juvenile chronic myelogeneous leukemia (JCML) were treated with cyclophosphamide 120 mg/kg, fractionated TBI 1320 cGy, and ATGAM 60 mg/kg; patients with bone marrow failure syndromes or metabolic disease were

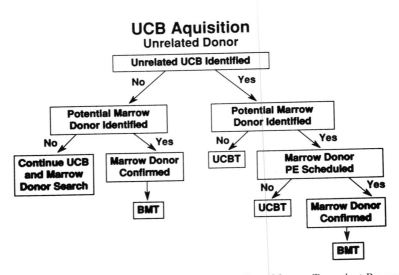

UCB Aquisition
Unrelated Donor

Figure 3. Algorithm used by the University of Minnesta Bone Marrow Transplant Program for selecting the source of unrelated donor hematopoietic stem cells (umbilical cord blood versus bone marrow). Abbreviations: UCBT, umbilical cord blood transplant; BMT, bone marrow transplant.

Table 4. Diagnosis and disease status of patients transplanted with unrelated donor umbilical cord blood at University of Minnesota as of December 1995

UPN#	Disease	Age/Sex	Wt	Prep Rx	HLA disparity
2051	ALL CR3	10.9/M	47.7	TBI/CY	6/6
2058	GLD	2.8/M	18.7	BU/CY/TBI	5/6 (DR)
M007	AML REL2	2.5/M	12.1	CY/TBI	5/6 (B)
2207	ALL REL3	10.5/M	35.3	TBI/CY	6/6
2214	Blackfan–Diamond	1.4/M	9.1	BU/CY/TBI	4/6 (B,DRB1)
2224	AML REL3	2.1/M	11.2	CY/TBI	6/6
2240	AML CR2	1.0/F	7.5	CY/TBI	4/6 (B,DRB1)
2249	ALL CR2	1.0/F	6.5	TBI/CY	5/6 (A)
2270	Osteopetrosis	0.1/M	3.3	BU/CY/TBI	5/6 (A)
2293	AML REL2	14.9/F	78.8	CY/TBI	6/6
2297	ALL REL1 Ph1+	10.0/F	29.0	TBI/CY	5/6 (DRB1)
2313	FA/RA	21.3/F	49.5	CY/TBI	3/6 (B,B,DRB1)
2316	JCML	1.1/F	10.0	CY/TBI	6/6

Abbreviations: Age, age in years; Wt, weight in kilograms; ALL, acute lymphocytic leukemia; Ph1+, Philadelphia chromosome positive; AML, acute myelocytic leukemia; GLD, globoid cell leukodystrophy; ALD, adrenoleukodystrophy; FA/RA, Fanconi anemia with refractory anemia; CR, complete remission; REL, relapse; TBI, total body irradiation; CY, cyclophosphamide; BU, busulfan.

treated with busulfan 320 mg/m², cyclophosphamide 120 mg/kg, TBI 750 cGy in a single fraction, and ATGAM 60 mg/kg. Prophylaxis for acute GVHD consisted of cyclosporine A in combination with methylprednisolone ($n = 11$) or methotrexate ($n = 2$).

Umbilical cord blood graft characteristics. Searches for potential unrelated donor umbilical cord blood grafts were performed by the New York Blood Center. Prior to transplantation, confirmatory HLA typing of patient and cryopreserved donor specimens were performed using standard serological techniques identifying all WHO-recognized specificities for HLA-A and B antigens. In addition, HLA-DR typing of all 13 donor–recipient pairs was performed using high-resolution DNA techniques. For this cohort of patients, the median time between date of initial search request and umbilical cord blood transplantation was 83 days (range: 52 to 152). Notably, the median time between date of initial search request and HLA confirmation of the donor graft was 40 days (range: 12 to 114).

The methods of umbilical cord blood collection and testing have been reported previously [35]. Briefly, the delivered placenta was suspended from a frame with the umbilical cord side down. After cleansing the umbilical cord with ethanol and iodine, the blood was collected by cannulating the umbilical vein with a 16-gauge needle. Blood was collected into a blood collection bag (Baxter) containing approximately 23 mL citrate phosphate dextrose-A (CPD-A). The blood was stored at room temperature and transported to the New York Blood Center for testing and cryopreservation. All grafts were cryopreserved in DMSO (10% final concentration).

Cryopreserved donor units were delivered to the University of Minnesota from the New York Blood Center via air transportation by overnight express. Prior to infusion, the umbilical cord blood graft was placed in a sterile bag and then thawed in a 38°C waterbath with gentle agitation. After thawing, an equal volume of dextran/albumin solution was added over 10 minutes, centrifuged at 250 g for 10 minutes at 10°C, and the supernatant removed. The cell pellet was resuspended in dextran/albumin and immediately infused into the patient over 30 minutes to four hours.

The median volume of UCB collected was 83.1 mL (range: 46.6–104 mL), and the median number of nucleated cells per kilogram recipient weight was 4.1×10^7 (range: 1.4 to 40.0).

Hematopoietic recovery and engraftment. Nine of 13 patients were considered evaluable for hematopoietic recovery (i.e., survival >30 days). The probability of donor-derived neutrophil recovery at 60 days after transplantation was 1.00 ± 0.00 with a median time to an ANC $\geq 5 \times 10^8/L$ of 29 days (range: 16 to 53). As reported for recipients of sibling donor umbilical cord blood, time to neutrophil recovery did not correlate with the number of nucleated cells infused (correlation coefficient: −0.135) based on recipient body weight. Insufficient data were available for a correlation of engraftment with numbers of granulocyte-macrophage colony forming cells infused.

Platelet recovery was delayed, as has been reported for recipients of sibling donor umbilical cord blood [25]. Of nine evaluable patients, seven became platelet transfusion independent. For these patients, the median time to achieve a platelet count $\geq 2 \times 10^{10}/L$ and $\geq 5 \times 10^{10}/L$ was 54 days (range: 39 to 130) and 67 days (range: 55 to 120) after transplantation, respectively.

Of 11 patients surviving to day 21 (day of marrow examination), all had evidence of myeloid and erythroid engraftment. Eight demonstrated complete chimerism and two demonstrated mixed chimerism with one patient having insufficient numbers of cells for evaluation. Mixed chimerism in one patient was due to persistent disease.

Graft-versus-host disease. For these recipients of HLA identical and HLA-1 to 3 antigen-disparate umbilical cord blood grafts, the probability of having grade II–IV acute GVHD by 100 days after transplantation was 0.50 ± 0.11. In two cases, however, the cutaneous disease recurred during steriod taper and required treatment with antithymocyte globulin. The probability of grade III–IV acute GVHD by 100 days after transplantation was 0.0 ± 0.0 in this series. Notably, the two recipients of HLA 2 antigen-disparate unrelated umbilical cord blood grafts had only grade II disease, with both responding to steroid therapy alone.

Survival. The probability of survival at three and six months after transplantation is 0.69 ± 0.10. Causes of death were early fungal sepsis ($n = 2$), chemotherapy-related toxicity/multiorgan failure ($n = 1$), and relapse ($n = 2$). Of the two patients relapsing after unrelated donor umbilical cord blood transplant, both had AML in relapse at the time of transplant with one having previously relapsed after autologous marrow transplantation.

Summary. Similar to the results observed in recipients of umbilical cord blood from sibling donors, a high rate of engraftment was observed after unrelated donor umbilical cord blood transplantation. In this study, all patients surviving at least 30 days demonstrated donor-derived hematopoiesis, with early evidence of hematopoietic recovery in three additional patients dying between days 21 and 28. These patients achieved an ANC $\geq 5 \times 10^8$/L at a median of 29 days, which is greater than that observed after sibling donor umbilical cord blood transplantation (median 22.5 days [25]) and unrelated donor bone marrow transplantation [34]. Platelet recovery, however, was markedly delayed, as observed in sibling donor umbilical cord blood transplant recipients. While longer follow-up is required for some patients enrolled in this trial, donor-derived hematopoiesis has been sustained, with late graft failure yet to be observed. Notably, Kurtzberg et al. [39] have observed graft failure in 2 of 19 evaluable recipients of unrelated donor umbilical cord blood. This result is particularly interesting in view of the disproportionate number of patients with HLA-2 and 3 antigen-disparate donors. A list of diseases treated by unrelated donor umbilical cord blood transplantation is shown in table 5.

Of note, engraftment was also observed in the largest recipient, who weighed 78.8 kilograms (figure 4). Rates of neutrophil and platelet recovery, however, were exceedingly slow. While trilineage hematopoiesis of donor

Table 5. Diseases treated by umbilical cord blood transplantation using unrelated donors

Malignant diseases	Nonmalignant diseases
Acute lymphocytic leukemia	Fanconi anemia
Acute myelocytic leukemia	Idiopathic aplastic anemia
Juvenile chronic myelogeneous leukemia	Amegakaryocytic thrombocytopenia
Chronic myelogeneous leukemia	Kostman syndrome
Myelodysplastic syndrome	Blackfan–Diamond syndrome
Neuroblastoma	Osteopetrosis
	Globoid cell leukodystrophy
	Adrenoleukodystrophy
	Lesch–Nyhan syndrome

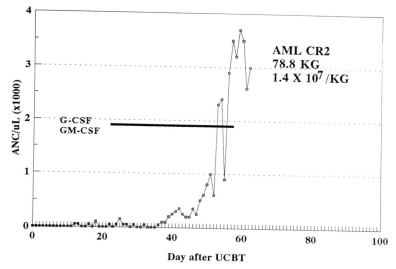

Figure 4. Hematopoietic recovery in a single patient weighing 78.8 kilograms.

origin was documented in the bone marrow as early as 21 days after transplantation, neutrophil recovery in the peripheral blood was not observed until day 40. Notably, no correlation between nucleated cell content of the umbilical cord blood graft and interval to neutrophil recovery could be discerned despite the wide range of cell doses infused in this cohort. Whether the marked delay in recovery in the single adult-size recipient will be a consistent finding remains to be determined.

The second major endpoint of this phase I clinical trial was to estimate the risk of grade II–IV and grade III–IV acute GVHD after unrelated donor umbilical cord blood transplantation. In this series, the incidence of grade II–IV GVHD was 50%. All patients, however, had disease limited to the skin and, in most cases, responsive to first-line therapy with methylprednisolone alone. These results compare favorably with those reported for young recipients of unrelated donor bone marrow [40,41]. Balduzzi et al. [41] have recently reported an incidence of grade III–IV acute GVHD of 37% and 63% in recipients of HLA matched ($n = 46$) and HLA mismatched ($n = 41$) unrelated donor bone marrow, respectively. While case-controlled studies must be performed to verify the benefit of unrelated donor umbilical cord blood in terms of GVHD risk, these results indeed prove that umbilical cord blood lymphocytes are capable of inducing a significant graft-versus-host response. Indeed, others have reported grade III and IV acute GVHD after unrelated donor umbilical cord blood transplantation. Detailed analysis of these patients is warranted to rule out the possibility of maternal lymphocyte contamination and unknown HLA disparities.

Umbilical cord blood collection, separation, and cryopreservation

Documentation of hematological reconstitution after myeloablative therapy and umbilical cord blood transplantation has resulted in considerable interest in the techniques of placental and umbilical cord blood collection and storage. While the individual procedures used are not novel, the collection and processing procedures for umbilical cord blood are not the same as those used for bone marrow. Unlike the typical bone marrow collection, the obstetrician and/ or hematologist cannot collect a predetermined volume of umbilical cord blood but rather are restricted to the finite amount available.

Using an open collection procedure detailed elsewhere [42], a variety of obstetricians nationwide have collected umbilical cord blood for purposes of hematopoietic stem cell transplantation. The volume of umbilical cord blood collected ranged from 42 mL to 240 mL, with a median volume of 103 ± 49 mL ($n = 38$). Needle aspirations of the placental veins produced an additional 8 mL to 85 mL, with a median volume of 31 ± 16 mL ($n = 31$). Of specimens ($n = 38$) sent by overnight courier express mail, the total number of nucleated cells contained in a single collection has ranged from 4.7×10^8 to 4.6×10^9 cells with a median value of $1.4 \times 10^9 \pm 0.96 \times 10^9$. The nucleated cell concentration varied significantly between patients (range: 3.1×10^6 cells/mL to 24.3×10^6 cells/mL). The numbers of day-14 colony forming unit-granulocyte/macrophage (CFU-GMs, colonies and clusters) ranged from 5.4×10^5 to 59.2×10^5 (median $21.5 \times 10^5 \pm 3.1 \times 10^5$ [standard error of measurement]). While these numbers of nucleated cells and CFU-GMs have subsequently been shown to be sufficient for engraftment, at least in smaller recipients, these numbers are far less than that expected for the typical bone marrow allograft regardless of recipient size.

A variety of collection methods (figure 5) have been proposed in order to optimize the collection volume and reduce the risks of microbial and maternal cell contamination [42–47]. While no single method has been proven to be substantially better than another, the collection of free-flowing umbilical cord blood into an open collection jar has several potential advantages, the most important being the ease of collection, which requires no training and little setup time. In contrast, closed systems utilizing catheters and needles are technically more challenging and not uniformly transferrable to obstetricians

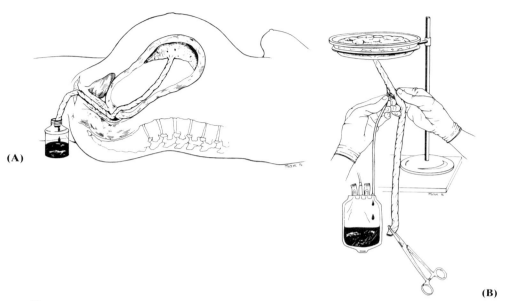

(A)

(B)

Figure 5. Examples of open (5A) and closed (5B) collection systems

or midwives who have not had the opportunity to evaluate the system prior to the umbilical cord blood collection. Closed collection systems have been principally utilized by designated umbilical cord blood collection centers with trained staff. While the open collection system may be technically easier, the most important disadvantage is the greater potential for microbial and maternal cell contamination.

Different procedures for umbilical cord blood collection, separation, and cryopreservation have been evaluated and reported in anticipation of large-scale banking projects proposed in the United States and Europe. Bertolini et al. [46] have reported on one of the most extensive evaluations of umbilical cord blood collection procedures thus far, comparing open and closed collection systems, the effect of vaginal versus Caesarian section delivery, and the recoveries of colony forming cells (CFCs) and high proliferative potential-colony forming cells (HPP-CFCs) after density-gradient centrifugation and gelatin sedimentation of both fresh and cryopreserved cell samples. Bertolini et al. failed to demonstrate any statistical differences in the collection volumes of umbilical cord blood recovered during vaginal delivery in utero, $n = 445$) or after Caesarian section deliveries (ex utero, $n = 82$). The median volume of blood collected was 72 ± 34 ml and 62 ± 19 ml, respectively. Furthermore, no significant difference in collection volume could be discerned between open and closed collection systems. Expectedly, there appeared to be a lower risk of bacterial contamination for samples collected by venipuncture into a blood collection bag as compared to the open collection method (4% versus 14%, respectively).

In this instance, where there are already limited numbers of nucleated cells and hematopoietic progenitors, manipulations that might further reduce the number of these cells in the umbilical cord blood graft must be avoided. Broxmeyer et al. [20] first reported significant losses in progenitor recovery with umbilical cord blood after density-gradient centrifugation (Ficoll-Hypaque, 1.077 g/ml, Sigma, St. Louis, MO). Broxmeyer et al. found that colony CFCs were lost by a variety of red cell separation techniques, suggesting that red cell depletion prior to clinical transplantation, even if the recipient and donor were ABO incompatible, should be carefully considered. Others [45–48], however, failed to observe the same substantial losses of progenitor cells as assessed by in vitro colony forming assays. Harris et al. [45] described a double Ficoll-Hypaque procedure in which the final preparation was virtually devoid of red cells and polymorphonuclear leukocytes but contained virtually all CFCs. Bertolini et al. [46] compared the double Ficoll-Hypaque method proposed by Harris et al. and a 3% gelatin sedimentation method proposed by Nagler et al. [49]. Umbilical cord blood separation using either Ficoll-Hypaque or gelatin sedimentation resulted in only 8% to 14% loss of CFCs and HPP-CFCs. However, Bertolini et al. also found that the effectiveness of either separation procedure was markedly reduced when umbilical cord blood was stored for more than 12 hours prior to the procedure. While the gelatin procedure took less time (1.5 hours versus 2.5 hours) relative to the Ficoll-Hypaque method, in one third of instances, the gelatin procedure failed to result in red cell depletion when performed at room temperature. This technical issue, however, was corrected simply by performing the procedure at 4°C. Rubinstein et al. [35] suggest that the umbilical cord blood graft be placed in a sterile bag and then thawed in a 38°C waterbath with gentle agitation. With an equal volume of dextran/albumin solution added after thawing, the cells are centrifuged gently and the supernatant is removed. Together, this procedure removes the bulk of red cell ghosts, free hemoglobin, and DMSO, thus reducing some of the risks associated with the procedure. These data suggest that red cell depletion by either density-gradient centrifugation or gelatin sedimentation results in only modest losses of hematopoietic progenitor cells.

Interest in the creation of large-scale unrelated umbilical cord blood banks worldwide make red cell separation a particularly important issue. Cryopreservation of mononuclear cell preparations would 1) reduce the risk of ABO-incompatible reactions (i.e., anaphylaxis and effects secondary to the infusion of free hemoglobin), 2) reduce the volume of the cord blood graft and thus significantly reduce the space required for banking, 3) potentially improve the ability to manipulate these cells after thawing (e.g., CD34+ selection and ex vivo progenitor cell expansion), and 4) reduce the risk of DMSO-related reactions. Importantly, both density-gradient centrifugation with Ficoll-Hypaque and gelatin sedimentation [7,8] of umbilical cord blood have been successfully used prior to clinical transplantation without deleterious effects on hematopoietic recovery and engraftment.

202

Characterization of umbilical cord blood progenitor cells

Characterization of the hematopoietic progenitor cell population circulating in umbilical cord blood has revealed similarities and differences with those in adult marrow. Saeland et al. [50] extensively characterized the CD34+ population in umbilical cord blood. Besides the lack of a distinct subpopulation of CD10+/CD34+ B-cell precursors typically found in adult marrow, expression of adhesion receptors (e.g., LFA-1, ICAM-1, LFA-3, H-CAM, LAM-1) and other differentiation antigens (e.g., CD33, HLA-DR) were remarkably similar between umbilical cord blood and adult marrow.

Through the use of a number of physical and immunological parameters, it has been possible to separate primitive from more committed progenitors. Immunofluorescent staining with anti-CD34 and anti-HLA-DR allows separation of more committed hematopoietic progenitors (CD34+/DR+ cells) from a more primitive (CD34+/DR–) subpopulation in adult marrow. Traycoff et al. [51] demonstrated that there is a higher proportion of HLA-DR– cells expressing the CD34+ phenotype in umbilical cord blood. Moreover, high proliferative potential colony-forming cells (HPP-CFCs) and long-term culture-initiating cells (LTC-ICs) in umbilical cord blood did not segregate with the HLA-DR– subpopulation of CD34+ cells. In marked contrast to adult marrow, the majority of HPP-CFCs were detected in the CD34+/DR+ subpopulation (ninefold greater than the number found in the DR– subpopulation) and the quantity of LTC-ICs, as measured by production of BFU-E and CFU-GM after five weeks in culture, were consistently higher in the CD34+/DR+ subpopulation. Similarly, Dugan et al. [52] have demonstrated that the frequency of LTC-ICs by limiting dilution analysis is identical between the two subpopulations of CD34+ cells segregated on the basis of HLA-DR expression (i.e., 1:100). In summary, these findings demonstrate that the primitive hematopoietic progenitor cells in umbilical cord blood express both CD34 and HLA-DR, which suggests that neonatal primitive progenitor cells do not share the same phenotypic properties of adult marrow primitive progenitors.

While HLA-DR expression identifies a very primitive progenitor population in umbilical cord blood in contrast to bone marrow, Hao et al. [53] and Cardoso et al. [54] have demonstrated that the CD34+CD38– immunophenotype defines a rare, quiescent subpopulation in both umbilical cord blood and bone marrow that can be distinquished functionally from the CD34+CD38+ population by sustained clonogenicity in extended (eight weeks) long-term culture assay. In contrast to CD34+CD38– bone marrow cells, Hao et al. showed that CD34+CD38– umbilical cord blood cells continue to proliferate well beyond five and eight weeks. They also reported a lower retroviral transduction frequency in the extended LTC-IC (5%) as compared to the standard five-week LTC-IC (40%–60%). These authors also found that umbilical cord blood CD34+CD38– cells proliferated more rapidly in response to cytokine stimulation in vitro than their marrow counterparts. Moreover, each CD34+ cell in umbilical cord blood generated a signficantly greater number of progeny.

In a comparison of the proliferative response of purified candidate stem cell populations in adult marrow, fetal liver, and umbilical cord blood, Lansdorp et al. [55] isolated cells with the CD34+CD45RA^{lo}CD71^{lo} phenotype. When cells were cultured in serum-free medium supplemented with a mixture of cytokines that included IL-3, IL-6, stem cell factor (SCF), and erythropoietin (EPO), large differences were observed between the number of CD34+ cells recovered from each of the cultures every 7 to 10 days. Throughout the culture, the number of CD34+ bone marrow cells remained relatively constant at input values, whereas CD34+ umbilical cord blood cells increased several hundred fold (and several thousand fold for CD34+ fetal liver cells). The purified cells also differed markedly in their response to growth factor. PKH26-labeled CD34+ cells from bone marrow remained brightly labeled after seven days in culture, whereas CD34+ cells from umbilical cord blood demonstrated markedly decreased fluorescence over the same time period. Together, these results indicate that marrow CD34+ cells are relatively quiescent during this time period, whereas umbilical cord blood CD34+ cells are highly proliferative. Such differences would have important implications for the use of umbilical cord blood over bone marrow stem cells in gene therapy and ex vivo expansion protocols.

Ex vivo expansion of hematopoietic cells in umbilical cord blood

Hematopoietic stem cells are defined as a population of cells that not only can give rise to each of the lymphohematopoietic lineages but can also maintain long-term hematopoiesis. Studies by Lansdorp et al. [55], Traycoff et al. [56], and Hao et al. [53] show an age-related difference in the functional capacity of hematopoeitic progenitors cells. During gestation, the total blood cell number is continuously expanding, whereas in adult life, maintenance of the blood cell number and not expansion is required. Data presented here and elsewhere suggest that the potential for stem cell expansion is greatest with CD34+ cell populations in fetal liver, intermediate with those in umbilical cord blood, and poorest with those from adult marrow. Although there is marked interest in determining the similarities and differences between stem cells in each tissue source, the single greatest impetus for exploring the ex vivo expansion potential of stem cells in umbilical cord blood is its limited availability. While marrow and peripheral blood from donors is relatively limitless, only a finite volume of blood can be extracted from a placenta after delivery. The clinical data presented above already indicate a prolonged interval to neutrophil and platelet recovery and force us to be concerned about the adequacy of this stem cell source for the largest adult recipients.

Broxmeyer et al. [57] have attempted to address the issue regarding the suitability of umbilical cord blood as a graft for adult recipients. Broxmeyer et al. reported that the total numbers of CFU-GM in a typical umbilical cord blood graft and unpurged autologous bone marrow graft are remarkably similar. While the numbers of nucleated cells and progenitors in cord blood specimens are lower than that expected for allogeneic bone marrow grafts, Broxmeyer et al. showed that that progenitors in umbilical cord blood had a greater capacity for expansion than bone marrow in short-term liquid culture in the presence of specific cytokines. Moreover, Moore et al. [58] reported that a marked expansion of umbilical cord blood progenitors could be achieved without expenditure of the primitive, LTC-IC compartment.

It has already been shown that umbilical cord blood CD34+ cells have a greater proliferative potential and have different growth factor requirements compared to adult marrow CD34+ cells. Traycoff et al. [51] reported that stem cell factor (SCF), interleukin-3 (IL-3), interleukin-6 (IL-6), and erythropoietin resulted in a 2500-fold increase in cell number at nine weeks, with peak production of CFU-GM and BFU-E at weeks 3 and 4 of long-term culture, respectively. Cardoso et al. [54] evaluated CD34+/CD38– umbilical cord blood cells in liquid suspension culture containing IL-3, IL-6, granulocyte-colony stimulating factor (G-CSF), SCF, and antitransforming growth factor (TGFβ). As reported with adult marrow, the CD34+/CD38– subpopulation was significantly more effective in generating CFU-GM, BFU-E, and CFU-GEMM after long-term culture than the CD38+ subpopulation. Notably, the total CFU-GM production of the CD34+/CD38– subpopulation of umbilical cord blood was 7.6-fold greater than the corresponding population in adult marrow.

Various investigators have demonstrated that culture of adult marrow CD34+ cells in the presence of multiple cytokines results in expansion of hematopoietic progenitors even in the absence of stroma. Although primitive progenitors can be induced to differentiate in such cultures, Verfaillie et al. [59,60] showed that maintenance and extensive proliferation of LTC-ICs from adult marrow is poor in stroma-free conditions but markedly improved by the presence of stroma-conditioned media supplemented by IL-3 and macrophage inhibitory protein-1α (MIP-1α). Using various starting populations and ex vivo culture conditions potentially useful for the expansion of primitive and committed hematopoietic progenitor cells in umbilical cord blood, Han et al. [61] evaluated the ability to expand the number of CFCs and LTC-ICs. As with adult marrow, the use of stroma-conditioned media supplemented by IL-3 and MIP-1α was superior to stroma-free conditions supplemented with various cytokines with regard to LTC-IC maintenance and progenitor expansion. In contrast, fold expansion of CFU-GMs was greatest for CD34+ umbilical cord blood cells cultured without stroma in the presence of SCF, IL3, IL-6, interleukin-1, G-CSF, and MIP-1α. While these data suggest that it is possible to expand both primitive and committed progenitors in umbilical cord blood, additional work is required utilizing clinically available reagents as well as determining the effect of prior cryopreservation. Transplants with umbilical cord blood cells previously in ex vivo expansion culture, however, must be performed in order to document safety of the expansion procedure and efficacy with regard to its effect on hematopoietic recovery and engraftment.

The data presented above suggest that there are indeed methods available for increasing the number of hematopoietic progenitor cells in umbilical cord blood and for potentially reducing the time to hematopoietic recovery after transplantation. Since it is not known how few stem cells are required for engraftment in any size recipient, only guesses can be made using surrogate markers (i.e., number of CFU-GMs or number of CD34+ cells per kilogram recipient body weight). While there is concern that umbilical cord blood grafts will contain too few cells for adult recipients, this question can only be definitively addressed by the transplantation of larger recipients.

Immunological properties of cord blood lymphocytes

The next critical question is whether umbilical cord blood has a decreased potential for effecting graft-versus-host disease. It has been hypothesized that umbilical cord blood lymphocytes are 'naive' and are 'functionally immature.' Clinical results thus far would suggest that allorecognition by umbilical cord blood lymphocytes may indeed be decreased. If this is true, then what is the mechanism for this decreased alloreactive response?

There are a number of important qualitative and quantitative differences between cord blood and adult peripheral blood lymphocytes. Rainaut et al. [62] have extensively investigated fetal and neonatal blood with regard to cell surface antigen expression. Relative to adult peripheral blood, umbilical cord blood has 1) a significantly greater absolute number of lymphocytes per milliliter (2- to 3-fold greater), 2) a significantly lower percentage of CD8+ T cells, and 3) a significantly greater CD4:CD8 ratio. Hannet et al. [63] further characterized umbilical cord blood lymphocytes using two-color flow microfluorometric analysis. Umbilical cord blood lymphocytes were found to have the phenotypic characteristics associated with T-cell 'immaturity'; the majority of CD4+ umbilical cord blood lymphocytes coexpressed CD45RA (91% as compared to 40% of adult CD4+ lymphocytes), fewer CD3+ T cells expressed IL-2 receptors (8% versus 18%) and fewer CD3+ T cells expressed the activation marker HLA-DR (2% versus 10%). Clement et al. [64] found that virtually all umbilical cord blood CD4+ T cells coexpressed CD38 (95%) and CD45RA (>90%). They demonstrated that CD4+/CD45RA+ (CD38+) cord blood T cells had no detectable helper function and their dominant immunoregulatory activity was suppression.

Acute GVHD involves the activation of donor-derived T lymphocytes recognizing alloantigens on host-antigen presenting cells, which in turn results in clonal expansion and proliferation. Secretion of proinflammatory cytokines, such as IL-2, TNF-α, and interferon-α, by these host reactive T cells mediates tissue damage either directly or via activation of other effector cells.

206

Roncarolo et al. [28] investigated the immunologic properties of umbilical cord blood lymphocytes. In this study, purified umbilical cord blood T cells were found to proliferate vigorously when activated by allogeneic antigens in primary mixed lymphocyte reactions (MLRs), indicating that umbilical cord blood cells responded normally to activation by alloantigens. In addition, strong proliferative responses were observed when the umbilical cord blood T cells were activated by cross-linked anti-CD3 monoclonal antibodies. Together, these data indicate that T cells in umbilical cord blood can be normally activated via their T-cell receptor (TcR) and that their proliferative response is normal. In contrast, umbilical cord blood cells had a reduced capacity to stimulate allogeneic cells in primary MLRs. The data suggest that this defect is related to a reduced antigen-presenting capacity. Umbilical cord blood monocytes expressed lower levels of HLA-DR, B7, and ICAM-1 compared to adult monocytes and produced lower levels of IL-10. The exact mechanism underlying the defect in the antigen-presenting capacity of umbilical cord blood, however, remains to be clarified. In addition, umbilical cord blood cells were also impaired in their capacity to generate allogeneic cytotoxic activity in primary MLRs. Whether this defect is intrinsic to the cytotoxic T cells or due to other cells or factors preventing the generation of alloantigen-specific cytotoxic T cells is not yet known.

Several investigators have reported reduced natural killer (NK) activity by umbilical cord blood cells. However, Roncarolo et al. [28] have recently shown that the NK activity of purified CD56+ umbilical cord blood NK cells against NK-sensitive targets is comparable to that observed with adult NK cells. As in bone marrow transplant recipients, the majority of circulating lymphocytes in the early posttransplant period express CD56 phenotype. Roncarolo et al. [28] also demonstrated that IL-2, IL-6, and TNF-α production by umbilical cord blood mononuclear cells following activation was comparable to that observed with peripheral blood mononuclear cells isolated from normal adult donors. In contrast, interferon-gamma and interleukin-10 production was significantly decreased, and interleukin-4 and interleukin-5 were absent. GM-CSF levels were in general higher in the supernatants of umbilical cord blood cells. Thus, umbilical cord blood mononuclear cells differ from adult peripheral blood cells at several levels: 1) decreased capacity to stimulate an allogeneic response, 2) impaired cytotoxic effector function, and 3) unique cytokine profile. Whether these properties account for the reduced capacity of transplanted umbilical cord blood cells to modulate GVHD remains to be determined.

Harris et al. [65] assessed the immunologic reactivity of umbilical cord blood cells with lymphocytes from various family members and analyzed the development of alloreactivity in the infant over the first year of life. At birth, umbilical cord blood cells were observed to be immunologically unreactive with cells from mother and minimally reactive with cells from father. Moreover, lymphocytes from the mother demonstrated a decreased ability to mediate NK lysis shortly after the time of delivery, as well as a depressed alloreactive response. While the neonatal blood was capable of mediating NK lysis, the infant did not develop the ability to generate an alloantigen-specific cytoxic response until sometime between birth and 6 months of age. The inability of umbilical cord blood to respond to parental lymphocytes as measured by mixed lymphocyte culture and by the inability to generate alloantigen-specific cytotoxic T cells suggests that umbilical cord blood might be partially tolerant, particularly with maternal antigens. The idea that the fetus may become partially tolerant to the noninherited maternal allele (NIMA) was first proposed on the basis of outcomes observed in recipients of parental renal allografts [66,67]. How such 'tolerance' develops is unknown, but such results are particularly intriguing in view of the clinical results observed in haploidentical sibling donor–recipient pairs. If the umbilical cord blood graft is tolerant to HLA antigens on the non-inherited maternal allele, this finding would have wide-reaching implications in defining an 'acceptable' donor. The differences between neonatal and adult lymphocytes are summarized in table 6.

While there is an impression that umbilical cord blood is less likely to induce a graft-versus-host reaction, it is clearly not absent. Severe or lethal GVHD has been reported. In some instances, the grafts were highly HLA disparate. Since it has already been shown that any HLA-A, B, DR disparity [40,41], including a disparity at the level of DRB1 [68], increases the risk of severe acute GVHD after unrelated donor bone marrow transplantation, the same degree of prospective HLA typing should be considered prior to umbilical cord blood transplantation. While unavailability of a closely matched marrow or umbilical cord blood donor may necessitate use of a highly mismatched umbilical cord blood graft, the idea that umbilical cord blood 'cannot cause GVHD' is not true. The recipient should be made aware of the donor types available and the degree of HLA disparity based on currently available techniques shown to impact the risks of graft failure, GVHD, and survival (i.e., class I by serology and class II by DNA techniques).

Table 6. Functional differences between neonatal and adult lymphocytes

Neonatal lymphocyte function	Comparison to adult lymphocyte function
1) T-cell activation	Same
2) T-cell proliferation to alloantigen	Same
3) Cytotoxic response to alloantigen	Reduced
4) Suppressor cell activity	Increased
5) CTLp frequency	Same
6) NK activity	Same
7) Antigen presenting cell activity	Reduced
8) Cytokine production: IL-2	Same
IL-4	Absent
IL-5	Absent
IL-10	Reduced
INF-α	Reduced

Unrelated donor umbilical cord blood banking

As a result of the early successes with umbilical cord blood transplantation using sibling donors, pilot programs for the banking of screened, unrelated donor umbilical cord blood have been proposed in many countries worldwide and initiated in the United States, France, United Kingdom, Germany, and Italy (table 7). As of December 1995, more than 5000 umbilical cord blood grafts have been collected, human-leukocyte-antigen (HLA) typed, tested for transmissible infectious diseases, and cryopreserved, with an additional 50 umbilical cord blood grafts processed each week. A primary objective of this pilot program is to test the feasibility of large-scale umbilical cord blood collection, testing, and storage. Therefore, it has been necessary to 1) optimize and standardize the umbilical cord blood collection procedure; 2) standardize quality assessment procedures (i.e., quantification of hemato-poietic progenitors, sterility, and detection of genetic and transmissible in-fectious diseases; 3) streamline large-scale histocompatibility testing using restricted volumes of the sample from the potential umbilical cord blood graft in mother; 4) develop repositories of viable cells, serum, and DNA on donor and mother for future testing; 5) optimize both the cryopreservation and thawing procedure to reduce cell loss and minimize infusion of DMSO and red

Table 7. Umbilical cord blood banking programs

New York Blood Center (New York) Pablo Rubinstein, M.D., Director FAX 212.570.9061	February 2, 1993 (inception) 5493 units (50 per week) 1854 search requests 136 transplants
Centro Transfusionale e di Immunologia del Traplanti (Milano) Girolamo Sirchia, M.D., Director FAX 011.39.2.545.81.29	February 10, 1993 (inception) 857 units (15 per week) 1027 search requests 12 transplants
CB-DI-GER (Dusseldorf) Peter Wernet, M.D., Director FAX 011.49.211.934.8435	August 14, 1993 (inception) 789 units (8 per week) 126 search requests 1 transplant (as of August 1995)
France Greffe de Moelle Colette Raffoux, M.D., Director FAX 011.33.14.803.02.02	January 1, 1995 (inception) 35 units (8 per week) 174 search requests 1 transplant
London Cord Blood Bank Marcela Contreras, M.D., Director FAX 011.181.200.6449	February 21, 1996 (inception) 61 total units (30 per week) 0 search requests 0 transplants
Northern Ireland Cord Blood Bank Chitra Bharucha, M.D., Director FAX 011.44.1232.439017	June 1, 1993 (inception) 192 total units (10 per week) 0 search requests 0 transplants

cell debris; and 6) establish a computer network for efficient data storage and retrieval. Once we have demonstrated that unrelated umbilical cord blood reduces the risks of allogeneic transplant therapy or that it can supplement the pool of unrelated marrow donors, particularly for certain ethnic/racial minorities, it is likely that these repositories of umbilical cord blood will be greatly expanded.

Autologous storage of umbilical cord blood

Umbilical cord blood as a source of hematopoietic stem and progenitor cells has both real and theoretical advantages and disadvantages over bone marrow. On the basis of the potential advantages, development of large repositories of autologous umbilical cord blood for future use has been proposed. Storage of the infant's own umbilical cord blood might be useful in several ways: 1) it might be an optimal source of tumor-free, virus-free stem cells if the child should develop a malignant condition or acquired bone marrow failure syndrome later in life, 2) it might be a source of HLA matched or closely matched stem cells for a sibling requiring transplant therapy at some point, and 3) it might be an optimal source of stem cells for gene therapy should such therapy be needed for the treatment of a genetic disorder in that child (e.g., Fanconi anemia, Hurler syndrome). It has been suggested that autologous storage of umbilical cord blood stem cells is a form of 'biological insurance.'

Biocyte Corporation was founded on the concept that umbilical cord blood would be useful in the treatment of a variety of disorders, including cancers, genetic disorders, and immune deficiency states. The company holds a U.S. patent [69] for the collection and cryopreservation of placental and umbilical cord. The validity of the patent, however, is being considered at this time.

Two companies currently offer this service for a fee to expectant parents, namely, ViaCord and Cord Blood Registry, Inc.

Ethical considerations

The collection of umbilical cord blood poses a number of ethical issues. If it is considered to be like any other organ or tissue, then consent must be obtained by the tissue donor. In the case of umbilical cord blood, the donor is always a minor, and therefore, consent must be obtained from the infant's mother. Therefore, the following questions arise. First, when should consent be obtained from the mother? Second, will the infant donor at 21 years of age have any rights to the umbilical cord blood that was previously given to the unrelated cord blood registry? While the second issue must be addressed by the legal agencies, current practice would dictate that consent from the donor's mother should be obtained prior to labor or at least some finite period of time after delivery.

Alternatively, umbilical cord blood may be considered to be discarded tissue. If so, consent is not required. The collection of umbilical cord blood from the delivered placenta poses no risk to mother or infant. However, if umbilical cord blood is to be considered discarded tissue and consent is not required, what do we do about the issue of HIV testing, and how do we protect the rights of individuals whose religious and cultural practices would not allow the collection and transplantation of placental blood? While umbilical cord blood offers several real and potential advantages as an alternate source of hematopoietic stem cells, it also opens a new set of issues that needs to be considered prior to large-scale collection of this tissue worldwide.

Other related issues that are beyond the scope of this review include 1) commercial aspects of umbilical cord blood collection and storage and 2) ability to 'backtrack' and perform additional donor testing prior to the use of an umbilical cord blood graft. By necessity, these and other issues need to be considered by medical ethicists and the physicians offering this treatment option.

Regulatory issues

Over the past five years, umbilical cord blood has moved from the status of 'biological waste' to a potentially important source of hematopoietic stem cells. Clinical experience has already demonstrated that placental and umbilical cord blood contains sufficient numbers of hematopoietic stem cells to engraft at least small recipients consistently. As a result, banks of umbilical cord blood have been developed or are being considered throughout the U.S. and Europe as well as in many countries in South America and Asia. Moreover, the potential for storing the child's own cord blood for future use as a form of 'biological insurance' has also been considered, resulting in the establishment of commercial banks. Hence, there has been an explosion of banking activity, making the need for standard policies and procedures particularly acute. It is likely that umbilical cord blood will be the first source of hematopoietic stem cells to be regulated by the U.S. Food and Drug Administration [70].

While there will be debate on the optimal procedures for handling umbilical cord blood, there is already extensive experience in handling blood and marrow. Many of the procedures for obtaining consent, collection, testing, cryopreservation, red cell depletion, histocompatibility testing, and sample labelling are likely to be extracted from existing operating manuals for blood. A major problem, however, will be in the definition of 'suitable' product. Moreover, the definition of 'suitable' product may vary depending upon the type of recipient — self, sibling, or unrelated. A list of key elements for a quality assurance program for an umbilical cord blood bank are shown in table 8 [71].

Table 8. Elements of quality assurance program for cord blood banking

---

Procedures
    Collection
    Processing (red cell depletion, CD34 selection, ex vivo expansion, etc.)
    Characterization of the graft (volume, red blood cell count, nucleated cell count,
        enumeration of CFU-GMs and LTC-ICs, quantitation of CD34 (subsets), quantitation of
        CD3 (subsets), maternal cell contamination, microbiologic assays
    Cryopreservation
    Transplantation

Personnel
    Qualifications
    Training

Although it is clear that umbilical cord blood should be considered a viable source of hematopoietic stem cells for transplantation, we are still in the 'learning phase.' Just as the transplant physician requires assurances that the umbilical cord blood graft product has been processed and stored properly, the director of the umbilical cord blood bank may require assurances that the transplant team will use the graft properly. Clinical outcome data may impact upon the bank's methods of processing and graft characterization. Policies for defining the qualifications of transplant teams and the appropriate use of umbilical cord blood should not be overlooked. In the past, similar issues had to be addressed by the National Marrow Donor Program. Perhaps existing societies, such as the International Society of Hematotherapy and Graft Engineering (ISHAGE) and The American Society of Bone Marrow Transplantation (ASBMT), will aid in addressing these difficult issues.

Summary

Interest in umbilical cord blood as an alternate source of hematopoietic stem cells is growing rapidly. Umbilical cord blood offers the clinician a source of hematopoietic stem cells that is rarely contaminated by latent viruses and is readily available. Moreover, the collection of umbilical cord blood poses no risk to the donor; there is no need for general anesthesia or blood replacement, and the procedure causes no discomfort. Whether cord blood lymphocytes are as likely to cause GVHD as lymphocytes from older individuals is unknown. Current clinical experience would suggest that the incidence may be low. Few of the patients transplanted with umbilical cord blood thus far have developed clinically significant GVHD, including recipients of HLA-disparate grafts. These results and associated laboratory findings pose intriguing possibilities for the future of umbilical cord blood stem cells in the setting of unrelated transplantation. With the marked incidence of grade 2–4 acute GVHD that is currently observed after unrelated bone marrow transplantation, a reduction in incidence or severity would be a major advancement in this field. In the setting of autologous trans-plantation, there are other intriguing possibilities; for example, cord blood may be an optimal source of pluripotential stem cells for gene therapy.

The large-scale collection and storage of cord blood stem cells has become a reality. Pilot programs for the banking of unrelated umbilical cord blood have already begun in the United States and Europe. Not only is there the potential for reducing the time from search initiation to the time of donor stem cell acquisition but also there is the potential for reducing the risks associated with unrelated bone marrow transplantation. There is also the hope of remedying the shortage of donors from ethnic and racial backgrounds that are currently underrepresented in most unrelated donor programs. Even with the creation of such banks, it should not be forgotten that the collection of umbilical cord bloods should at least be considered when a child with leukemia, lymphoma, neuroblastoma, marrow failure syndrome, immunodeficiency state, or inborn error of metabolism has a mother who is pregnant. The clinical results to date in small recipients would suggest that it is at least as good as bone marrow; but additional patients and more time will be needed to finalize this conclusion.

Acknowledgments

The author wishes to express his gratitude to Professor Edward Boyse and Ms. Judith Bard for graciously sharing their data on the early experiments with murine fetal and neonatal blood and to Ms. Judith Bard for her careful review of the manuscript. Without their foresight and that of Dr. Hal Broxmeyer, it is not likely that anyone would be using umbilical cord blood as a source of stem cells for transplantation today.

This work was supported in part by grants from the Childrens Cancer Research Fund, National Institutes of Health Grant Nos. P01-CA65493 and P01-CA21737, and American Cancer Society Career Development Award No. 91-56.

References

1. Gluckman E, Broxmeyer HE, Auerbach AD, et al. Hematopoietic reconstitution in a patient with Fanconi's anemia by means of umbilical cord blood from an HLA-identical sibling. N Engl J Med 321:1174–1178, 1989.
2. Broxmeyer HE, Kurtzberg J, Gluckman E, et al. Umbilical cord blood hematopoietic stem and repopulating cells in human clinical transplantation. Blood Cells 17:313–329, 1991.
3. Wagner JE, Broxmeyer HE, Byrd RL, et al. Transplantation of umbilical cord blood after myeloablative therapy: analysis of engraftment. Blood 79:1874–1881, 1992.
4. Vilmer E, Sterkers G, Rahimy C, et al. HLA-mismatched cord blood transplantation in a patient with advanced leukemia. Transplantation 53:1155–1157, 1992.

5. Vanlemmens P, Plouvier E, Amsallem D, et al. Transplantation of umbilical cord blood in neuroblastoma. Nouv Rev Fr Hematolol 34:243–246, 1992.
6. Kernan NA, Schroeder ML, Ciavarella D, et al. Umbilical cord blood infusion in a patient for correction of Wiskott–Aldrich syndrome. Blood Cells 20:242–244, 1994.
7. Kurtzberg J, Graham M, Casey J, et al. The use of umbilical cord blood in a mismatched related and unrelated hematopoietic stem cell transplantation. Blood Cells 20:275–284, 1994.
8. Pahwa RN, Fleischer A, Than S, et al. Successful hematopoietic reconstitution with transplantation of erythrocyte-depleted allogeneic human umbilical cord blood cells in a child with leukemia. Proc Nat Acad Sci 91:4485–4488, 1994.
9. Bogdanic V, Nemet D, Kastelan A, et al. Umbilical cord blood transplantation in a patient with Philadelphia-chromosome positive chronic myeloid leukemia. Transplantation 56:477–479, 1993.
10. Vowels MR, Lam-PO-Tang R, Berdoukas V, et al. Brief report: correction of X-linked lymphoproliferative disease by transplantation of cord-blood stem cells. N Engl J Med 329:1623–1625, 1993.
11. Kohli-Kumar M, Shahidi NT, Broxmeyer HE, et al. Haematopoietic stem/progenitor cell transplant in Fanconi anaemia using HLA-matched sibling umbilical cord blood cells. Br J Haematol 85:419–422, 1993.
12. Issaragrisil S, Visuthisakchai S, Suvatte V, et al. Transplantation of cord blood stem cells into a patient with severe thalassemia. N Engl J Med 332:367–369, 1995.
13. Neudorf SML, Blatt J, Corey S, et al. Graft failure after an umbilical cord blood transplant in a patient with severe aplastic anemia (letter). Blood 85:2991–2992, 1995.
14. Miniero R, Busca A, Roncarolo MG, et al. HLA haploidentical umbilical cord blood stem cell transplantation in a child with advanced leukemia: clinical outcome and analysis of hematopoietic recovery. Bone Marrow Transplant 16:229–240, 1995.
15. Tavian M, Coulombel L, Luton D, et al. Aorta-associated CD34+ hematopoietic cells in the early human embryo. Blood 87:67–72, 1996.
16. Moore MAS, Metcalf D. Ontogeny of the haematopoietic system: yolk sac origin in vivo and in vitro colony forming cells in the developing mouse embryo. Br J Haematol 18:279–285, 1970.
17. Nathan DG, Housman DE, Clarke BJ. The anatomy and physiology of hematopoiesis. In Nathan DG, Oski FA (eds), Hematology of Infancy and Childhood. Philadelphia: W.B. Saunders Co., 1981, pp. 144–167.
18. Knudtzon S. In vitro growth of granulocyte colonies from circulating cells in human cord blood. Blood 43:357–361, 1974.
19. Gabutti V, Foa R, Mussa F, Aglietta M. Behavior of human hematopoietc stem cells in cord and neonatal blood. Haematologica (Roma) 4:60–68, 1975.
20. Broxmeyer HE, Douglas GW, Hangoc G, et al. Human umbilical cord blood as a potential source of transplantable hematopoietic stem/progenitor cells. Proc Natl Acad Sci USA 86:3828–3832, 1989.
21. Broxmeyer HE, Hangoc G, Cooper S, et al. Growth characteristics and expansion of human umbilical cord blood and estimation of its potential for transplantation in adults. Proc Natl Acad Sci USA 89:4109–4113, 1992.
22. Boyse EA. Personal communication.
23. Linch DC, Brent L. Can cord blood be used? (letter). Nature 340:676, 1989.
24. Nathan DG. The beneficence of neonatal hematopoiesis. N Engl J Med 321:1190–1191, 1989.
25. Wagner JE, Kernan NA, Steinbuch M, Broxmeyer HE, Gluckman E. Allogeneic sibling umbilical-cord-blood transplantation in children with malignant and non-malignant disease. Lancet 346:214–219, 1995.
26. Weisdorf D, Haake R, Blazar BR, et al. Risk factors for acute graft-versus-host disease in histocompatible donor bone marrow transplantation. Transplantation 51:1197–1203, 1991.
27. Gale RP, Bortin MM, van Bekkum DW, et al. Risk factors for acute graft-versus-host disease. Br J Haematol 67:397–406, 1987.

214

28. Roncarolo MG, Bigler M, Ciuti E, Martino S, Tovo P-A. Immune responses by cord blood cells. Blood Cells 20:573–586, 1984.
29. Deacock SJ, Schwarer AP, Bridge J, et al. Evidence that umbilical cord blood contains a higher frequency of HLA Class II specific alloreactive T cells than adult peripheral blood: a limiting dilution analysis. Transplant 53:1128–1134, 1992.
30. Bensussan A, Gluckman E, El Marsafy S, et al. BY55 monoclonal antibody delineates within human cord blood and bone marrow lymphocytes distinct subsets mediating cytotoxic activity. Proc Nat Acad Sci 91:9136–9140, 1994.
31. Risdon G, Gaddy J, Stehman FB, Broxmeyer HE. Proliferative and cytotoxic responses of human umbilical cord blood T lymphocytes following allogeneic stimulation. Cell Immunol 154:14–24, 1994.
32. Socié G, Gluckman E, Carosella E, Brossard Y, Lafon C, Brison O. Search for maternal cells in human umbilical cord blood by polymerase chain reaction by amplification of two minisatellite sequences. Blood 83:340–344, 1984.
33. Hall J, Lingenfelter P, Adams S, Bean MA, Hansen JA. Detection of maternal T-cells in human umbilical cord blood using FISH. Blood 84(suppl. 1):97a, 1994.
34. Kernan NA, Bartsch G, Ash RC, et al. Analysis of 462 unrelated marrow transplants facilitated by the National Marrow Donor Program. N Engl J Med 328:593–602, 1993.
35. Rubinstein P, Rosenfield RE, Adamson JW, Stevens CE. Review: stored placental blood for unrelated bone marrow reconstitution. Blood 81:1679–1690, 1993.
36. Gluckman E, Wagner J, Hows J, Kernan N, Bradley B, Broxmeyer HE. Cord blood banking for haematopoitic stem cell transplantation: an international cord blood transplant registry. Bone Marrow Transplant 11:199–200, 1993.
37. Stagno S, Pass RF, Cloud G, et al. Primary cytomegalovirus infection in pregnancy. J Am Med Assoc 256:1904–1908, 1986.
38. Chang RS, Seto DSY. Perinatal infection by Epstein–Barr virus. Lancet 2:201–205, 1979.
39. Kurtzberg J, Laughlin M, Smith C, et al. Umbilical cord blood: an alternative source of hemopoietic stem cells for bone marrow reconstitution in unrelated donor transplantation (abstract). Blood 86:290, 1995.
40. Davies SM, Shu XO, Blazar BR, et al. Unrelated donor bone marrow transplant: influence of HLA-A and B incompatibility on outcome. Blood 86:1636–1642, 1995.
41. Balduzzi A, Gooley T, Anasetti C, et al. Unrelated donor bone marrow transplantation in children. Blood 86:3247–3256, 1995.
42. Wagner JE, Broxmeyer HE, Cooper S. Umbilical cord and placental blood hematopoietic stem cells: collection, cryopreservation and storage. J Hematother 1:167–173, 1992.
43. Traineau R, Thierry D, Djenandar B, Benbunan M, Gluckman E. Collection of sibling cord blood for hematopoietic stem cell transplantation. J Hematother 2:231–232, 1993.
44. Turner CW, Luzins J, Hutcheson C. A modified harvest technique for cord blood hematopoietic stem cells. Bone Marrow Transplant 10:89–91, 1992.
45. Harris DT, Schumacher MJ, Rychlik S, et al. Collection, separation and cryopreservation of umbilical cord blood for use in transplantation. Bone Marrow Transplant 13:135–143, 1994.
46. Bertolini F, Lazzari L, Lauri E, et al. A comparative study of different procedures for the collection and banking of umbilical cord blood. J Hematother 4:29–38, 1995.
47. Newton I, Charbord P, Schaal JP, Herve P. Toward cord blood banking: density separation and cryopreservation of cord blood progenitors. Exp Hematol 21:671–674, 1993.
48. Nicol A, Nieda M, Donaldson C, Denning-Kendall P, Bradley B, Hows J. Analysis of cord blood CD34+ cells purified after cryopreservation. Exp Hematol 23:1589–1594, 1995.
49. Nagler A, Peacock M, Tantoco M, Lamons D, Okcarma TB, Okrongly DA. Separation of hematopoietic progenitor cells from human umbilical cord blood. J Hematother 2:243–245, 1993.
50. Saeland S, Duvert V, Caux C, et al. Distribution of surface-membrane molecules on bone marrow and cord blood CD34+ hematopoietic cells. Exp Hematol 20:24–33, 1992.
51. Traycoff CM, Abboud MR, Laver J, et al. Evaluation of the in vitro behavior of phenotypi-

cally defined populations of umbilical cord blood hematopoietic progenitor cells. Exp Hematol 22:215–221, 1994.

52. Dugan M, Han CS, McGlave PB. Committed and primitive progenitor content of umbilical cord blood CD34+ subpopulations (abstract). Exp Hematol 22:791, 1994.

53. Hao QH, Shah AM, Thiermann FT, Smogorzewska EM, Crooks GM. A functional comparison of CD34+CD38– cells in cord blood and bone marrow. Blood 86:3745–3753, 1995.

54. Cardoso AA, Li ML, Hatzfeld A, et al. Release from quiescence of CD34+CD38– human umbilical cord blood cells reveals their potentiality to engraft adults. Proc Nat Acad Sci USA 90:8707–8712, 1993.

55. Lansdorp PM, Dragowska W, Mayani H. Ontogeny-related changes in proliferative potential of human hematopoietic cells. J Exp Med 178:787–791, 1993.

56. Traycoff CM, Kosak ST, Grigsby S, Srour EF. Evaluation of ex vivo expansion of cord blood and bone marrow hematopoietic progenitor cells using cell tracking and limiting dilution analysis. Blood 85:2059–2068, 1995.

57. Broxmeyer H, Hangoc G, Cooper S, et al. Growth characteristics and expansion of human umbilical cord blood and estimation of its potential for transplantation in adults. Proc Natl Acad Sci USA 89:4109–4113, 1992.

58. Moore MAS. Ex vivo expansion and gene therapy using cord blood CD34+ cells. J Hematother 2:221–224, 1993.

59. Verfaillie CM. MIP-1α combined with IL-3 conserves primitive human LTBMC-IC for at least 8 weeks in ex vivo 'stoma non-contact' cultures. J Exp Med 179:643–649, 1994.

60. Verfaillie CM. Soluble factor(s) produced by human bone marrow stroma increase cytokine induced proliferation and maturation of primitive hematopoietic progenitors while preventing their terminal differentiation. Blood 82:2045–2054, 1993.

61. Han CS, Dugan MJ, Verfaillie CM, Wagner JE, McGlave PB. In vitro expansion of umbilical cord blood committed and primitive progenitors (abstract). Exp Hematol 22:723, 1994.

62. Rainaut M, Pagniez M, Hercend T, Dafos F, Forestier F. Characterization of mononuclear cell subpopulations in normal fetal peripheral blood. Human Immunol 18:331–337, 1987.

63. Hannet I, Erkeller-Yuksel F, Lydyard P, Deneys V, DeBruyere M. Developmental and maturational changes in human blood lymphocyte subpopulations. Immunol Today 13:215–218, 1992.

64. Clement LT, Vink PE, Bradley GE. Novel immunoregulatory functions of phenotypically distinct subpopulations of CD4+ cells in the human neonate. J Immunol 145:102–108, 1990.

65. Harris DT, Schumacher MJ, LoCascio J, Booth A, Bard J, Boyse EA. Immunoreactivity of umbilical cord blood and postpartum maternal peripheral blood with regard to HLA-haploidentical transplantation. Bone Marrow Transplant 14:63–68, 1994.

66. van Rood JJ, Class FHJ. The influence of allogeneic cells on the human T and B cell repertoire. Science 248:1388–1393, 1990.

67. Claas FHJ, Gijbels Y, van der Velden-de Munck J, van Rood JJ. Induction of B cell unresponsiveness to noninherited maternal HLA antigens during fetal life. Science 241:1815–1817, 1988.

68. Petersdorf EW, Longton GM, Anasetti C, et al. The significance of HLA-DRB1 matching on clinical outcome after HLA-A, B, DR identical unrelated donor marrow transplantation. Blood 86:1606–1613, 1995.

69 Boyse EA. Broxmeyer HE, Douglas GW. Preservation of fetal and neonatal hematopoietic stem and progenitor cells of the blood. U.S. Patent 5,004,681 issued April 2, 1991; assigned to Biocyte Corporation.

70. Federal Register docket no. 96N-0002. February 26, 1996.

71. McCullough J, Clay ME, Fautsch S, et al. Proposed policies and procedures for the establishment of a cord blood bank. Blood Cells 20:609–626, 1994.

10. The use of unrelated donors for bone marrow transplantation

Guido Tricot

The search for an unrelated donor

Histocompatibility

Allogeneic bone marrow transplantation has curative potential in hematologic malignancies, bone marrow failure syndromes, and congenital disorders of the hematopoietic and/or lymphoid system. Suitable donors have been human leukocyte antigen (HLA) genotypically identical siblings. Given the current average family size, less than 30% of patients in North America have an HLA-matched sibling donor. This percentage can be increased by 3% to 5% if partially matched relatives (one antigen-mismatch) are included. As the precision of HLA typing increased, it became possible to identify unrelated donors who are HLA matched with the patient. A relation between the registry size and the probability of finding an HLA-matched donor for a random patient cannot be derived from theoretical calculations, because it depends on the frequency of HLA haplotypes in donor and recipient populations. Models have been designed to solve this problem, showing that the relation of the probability of finding a matching donor to the registry size is sigmoidal, with small increases in probability at the extremes of the registry size but a middle range of registry size within which the probability of matching increases sharply [1]. Because of genetic disequilibrium, a small number of common HLA haplotypes comprises most of the registry population. It has been calculated that for a registry size of 100,000 volunteers, the 17% of patients with the most common haplotypes have a greater than 90% chance of finding a donor. In contrast, the 48% with unusual haplotypes have a less than 10% chance of identifying a donor [2]. As of April 1, 1995, more than 1.5 million potential donors of known HLA-A and B type have been listed in the National Marrow Donor Program. An increasing number of donors are being typed for HLA-DR, which should shorten the time required to identify a suitable donor. With the present size, the probability of finding a matching donor is approximately 75% for Caucasian patients [3]. However, since the NMDP contains predominantly Caucasian volunteers, the odds of finding a donor for a patient of another racial group are dramatically decreased.

Jane N. Winter (ed.) BLOOD STEM CELL TRANSPLANTATION. 1997. Kluwer Academic Publishers. ISBN 0-7923-4260-7. All rights reserved.

Table 1. Unrelated donor transplant: degrees of matching

Degree of matching	HLA-A, B		HLA-DR
Perfect match	Serologically identical		Serologically identical Molecular typing identical
Minor match	One antigen NOT identical but belongs to same cross-reactive group		Serologically identical Molecular typing identical
		OR	
	Serologically identical		Serologically identical Molecular typing different
Major mismatch	One antigen NOT identical and belongs to noncross-reactive group		Serologically identical Molecular typing identical
		OR	
	Identical		One antigen serologically not identical

As improvements in HLA typing have increased the sensitivity of histocompatibility testing, the definition of a matching donor has changed. Before molecular techniques were available, typing was limited to serologic methods (phenotypic identity). Using SSOP/PCR (sequence-specific oligonucleotide probes), genotypes for DR, DQ, and DP loci can be defined. Molecular analysis for HLA-A, B, and C is feasible, but is not performed routinely. Typing for class I antigens is still based solely on serologic typing and occasionally on immuno-electro focusing (IEF) to identify variants not recognizable by serology. IEF, however, cannot identify all molecular variants. Therefore, definite matching for HLA-A, B, and C is not possible until molecular typing for class I alleles is performed routinely.

Different degrees of matching are now recognized (see table 1): 1) a perfect matching donor is serologically identical for HLA-A and B and genotypically identical for DR; 2) a minor mismatch has one HLA-A or B antigen that is not identical, but belongs to the same cross-reactive group, while molecular typing for DR is identical *or* HLA-A, B, and DR are identical serologically, but the HLA-DR differs by SSOP/PCR; and 3) a major mismatch is defined as follows: one HLA-A or B antigen is distinctly different and noncross-reactive *or* one DR antigen that is different by serology. In addition to classifying matching according to the degree of overall disparity for each locus, matching should also be described in terms of the vector of incompatibility: incompatibility in the donor defines the risk of rejection; incompatibility in the recipient defines the risk of graft-versus-host disease (GVHD). The distinction is relevant when either patient or donor are homozygous for one HLA-A, B, or DR locus.

Recommendations and requirements to perform unrelated transplants

As discussed later, unrelated donor transplants are associated with a higher risk of morbidity and mortality. Therefore, some limitations have been pro-

Table 2. Malignant diseases treatable by unrelated donor transplant

---

Standard of care
Acute lymphoblastic leukemia
  First complete remission, high risk
  Second or subsequent complete remission
Acute myeloid leukemia
  First complete remission, high risk
  Second or subsequent complete remission
Chronic myelogenous leukemia
  Chronic phase, accelerated phase, second chronic phase
Myelodysplasia
  Refractory anemia (with or without sideroblasts) and rapidly increasing cytopenias
  Refractory anemia with excess blasts (or in transformation)
Lymphoma — after relapse with either bone marrow involvement or insufficient stem cell
  reserve
Myeloma — with poor response to autotransplantation or high-risk features (Ig isotype,
  cytogenetics)

On an IRB-approved research protocol
Acute leukemia in relapse
Chronic myelogenous leukemia in blastic crisis

Table 3. Nonmalignant diseases treatable by unrelated donor transplant

---

Standard of care
  Very severe aplastic anemia (SAA), refractory to immunosuppressive therapy
  Inborn errors/immunodeficiencies
  Severe combined immune deficiency
  Combined immunodeficiency
  Leukocyte adhesion deficiency
  Wiskott–Aldrich syndrome
  Chediak–Higashi syndrome
  Familial erythrophagocytotic lymphohistiocytosis
  Fanconi anemia and other congenital marrow failures
  Mucopolysaccharidosis I (Hurler disease)
  Mucopolysaccharidosis VI (Maroteaux–Lamy syndrome)
  Gaucher's disease
  Osteopetrosis

On an IRB-approved research protocol:
  Thalassemia
  Sickle cell disease

---

posed on the use of unrelated donor transplants [4,5]. Adequate experience of the transplant center is required and is defined as having been operational for at least two years with at least ten allogeneic transplants performed annually. Patients will generally be eligible for an unrelated transplant up to the age of 50 years. They should have a malignant disease (see table 2), such as high-risk leukemia, myelodysplastic syndrome (MDS), lymphoma, or myeloma, or a life-threatening nonmalignant disease (see table 3), such as severe aplastic anemia not responding to immunosuppressive therapy, severe combined immune deficiency, leukocyte adhesion deficiency, Wiskott–Aldrich and

Chediak–Higashi syndrome, Fanconi anemia, mucopolysaccharidosis, Gaucher's disease, or osteopetrosis. It is recommended that donor and patient are serologically identical for class I loci and molecularly identical for DR. If a serologically identical unrelated donor is not available, an unrelated donor with a minor mismatch for one HLA-A, B, or DR locus can be used. Donors should be 18 to 55 years old and are counseled about the requirement for virological testing, donation of autologous blood, the possibility of needing an allogeneic blood transfusion, and the risks of anesthesia and harvest procedure. Donors who are HIV or HTLV-1 positive or pregnant are excluded from donations. Marrow collections are performed at an accredited marrow collection center, near the donor's normal residence. General anesthesia is recommended for the marrow collection, but spinal or epidural anesthesia is acceptable if the donor and medical team agree. The marrow is aspirated from the posterior and, if required, anterior iliac crest. The sternum should only be used if the donor has agreed in advance. The total volume of bone marrow collected should be 1000 to 1200 ml and only under exceptional circumstances increased to 1500 ml. Every effort should be made to avoid the transfusion of allogeneic blood. If its use is essential, the blood should be irradiated (>20 Gy). Maintenance of donor confidentiality is essential. The National Marrow Donor Program accepts the principle that donor and recipient may meet 12 months after a successful transplant, provided that both individuals have consented.

Donor complications

While the incidence of serious morbidity as a result of bone marrow donation is rare, the incidence of lesser complications and the long-term consequences of bone marrow donation have not been studied routinely. The National Marrow Donor Program has analyzed the results of the first 493 patients who donated bone marrow [6]. The median age of the donors was 38 years (range 19–55). The median volume of marrow collected was 1050 ml (180–2983 ml). Only three donors received allogeneic blood, while 90% of donors were transfused with autologous RBCs. As a result of the marrow collection procedure, 6% of the donors experienced acute complications, such as hypotension, pain and bleeding at the site of aspiration, febrile episodes, headaches in patients who received spinal or epidural anesthesia, prologed nausea, phlebitis at the site of a peripheral intravenous catheter, skin rashes related to medication, and hematuria in one patient. One donor experienced an apneic episode during spinal anesthesia. This complication resolved completely, and the marrow was collected successfully. Two days after the collection, 75% of the donors experienced fatigue, 68% complained of pain at the collection site, and 52% had lower back pain. The mean recovery time of these complaints was 16 days. Ten percent of the donors recovered fully only after 30 days or more. The duration of the postcollection complaints and recovery time correlated well with the duration of the collection procedure.

When the psychosocial effects of bone marrow donation were investigated, 87% of the donors felt their marrow donation was very worthwhile and 91% would be willing to donate again in the future [7]. Marrow donors were more likely to feel better about themselves as a result of the donation than kidney donors. Donors with longer collection times were in general less positive about their bone marrow donation.

Results of unrelated donor transplants

Engraftment

Patients with hematologic malignancies receiving cyclophosphamide (CY) and total body irradiation (TBI) prior to transplantation have a 98% probability of achieving sustained engraftment when transplanted from a genotypically HLA-identical sibling donor and when the bone marrow is not depleted of T cells, compared to 88% of patients transplanted from an HLA-haploidentical donor, with variable matching for the HLA antigens of the nonshared haplotype [8]. A higher risk of graft failure was observed in haploidentical transplants with a positive antidonor T-cell or B-cell cross-match (62% versus 7%; $p = 0.001$). The risk of graft failure for a fully matched unrelated donor was 1.6% (3/187) and 2.5% (2/80) when a minor mismatch was present. The use of bone marrow depleted of T cells increases the risk of secondary graft

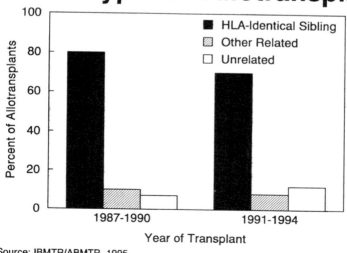

Source: IBMTR/ABMTR, 1995

Figure 1. An increasing percentage of allogeneic bone marrow transplants involve unrelated donors.

failure to 14% [9], although T-cell depletion was not a risk factor for primary nonengraftment [10]. To reduce the increased risk of secondary graft failure with T-cell-depleted transplants, conditioning regimens have been intensified by adding thiotepa and antithymocyte globulin to the pretransplant regimen and G-CSF and methylprednisolone following transplantation. With this regimen, very few graft failures are seen [11]. The incidence of graft failure also appears to increase if non-TBI conditioning regimens such as busulfan and cyclophosphamide are used [2,13]. In one series, only 2 of 5 patients engrafted [12]; in another series, 6 of 33 experienced graft failure [13]. The increased risk of graft failure associated with non-TBI-containing conditioning regimens may by overcome by the addition of total lymphoid irradiation and antithymocyte globulin [14].

Acute graft-versus-host disease (GVHD)

Unrelated donor transplants are associated with a higher risk of moderate to severe acute GVHD (grades II–IV) when compared to sibling donor transplants (79% versus 36%; $p < 0.001$) [15]. The incidence of severe GVHD (grades III–IV) is increased from 14% to 35% ($p = 0.002$) [15]. The risk of acute GVHD is further increased if minor mismatched donors are compared to matching unrelated donors: 95% versus 78% ($p < 0.001$) for grades II–IV GVHD and 51% versus 36% for grades III–IV GVHD [16]. Acute GVHD grades II–IV occurred in 91% of A-locus mismatched, 82% of B-locus mismatched, and 94% of DR mismatched transplants ($p < 0.05$). Acute GVHD grades III–IV was seen in 62% of A-locus mismatched, 57% of B-locus mismatched, and 58% of DR mismatched transplants ($p = 0.33$) [8].

The significance of HLA-DP matching has been analyzed in 129 patients who underwent marrow transplantation from HLA-A, B, DR, and DQ matched unrelated donors [17]. In 22% of these pairs there was no DP incompatibility; one DP mismatch was present in 56% and two DP mismatches in 22%. This study shows that incompatibility for DP does not influence the risk of acute GVHD and therefore, HLA-DP disparity should not be used as an exclusion criterion for donor selection in unrelated marrow transplantation.

Clinical GVHD results from an immune reaction of mature donor T lymphocytes contained in the bone marrow inoculum against histocompatibility determinants of the recipient. Therefore, T-cell depletion of the donor bone marrow should reduce the risk of severe GVHD. Indeed, the risk of grades III–IV acute GVHD in 196 consecutive unrelated donor marrow transplants was 60% in recipients of unmanipulated bone marrow, compared to 20% ($p = 0.0003$) in those who received T-cell depleted transplants [18]. In patients receiving unmanipulated unrelated donor transplants, the combination of methotrexate and cyclosporin A as GVHD prophylaxis is superior to monotherapy [19]. No benefit was derived by adding methylprednisolone to cyclosporin–methotrexate [20]. A study performed by Ringden et al. suggests that if patient and unrelated donor are perfectly matched by serologic and molecular techniques, the incidence of grades II–IV acute GVHD is not different from that seen in HLA-identical siblings (15%) [21]. In a larger study from Seattle, however, the incidence of grades III–IV acute GVHD was still 48% if patient and donor were perfect matches, but this was lower than the 70% seen in mismatched patients ($p < 0.01$) [22]. Acute GVHD following unrelated donor marrow transplantation is much more resistant to standard treatment with prednisone [23]. Of the 89 patients who received an unrelated donor marrow transplant at the University of Minnesota, 49 developed acute GVHD. Seven were excluded from analysis for different reasons. Of the remaining 42 patients treated for acute GVHD, only nine (21%) achieved a complete and continuing response by day +100, suggesting that more aggressive treatment modalities such as antibodies against the interleukin-1 or the interleukin-2 receptor may be required to control GVHD [23,24].

Chronic graft-versus-host disease

The probability of extensive chronic GVHD after an unrelated donor transplant is 55% to 75% [8,26–28]. The Seattle group analyzed 146 unrelated donor transplants who received cyclosporin and methotrexate for GVHD prophylaxis, who survived more than 100 days, and who remained relapse-free [8]. In only 15% of these patients was no clinical or pathological evidence of chronic GVHD found. Immunosuppressive therapy could be discontinued within six months after transplantation. The mortality rate in the group was 15%. In 8% of patients, chronic GVHD remained subclinical and was detected only by an abnormal biopsy of skin or lip or by limited manifestations of skin or liver GVHD. Extensive chronic GVHD occurred in 77% of patients in one of the following patterns: 1) acute GVHD never resolving and progressing to chronic GVHD (30%); 57% of these patients died, usually from opportunistic infections (mainly CMV and *Aspergillus*); 2) acute GVHD subsiding before the onset of chronic GVHD (40%); 33% of these patients died; and 3) chronic GVHD developing de novo in 7% of patients; 15% of these patients died. For surviving patients, the median time to successful withdrawal of immunosuppressive therapy was 18 months; 3% of patients continued to require immunosuppressive therapy five years or more after transplantation. The incidence of extensive chronic GVHD can be decreased significantly by depleting the bone marrow T cells ($p = 0.001$) [9,18].

Opportunistic infections

Repopulation by mature T cells and recovery of immunoglobulin production are extremely slow after unrelated donor transplants. Immune reconstitution is further delayed in patients with acute and chronic GVHD on prolonged immunosuppressive therapy and in patients receiving T-cell-depleted allografts, in whom functional T cells remain absent for 6 to 12 months. The severe and prolonged immune deficiency predisposes patients to opportunistic infections, predominantly with *Aspergillus*, yeast, and cytomegalovirus (CMV). Disseminated *Aspergillus* infection occurs in approximately 15% of unrelated transplants and has a greater than 90% mortality [29]. No major improvement in prevention or treatment of *Aspergillus* infections has been observed during the last five years. Prophylaxis with low-dose amphotericin B has not decreased the risk of *Aspergillus*. Itraconazole, although active against *Aspergillus*, is poorly absorbed in patients with poor food intake on antacids, especially in the presence of diarrhea or malabsorption as frequently seen in active or chronic GVHD. Serious CMV infections are more common in unrelated donor transplants than in sibling transplants [26]. Ganciclovir can prevent CMV disease in CMV-seropositive recipients of unrelated donors [30]. However, in patients receiving T-cell-depleted grafts, ganciclovir prophylaxis may lead to delayed hematopoietic recovery or persistent cytopenia. Serious viral infections not caused by CMV are also more common in unrelated donor transplants [16]. Most of these infections occur before day 100 and are often fatal.

Relapse

The incidence of relapse is significantly lower in unrelated donor transplants when compared to related donors [28]. Even after adjusting for acute GVHD grades II to IV, the decreased risk of relapse remains [28]. The risk of relapse in comparable groups of patients was approximately 15% in unrelated donor transplants compared to 40% in sibling transplants ($p = 0.03$) [28]. The same trend was reported by the Seattle group [15]. Although recipients of HLA-identical marrow depleted of T cells for the treatment of advanced acute leukemia or chronic myeloid leukemia are at increased risk of relapse after transplantation, recipients of T-cell-depleted marrow from unrelated donors do not appear to be at a similar increased risk of relapse [9]. The low probability of relapse suggests that transplants from unrelated donors may offer a considerable graft-versus-leukemic effect.

Quality of life

The University of Minnesota compared the quality of life of 31 unrelated donor transplant recipients to that of 52 related donor recipients matching for age and year of transplant and surviving at least two years after transplant [28]. Both groups generally judged their quality of life to be good, with only one of the unrelated transplants being unable to perform normal activity. Overall, there were no significant differences between unrelated and related donor transplants. Of the 31 unrelated donor transplants, 28 were working full-time or were attending school. The Hammersmith group reported 14 of their 25 surviving unrelated transplants having a normal performance status, whereas seven have a performance status of 80 or less [26]. Of the 11 unrelated donor

224

transplants with an abnormal performance status, nine had significant GVHD and only four were working at their normal jobs.

Survival

The Seattle group showed that the probability of relapse-free survival appeared similar in unrelated donor transplant patients and in disease, disease-stage, and age-matched controls (41% vs. 46% at one year) [15]. The same group subsequently demonstrated comparable survival for phenotypically identical and minor mismatched unrelated donors [16]. In the Hammersmith study, the probability of leukemia-free survival at two years in CML patients was 72% for the sibling donor group versus 42% for the unrelated donor group ($p = 0.05$) [26]. A recent report from the Minnesota group compared the outcome of 142 unrelated donor transplants to that of 142 sibling transplants [28]. The pairs were matched for diagnosis, stage of disease, age, and year of transplant. The difference in survival between the two groups was insignificant for recipients of fully matched unrelated donor marrow ($p = 0.17$) at three years, but significantly inferior for HLA-A or B mismatched unrelated donor recipients (three-year survival, 0.26 versus 0.52; $p = 0.00001$) [28]. Among patients with acute leukemia in first or second remission, the probability of disease-free survival at two years was 45%, superior to that of patients with more advanced disease (19%; $p < 0.001$) [9]. In patients with congenital disorders, the probability of survival at two years was 52% [9]. In a multivariate analysis performed by the National Marrow Donor Program, younger age was the most significant favorable variable for disease-free survival in leukemia patients receiving unrelated donor marrow [9]. This observation was confirmed by the Minnesota [28] and Seattle groups [8].

Causes of death

A review by the National Marrow Donor Program of the primary and secondary causes of death in 307 unrelated transplant patients showed that infection (37%) and acute and chronic GVHD (33%) were the leading causes of mortality, followed by interstitial pneumonia (21%), hemorrhagic complications (15%), toxicity related to chemoradiotherapy (14%), relapse (14%), and graft failure (11%) [9]. Lymphoproliferative disorders were more common in patients who received T-cell-depleted transplants, but were also seen in patients who received unmanipulated marrows [9].

Conclusions

Unrelated donor transplants are associated with an increased risk of engraftment problems and acute and chronic GVHD. These problems are related partly to disparities for HLA determinants. Molecular typing for class I antigens has just started [31,32] and should help in identifying the best possible unrelated donor, resulting in a decrease in graft failure and GVHD. However, improvements in molecular typing will make it more difficult to find perfect matches, and a certain degree of genetic disparity will have to be allowed for. Since mortality due to GVHD is substantial, especially in patients over 20 years of age, and since T-cell-depleted marrow grafts are associated with more rapid engraftment and a decrease in the incidence and severity of GVHD, T-cell depletion should be strongly considered in older unrelated donor transplants. The risk of graft failure associated with T-cell depletion can be drastically reduced by a more intensive conditioning regimen including thiotepa, antithymocyte globulin pretransplantation, and hematopoietic growth factors post-transplantation. The risk of relapse in unrelated transplants is not increased with T-cell depletion. The major problems with T-cell depletion and the more intensive immunosuppressive anti-GVHD regimens are related to the profound and prolonged immune deficiency resulting in a substantial risk of opportunistic infections. Although mortality due to CMV infections has been reduced significantly with the administration of prophylactic ganciclovir and the availability of techniques that allow early detection of CMV, no decrease in mortality due to fungal and yeast infections has yet been seen. The administration of low numbers of T cells at a time that some degree of tolerance to donor cells has been established may restore the immune function without the need for prolonged and intensive immunosuppressive therapy. It will also eliminate the risk of lymphoproliferative disorders and will induce an antitumor effect.

The major challenge for the future is to better deal with the profound and prolonged immune suppression. If this can be achieved, unrelated donor transplants should be associated with a morbidity and mortality rate that is no higher than that seen in sibling transplants.

References

1. Sonnenberg FA, Eckman MH, Pauker SG. Bone marrow donor registries: the relation between registry size and probability of finding complete and partial matches. Blood 74:2569–2578, 1989.
2. Beatty PG, Dahlber S, Michelson EM, Nisperos B, Opetz G, Martin PJ, Hansen JA. Probability of finding HLA matched unrelated donors. Transplantation 45:714–718, 1988.
3. Beatty PG. Marrow transplantation using volunteer unrelated donors in a comparison of mismatched family donor transplants: a Seattle perspective. Bone Marrow Transplant 14(Suppl 4):39–41, 1994.
4. Executive Committee of the World Marrow Donor Association. Bone marrow transplants using volunteer donors — recommendations and requirements for a standardized practice throughout the world. Bone Marrow Transplant 10:287–291, 1992.
5. Goldman JM, for the WMDA Executive Committee. A special report: bone marrow transplants using volunteer donors — recommendations and requirements for a standardized practice throughout the world — 1994 update. Blood 84:2833–2839, 1994.
6. Stroncek DF, Holland PV, Bartch G, Bixby T, Simmons RG, Antin JH, Anderson KC, Ash RC, Bolwell BJ, Hansen JA, Heal JM, Henslee-Downey PJ, Jaffe ER, Klein HG, Lau PM,

Perkins HA, Popovsky MA, Price TH, Rowley SD, Stehling LC, Weiden PL, Wissel ME, McCullough J. Experiences of the first 493 unrelated marrow donors in the National Marrow Donor Program. Blood 81:1940–1946, 1993.

7. Butterworth VA, Simmons RG, Bartsch G, Randall B, Schimmel M, Stroncek DF. Psychosocial effects of unrelated bone marrow donation: experiences of the National Marrow Donor Program. Blood 81:1947–1959, 1993.

8. Hansen JA, Petersdorf EW, Choo SY, Martin PJ, Anasetti C. Marrow transplantation from HLA partially matched relatives and unrelated donors. Bone Marrow Transplant 15(Suppl 1):128–139, 1995.

9. Kernan NA, Bartsch G, Ash RC, Beatty PG, Champlin R, Filipovich A, Gajewski J, Hansen JA, Henslee-Downey J, McCullough J, McGlave P, Perkings HA, Phillips GL, Sanders J, Stroncek D, Thomas ED, Blume KG. Analysis of 462 transplantations from unrelated donors facilitated by the National Marrow Donor Program. N Engl J Med 328:593–602, 1993.

10. McGlave PB, Beatty P, Ash R, Hows JM. Therapy for chronic myelogenous leukemia with unrelated donor bone marrow transplantation: results in 102 cases. Blood 75:1728–1732, 1990.

11. Kernan NA. Strategies to prevent graft rejection following T-cell depleted unrelated marrow transplantation. Bone Marrow Transplant 15 (Suppl 1): 92–93, 1995.

12. Mehta J,Powles RL, Mitchell P, Rege K, De Lord C, Treleaven J. Graft failure after bone marrow transplantation from unrelated donors using busulphan and cyclophosphamide for conditioning. Bone Marrow Transplant 13:583–587, 1994.

13 Gajewski J, Sahebi F, Crilley P, Bolwell B, Copelan E. Use of the Ohio state busulfan/cyclophosphamide regiment in recipients of matched unrelated donor transplants. Bone Marrow Transplant 15 (Suppl 1):88–91, 1995.

14. Kanfer EJ, Macdonald IK, Hall G, Ward H, Smith J, Evans M, Taylor J, Camba L, Glaser MG, Samson DM, McCarthy DM. Poor prognosis acute myeloid leukaemia treated by matched unrelated donor marrow transplant without preceding total body irradiation. Bone Marrow Transplant 9:67–69, 1992.

15. Beatty PG, Hansen JA, Longton GM, Thomas ED, Sanders JE, Martin PJ, Bearman SI, Anasetti C, Petersdorf EW, Mickelson EM, Pepe MS, Appelbaum FR, Buckner CD, Clift RA, Petersen FB, Stewart PS, Storb RF, Sullivan KM, Tesler MC, Witherspoon RP. Marrow transplantation from HLA-matched unrelated donors for treatment of hematologic malignancies. Transplantation 51:443–447, 1991.

16. Beatty PG, Anasetti C, Hansen JA, Longton GM, Sanders JE, Martin PJ, Mickelson EM, Choo SY, Petersdorf EW, Pepe MS, Appelbaum FR, Bearman SI, Buckner CD, Clift RA, Petersen FB, Singer J, Stewart PS, Storb RF, Sullivan KM, Tesler MC, Witherspoon RP, Thomas ED. Marrow transplantation from unrelated donors for treatment of hematologic malignancies: effect of mismatching for one HLA locus. Blood 81:249–253, 1993.

17. Petersdorf EW, Smith AG, Mickelson EM, Longton GM, Anasetti C, Choo SY, Martin PJ, Hansen JA. The role of HLA-DPB1 disparity in the development of acute graft-versus-host disease following unrelated donor marrow transplantation. Blood 81:1923–1932, 1993.

18. McGlave P, Bartsch G, Anasetti C, Ash R, Beatty P, Gajewski J, Kernan NA. Unrelated donor marrow transplantation therapy for chronic myelogenous leukemia: initial experience of the National Marrow Donor Program. Blood 81:543–550, 1993.

19. Ringden O, Klaesson S, Sundberg B, Ljungman P, Lonnqvist B, Persson U. Decreased incidence of graft-versus-host disease and improved survival with methotrexate combined with cyclosporin compared with monotherapy in recipients of bone marrow from donors other than HLA identical siblings. Bone Marrow Transplant 9:19–25, 1992.

20. Leelasiri A, Greer JP, Stein RS, Goodman S, Brandt SA, Edwards JR, Wolff SN. Graft-versus-host disease prophylaxis for matched unrelated donor bone marrow transplantation: comparison between cyclosporine-methotrexate and cyclosporine-methotrexate-methylprednisolone. Bone Marrow Transplant 15:401–405, 1995.

21. Ringden O, Remberger M, Persson U, Ljungman P, Aldener A, Andstrom E, Aschan J, Bolme P, Dahllof G, Dalianis T, Gahrton G, Hagglund H, Lonnqvist B, Olerup O, Shanwell A, Sparrelid E, Winiarski J, Moller E, Oberg M. Similar incidence of graft-versus-host disease

using HLA-A, -B and -DR identical unrelated bone marrow donors as with HLA-identical siblings. Bone Marrow Transplant 15:619–625, 1995.

22. Petersdorf EW, Longton GM, Anasetti C, Martin PJ, Mickelson EM, Smith AG, Hansen JA. The significance of HLA-DRB1 matching on clinical outcome after HLA-A, B, DR identical unrelated donor marrow transplantation. Blood 86:1606–1613, 1995.

23. Roy J, McGlave PB, Filipovich AH, Miller WJ, Blazar BR, Ramsay NK, Kersey JH, Weisdorf DJ. Acute graft-versus-host disease following unrelated donor marrow transplantation: failure of conventional therapy. Bone Marrow Transplant 10:77–82, 1992.

24. Antin JH, Weinstein HJ, Guinan EC, McCarthy P, Bierer BE, Gilliland G, Parsons SK, Ballen KK, Rimm IJ, Falzarano G, Bloedow DC, Abate L, Lebsack M, Burakoff SJ, Ferrara JLM. Recombinant human interleukin-1 receptor antagonist in the treatment of steroid-resistant graft-versus-host disease. Blood 84:1342–1348, 1994.

25. Anasetti C, Hansen JA, Waldmann TA, Appelbaum FR, Davis J, Deeg HJ, Doney K, Martin PJ, Nask R, Storb R, Sullivan KM, Witherspoon RP, Binger M-H, Chizzonite R, Hakimi J, Mould D, Satoh H, Light SE. Treatment of acute graft-versus-host disease with humanized anti-tac: an antibody that binds to the interleukin-2 receptor. Blood 84:1320–1327, 1994.

26. Marks DI, Cullis JO, Ward KN, Lacey S, Szydlo R, Hughes TP, Schwarer AP, Lutz E, Barrett AJ, Hows JM, Batchelor R, Goldman JM. Allogeneic bone marrow transplantation for chonic myeloid leukemia using sibling and volunteer unrelated donors. Ann Intern Med 119:207–214, 1993.

27. Nademanee A, Schmidt GM, Parker P, Dagis AC, Stein A, Snyder DS, O'Donnell M, Smith EP, Stepan DE, Molina A, Wong KK, Margolin K, Somlo G, Littrell B, Woo D, Sniecinski I, Niland JC, Forman SJ. The outcome of matched unrelated donor bone marrow transplantation in patients with hematologic malignancies using molecular typing for donor selection and graft-versus-host disease prophylaxis regimen of cyclosporine, methotrexate, and prednisone. Blood 86:1228–1234, 1995.

28. Davies SM, Shu XO, Blazar BR, Filipovich AH, Kersey JH, Krivit W, McCullough J, Miller WJ, Ramsay NKC, Segall M, Wagner JE, Weisdorf DJ, McGlave PB. Unrelated donor bone marrow transplantation: influence of HLA A and B incompatibility on outcome. Blood 86:1636–1642, 1995.

29. Anasetti C, Etzioni R, Petersdorf EW, Martin PJ, Hansen JA. Marrow transplantation from unrelated volunteer donors. Annu Rev Med 46:169–179, 1995.

30. Lanino E, Anasetti C, Longton G, Etzioni R, Bowden R, Hansen JA. Prevention of cytomegalovirus disease with ganciclovir in recipients of marrow transplants from unrelated donors. Blood 82(Suppl 1):344a, 1993.

31. Blasczyk R, Hahn U, Wehling J, Huhn D, Salama A. Complete subtyping of the HLA-A locus by sequence-specific amplification followed by direct sequencing or single-strand conformation polymorphism analysis. Tissue Antigens 46:86–95, 1995.

32. Petersdorf EW, Hansen JA. A comprehensive approach for typing the alleles of the HLA-B locus by automated sequencing. Tissue Antigens 46:73–85, 1995.

III

Reducing the Toxicity Associated with Hematopoietic Stem Cell Transplantation

11. Supportive care in bone marrow transplantation: pulmonary complications

Stephen W. Crawford

Pulmonary complications after marrow transplantation

Incidence and significance

Overall, 40% to 60% of patients develop pulmonary disease at some time after marrow transplantation, and 24% to 40% require intensive care [1,2]. Characteristics such as increased HLA disparity with the donor source, high-dose conditioning regimens, active malignancy, and advanced age of the patient are associated with increased incidence of complications [3,4]. The incidence among patients who receive total body irradiation (TBI) for conditioning is higher than that of patients who receive only chemotherapy. Pneumonia as a clinical syndrome is the leading infectious cause of death, and until recently, Cytomegalovirus (CMV) was the most common cause of fatal pulmonary infection [5]. The incidence of some pulmonary infections, such as Pneumocystis carinii and perhaps bacterial pneumonia, has decreased due to the routine use of prophylactic antimicrobial agents. However, diffuse 'idiopathic' pulmonary injury continues, with mortality rate exceeding 60%. Newer understanding of idiopathic lung injury has led to the delineation of the recently coined 'idiopathic pneumonia syndrome' [6].

Significant pulmonary dysfunction persists or develops in some long-term survivors months and even years after successful marrow transplantation. Airflow obstructive defects occur in at least 10% of patients with chronic GVHD and have been seen, albeit rarely, in recipients of autologous marrow [7–9]. Obliterative bronchiolitis is the most commonly identified obstructing lesion and may progress to profound respiratory insufficiency and death [7]. Progressive restrictive lung disease may be seen as a complication of transplantation occurring years after the procedure. Little is currently known about the incidence and risks of these long-term processes.

Temporal sequence of pulmonary disease syndromes

Specific complications tend to occur within well-defined periods that correspond to the state of immune reconstitution [10]. These complications may be

Jane N. Winter (ed.) BLOOD STEM CELL TRANSPLANTATION. 1997. Kluwer Academic Publishers. ISBN 0-7923-4260-7. All rights reserved.

grouped according to the time of presentation relative to the day of marrow transplantation [11]. The groupings are based in part on the fact that chronic GVHD occurs approximately at or beyond day 100 after allogeneic transplant, delimiting a 'late' from an 'early' period.

Complications within the first 30 days are dominated by regimen-related toxicities. A period of pancytopenia is the rule, although administration of hematopoietic colony stimulating factors may shorten the duration [12]. Pulmonary edema syndromes due to excess fluid administration have been reported in up to half of marrow transplantation recipients, but should be expected less frequently with appropriate attention to fluid management [13]. Also, congestive heart failure due to cardiotoxic chemotherapy, adult respiratory distress syndrome (ARDS) due to chemoradiotherapy injury or sepsis, and pulmonary hemorrhage in the presence of thrombocytopenia contribute to diffuse infiltrates. These patients frequently suffer from multiorgan disease with regimen-related toxicities or, among allogeneic marrow recipients, grade II–IV (moderate-severe) acute GVHD. Severe oral mucositis is common and may result in recurrent aspiration of oral secretions. Secondary infection of the denuded oral mucosa with Herpes simplex virus (HSV) or Gram-negative bacilli may delay healing and increase the risk of pneumonia. During this period, diffuse pulmonary infiltrates rarely are infectious, and opportunistic infections are not prevalent [14].

During days 30 to 100–150, granulocyte number and function usually have returned to normal, but defects in humoral and cell-mediated immunity persist. Both opportunistic and idiopathic pneumonias occur in this period. Historically, viral pneumonias, especially CMV, were the most frequent causes for diffuse pulmonary infiltrates. More recently, the advent of effective prophylaxis and early treatment strategies has markedly decreased the incidence of CMV and HSV pneumonia [15–17].

Impact of transplant techniques (PBSCs, growth factors)

The primary differences in pulmonary complications between autologous and allogeneic marrow transplantation are the incidence of infections and late airflow obstructive defects. Viral pneumonia is significantly less common among autologous marrow recipients, presumably due to less suppression of cytotoxic T lymphocytes (CTLs) from graft-versus-host disease and its treatment and prophylaxis. CMV pneumonia occurs in 4% or less of autologous recipients [18]. Additionally, invasive fungal disease after the initial period of neutropenia appears less common for similar reasons [19].

Idiopathic lung injury, associated with chemoirradiation or sepsis syndrome, occurs after both autologous and allogeneic marrow transplantation with similar frequency. We have recently shown that there is no statistical difference in the incidence of idiopathic injury within the first four months: 7.6% for allogeneic and 5.7% for autologous [20].

The use of alternative hematopoietic precursor sources, such as mobilized

232

peripheral blood stem cells, and cytokines, such as hematopoietic cell colony stimulating factors, have shortened the time to engraftment [12]. The shorter period of neutropenia would be expected to decrease the incidence of pulmonary complications through several avenues. First, marrow recipients should be at reduced risk of opportunistic infections due both to the improved granulocyte numbers and to the shortened duration of hospitalization. Second, improved platelet counts should decrease hemorrhage associated with lung injury.

However, the risks for lung injury associated with chemoirradiation therapy may be unchanged by the hematopoietic precursor source. Idiopathic lung injury remains a danger. At present, few data exist to convincingly demonstrate that the incidence of pulmonary complications is lower with the newer transplant techniques. It is likely that opportunistic infections will decrease but idiopathic injury will be unchanged, similar to the experience with autologous marrow transplantation.

Surveillance for pulmonary complications

Pulmonary function testing

Pretransplant. Pulmonary function testing (PFT) is a standard part of the pretransplant evaluation at many centers. The results form baseline data for comparison with later testing and have been used as an indication to exclude a candidate from transplant. Abnormalities in the measures of airflow, lung volume, and diffusing capacity have been associated with increased risk of pulmonary complications after transplant [21,22].

Abnormal pretransplant PFT results are predictive of mortality [23]. After other clinical characteristics associated with death after transplantation (age, relapsed malignancy, HLA-mismatched graft, etc.) have been accounted for, restrictive lung defect (decreased total lung capacity), hypoxemia, and reduced diffusing capacity are associated with statistically increased risk of death, especially within the first few months after transplant (figure 1). In this study, the risks associated with these PFT results were applicable to autologous as well as allogeneic marrow recipients, suggesting that the risks predicted mortality due to treatment-related toxicities. Surprisingly, hypoxemia and reduced diffusing capacity were independently associated with death, each carrying risk. It was initially assumed that these two physiologically linked measurements would provide similar information regarding mortality risk. However, reduced diffusing capacity appears to predict death by means other than respiratory failure. It is likely that reduced diffusing capacity is associated with an increased risk of fatal hepatic veno-occlusive disease (data unpublished). Systemic endothelial injury due to previous chemotherapy may account for both the diffusing capacity abnormalities and fatal liver failure.

While pretransplant PFT results are statistically associated with complica-

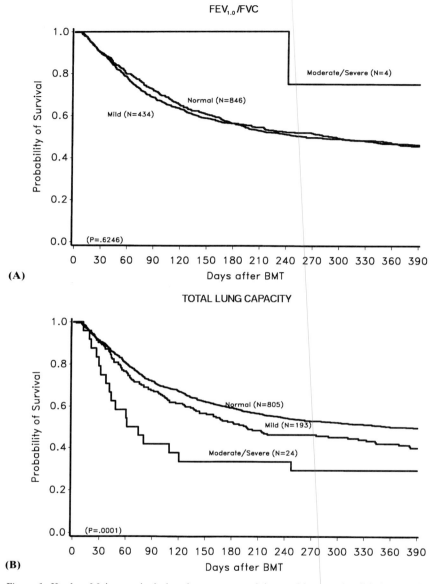

Figure 1. Kaplan–Meier survival plots for marrow recipients with normal, mild abnormalities or moderate-severe abnormalities in PFT before marrow transplantation. Log-rank *p*-values are indicated in parentheses. **(A)** FEV_1/FVC; normal ≥80%, mild <80% and ≥60%, moderate/severe <60%. **(B)** Total lung capacity (TLC); normal ≥80% of predicted, mild <80% and ≥60% of predicted, moderate/sever <60% of predicted. **(C)** Diffusing capacity (D_LCO_{sb}); normal ≥80% of predicted, mild <80% and ≥60% of predicted, moderate/severe <60% of predicted. **(D)** Alveolar-arterial pO_2 gradient ($P(A-a)O_2$); normal ≤20 mmHg, mild >20 mmHg and ≤30 mmHg, moderate/severe >30 mmHg. (From Crawford SW, Fisher L. Predictive value of pulmonary function tests before marrow transplantation. Chest 101:1257–64, 1992, with permission.)

234

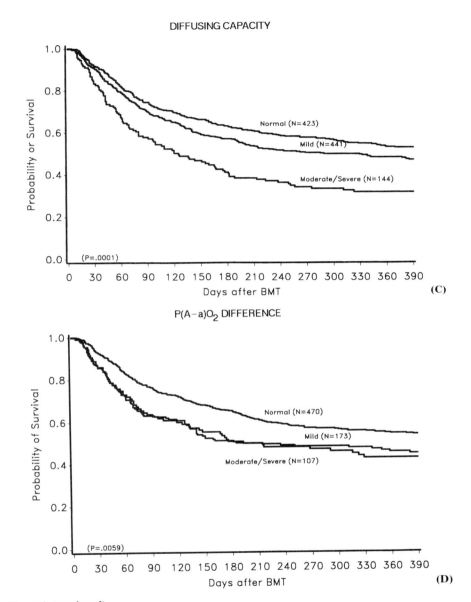

DIFFUSING CAPACITY

Normal (N=423)

Mild (N=441)

Moderate/Severe (N=144)

(P=.0001)

Days after BMT

(C)

P(A−a)O$_2$ DIFFERENCE

Normal (N=470)

Mild (N=173)

Moderate/Severe (N=107)

(P=.0059)

Days after BMT

(D)

Figure 1 (continued)

tions and death, there are no absolute values for these tests that predict these
outcomes with specificity (figure 2). On average, a total lung capacity or
diffusing capacity value (corrected for hemoglobin content) below the lower
limits of normal may be associate with a 20% decrease in the probability of
survival. Such information should not be used as an absolute contraindication

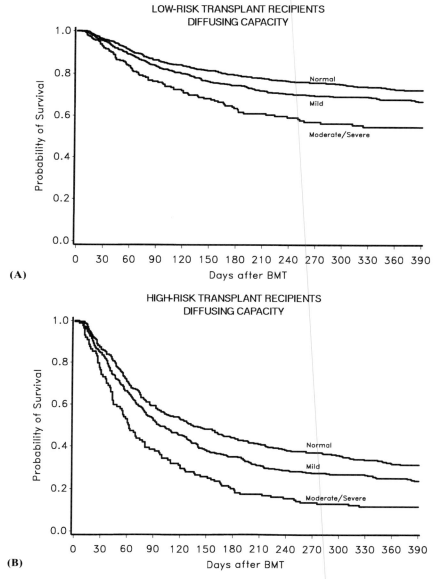

Figure 2. Kaplan–Meier survival plots estimated from the Cox proportional hazards regression model for 'low-risk' patients compared to those for 'high-risk' patients for various degrees of D_LCO_{sb} abnormality. **(A)** 'Low-risk' patients were less than 21 years old with malignancy in remission and received HLA-identical marrow grafts. **(B)** 'High-risk' patients were more than 21 years old with malignancy in relapse and received HLA-nonidentical marrow grafts. (From Crawford SW, Fisher L. Predictive value of pulmonary function tests before marrow transplantation. Chest 101:1257–64, 1992, with permission.)

236

to transplantation, but rather in combination with other known risks for transplant-related mortality to fully assess the risks.

Posttransplant. There are both acute and long-term decrements in pulmonary function after intensive chemotherapy and irradiation as utilized in marrow transplantation [24–33]. Reductions in lung volumes, diffusing capacity, and exercise tolerance were documented after treatment for leukemia in children as well and were thought largely secondary to chemotherapy [34]. PFT abnormalities have been reported to include declines in lung volumes, gas diffusion, and airflow. Reductions in lung volumes and diffusing capacity are common 'early' (i.e., months) after marrow transplant. The declines in lung volumes may be at least partially reversible within two years after transplantation, while the low diffusing capacity reportedly persists for several years. Development of airflow obstruction has been seen in approximately 10% of allogeneic marrow recipients in the presence of chronic graft-versus-host disease (GVHD) and most often is related to obliterative bronchiolitis [7,8,35].

Few reports have examined abnormalities in other PFT results for association with increased mortality. Badier et al. noted that both relapse of malignancy and overall mortality were correlated with falls in lung volumes and diffusion one year after marrow transplantation [33].

In order to investigate the clinical significance of declines in pulmonary function early after marrow transplantation, we recently reviewed prospective, nonrandomized PFT results of all 960 marrow recipients who performed PFT between days 60 and 120 after marrow transplantation over an eight-year period for association with nonrelapse mortality [36]. At three months after transplantation, the mean values for total lung capacity (TLC) and diffusing capacity decreased, and restrictive ventilatory defects (TLC < 80% of predicted) were noted in 34% of the cohort. Airflow rates (FEV_1/FVC) were unchanged. A restrictive lung defect at three months after transplant or a significant decline ($\geq 15\%$) in TLC from baseline despite remaining within the normal range were associated with a twofold increased risk of nonrelapse mortality. Neither airflow obstruction nor impairment in diffusing capacity were associated with an increased risk (figure 3). Abnormalities of the TLC at three months after transplant were associated with death with respiratory failure, but not with an increased risk of chronic GVHD.

These data support an increase in the nonrelapse mortality rate associated with either the presence of a restrictive defect three months after marrow transplantation or a significant decline in lung volume compared to baseline. This effect is most pronounced more than one year after marrow transplant and appears to be due to an increase in the rate of death with respiratory failure, not chronic GVHD. On the basis of these results, we routinely evaluate lung function three months and then yearly after marrow transplantation.

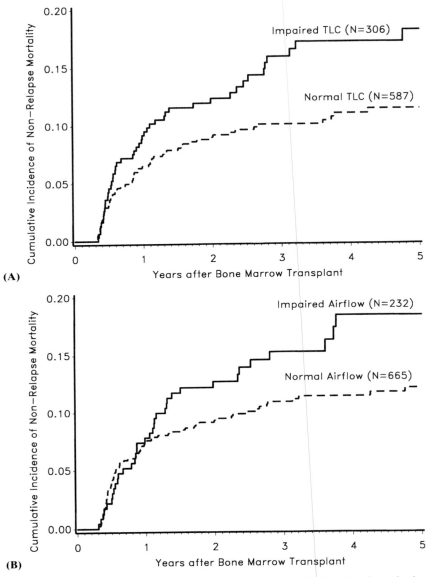

Figure 3. Estimates of the cumulative probabilities of nonrelapse death as functions of pulmonary function test results three months after marrow transplantation. **(A)** total lung capacity ($p = 0.004$, logrank); **(B)** FEV$_1$/FVC ($p = 0.08$, logrank); and **(C)** diffusing capacity ($p > 0.05$, logrank). In each plot, the solid curve corresponds to marrow recipients with pulmonary function test result impairment and the dashed curve to those with normal pulmonary function test results. (From Crawford SW, Pepe M, Lin D, Benedetti F, Deeg HJ. Abnormalities of pulmonary function tests after marrow transplantation predict non-relapse mortality. Am J Respir Crit Care Med 152:690–695, 1995, with permission.)

238

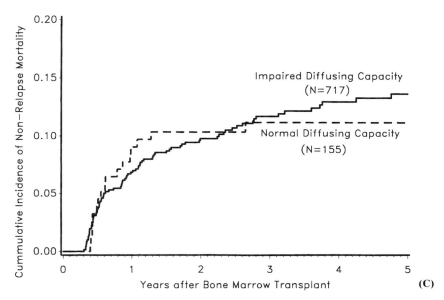

Figure 3 (continued)

Radiographs. Attention to radiographic abnormalities of the chest is crucial to avoid unnecessary complications. Focal abnormalities frequently represent opportunistic infection in neutropenic hosts and those with malignancy, even in the absence of symptoms. In our experience, focal lesions evident on chest radiography in patients with recent chemotherapy or hematological malignancy were infectious in over 80% of cases. Stanford investigators noted that focal lung lesions in patients with non-Hodgkin's and Hodgkin's lymphoma are most often parenchymal lymphoma [37,38]. However, fungal pneumonia may present after chemotherapy and be indistinguishable radiographically from malignancy [39]. Additionally, tuberculosis after transplantation most often occurs in patients with evidence of prior parenchymal lung disease [40].

Suspicion of focal lesions on chest radiography should prompt aggressive diagnostic evaluation before transplantation. Computerized tomographic examination may help localize and anatomically define the lesion(s). Depending upon the number, size, and location of the lesions, diagnostic procedures are warranted for treatment planning. Bronchoscopy, percutaneous needle aspiration, and/or lung resection should generally follow radiographic identification.

Predictors of mortality with respiratory failure

Predicting respiratory failure

It can be predicted which patients are at risk to require mechanical ventilatory support. The risk factors present at time of transplantation for subsequent

239

respiratory failure are receipt of an HLA-nonidentical donor marrow, active phase of malignancy, and older age (>21 years) [41]. The incidence of respiratory failure increases from 10% to 13% with none of these risk factors to over 50% when all three are present.

It is important that transplant units and patients have adequate information to assess the risks associated with marrow transplantation. Such information is crucial to discussions of advanced-care directives and cost containment. Given the difficulty in assessing medical futility in the marrow transplant recipient with respiratory failure, autonomous decisions by the patient should be followed [42]. Advanced-care directives should be obtained prior to marrow transplantation from marrow recipients at risk for respiratory failure, and the estimated risk of complications should be used in counseling before marrow transplantation.

Predicting outcome

Studies of intensive care for respiratory failure of patients with cancer [43–45], hematological malignancies [46,47], and marrow transplantation have reported low survival rates. In reports from our center, the University of Minnesota, and others, approximately 3% of marrow recipients receiving mechanical ventilation survived to six months after transplantation [1,48–51]. Recent studies of pediatric marrow transplant recipients find the same poor prognosis as noted among adults [52]. In addition, intensive care for marrow recipients with respiratory failure utilizes inordinate medical resources. In a study of 50 patients by Denardo et al., nonsurvivors of respiratory failure utilized the vast majority of blood products administered in the intensive care unit [51].

The results of these studies can be viewed in various ways. The low incidence of long-term survivors can be taken to mean that 'the prognosis is uniformly grim.' Such a conclusion may imply that medical intervention would be futile. However, given the controversy surrounding the meaning of medical futility, a low probability of survival alone may not be a valid argument for withholding mechanical ventilation from the marrow transplant recipient.

Another view of the data would be that long-term survival is possible. The decision regarding continued treatment should be made by the patient (or surrogate) on the basis of the probabilities and likely burdens imposed by the treatment. Given the relatively young age of many of the marrow transplant recipients and the prospects for long-term survival, optimism may be an appropriate view to take of the data. Early identification of patients destined to die despite life support, without compromising the chances of potential survivors, is clearly needed.

In recent work at the Fred Hutchinson Cancer Research Center, we have identified specific predictors of nonsurvival in mechanically ventilated marrow transplant recipients [53]. A nested case–control study of all survivors ($n = 53$) and a cohort of matched nonsurvivors ($n = 106$) were selected from

Table 1. Estimated probability of survival after mechanical ventilation in marrow transplant recipients

Clinical condition during support	Estimated survival[a] (95% CI)
Severe lung injury[b]	1.3% (0.5, 3.0)
Hepatic–renal dysfunction[c]	2.0% (0.1, 4.0)
Hypotension[d]	0.5% (0.06, 1.7)
Severe lung injury and Hepatic–renal dysfunction or Hypotension	0% (0, 2.0)

[a] Survival defined as alive 30 days after extubation and discharge from hospital.
[b] $F_1O_2 > 0.6$ or PEEP > 5 cm H_2O after initial 24 hours of support.
[c] Bilirubin > 4 mg/dl and creatinine > 2 mg/dL.
[d] Requirement of more than four hours of vasopressor support of more than 5 ug/kg/min of dopamine.

all mechanically ventilated marrow transplant recipients (n = 865) from January 1980 to July 1992. Patients mechanically ventilated less than 24 hours after a procedure or after a second marrow transplant were excluded. Survival was defined as alive 30 days after extubation and discharge from hospital.

Survival was statistically associated with younger age, lower APACHE III score, and a shorter time from transplant to intubation, but these measures lacked sensitivity for clinical use. However, there were *no* survivors among an estimated 398 patients who had severe lung injury ($F_1O_2 > 0.6$ or PEEP > 5 cm H_2O) who also required more than four hours of vasopressor support or had sustained combined hepatic and renal insufficiency (table 1). Using these factors, an accurate prediction of death could be made within four days of mechanical ventilation in 90% of nonsurvivors. Over the last five years of the review, there was a statistically significant improvement in survival rates (from 5% to 16%) ($p = 0.008$) that was not explained by a change in patient age, the intubation rate or timing, or the percentage of HLA-nonidentical allogeneic transplants.

These data appear to conflict with those presented by Faber–Langendoen et al., where among 191 marrow recipients requiring mechanical ventilation, age over 40 years and respiratory failure within 90 days of transplant were generally associated with fatality [48]. The bases for the differences in the data are unclear. The Fred Hutchinson Cancer Research Center data were largely confined to several months after transplant, while the University of Minnesota experience included patients several years after transplant. Regional differences in patient care may also contribute. Regardless, the Faber-Langendoen et al. report does not dispute that severe multiorgan failure with mechanical ventilation after marrow transplantation is highly fatal.

We concluded that severe lung injury combined with hemodynamic insta-

241

bility or hepatic–renal insufficiency are sensitive and highly specific predictors of nonsurvival in mechanically ventilated marrow transplant recipients. These overwhelmingly negative results in the largest cohort assembled — nearly equal in size to the total published experience — justify a standard of care for certain mechanically ventilated bone marrow transplant patients that restricts prolonged intensive care. We use such information to counsel patients and families to the expected outcomes of such situations, and will withdraw life-support on the basis of these data.

Noninfectious lung disease

Idiopathic pneumonia syndrome

Incidence and epidemiology. While 40% to 60% of patients develop pneumonia after allogeneic marrow transplantation, no infectious etiology is identified in 30% to 45% of cases with nonbacterial pneumonia [3,54]. These episodes are referred to as idiopathic pneumonias (or idiopathic interstitial pneumonias) to indicate the lack of documented infection and uncertainty regarding the precise etiologies. Several studies have reported the incidence of idiopathic pneumonia to be 11% to 17% after allogeneic marrow transplantation, with a median onset of 39 to 52 days and associated mortality rates of 60% to 70% [3,4,55].

The risk factors associated with idiopathic pneumonia in most studies were transplantation for malignancy and age greater than 20 years. Suggested etiologies for the apparently noninfectious lung injury after marrow transplantation have included chemoirradiation damage [55–57], occult Cytomegalovirus infection [58], and a graft-verus-host reaction [59].

Clinical presentation and course. The usual clinical presentation of 'interstitial pneumonia' is described as diffuse radiographic infiltrates, fever, dyspnea, and hypoxemia [3,4]. However, this presentation also describes viral pneumonia. There is no apparent distinction in presentation for idiopathic processes. The diagnosis of idiopathic pneumonia is one of exclusion of infection. Large studies of pneumonia after marrow transplantation by Meyers et al. [3] and Wingard et al. [4] therefore have required examination of lung tissue either from lung biopsy or autopsy for the diagnosis.

A recent description of the clinical course of idiopathic pneumonia diagnosed by lung biopsy is found in a review of 41 allogeneic marrow transplant recipients with an open lung biopsy between 1983 and 1988 that did not reveal infection [60]. The onset of pneumonia was 11 to 143 days after transplant (mean = 35), and 93% of cases displayed diffuse pulmonary infiltrates. Overall in-hospital mortality was 71% (n = 29). The case-fatality rate was 59% (n = 24). Thirteen patients (32%) died with progressive respiratory failure. The other 11 fatalities (27%) died either with recurrent respiratory failure after initial

242

Table 2. Definition of idiopathic pneumonia syndrome

1) Evidence of widespread alveolar injury:
   • multilobar infiltrates on chest radiograph or computed tomography
   • symptoms and signs of pneumonia
   • evidence of abnormal physiology
and
2) Absence of active lower respiratory tract infection, documented by
   • negative bronchoalveolar lavage, lung biopsy, or autopsy with examination of stains and cultures for bacteria, fungi, and viruses, including cytomegalovirus (CMV) centrifugation culture, cytology for viral inclusions and Pneumocystis carinii, and immunofluorescence monoclonal antibody staining for CMV, respiratory syncytial virus, influenza virus, parainfluenza virus, and adenovirus

improvement ($n = 7$) or due to nonpulmonary causes without resolution of pneumonia ($n = 4$). Infection was a major complication and was present at autopsy in 11 of 16 cases (69%). Six of 12 patients discharged from the hospital died within one year, most commonly with relapse of malignancy.

On the basis of this review of lung biopsies, the overall mortality of idiopathic pneumonia after allogeneic marrow transplantation is high, but less than one third of patients die of progressive respiratory failure, and infection is commonly associated with death despite a previous negative lung biopsy.

Definition of IPS. The results of a recent National Institutes of Health workshop addressed the issues of definitions and diagnostic criteria for idiopathic pneumonia after marrow transplantation [6]. That workshop recommended that the process be referred to as 'idiopathic pneumonia syndrome' (IPS) to reflect the diversity of clinical presentations and likely multifactorial etiologies of the apparently noninfectious diffuse lung injuries. IPS was defined as 'evidence of widespread alveolar injury in the absence of active lower respiratory tract infection' after marrow transplantation (table 2). Bronchoalveolar lavage, rather than lung biopsy, was recommended as the primary diagnostic approach.

At the Fred Hutchinson Cancer Research Center, we sought to determine whether this newly defined IPS occurs with the same incidence or with the same risk factors as described in the past for idiopathic pneumonia. Ready access to minimally invasive and highly sensitive diagnostic techniques (such as bronchoalveolar lavage and centrifugation viral culture) may have increased the recognition (and thus the reported incidence) of lung injury [61]. In addition, it is probable that the spectrum of lung injury in marrow recipients has changed over time, with modification in infection prophylaxis, methods and intensity of cytoreduction, and immune suppression.

Among 1165 consecutive marrow recipients from 1988 to 1991, IPS was documented in 85 marrow recipients by bronchoalveolar lavage ($n = 68$), open lung biopsy ($n = 3$), or autopsy ($n = 14$). The incidence estimate for IPS within 120 days of transplantation was 7.7%. Median time to onset was 21 days (mean 34 ± 30). Similar to previous studies, hospital mortality was 79%. Fifty-three transplant recipients (62%) died with progressive respiratory failure. IPS resolved in 22 patients (26%), and 18 (21%) survived to discharge. Mechanical ventilation was required by 59 marrow recipients (69%) within a median of two days of onset of infiltrates, and two (3%) of these patients survived to discharge. Pulmonary infection (predominantly fungal) was noted in 7 of 25 (28%) marrow recipients who had an autopsy. Potential risk factors for IPS were assessed in univariate and multivariate logistic regression analyses. Although the difference in incidence was not significantly different between autologous (5.7%) and allogeneic marrow recipients (7.6%), risks were identified only for the latter, namely, malignancy other than leukemia and grade 4 graft-versus-host disease. No factors were associated with recovery.

Based on this recent study, the incidence of IPS appears lower, the onset earlier, and the risk factors changed from those previously reported for idiopathic pneumonia. The major risks appear to be regimen-related toxicity and multiorgan dysfunction associated with alloreactive processes.

Pulmonary hemorrhage

Epidemiology, clinical presentation, and course. Robbins et al. described a syndrome of diffuse pulmonary infiltrates, fever, hypoxemia, thrombocytopenia, and renal insufficiency occurring within the first few weeks after autologous marrow transplantation for solid tumors [62]. The hallmark of the syndrome was progressively bloodier return from bronchoalveolar lavage (BAL) and the absence of infection in the lungs. This diffuse alveolar hemorrhage (DAH) syndrome was associated with a very high mortality — over 90%. DAH appeared unrelated to the platelet count, but correlated with increased requirements for platelet transfusion.

Initially seen in 29% of the patients at the University of Nebraska, the incidence of the syndrome declined significantly, to less than 7%, presumably due to alterations in either patient selection or transplant conditioning regimens. Among marrow recipients with lymphoma at the Memorial Sloan Kettering Cancer Center, the reported incidence was 8% [63]. All centers reporting the syndrome note mortality rates over 67%.

Recent European studies of alveolar hemorrhage suggest that the finding of blood in BAL fluid may not represent a specific syndrome. DeLassence et al. reported that among a cohort of 194 immunosuppressed patients undergoing bronchoalveolar lavage, detection of alveolar bleeding by the presence of alveolar siderophages did not correlate with specific lung pathology, presence of infection, or clinical outcome [64]. Siderophages did correlate with uremia, thrombocytopenia, coagulopathies, and a long history of tobacco smoking. This quantitative measure of alveolar bleeding circumvents the subjective nature of recognizing 'progressively bloodier' BAL. The correlations support a contention that alveolar blood is a *sign* of disease, and not a specific diagnostic category. Spanish investigators noted that there was poor correlation between the presence of blood in the lungs at autopsy and BAL results during life in patients after allogeneic marrow transplant or hematological malignancy, further questioning the specificity of the BAL findings as representing a specific syndrome [65].

Pathogenesis and pathology. All cases of DAH that have come to autopsy have demonstrated diffuse alveolar damage, alveolar desquamation, and hyaline membrane formation, typical of ARDS. Because the incidence of the syndrome tended to correlate with the recovery of circulating granulocytes in affected patients, the Nebraska investigators proposed that neutrophilic inflammation played a pathogenic role [66]. Supporting this contention, visual evidence of airway inflammation (ascertained by a bronchitis index) before transplant was associated with the syndrome.

The timing and pathology of the syndrome suggest that chemoradiation injury to multiple organs is central. It remains unclear whether the hemorrhage is a key element to the pathogenesis and outcome, or merely an expected consequence of diffuse lung injury in the presence of a coagulopathy.

Treatment. There are no controlled studies of the treatment of DAH. Retrospective data from Nebraska and anecdotal reports of four cases from Stanford suggest that high-dose corticosteroids may improve the survival rates [67,68]. Doses of methylprednisolone ranging from greater than 30 mg/day to 1 gram/day have been associated with survival. Metcalf et al. reported mortality rates improved from more than 90% to 67% with the routine addition of corticosteroids in the treatment plan [67]. Clouding the interpretation of this finding was the simultaneous declining incidence of the syndrome at the authors' center, suggesting that unidentified factors influencing the course and severity of the disease may have been altered as well.

Airflow obstruction and bronchiolitis

Epidemiology. Several centers report that 6% to 10% of allogeneic marrow recipients develop chronic airflow obstruction. Most of these cases are among long-term survivors with chronic GVHD. Schultz et al. recently reported a higher incidence in children transplanted at the center in Vancouver, Canada [69]. It is unclear whether this represents a regional difference or an age-related effect.

In 70% of the reported cases, the histology of the lungs was obliterative bronchiolitis [7]. The obliterative bronchiolitis lesions in the lungs of marrow transplantation recipients are occasionally, but not invariably, accompanied by interstitial infiltrates of mononuclear cells. However, interstitial fibrosis and bronchitis, without obliteration, have also been noted among patients with airflow obstructive physiology. Recently, airflow obstruction with obliterative bronchiolitis has been reported in two patients after autologous marrow transplantation [9]. On the basis of these findings, new onset airflow obstruction is

245

the hallmark of this problem, not the presence of obliterative bronchiolitic lesions.

Pathogenesis. The etiology of obliterative bronchiolitis after marrow transplantation is unknown. Those causes recognized in otherwise normal hosts, such as recurrent aspiration, viral infection with influenza, adenovirus or measles, and bacterial or mycoplasma infection, have not been found consistently in marrow recipients with obliterative bronchiolitis. Immunological mechanisms inducing bronchial epithelial injury are suggested by the strong association between chronic GVHD and the development of obliterative bronchiolitis [7,8,70]. Factors associated with the increased risk of GVHD, such as increasing age and HLA-nonidentical marrow grafts, are not independent risk factors for the development of obliterative bronchiolitis. The lung epithelium may be the target of immune mediated injury in chronic GVHD through the expression of Ia antigens and subsequent activation of donor cytotoxic T cells. The reported association with the administration of methotrexate also raises the possibility of direct drug-related injury to the pulmonary bronchial epithelium [8]. Also, there is a higher incidence of decreased levels of IgG among patients with obliterative bronchiolitis than that seen in other marrow recipients [70]. This hypogammaglobulinemia may be a manifestation of the immunological lesion responsible for the airway disease or merely may be related to the presence of chronic GVHD [71].

Airflow obstruction is occasionally seen within 100 days of transplant. Histology is available for fewer of these cases, and the defect is possibly related to airway infection. This early presentation is often associated with acute GVHD.

Clinical presentation and course of disease. Typical manifestations of airflow obstruction due to obliterative bronchiolitis after marrow transplantation are insidious progression of tachypnea, dyspnea on exertion, and dry, nonproductive cough. Fever is not common [35]. Physical findings may be minimal. Scattered expiratory wheezing and occasionally diffuse inspiratory crackles may be heard, but chest auscultation is sometimes normal. The chest radiograph is commonly interpreted as normal; however, recent studies reveal that almost all affected children have typical abnormalities noted on high-resolution chest CT scans [72].

The diagnosis of airflow obstruction is made among marrow transplantation recipients by routine pulmonary function testing When the presentation is more than 150 days after marrow transplantation, evidence of chronic GVHD is usually present, although the condition may occur at any time after transplantation.

The syndrome is often progressive and results in death due to respiratory failure. A more rapid onset and faster rate of progression is associated with worse outcome [35]. Control of chronic GVHD with increased immunosuppression may achieve stabilization of the airway disease. Patients with gradual declines in airflow tend to have more benign courses. Marrow recipients with the onset of airflow obstruction beyond 150 days after transplantation tend to have a more gradual decline in lung function. Airflow may stabilize in 50% of these patients. Reversal of the obstruction is reported in only 8% of cases [7].

Treatment. There are no prospective studies of the treatment of new onset airflow obstruction after marrow transplantation. Obstructive airflow in the presence of chronic GVHD is managed primarily by controlling the GVHD with increased immunosuppression. Airflow obstruction has improved in some patients with increased immunosuppression [73]. Experience with obliterative bronchiolitis among the recipients of heart–lung transplant suggests that the addition of azathioprine (1.0–1.5 mg/kg/day) to cyclosporine may be effective in arresting the decline in airflow in these patients [74]. In addition, aerosolized bronchodilator treatment for symptomatic patients is appropriate. Early and aggressive antibiotic treatment for any potential lower respiratory infection should be initiated. Prophylactic trimethaprim-sulfamethoxazole (or other form of anti-Pneumocystis prevention) should be continued for the duration of immune suppression. Routine intravenous replacement of immunoglobulin for those with low class or subclass levels is usual [75].

Similar immunosuppressive management is recommended for airflow obstruction that develops early in the transplant course in the absence of chronic GVHD. Evaluation for possible airway infection by respiratory viruses or fungus should be undertaken in rapidly developing obstruction, especially in the presence of acute GVHD.

Early recognition and treatment may improve outcome. Therefore, routine spirometry after marrow transplantation among patients with chronic GVHD is encouraged to detect the insidious onset of this process.

Diagnostic approaches

Bronchoscopy

Fiberoptic bronchoscopy with bronchoalveolar lavage (BAL) is the procedure of choice to evaluate diffuse infiltrates after marrow transplantation (table 3). Rapid virological and microbiological detection methods permit sensitive and specific detection of viral as well as bacterial and Pneumocystis carinii infections. Fluorescent antibody staining with monclonals has increased sensitivity over cytology alone [76]. Rapid centrifugation (shell vial) culture appears to be an even more sensitive method of detecting viral infection [77]. PCR detection of viral nucleic acids may further increase the sensitive of detection.

BAL is safe in marrow transplantation recipients and may be performed in profoundly thrombocytopenic patients with little risk of bleeding or infection,

Table 3. Routine laboratory evaluation of bronchoalveolar lavage specimens in marrow and stem cell transplant recipients

---

Pathology[a]
  Wright–Giemsa stain
  Papanicolaou stain
  Silver stain
  Modified Jimenez stain (or other suitable for detecting Legionella)

Consider in exceptional setting: Monoclonal fluorescent antibody stain for Pneumocystis

Microbiology
  Stains:
    Gram
    Wet mount KOH or calcofluor white
    Modified acid-fast
    Fluorescent antibody stain for Legionella
  Culture:
    Bacterial (aerobic), semiquantitative method
    Fungal
    Legionella (chocolate yeast extract)
    Acid fast

Virology
  Fluorescent antibody stains:[b]
    CMV
    HSV
    RSV, parainfluenza and influenza viruses pooled antibodies[c,d]
  Culture (rapid centrifugation technique preferred):[e]
    CMV
    HSV
    Adenovirus
    RSV, parainfluenza and influenza viruses (in appropriate clinical setting)

---

[a] Studies usually reviewed by a pathologist.
[b] Studies may be performed in a virology or pathology laboratory.
[c] Separate studies for each virus should be performed if the study with pooled antibodies is positive.
[d] Fluorescent antibody stains may be supplemented or replaced by enzyme-immunoassays (EIAs) as available.
[e] If accessible. Culture may be replaced with fluorescent antibody stains or EIAs alone if culture facilities are unavailable.

even when performed via the transnasal route [78]. Although BAL can document the presence of viral and bacterial infection, negative results do not exclude the presence of fungal infection nor confirm the diagnosis of idiopathic pneumonia. The use of additional invasive procedures must be individualized on the basis of the likelihood of undiagnosed treatable infection. The yield in Pneumocystis carinii infection is unclear; however, we have never confirmed the presence of the organism by any other means after BAL failed to detect an infection. Transbronchial lung biopsy does not appear to improve the diagnostic yield in marrow recipients with diffuse infiltrates [79], is not specific for idiopathic processes [80,81], and may be unsafe in thrombocytopenic patients.

Most reports note that thoracotomy may be undertaken with acceptable morbidity and mortality, even in severely immunosuppressed patients, as long as the platelet count is adequate (usually >50,000/mm^3) [82–84]. Open lung biopsy has the highest probability of rendering a specific diagnosis of the procedures available and had been the mainstay of diagnosis for diffuse pulmonary infiltrates prior to the advent of rapid and sensitive virological diagnostic techniques applied to bronchoscopy specimens.

The morbidity of lung biopsy may be diminished in the hands of a surgeon who is skilled in the use of a thoracoscope. Thorascopically directed biopsy permits diagnostic tissue to be obtained without a formal thoracotomy incision. In most patients, the postoperative recovery is faster with less incisional pain [85,86]. Access to thorascopic lung biopsy has increased our willingness to subject marrow transplant recipients to surgery. One limitation to the procedure is the requirement for bilateral bronchial intubation to permit deflation of the involved lung. Patients with little pulmonary reserve or severe bilateral disease may tolerate this procedure poorly.

Thorascopic lung biopsy also has a role in the diagnosis and management of focal lung lesions, especially those close to the pleural surface. Surgical resection of a focal fungal lesion may be curative while also diagnostic. Caution must be exercised, however, in discounting fungal disease on the basis of a negative open lung biopsy. Despite the relatively large tissue specimen that can be sampled, the diagnosis may not be evident in the pathological examination. Invasive filamentous fungi, by their focal nature and accompanying large degree of tissue infarction and hemorrhage, may not be seen in as many as 20% of cases in which they are present. Therefore, it is difficult to withdraw or withhold empirical antifungal therapy in the neutropenic patient despite "negative" results.

Conclusions

The number of transplant procedures continues to increase as the indications expand and the sources of donor stem cells enlarge. More patients are at risk for complications and require supportive care. To a large extent, support for these patients is similar to that for others receiving intensive induction chemotherapy regimens. Distinctions include the severe degree of immune suppression, the predictable rate and pattern of reconstitution of immunity that follows transplantation, and the presence of GVH reactions among allogeneic recipients.

Increasingly, we are able to predict with more precision patients at risk for complications. Among the tools are pulmonary function tests, both before and after transplantation. In addition, the prognosis for patients with respiratory failure is clearer. The dilemma of identifying those patients who will not survive is being unravelled.

Diagnostic and treatment procedures clearly can be undertaken in these patients with acceptable risks. Bronchoalveolar lavage and thorascopic lung biopsy yield results in patients previously thought to be at high risk for such procedures. Further analyses will continue to define situations where these modalities produce the highest yields, as well as the limitations of such approaches.

References

1. Afessa B, Tefferi A, Hoagland HC, Letendre L, Peters SG. Outcome of recipients of bone marrow transplants who require intensive-care unit support. Mayo Clin Proc 67:117–122, 1992.
2. O'Quin T, Moravec C. The critically ill bone marrow transplant patient. Semin Oncol Nursing 4:25–30, 1988.
3. Meyers JD, Flournoy N, Thomas ED. Nonbacterial pneumonia after allogeneic marrow transplantation: a review of ten years' experience. Rev Infect Dis 4:1119–1132, 1982.
4. Weiner RS, Bortin MM, Gale RP, et al. Interstitial pneumonitis after bone marrow transplantation: assessment of risk factors. Ann Intern Med 104:168–175, 1986.
5. Ljungman P. Cytomegalovirus pneumonia: presentation, diagnosis and treatment. Semin Respir Infect, in press.
6. Clark JG, Hansen JA, Hertz MI, Parkman R, Jensen L, Peavy H. NHLBI Workshop Summary: Idiopathic pneumonia syndrome following bone marrow transplantation. Am Rev Respir Dis 147:1601–1606, 1992.
7. Chan CK, Hyland RH, Hutchen MA, et al. Small-airways disease in recipients of allogeneic bone marrow transplants. Medicine 66:327–340, 1987.
8. Clark JC, Schwartz DA, Flournoy N, Sullivan KM, Crawford SW, Thomas ED. Risk factors for airflow obstruction in recipients of bone marrow transplants. Ann Intern Med 107:648–656, 1987.
9. Paz HL, Crilley P, Patchefsky A, Schiffman RL, Brodsky I. Bronchiolitis obliterans after autologous bone marrow transplantation. Chest 101:775–778, 1992.
10. Meyers JD. Infection in bone marrow transplant recipients. Am J Med 81(Suppl 1A):27–38, 1986.
11. van der Meer JWM, Guiot HFL, van den Broek PJ, van Furth R. Infections in bone marrow transplant recipients. Semin Hematol 21:123–140, 1984.
12. Hansen F. Hematopoietic growth and inhibitory factors in treatment of malignancy. A review. Acta Oncol 34:453–468, 1995.
13. Dickout WJ, Chan CK, Hyland RH, et al. Prevention of acute pulmonary edema after bone marrow transplantation. Chest 92:303–309, 1987.
14. Crawford SW, Hackman RC, Clark JG. Open lung biopsy diagnosis of diffuse pulmonary infiltrates after marrow transplantation. Chest 94:949–953, 1988.
15. Goodrich JM, Bowden RA, Fisher L, Keller C, Schoch G, Meyers JD. Ganciclovir prophylaxis to prevent cytomegalovirus disease after allogeneic marrow transplant. Ann Intern Med 118:173–178, 1993.
16. Schmidt GM, Horak DA, Niland JC, Duncan SR, Forman SJ, Zaia JA. A randomized, controlled trial of prophylactic ganciclovir for cytomegalovirus pulmonary infection in recipients of allogeneic bone marrow transplantation. N Engl J Med 324:1005–1011, 1991.
17. Winston D, Ho W, Bartoni K, et al. Ganciclovir prophylaxis of cytomegalovirus infection and disease in allogeneic bone marrow transplant recipients. Ann Intern Med 118:179–184, 1993.
18. Ljungman P, Biron P, Bosi A, Cahn JY, Goldstone AH, Gorin NC, Link H, Messina C,

Michallet M, Richard C. Cytomegalovirus interstitial pneumonia in autologous bone marrow transplant recipients. Infectious Disease Working Party of the European Group for Bone Marrow Transplantation. Bone Marrow Transplant 13:209–212, 1994.

19. McWhinney PH, Kibbler CC, Hamon MD, Smith OP, Gandhi L, Berger LA, Walesby RK, Hoffbrand AV, Prentice HG. Progress in the diagnosis and management of aspergillosis in bone marrow transplantation: 13 years' experience. Clin Infect Dis 17:397–404, 1993.

20. Kantrow SP, Hackman RC, Boeckh M, Myerson D, Crawford SW. Idiopathic pneumonia syndrome after bone marrow transplantation. Am Rev Respir Dis 149:A1030, 1994.

21. Carlson K, Backlund L, Smedmyr B, Oberg G, Simonsson B. Pulmonary function and complications subsequent to autologous bone marrow transplantation. Bone Marrow Transplant 14:805–811, 1994.

22. Ghalie R, Szidon JP, Thompson L, Nawas YN, Dolce A, Kaizer H. Evaluation of pulmonary complications after bone marrow transplantation: the role of pretransplant pulmonary function tests. Bone Marrow Transplant 10:359–365, 1992.

23. Crawford SW, Fisher L. Predictive value of pulmonary function tests before marrow transplantation. Chest 101:1257–1264, 1992.

24. Springmeyer SC, Flournoy N, Sullivan KM, Storb R, Thomas ED. Pulmonary function changes in long-term survivors of allogeneic marrow transplantation. In Recent Advances in Bone Marrow Transplantation. New York: Alan R. Liss, Inc., 1983, pp. 343–353.

25. Springmeyer SC, Silvestri RC, Flournoy N, Kosanke W, Peterson DL, Huseby JS, Hudson LD, Storb R, Thomas ED. Pulmonary function of marrow transplant patients: I. Effects of marrow infusion, acute graft-versus-host-disease, and interstitial pneumonitis. Exp Hematol 12:805–810, 1984.

26. Sutedja TG, Apperley JF, Hughes JMB, Aber VR, Kennedy HG, Nunn P, Jones L, Hopper L, Goldman JM. Pulmonary function after bone marrow transplantation for chronic myeloid leukaemia. Thorax 43:163–169, 1988.

27. Tait RC, Burnett AK, Robertson AG, McNee S, Riyami BMS, Carter R, Stevenson RD. Subclinical pulmonary function defects following autologous and allogeneic bone marrow transplantation: relationship to total body irradiation and graft-versus-host disease. Int J Radiat Oncol Biol Phys 20:1219–1227, 1991.

28. Prince DS, Wingard JR, Saral R, Santos GW, Wise RA. Longitudinal changes in pulmonary function following bone marrow transplantation. Chest 96:301–306, 1989.

29. Link H, Reinhard U, Blaurock M, Ostendorf P. Lung function changes after allogeneic bone marrow transplantation. Thorax 41:508–512, 1986.

30. Sorensen PG, Ernst P, Panduro J, Moller J. Reduced lung function in leukemia patients undergoing bone marrow transplantation. Scand J Haematol 32:253–257, 1984.

31. Depledge MH, Barrett A, Powles RL. Lung function after bone marrow grafting. Int J Radiat Oncol Biol Phys 9:145–151.

32. Hatta Y, Baba M, Aizawa S, Itoh T, Shida M, Yamazaki T, Sawada U, Ohshima T, Sawada S, Horie T. Changes of pulmonary function in patients treated with bone marrow transplantation after total body irradiation. Acta Haematol Jpn 53:923–930, 1990.

33. Badier M, Guillot C, Delpierre S, Vanuxem P, Blaise D, Maraninchi D. Pulmonary function changes 100 days and one year after bone marrow transplantation. Bone Marrow Transplant 12:457–461, 1993.

34. Jenney ME, Faragher EB, Jones PH, Woodcock A. Lung function and exercise in survivors of childhood leukemia. Med Pediat Oncol 24:222–230, 1995.

35. Clark JG, Crawford SW, Madtes DK, Sullivan KM. Obstructive lung disease after allogeneic marrow transplantation: clinical presentation and course. Ann Intern Med 111:368–376, 1989.

36. Crawford SW, Pepe M, Lin D, Benedetti F, Deeg HJ. Abnormalities of pulmonary function tests after marrow transplantation predict non-relapse mortality. Am J Respir Crit Care Med 152:690–695, 1995.

37. Caterall JR, McCabe RE, Brooks, Remington JS. Open lung biopsy in patients with Hodgkin's disease and pulmonary infiltrates. Am Rev Respir Dis 139:1274–1279, 1989.

38. McCabe RE, Brooks, Caterall JR, Remington JS. Open lung biopsy in patients with non-Hodgkin's lymphoma and pulmonary infiltrates. Chest 96:319–324, 1989.
39. Roth B, Crawford SW. Fungal infection with non-Hodgkin's lymphoma. Chest 98:512, 1990.
40. Navari RM, Sullivan KM, Springmeyer SC, Siegel MS, Meyers JD, Buckner CD, Sanders JE, Stewart PS, Clift RA, Fefer A, Storb R, Thomas ED. Mycobacterial infections in marrow transplant patients. Transplantation 36:509–513, 1983.
41. Crawford SW, Schwartz DA, Petersen FB, Clark JG. Mechanical ventilation after marrow transplantation: risk factors and clinical outcome. Am Rev Respir Dis 137:682–687, 1988.
42. Schneiderman LJ, Arras JD. Counseling patients to counsel physicians on future care in the event of patient incompetence. Ann Intern Med 102:693–698, 1985.
43. Hauser MJ, Tabak J, Baier H. Survival of patients with cancer in a medical intensive care unit. Arch Intern Med 142:527–529, 1982.
44. Snow RM, Miller WC, Rice DL, Ali MK. Respiratory failure in cancer patients. J Am Med Assoc 241:2039–2042, 1979.
45. Ewer MS, Ali MK, Atta MS, Morice RC, Balakrishnan PV. Outcome of lung cancer patients requiring mechanical ventilation for pulmonary failure. J Am Med Assoc 256:3364–3366, 1986.
46. Schuster DP, Marion JM. Precedents for meaningful recovery during treatment in a medical intensive care unit: outcome in patients with hematological malignancy. Am J Med 75:402–408, 1983.
47. Peters SG, Meadows JA, Gracey DR. Outcome of respiratory failure in hematological malignancy. Chest 94:99–102, 1988.
48. Faber-Langendoen K, Caplan AL, McGlave PB. Survival of adult bone marrow transplant patients receiving mechanical ventilation: a case for restricted use. Bone Marrow Transplant 12:501–507, 1993.
49. Crawford SW, Schwartz DA, Petersen FB, Clark JG. Mechanical ventilation after marrow transplantation: risk factors and clinical outcome. Am Rev Respir Dis 137:682–687, 1988.
50. Crawford SW, Petersen FB. Long-term survival from respiratory failure after marrow transplantation. Am Rev Respir Dis 145:510–514, 1992.
51. Denardo SJ, Oye RK, Bellamy PE. Efficacy of intensive care for bone marrow transplant patients with respiratory failure. Crit Care Med 17:4–6, 1989.
52. Bojko T, Notterman DA, Greenwald BM, DeBruin WJ, Magid MS, Godwin T. Acute hypoxemic respiratory failure in children following bone marrow transplantation: an outcome and pathologic study. Crit Care Med 23:755–759, 1995.
53. Rosenfeld GD, Crawford SW. Withdrawing life support from mechanically ventilated recipients of bone marrow transplants: a case for evidence-based guidelines. Annals Intern Med 125:625–633, 1996.
54. Krowka MJ, Rosenow EC, Hoagland HC. Pulmonary complications of bone marrow transplantation. Chest 87:237–246, 1985.
55. Wingard JR, Mellits ED, Sostrin MB, Chen DY-H, Burns WH, Santos GW, Vriesendorp HM, Beschorner WE, Saral R. Interstitial pneumonia after allogeneic marrow transplantation. Medicine (Baltimore) 67:175–186, 1988.
56. Hackman RC. Lower respiratory tract. In Sale GE, Shulman HM (eds), The Pathology of Bone Marrow Transplantation. New York: Masson, 1984, pp. 156–170.
57. Appelbaum FR, Sullivan KM, Buckner CD, et al. Treatment of malignant lymphoma in 100 patients with chemotherapy, total body irradiation, and marrow transplantation. J Clin Oncol 5:1340–1347, 1987.
58. Sloane JP, Depledge MH, Powles RL, Morgenstern GR, Trickey BS, Dady PJ. Histopathology of the lung after bone marrow transplantation. J Clin Pathol 36:546–554, 1983.
59. Beschorner WE, Saral R, Hutchin GM, et al. Lymphocytic bronchitis associated with graft-versus-host disease in recipients of bone marrow transplants. N Engl J Med 299:1030–1036, 1978.

60. Crawford SW, Hackman RC. Clinical course of idiopathic pneumonia after marrow transplantation. Am Rev Respir Dis 147:1393–1400, 1993.
61. Crawford SW, Bowden RA, Hackman RC, Gleaves CA, Meyers JD, Clark JG. Rapid detection of cytomegalovirus pulmonary infection by bronchoalveolar lavage and centrifugation culture. Ann Intern Med 108:180–185, 1988.
62. Robbins RA, Linder J, Stahl MG, Thompson AB, Haire W, Kessinger A, Armitage JO, Arneson M, Woods G, Vaughn WP, Rennard SI. Diffuse alveolar hemorrhage in autologous bone marrow transplant recipients. Am J Med 87:511–518, 1989.
63. Jules-Elysee K, Stover DE, Yahalom J, White DA, Gulati SC. Pulmonary complications in lymphoma patients treated with high-dose therapy and autologous bone marrow transplantation. Am Rev Respir Dis 146:485–491, 1992.
64. DeLassence A, Fleury-Feith J, Escudier E, Beaune J, Bernaudin J-E, Cordonnier C. Alveolar hemorrhage: diagnostic criteria and results in 194 immunocompromised hosts. Am J Respir Crit Care Med 151:151–163, 1995.
65. Agusti C, Ramirez J, Picado C, Xaubet A, Carreras E, Ballester E, Torres A, Battochia C, Rodriquez-Roisin R. Diffuse alveolar hemorrhage in allogeneic bone marrow transplantation: a post-mortem study. Am J Respir Crit Care Med 151:1006–1006, 1995.
66. Sisson JH, Thompson AB, Anderson JR, Robbins RA, Spurzem JR, Spence PR, Reed EC, Armitage JO, Vose JM, Arneson MA, Vaughn WP, Rennard SI. Airway inflammation predicts diffuse alveolar hemorrhage during bone marrow transplantation in patients with Hodgkin's disease. Am Rev Respir Dis 146:439–443, 1992.
67. Metcalf JP, Rennard SI, Reed EC, Haire WD, Sisson JH, Walter T, Robbins RA. Corticosteroids as adjunctive therapy for diffuse alveolar hemorrhage associated with bone marrow transplantation. Am J Med 96:327–334, 1994.
68. Chao NJ, Duncan SR, Long GD, Horning SJ, Blume KG. Corticosteroid therapy for diffuse alveolar hemorrhage in autologous bone marrow transplant recipients. Ann Intern Med 114:145–146, 1991.
69. Schultz KR, Green GJ, Wensley D, Sargent MA, Magee JF, Spinelli JJ, Pritchard S, Davis JH, Rogers PC, Chan KW, et al. Obstructive lung disease in children after allogeneic bone marrow transplantation. Blood 84:3212–3220, 1994.
70. Holland HK, Wingard JR, Beschorner WE, Saral R, Santos GW. Bronchiolitis obliterans in bone marrow transplantation and its relationship to chronic graft-v-host disease and low serum IgG. Blood 72:621–627, 1988.
71. Witherspoon RP, Storb R, Ochs HD, et al. Recovery of antibody production in human allogeneic marrow graft recipients: influence of time post-transplantation, presence or absence of chronic graft-versus-host disease, and antithymocyte globulin treatment. Blood 58:360–368, 1981.
72. Sargent MA, Cairns RA, Murdoch MJ, Nadel HR, Wensley D, Schultz KR. Obstructive lung disease in children after allogeneic bone marrow transplantation: evaluation with high-resolution CT. Am J Roentgen 164:693–696, 1995.
73. Urbanski SJ, Kossakowska AE, Curtis J, et al. Idiopathic small airways pathology in patients with graft-versus-host disease following allogeneic bone marrow transplantation. Am J Surg Pathol 11:965–971, 1987.
74. Glanville AR, Baldwin JC, Burke CM, et al. Obliterative bronchiolitis after heart–lung transplantation: apparent arrest by augmented immunosuppression. Ann Intern Med 107:300–304, 1987.
75. Sullivan KM, Kopecky KJ, Jocom J, Fisher L, Buckner CD, Meyers JD, Counts GW, Bowden RA, Petersen FB, Witherspoon RP, Budinger MD, Schwartz RS, Appelbaum FR, Clift RA, Hansen JA, Sanders JE, Thomas ED, Storb R. Immunomodulatory and antimicrobial efficacy of intravenous immunoglobulin in bone marrow transplantation. N Engl J Med 323:705–712, 1990.
76. Crawford SW, Bowden RA, Hackman RC, Gleaves CA, Meyers JD, Clark JG. Rapid detection of cytomegalovirus pulmonary infection by bronchoalveolar lavage and centrifugation culture. Ann Intern Med 108:180–185, 1988.

77. Emanuel D, Peppard J, Stover D, Gold J, Armstrong D, Hammerling U. Rapid immunodiagnosis of cytomegalovirus pneumonia by bronchoalveolar lavage using human and murine monoclonal antibodies. Ann Intern Med 104:476–481, 1986.

78. Weiss SM. Hert RC, Gianola FJ, Clark JG, Crawford SW. Complications of fiberoptic bronchoscopy in thrombocytopenic patients. Chest 104:1025–1028, 1993.

79. Springmeyer SC, Silvestri RC, Sale GE, et al. The role of transbronchial biopsy for the diagnosis of diffuse pneumonias in immunocompromised marrow transplant recipients. Am Rev Respir Dis 126:763–765, 1982.

80. Nishio JN, Lynch JP. Fiberoptic bronchoscopy in the immunocompromised host: the significance of a 'nonspecific' transbronchial biopsy. Am Rev Respir Dis 121:307–312, 1980.

81. Haponik EF, Summer WR, Terry PB, Wang KP. Clinical decision making with transbronchial lung biopsies: the value of nonspecific histologic examination. Am Rev Respir Dis 125:524–529, 1982.

82. Ellis ME, Spence D, Bouchama A, Antonius J, Bazarbashi M, Khougeer F, De Vol EB. Open lung biopsy provides a higher and more specific diagnostic yield compared to bronchoalveolar lavage in immunocompromised patients. Scand J Infect Dis 27:157–162, 1995.

83. Bove P, Ranger W, Pursel S, Glover J, Bove K, Bendick P. Evaluation of outcome following open lung biopsy. Am Surg 60:564–570, 1994.

84. Wagner JD, Stahler C, Knox S, Brinton M, Knecht B. Clinical utility of open lung biopsy for undiagnosed pulmonary infiltrates. Am J Surg 164:104–108, 1992.

85. Rubin JW. Video-assisted thoracic surgery: the approach of choice for selected diagnosis and therapy. Eur J Cardio-Thorac Surg 8:431–435, 1993.

86. Schwarz CD, Lenglinger F, Eckmayr J, Schauer N, Hartl P, Mayer KH. VATS (video-assisted thoracic surgery) of undefined pulmonary nodules. Preoperative evaluation of video-endoscopic resectability. Chest 106:1570–1574, 1994.

12. Recombinant cytokines and hematopoietic growth factors in allogeneic and autologous bone marrow transplantation

Hillard M. Lazarus

In 1991, the United States Food and Drug Administration (FDA) approved the commercial sale of colony-stimulating factors for use in cancer patients receiving cytotoxic agent therapy. Many of the data to support the licensure of the two approved agents, G-CSF (filgrastim) and GM-CSF (sargramostim), were derived from studies conducted in patients undergoing bone marrow transplantation. This group of agents, predominantly glycoproteins in nature, controls the survival, proliferation, and differentiation of the various hematopoietic blood cell lineages [1–5]. These agents act on both early and committed progenitors and enhance the function of mature effector cells [6].

Since early clinical trials, the use of colony-stimulating factors has nearly revolutionized the conduct of bone marrow and hematopoietic progenitor cell transplantation. While the numbers of patients undergoing allogeneic and autologous bone marrow transplantation has increased dramatically in recent years, this treatment modality still carries a significant risk of infection and bleeding and generally requires a prolonged hospitalization [7,8]. Use of hematopoietic growth factors has significantly reduced the morbidity, mortality, and financial cost of this procedure. This chapter will address the use of recombinant hematopoietic growth factors after infusion of hematopoietic stem cells in patients undergoing high-dose cytotoxic therapy for cancer. The clinical experience with cytokines that are commercially available for clinical use and those which remain investigational will be described (table 1).

Rationale for exogenous cytokine administration

While high doses of cytotoxic therapy may be associated with improved anti-tumor activity, morbidity and mortality are increased. This increased risk, to a large extent, reflects the injury to host hematopoietic tissue induced by cytotoxic therapy. The fact that successful marrow engraftment and expansion take place after intensive chemoradiation therapy implies that either the regulatory systems controlling hematopoiesis are resistant to myeloabative therapy or the infused marrow itself contains populations of cells able to provide the necessary proliferative signals for hematopoietic tissue [9,10]. Despite infusion

Jane N. Winter (ed.) BLOOD STEM CELL TRANSPLANTATION. 1997. Kluwer Academic Publishers. ISBN 0-7923-4260-7. All rights reserved.

Table 1. Cytokines approved for clinical use and those evaluated clinically but not yet approved

---

Approved
   Erythropoietin
   Granulocyte-macrophage colony-stimulating factor (GM-
      CSF)
   Granulocyte-colony-stimulating factor (G-CSF)
   Interleukin-2 (IL-2)

Under clinical investigation
   Macrophage colony-stimulating factor (M-CSF)
   Interleukin-1 (IL-1)
   Interleukin-3 (IL-3)
   Interleukin-6 (IL-6)
   Interleukin-11 (IL-11)
   Pixy 321 (fusion molecule IL-3/GM-CSF)
   Stem cell factor (SCF)
   Thrombopoietin

---

of large numbers of autologous or allogeneic hematopoietic progenitor cells, prolonged and profound neutropenia and thrombocytopenia ensue. The patient is placed at great danger due to an increased probability of life-threatening infection and/or hemorrhage. The neutropenia and thrombo-cytopenia that result are strong stimuli that release endogenous cytokines to correct these problems. Yamasaki et al. [11] described growth-supporting, growth-promoting, and growth-factor-like activities in the plasma, which peak 7 to 21 days after marrow transplant. Subsequently, other investigators re-ported the detection of substances that could be characterized as G-CSF and IL-3. These factors and possibly others, detectable only in extremely low concentrations in the blood in steady state, often increase dramatically during the period of cytopenias associated with hematopoietic stem cell transplanta-tion [11–18]. However, concentrations of endogenous colony-stimulating fac-tors such as G-CSF may be detectable in only 35% of patients during transplantation, and serum concentrations of endogenous GM-CSF do not appear to be elevated in the plasma during post-transplant neutropenia [17]. In these patients, exogenous administration of cytokines may be important for enhancing recovery of peripheral blood counts.

In representative series that did not utilize exogenous colony-stimulating factors, the median time to recover peripheral blood neutrophils more than 500/μL after marrow infusion was approximately 21 days or longer; the median time to independence from platelet transfusions, depending on the high-dose chemotherapy regimen and source of hematopoietic stem cell infusion, may be 60 days or more [19–21]. It was postulated, and subsequently demonstrated, that the use of exogenous colony-stimulating factors after administration of high-dose chemoradiation therapy and infusion of hematopoietic stem cells will speed marrow regeneration. Hematopoiesis provides for both ongoing replenishment of blood progenitors, which in many cases have a short half-life, and differentiation of target cells to correct cytopenias. This complex process is tightly regulated by a series of hematopoietic growth factors that only now is beginning to be understood. The colony-stimulating factors induce proliferation of progenitor cells, activate mature blood cells, and initiate production of other hematopoietic growth factors [6,22–26].

Cytokines in engraftment failure

In preclinical trials, GM-CSF and G-CSF were effective in augmenting antibacterial and antifungal host activity [27–29]. Colony-stimulating factor trials conducted in nonhuman primates demonstrated enhanced levels of circulating neutrophils and monocytes and increased regeneration of cellular elements following bone marrow transplantation [30,31]. For a variety of reasons, significant delays in marrow recovery or rejection of allogeneic donor cells may occur in up to 10% of patients undergoing bone marrow transplantation (table 2) [9,32,33]. Despite second marrow infusions, these patients often die of marrow aplasia [34].

Phase I trials to assess the efficacy of colony-stimulating factors after transplant were successful as compassionate treatment in patients who had failed to engraft (table 3). These trials used recombinant GM-CSF over various dose ranges. Nemunaitis et al. [35] demonstrated the utility of this approach after either autologous or allogeneic marrow infusion, although patients who received autologous bone marrow purged in vitro did not respond. Brandwein and associates [36] showed that GM-CSF had a transient effect on marrow recovery after failed or delayed engraftment in some autotransplant patients. Sierra et al. [37] showed benefit in both allogeneic and autologous marrow transplantation, but only in secondary rather than primary engraftment failure in the former situation. Ippoliti and coworkers [38] noted that GM-CSF was effective in most patients, even in lower doses. Vose et al. [39] and Klingemann et al. [40] also demonstrated the benefit of recombinant GM-CSF after marrow infusion. Several years later, Weisdorf et al. [34] compared

Table 2. Causes of primary and secondary engraftment failure after bone marrow transplantation

---

Disease relapse
Posttransplant infections, i.e., cytomegalovirus, herpesvirus 6, etc.
Low numbers of infused hematopoietic stem cells
Cytotoxic effect of ex vivo marrow purging
Extensive chemotherapy prior to marrow collection
Graft-versus-host disease
Drug toxicity, i.e., ganciclovir, trimethoprim-sulfamethoxazole
Use of matched unrelated or mismatched related allogeneic donor marrow
T-cell-depletion of donor marrow

Table 3. Summary of phase I and II trials using GM-CSF for engraftment failures during autologous and allogeneic bone marrow transplantation

Ref.	No. pts	Marrow type	Diseases	Type/ glycosylated	No. pts with enhanced neutrophil recovery[a]	Severe toxicities	Comment
35	22	Auto[c]	AML, ALL, CML, HD, NHL, NBL, Brst, Ovary	Mammalian/ yes	12/22	One pericardial effusion	Ineffective in purged marrow transplants
36	6	Auto	HD, NHL, AML	E.coli/no	3/6	None	Effect transient
35	15	Allo	AML, ALL, CML, HD, NHL, AA	Mammalian/ yes	7/15	None	No increase or exacerbation of GVHD
37	7	Auto	AML, ALL	E.coli/no	3/7	None	—
37	18	Allo	AML, ALL, CML, MM, MF	E.coli/no	11/18	'Capillary leak'	Effective only in secondary rather than primary failure
38	26[b]	Auto	Leuk, NHL, HD, MM, Brst, Ovary	E.coli/no	22/26	'Capillary leak', increased bilirubin	Low doses effective in some patients
39	12	Auto	NHL, HD	Mammalian/ yes	10/12	None	Decreased infections compared to historic controls
40	3	Allo	ALL, CML	E.coli/no	2/3	None	No increase in GVHD
40	6	Auto	AML, NHL, MM, NBL, Brst	E.coli/no	4/6	None	—

[a] Refers to those patients who had a significant increase compared to baseline, i.e., at least doubling neutrophil count and >500/μL.
[b] Peripheral blood progenitor cells given alone or in conjunction with marrow in nine patients.
[c] includes one syngeneic bone marrow transplant patient.
Abbreviations: Auto, autologous; allo, allogeneic; AML, acute myeloid leukemia; ALL, acute lymphoblastic leukemia; CML, chronic myeloid leukemia; NHL, non-Hodgkin's lymphoma; HD, Hodgkin's disease; AA, aplastic anemia; NBL, neuroblastoma; Brst, breast cancer; Ovary, ovarian cancer; MF, myelofibrosis; Leuk, leukemia, not otherwise specified.

G-CSF versus the sequence GM-CSF/G-CSF in patients who failed to engraft (see Combination Trials below). They noted no advantage for the sequential combination compared to the use of the single agent GM-CSF.

Cytokine graft-enhancement phase I and II trials

Phase I protocols were begun that systematically examined the toxic effects (and possible benefit) of colony-stimulating factors after transplantation. The initial trials examined patient groups who received autologous bone marrow (table 4); trials of hematopoietic growth factors in patients undergoing allogeneic bone marrow transplantation, in general, were not addressed until later (table 5). This decision related, in part, to the fact that cytokines may indirectly activate T cells through the release of tumor necrosis factor and IL-1 by macrophages that can be stimulated by GM-CSF, for example, causing or exacerbating graft-versus-host disease (GVHD) [41–49]. Furthermore, allogeneic transplantation is thought to be a more complex undertaking [42].

The phase I and II studies undertaken in patients undergoing autologous bone marrow transplantation are summarized in table 4. These studies, in general, employed recombinant GM-CSF (mammalian, yeast, and E. coli preparations) and G-CSF (E. coli), although one study used purified urine, subsequently demonstrated to be M-CSF [50–52]. These early studies were important, since they identified many toxic effects of the preparations and suggested efficacy, setting the stage for definitive phase III trials. Not only were the molecule (GM-CSF versus G-CSF) and dose determined to be important but also the route of administration and type of preparation (nonglycosylated, i.e., E. coli, versus glycosylated, i.e., mammalian or yeast) were found to be important variables. In the latter situation, glycosylation was thought to have effects on the biologic activities and toxicity of the various preparations, i.e., not all forms of one class of cytokine are equivalent in toxicity and efficacy [53–55].

Table 4 lists the results of 15 phase I–II studies using either GM-CSF ($N = 10$) or G-CSF ($N = 5$). Trials included 25 or fewer patients, usually subjects who had hematologic malignancies. In all trials, the use of a recombinant cytokine was associated with a significantly faster neutrophil recovery when compared to historic control data [56–71]. Toxicities identified in the lower and intermediate dose ranges were similar to those side effects observed in patients who received chemotherapy in conventional doses, including fever, nausea, vomiting, diarrhea, abdominal pain, and abnormalities in serum tests of liver function. At the highest doses examined, some patients developed a syndrome referred to as the 'capillary-leak' syndrome, characterized by dyspnea, and pleural, pericardial, or peritoneal effusions; some patients developed renal failure and hypotension. These effects appeared to be rapidly reversible with cessation of the colony-stimulating factor therapy or with dose

Table 4. Summary of phase I and II trials for GM-CSF and G-CSF after autologous bone marrow transplantation

Ref.	No. pts	Diseases	Cytokine	Type/glycosylated	Enhance neutrophil recovery[a]	Significant Toxicities	Comment
56	19	Breast, Melanoma	GM-CSF	Mammalian/yes	Yes	'Capillary leak' at higher doses[b]	Decreased renal & hepatic toxicity of chemotherapy
57	25	NHL, ALL	GM-CSF	Yeast/yes	Yes	One deep venous thrombosis	GM-CSF effective when infused with adequate # in vitro purged progenitors
58	10	NBL, ALL, Sarcomas	GM-CSF	Yeast/yes	Yes	None	None
59	18	HD	GM-CSF	E.coli/no	Yes	None	None
60	15	NHL, HD, ALL, Germ cell	G-CSF	E.coli/no	Yes	None	Significantly fewer days parenteral antibiotics
61, 62	15	NHL, ALL	GM-CSF	Yeast/yes	Yes	None	Enhanced platelet recovery
63	26	NHL	GM-CSF	Yeast/yes	Yes	Generalized edema & serositis common	Persistent fever common
64	20	ALL, NHL	GM-CSF	E.coli/no	Yes	None	GM-CSF speeded neutrophil recovery with purged marrow
65	12	HD	GM-CSF	Yeast/yes (N = 9) E.coli/no (N = 3)	Yes	Rare	Both yeast & E. coli forms active
66	16	NHL	GM-CSF	Mammalian/yes	Yes	None	Marked drop in neutrophils when GM-CSF stopped
67	10	HD	GM-CSF	Mammalian/yes	Yes	Severe dyspnea in 3 patients	24-hr infusion had faster marrow recovery but more toxicity
68	16	AML, ALL, CML, AA, NHL, MDS	G-CSF	Mammalian/yes	Yes	None	Doses up to 20µg/kg/day given
69	14	NHL	G-CSF	E.coli/no	no[c]	None	G-CSF given after infusion of in vitro purged bone marrow
70	22	Breast	G-CSF	E.coli/no	Yes	None	Acceleration of neutrophil recovery after purged marrow infusion
71	23	NHL	G-CSF	E.coli/no	Yes	None	Acceleration of neutrophil recovery after purged infusion marrow

[a] Refers to statistically significant change compared to historic control population.
[b] 'Capillary leak' included generalized edema, pleural and pericardial effusions.
[c] Comparison made with previously published report from another group.
Abbreviations: Breast, breast cancer; melanoma, malignant melanoma; ALL, acute lymphoblastic leukemia; NHL, non-Hodgkin's lymphoma; AML, acute myeloid leukemia; CML, chronic myeloid leukemia; AA, aplastic anemia; MDS, myelodysplastic syndrome; CLL, chronic lymphocytic leukemia; NBL, neuroblastoma.

Table 5. Summary of phase I and II trials using GM-CSF and G-CSF during allogeneic bone marrow transplantation

Ref.	No. pts	Diseases	Cytokine & dose	Type/glycosylated	Enhance neutrophil recovery[a]	Severe toxicities	Comment	Exacerbate GVHD
68	46	AML, ALL, CML, AA, NHL, MDS	G-CSF	Mammalian/yes	Yes	None	Up to 20µg/kg per day given	No
72	47	AML, ALL, CML, CLL, NHL, HD, MDS, MM	GM-CSF	Mammalian/yes	Yes[b]	'Capillary leak'	Optimal dose 250µg/m²	No
73	34	AML, ALL, CML, AA, NHL	G-CSF	E.coli/no	Yes[b]	None	Up to 800µg/m²/day given	No
74	10	ALL, NHL	GM-CSF	E.coli/no	Yes	'Capillary leak' in 2 pts	3 pts with grade IV GVHD	Yes
75, 76, 77	40	AML, ALL, CML, AA, NHL, MDS	GM-CSF	Mammalian/yes	Yes	One pericardial effusion	All unrelated donors	No
78	50	AML, ALL, CML, AA, NHL	G-CSF	E.coli/no	Yes[b]	None	20 matched unrelated donors used	No
79	13	AML, ALL, CML, MM, MDS, HD	G-CSF	Mammalian/yes	Yes	None	MTX GVHD prophylaxis blunted recovery	No
80	2[c]	AML, ALL	G-CSF	Mammalian/yes	Yes	None	Decrease in WBC count when stopped	No

[a] Refers to statistically significant change compared to historic control population.
[b] Benefit noted only when methotrexate was not given as part of the graft-versus-host disease prophylaxis regimen.
[c] Includes one syngeneic bone marrow transplant patient.

Abbreviations: ALL, acute lymphoblastic leukemia; NHL, non-Hodgkin's lymphoma; AML, actue myeloid leukemia; CML, chronic myeloid leukemia; AA, aplastic anemia; MDS, myelodysplastic syndrome; CLL, chronic lymphocytic leukemia; MM, multiple myeloma; MTX, methotrexate.

reduction. Some patients experienced a marked reduction in bacterial infections and less renal, hepatic, and pulmonary dysfunction often attributed to the high-dose chemotherapy preparative regimen, although these findings were not primary study objectives. These findings are thought to reflect early eradication of bacterial infection, attributed to more rapid neutrophil recovery. Several studies reported an earlier hospital discharge when compared to historic control subjects. In addition, 3 of 4 studies illustrated the potential benefit of G-CSF and GM-CSF therapy in enhancing neutrophil recovery when given after infusion of bone marrow purged in vitro [57,69–71]. Furthermore, tumor growth was not detected despite the fact that malignant cells may express receptors for colony-stimulating factors. Except for one study by Nemunaitis et al. [61], in which GM-CSF appeared to reduce the time to platelet transfusion independence from 38 to 29 days, neither G-CSF nor GM-CSF appeared to speed the recovery of platelet counts.

Similar results were noted in eight studies presented in table 5 for those patients undergoing allogeneic bone marrow transplantation followed by administration of recombinant hematopoietic growth factors GM-CSF ($N = 3$) and G-CSF ($N = 5$) [68,72–80]. As noted for the autologous bone marrow transplantation efforts, all studies noted enhancement of neutrophil recovery in most patients who received either of these colony-stimulating factors. On the other hand, patients given methotrexate as part of the regimen as prophylaxis against GVHD did not benefit to the extent seen without use of this cytotoxic agent. Of additional note, more patients appeared to developed pericardial effusions or other evidence of the 'capillary leak' syndrome than was observed in the autotransplant setting. Finally, Atkinson and associates [74], who transplanted ten leukemia and lymphoma patients using HLA-identical sibling donor marrow followed by recombinant GM-CSF (E. coli) reported that 6 of 8 evaluable patients experienced grade II–IV GVHD (three grade IV), a significantly higher percentage than the historic control group. The authors raised a cautionary note concerning the use of GM-CSF after allogeneic transplant. On the other hand, both Nemunaitis et al. [75–77] and Schriber et al. [78] studied unrelated matched allogeneic donors and did not observe this problem. As observed in the phase I–II autologous bone marrow transplant setting, neither G-CSF nor GM-CSF appeared to accelerate recovery of platelet counts.

Phase III randomized trials in autologous and allogeneic bone marrow transplantation

To assess the true benefit of recombinant hematopoietic growth factor therapy in the course of bone marrow transplantation, single-agent phase I–II studies must be confirmed by phase III clinical investigations. Such trials are necessary because there are many factors that can influence hematologic recovery in the course of transplantation (table 6).

262

Table 6. Factors influencing hematologic recovery after allogeneic and autologous bone marrow infusion

---

Allogeneic bone marrow
    Pretransplant conditioning regimen
    Histocompatibility of patient and donor
    Hematopoietic stem cell dose
    Posttransplant GVHD prophylaxis therapy
    Use of and type of hematopoietic growth factors
      posttransplant

Autologous bone marrow
    Previous myelosuppressive treatment
    Pretransplant treatment regimen
    Hematopoietic stem cell dose
    Use of in vitro purging
    Use of and type of hematopoietic growth factors
      posttransplant

Table 7 illustrates the results from 14 phase III randomized trials conducted in autologous bone marrow transplant patients to whom either GM-CSF ($N = 9$) or G-CSF ($N = 5$) were administered [81–95]. In all studies, the CSF chosen was shown to be effective in statistically shortening the time to neutrophil recovery after transplant. Less agreement was noted among trials with respect to lowering the prevalence of infection, reducing the duration of antibacterial agent therapy, and shortening the length of hospital stay. Similar data were noted for patients undergoing phase III placebo-controlled trials using GM-CSF ($N = 3$) or G-CSF ($N = 4$) after allogeneic bone marrow infusion (table 8) [91,93,95–101]. Neutrophil recovery was enhanced in all but one trial [93]. As was the case in the autotransplant setting, the studies did not provide a consistent statement regarding the benefit of recombinant colony-stimulating factors with respect to the prevalence of infection, the duration of antibacterial agent therapy, and length of hospital stay. In no instance was the use of the recombinant hematopoietic growth factors G-CSF and GM-CSF thought to stimulate growth of malignancy.

In these studies (table 7 and 8), the use of G-CSF and GM-CSF did not appear to enhance the recovery of peripheral blood platelet counts. On the other hand, the dramatic acceleration of neutrophil recovery in the course of transplantation improved the therapeutic index of the procedure by lowering early mortality; G-CSF and GM-CSF therapy became an integral part of the posttransplant treatment supportive care approach.

Erythropoietin

Erythropoietin, identified more than 40 years ago, was the first cytokine to be cloned and studied in clinical trials. Erythropoietin is a circulating, polypeptide hormone that induces and maintains the proliferation and differentiation

Table 7. Summary of randomized, vehicle-controlled phase III trials[a] for GM-CSF and G-CSF after autologous bone marrow transplantation

Ref.	No. pts	Diseases	Cytokine	Type/glycosylated	Enhance neutrophil recovery[b]	Fewer infections[b]	Fewer antibacterials day[b]	Shorter hospital stay[b]
81, 82	128	NHL, HD, ALL	GM-CSF	Yeast/yes	Yes	No	Yes	Yes
83	69[c]	NHL, HD	GM-CSF	E.coli/no	Yes	Yes	NA	No
84	24	HD	GM-CSF	E.coli/no	Yes	No	NA	Yes
85	91	NHL	GM-CSF	E.coli/no	Yes	No	No	Yes
86	79	NHL, ALL	GM-CSF	E.coli/no	Yes	Yes	No	No
87	231	AML, ALL, NHL, solid tumors	GM-CSF	E.coli/no	Yes	No	No	Yes
88	58	NHL, HD	GM-CSF	E.coli/no	Yes	No	No	No
89	53	ALL, AA, other	GM-CSF	E.coli/no	Yes	No	NA	Yes[d]
90	25	NHL, HD	G-CSF	E.coli/no	Yes	NA	No	No
91	245	NHL, HD, MM, ALL, solid tumors	G-CSF	Mammalian/yes	Yes	Yes	Yes	Yes
92	43	NHL, HD	G-CSF	E.coli/no	Yes	No	No	No
93	20	ALL	G-CSF	E.coli/no	Yes	NA	No	Yes
94	16	NBL	GM-CSF	E.coli/no	Yes	No	Yes	Yes
95[a]	102	NHL, HD, MM, ALL, solid tumors	G-CSF	Mammalian/yes	Yes	No	No	Yes

[a] Phase II single-blind randomized parallel group vehicle-controlled dose ranging study.

[b] Refers to statistically significant change.

[c] 39 patients received autologous peripheral blood progenitor cells alone or in conjunction with autologous bone marrow.

[d] Significantly shorter stay in laminar-air-flow isolation.

Abbreviations: NHL, non-Hodgkin's lymphoma; HD, Hodgkin's disease; ALL, acute lymphoblastic leukemia; MM, multiple myeloma; NBL, neuroblastoma; NA, not available.

Table 8. Summary of randomized, vehicle-controlled phase III trials[a] for GM-CSF and G-CSF after allogeneic bone marrow transplantation

Ref.	No. pts	Diseases	Cytokine	Type/glycosylated	Enhance neutrophil recovery[b]	Fewer infections[b]	Fewer antibacterials days[b]	Shorter hospital stay[b]
91	70	NHL, HD, MM, ALL, solid tumors	G-CSF	Mammalian/yes	Yes	Yes	Yes	Yes
93	24	ALL	G-CSF	E.coli/no	No	NA	Yes	No
95[a]	19	NHL, HD, MM, ALL, solid tumors	G-CSF	Mammalian/yes	Yes	No	No	Yes
96[c]	57	AML, ALL, CML, CLL, AA, MDS, MM	GM-CSF	Mammalian/yes	Yes	Yes	No	No
97, 98, 99	40	AML, ALL, CML	GM-CSF	Mammalian/yes	Yes	No	Worse[d]	No
100	84	AML, CML, NHL, MDS, MM	GM-CSF	Mammalian/yes	Yes	NA	NA	NA
101	70	AML, ALL, CML, AA, NHL	G-CSF	E.coli/no	Yes	No	No	No

[a] Phase II single-blind randomized parallel group vehicle-controlled dose ranging study.
[b] Refers to statistically significant change.
[c] Use of T-depleted allogeneic marrow.
[d] GM-CSF group had more antibiotic days.

Abbreviations: ALL, acute lymphoblastic leukemia; NHL, non-Hodgkin's lymphoma; AML, acute myeloid leukemia; CML, chronic myeloid leukemia; AA, aplastic anemia; MDS, myelodysplastic syndrome; CLL, chronic lymphocytic leukemia; MM, multiple myeloma; NA, not available.

265

of bone marrow erythroid progenitor cells into mature red blood cells [102–108]. Recombinant erythropoientin has an extremely restricted range of target activity; in vivo, it affects erythroid precursors predominantly [107–109]. In addition, erythropoietin has a 25% amino acid sequence homology with thrombopoietin, and the respective receptors are quite similar, leading to positive effects on megakaryocytopoiesis in vitro [110–115].

Anemia arising during bone marrow transplantation is multifactorial and includes inadequate red cell production, blood loss due to organ damage, thrombocytopenia, or infection, and hemolysis due to ABO incompatibility, microangiopathy from drugs such as cyclosporine, or idiopathic hemolytic–uremic syndrome [116]. Circulating blood and bone marrow erythroid progenitor cells may require at least 12 months to recover after marrow transplantation [117–119].

Endogenous erythropoietin

A number of allogeneic and autologous bone marrow transplant studies have consistently but paradoxically demonstrated that endogenous serum erythropoietin concentrations increase dramatically within days of completing chemotherapy or chemoradiation therapy [120–131]. It is unclear whether this increase reflects a direct effect of cytotoxic drugs on erythropoietin production by the kidney, a reduction in erythropoietin utilization due to the depletion of erythropoietin receptor-bearing erythroid precursors from bone marrow, or a reduction in renal blood flow; there is no stored reserve for erythropoietin in humans, and enhanced release cannot be a factor [122,123,132]. Erythropoietin concentrations fall to inappropriately low levels during the period of anticipated marrow recovery [118,126,128,131,133–136].

Exogenous erythropoietin administration

Several small retrospective studies and case reports evaluated recombinant erythropoietin therapy after bone marrow transplant [137–146]. Several showed an increase in reticulocyte count and decreased red cell transfusion requirement in some patients, but such findings were not uniform among these studies. Vannucchi and associates [141] prospectively compared exogenous erythropoietin therapy in 21 marrow transplant patients. The eight erythropoietin-treated patients experienced earlier red cell engraftment and required fewer red cell transfusions than the 11-patient control group. Finally, Steegmann and colleagues [142] reported similar results in a prospective, randomized trial; 13 erythropoietin-treated patients exhibited earlier appearance of reticulocytes and required fewer red cell transfusions than a control group of 11 patients. The response to erythropoietin after transplantation may occur even in the setting of adequate or high endogenous erythropoietin

266

serum concentrations, suggesting that high doses of exogenously administered erythropoietin may stimulate production of erythroid precursors and overcome circulating inhibitors if these are present [146].

In the most comprehensive investigation conducted to date, Link and associates [147] reported the use of recombinant erythropoietin in a prospective, randomized, placebo-controlled trial. They administered recombinant erythropoietin 150 units/kg/day as a continuous 24-hour intravenous infusion until patients demonstrated independence from erythrocyte transfusions for seven consecutive days with stable hemoglobin level ≥ 9.0 g/dL. Treatment was given to 106 allogeneic BMT pts, while 109 received placebo. Fifty-seven autologous transplant patients were given recombinant erythropoietin, and 57 received placebo. No major differences were noted in side effects or complications between the erythropoietin-treated and placebo-treated subjects. In the allogeneic group, independence from red blood cell transfusions occured a median of 19 days postreinfusion in the erythropoietin-treated group and 27 days in the placebo group ($p < 0.003$). Acute graft-versus-host disease, major ABO incompatibility, patient age of more than 35 years, and hemorrhage significantly increased the number of transfusions. At 20 days after transplant, however, erythropoietin significantly reduced the number of erythrocyte transfusions in these high-risk groups. Furthermore, for the whole study period, erythropoietin reduced the mean red cell transfusion requirement in grade 3 and 4 graft-versus-host disease from 18.4 ± 8.6 to 8.5 ± 6.8 units ($p = 0.05$). In the autologous transplant group, there were no differences in the time to independence from red blood cell transfusions and the regeneration of reticulocytes between the erythopoietin- and placebo-treated groups. Recombinant erythropoietin therapy had no effect on thrombopoiesis.

Other uses of erythropoietin in marrow transplantation

York and associates [148] reported the use of recombinant erythropoietin in the treatment of allogeneic bone marrow donors before marrow procurement. Therapy consisted of erythropoietin 100 units/kg subcutaneously daily in advance of the transplant along with oral iron supplementation. Erythropoietin was given at a dose of 150 units/kg thrice weekly until 2 to 3 weeks after marrow harvest. This approach was well tolerated and may be advantageous for children donors, in whom autologous blood donation is not routine.

Macrophage colony-stimulating factor (M-CSF)

One of the earliest bone marrow transplant studies using cytokines to enhance marrow recovery involved 37 allogeneic and 14 autologous bone marrow transplant patients given colony-stimulating factors purified from human urine [50]. These investigators reported enhancement of neutrophil recovery and, in the allograft setting, observed no increase in graft-versus-host disease when compared to historic controls [149]. Later, this cytokine was demonstrated to be M-CSF [51–52].

At high concentrations, M-CSF is a potent stimulator of human monocyte progenitor cells and, at clinically achievable concentrations, significantly increases monocyte cytotoxicity [150–151]. Fungal infection is a major cause of morbidity and mortality in patients undergoing marrow transplantation [152–155]. Neutrophils are not detected early after transplant and, when present, exhibit defects in killing microorganisms which may not be corrected by cytokine stimulation [26,156,157]. As a result, macrophages play an important role in host defense after bone marrow transplantation; without neutrophils, tissue macrophages may be the sole defense against infection. This speculation is supported indirectly by data demonstrating that after bone marrow transplantation endogenous M-CSF levels are elevated in early stage fungemia [158]. After allogeneic bone marrow transplant, macrophages are of host origin and repopulate various organs as hepatic Kupffer cells, alveolar macrophages, pleural and peritoneal macrophages, and microglial cells of the brain [159,160]. Three studies reported that exogenous administration of the cytokines GM-CSF and M-CSF after bone marrow transplantation will activate monocyte function [161,163]. On the other hand, Fabian et al. [164] noted no deficit in functional activity of monocytes after bone marrow transplant, and IL-3, GM-CSF, and M-CSF did not modulate functional activity of these cells. Nonetheless, as a result of such observations, M-CSF has been studied as an antifungal agent in bone marrow transplant patients who have established invasive fungal infections. In one of the few published trials using recombinant M-CSF, Nemunaitis and coworkers [165,166] reported a phase I study in which recombinant M-CSF 100–2000/µg/m²/d was given to 46 patients who had hematologic disorders or had undergone bone marrow transplantation. Toxic effects appeared to be limited to thrombocytopenia, affecting 11 patients, which responded to dose reduction. Although neutrophil, monocyte, and lymphocyte numbers were not increased, this therapy appeared effective, since 12 patients remained alive and free of fungal infection. When compared with historic controls who received antifungal agents only, a statistically significant survival advantage at two years was noted (27% versus 5%, $p = 0.027$) for treated patients. Similar results were noted in a randomized, phase II preliminary communication by Schiller et al. [167]. Despite these positive findings, at this time M-CSF's role in bone marrow transplantation is unclear.

Platelet recovery after marrow transplantation

Platelet transfusions, a necessary element of supportive care for preventing the spontaneous hemorrhagic manifestations of severe thrombocytopenia, may be associated with significant febrile and allergic reactions, transfusion-associated bacterial sepsis, and other infections [168,169]. Furthermore, plate-

Table 9. Cytokines that have the potential to enhance platelet recovery after bone marrow transplantation

---

Interleukin-1 (IL-1)
Interleukin-3 (IL-3)
Interleukin-6 (IL-6)
Interleukin-11 (IL-11)
Pixy 321 (fusion molecule IL-3/GM-CSF)
Stem cell factor (SCF)
Thrombopoietin

---

let concentrates stored in vitro prior to infusion may contain cytokines that paradoxically can further suppress hematopoiesis [170,171]. The cost and inconvenience of frequent platelet transfusions are not insignificant clinical and health-care problems. The use of thrombopoietic growth factors could have a major impact on decreasing platelet transfusions in this setting [172,173]. The colony-stimulating factors presently in use in clinical practice appear to have little effect on platelet recovery, and prolonged periods of thrombocytopenia after bone marrow transplantation remain a significant obstacle [4,174–176]. A number of agents that have recently entered clinical trials have the potential for stimulating platelet generation. Agents that may enhance platelet recovery are shown in table 9.

Interleukin-6 (IL-6)

IL-6 is a pleiotropic cytokine that has been demonstrated in preclinical studies to promote maturation of megakaryocytes, increases in size and ploidy, and thrombopoiesis [177,186]. In a dog model, rhIL-6 treatment was associated with production of larger platelets and greater sensitivity of platelets to activation by thrombin, both effects that potentially provide greater hemostatic benefit, especially after myeloablative therapy [187,188].

IL-6 can be given in doses up to $100.0\,\mu g/m^2$ in untreated cancer patients or those given conventional chemotherapy [189,190]. In a preliminary communication, Colwill and coworkers [191] administered IL-6 $1.0–2.5\,mg/m^2$/day after high-dose etoposide and melphalan and ABMT to six relapsed or refractory Hodgkin's disease patients. They observed a lower median number of platelet transfusions than in historical controls treated with GM-CSF, but no enhancement of platelet recovery. Lazarus and colleagues [192] treated 20 breast cancer patients in a phase I fashion using IL-6 $0.3–3.0\,\mu g/m^2$ after high-dose chemotherapy and autologous bone marrow reinfusion. Reversible hepatic toxicity manifested by hyperbilirubinemia was the dose-limiting toxicity at $3.0\,\mu g/m^2$, which established $1.0\,\mu g/m^2$ to be the phase II dose. Zone 3 microsteatosis was noted to be the histopathologic lesion, a finding also reported by Weber et al. [190] when higher doses of IL-6 were given after conventional chemotherapy. Other toxic effects included fever, chills, rash, nausea, vomiting, and diarrhea; these effects may reflect the complex interactions of IL-6 with endogenous IL-1 and tumor necrosis factor during the transplant [193–198]. Neutrophil recovery was quite slow, similar to those transplant patients who did not receive hematopoietic growth factors and consistent with the fact that IL-6 has little effect on myelopoiesis and neutrophil recovery after bone marrow transplantation [185,199,200]. Six of 20 treated patients had more rapid recovery of platelet counts. IL-6 currently is in phase II trials in combination with GM-CSF and other agents (see below).

Interleukin-3 (IL-3)

IL-3, also known as multi-CSF, appears to regulate both early and intermediate stages of hematopoiesis and promotes proliferation and differentiation of myeloid, erythroid, and megakaryocyte cell lineages [201–208]. IL-3 appears to act on bone marrow cells earlier in development than later-acting cytokines such as GM-CSF and G-CSF, which predominantly affect mature marrow elements. The functional activities of neutrophils and monocytes also are enhanced, to some extent, after exposure to IL-3 [209–211]. Studies using bone marrow in vitro have shown that recombinant human IL-3, alone or in combination with sequentially or simultaneously administered GM-CSF, stimulates the growth of both myeloid and megakaryocyte lineage cells [212–214]. Similarly, in preclinical animal models, recombinant human IL-3 alone or together with other cytokines has been shown to stimulate both neutrophil and platelet production [215–219]. In an effort to improve upon current methods, this agent has been administered prior to bone marrow and peripheral blood progenitor cell collection to quantitatively enhance cellular yield [220–222]. While these efforts were generally unsuccessful, IL-3 has been used effectively alone and in combination (sequentially) in bone marrow failure states and after bone marrow transplantation to enhance marrow recovery [223–227]. In bone marrow failure states, IL-3 therapy resulted in an increase in bone marrow cellularity, reticulocytes (up to fourfold), neutrophils (up to threefold), and platelets (up to 14-fold), although the effect usually was not long-lasting.

Nemunaitis and associates conducted a phase I trial [228] designed to examine the use of IL-3 as a single agent on bone marrow recovery after autologous bone marrow transplantation. Thirty lymphoma patients received IL-3 therapy by vein over two hours at doses of 1–10 μg/kg/day for 21 days after marrow infusion. Toxic effects attributed to IL-3 included malaise, confusion, fever, and headache. The authors did not observe earlier hematopoietic reconstitution compared to a similar cohort of historic controls treated with GM-CSF. These investigators noted no enhancement of either neutrophil or platelet count compared to placebo or GM-CSF (table 10). In a phase I/II study, Fibbe and associates [229] administered nonglycosylated E. coli IL-3 0.25–15.0 μg/kg/day for 14 days to 22 patients who were undergoing autologous bone marrow transplant for lymphoma. Toxic effects, including facial flushing,

270

Table 10. Influence of single agent and combinations of recombinant hematopoietic growth factors on recovery of peripheral blood counts during autologous bone marrow transplantation for lymphoid malignancies

Ref.	Cytokine therapy	Number of patients	Median day neutrophils ≥1000/μL	Median day platelets ≥20,000/μL
82	None	63	33	29
82	GM-CSF	65	26	26
95	G-CSF	49	17	33
228	IL-3	30	24	27
229	IL-3	8	17	19
240	PIXY 321	11	19	17
335	IL-3/GM-CSF (sequential)	37	16	15

Abbreviation: PIXY 321, GM-CSF/IL-3 fusion protein.

headache, and fever, were tolerable at all but the highest dose level. Eight patients who received the 10 μg/kg/day dose attained neutrophil and platelet recovery a median of 17 (range: 11–25) days and 19 days (range: 13–35 days) posttransplant, respectively. Subsequently, Fibbe et al. [230] reported preliminary data from a phase III randomized, placebo-controlled, multicenter trial in which they examined the use of subcutaneously administered E. coli IL-3 10 μg/kg/day after autologous bone marrow transplantation in lymphoma patients. They demonstrated that IL-3 treatment was superior to placebo for neutrophil and platelet recovery and that neutrophil recovery was similar to that observed in other studies using GM-CSF. The fact that platelet recovery appeared to be enhanced and that toxic effects were tolerable led to studies of IL-3 in combination with other cytokines (see below).

PIXY 321 (IL-3/GM-CSF fusion molecule)

PIXY 321 is a recombinant protein that combines both IL-3 and GM-CSF by the use of an amino acid linker protein [231]. This molecule was synthesized to combine the early, rapid-onset action of GM-CSF on committed late neutrophil progenitors with the slower, sustained, late-onset effect of IL-3 on earlier and intermediate progenitors of many lineages [232]. In preclinical animal studies, the activities of IL-3 and GM-CSF were preserved in this hybrid molecule [233]. In in vitro and preclinical studies, PIXY 321 demonstrated at least a tenfold greater specific activity compared to GM-CSF and/or IL-3 [231,234,235]. Williams and coworkers [236] and Mac Vittie et al. [237] treated normal primates with PIXY 321. All animals responded with marked increases (compared to baseline) in neutrophil and platelet counts after 7 to 10 consecutive days of PIXY 321, GM-CSF, IL-3, and GM-CSF plus IL-3 [237]. In irradiated primates (450 cGy total body irradiation), however, only animals

271

given PIXY 321 (50µg/kg/d) experienced significant enhancement of both platelets and neutrophils compared to albumin infusions (control); GM-CSF stimulated acceleration only of neutrophils, while IL-3 therapy stimulated only platelet recovery. While PIXY 321 appears to accelerate both neutrophil and platelet recovery after conventional-dose chemotherapy, few data are available on the use of this agent in bone marrow transplantation [238,239]. Vose and associates [240] reported that PIXY 321 administered after infusion of autologous bone marrow shortened the time to platelet transfusion independence in lymphoid malignancy patients from 26 days (historic controls) to 17 days. PIXY 321 also has been shown to be an effective agent for mobilizing hematopoietic progenitor cells for transplantation from peripheral blood [232,241]. A number of trials exploring the use of this promising agent in bone marrow and peripheral blood progenitor cell transplantation are under way.

Interleukin-1 (IL-1)

Interleukin-1 (IL-1), formerly known as hemopoietic-1, represents two polypeptide cytokines (IL-1α and IL-1β) that have an extremely broad range of biologic functions, including diverse effects on the immunologic and hematopoietic systems [242–249]. IL-1 induces expression of a number of hematopoietic growth factors, including G-CSF, GM-CSF, IL-3, IL-6, and SCF, which enhance survival of early hematopoietic progenitor cells and increase multipotential colony formation. As a single agent in vitro, however, IL-1 has no colony-stimulating activity. IL-1 activates lymphocytes, regulates B-cell differentiation, and protects cells through its activity as a free radical scavenger. In animals, administration of IL-1 has been associated with an increase in peripheral blood red blood cells, neutrophils, lymphocytes, and platelets; furthermore, use of this agent has been associated with prolongation of survival in animals exposed to chemotherapy and total body irradiation, in part by augmenting host antimicrobial defenses and enhancing immunologic function [250–259].

Although on theoretical grounds the use of an early-acting cytokine might be useful, experience using IL-1 after bone marrow transplantation is limited. Nemunaitis and coworkers [260] conducted a phase I dose-escalation trial in 17 acute myeloid leukemia patients in which recombinant human IL-1β (0.01–0.05 µg/kg/day) was administered as a 30-minute intravenous infusion for five days beginning the day of autologous bone marrow reinfusion. Moderate toxicity was noted, since fever, chills, and hypotension occured in nearly all patients; the authors concluded that the 0.05 µg/kg/day dose was the maximum tolerated dose. Compared to 74 historic controls who did not receive colony-stimulating factors after autotransplant, recovery of neutrophil count in excess of 500/µL occured faster (25 versus 34 days), the incidence of infection was reduced (12% versus 28%), and patient survival was improved (30% versus

20%) in the group that received IL-1β (all three variables of statistical significance). Platelet recovery and days of hospitalization did not differ between the two groups.

Another group conducted a phase I study evaluating the use of a 14-day course of IL-1α (0.1–10.0 μg/m²/day) given as a six-hour daily intravenous infusion beginning the day of bone marrow ($N = 7$) or peripheral blood progenitor cell ($N = 7$) infusion [261]. Forty Hodgkin's or non-Hodgkin's lymphoma patients were treated. Toxic effects occured in most patients and included fever, fatigue, severe chills, and hypotension (at 10.0 μg/m²/day); the maximum tolerated dose appeared to be 3.0 μg/m²/day. I patients who received IL-1α 3.0 μg/m²/day, median time to neutrophil count recovery (12 versus 27 days) and hospital discharge (25 versus 37 days) occured statistically earlier when compared to historic controls or to those subjects who received IL-1α at a dose less than 3.0 μg/m²/day. This group also demonstrated enhanced immunologic activation induced by IL-1α therapy, which could provide cytolytic therapy in the posttransplant period and lead to decreasing relapse rates [262].

IL-1 is still under investigation. It is unclear if the moderate clinical toxicities are outweighed by the hematologic and immunologic benefits when used after bone marrow transplantation.

Stem cell factor (SCF)

This cytokine has been referred to as stem cell factor (SCF), mast cell growth factor, steel factor, and c-kit ligand. SCF is a potent cytokine that acts on the earliest and most immature hematopoietic progenitors [263,264]. SCF exhibits pleiotropic effects on hematopoietic progenitor and stem cells and has been synergistic with other cytokines in vitro and in preclinical animal models for bone marrow transplantation [265–268]. SCF has many potential clinical uses, including treatment of bone marrow failure states, ex vivo expansion of hematopoietic progenitor and stem cells for marrow transplantation, gene transfer therapy, or both, and in vivo mobilization of peripheral blood progenitor and hematopoietic stem cells [267–270]. Given as a single agent at low doses to lung cancer patients, SCF appeared to have somewhat limited activity, yet at higher doses caused symptoms including wheezing and shortness of breath associated with mast cell activation [271]. In combination, however, this agent appears to be an extremely potent costimulatory factor that synergistically increases the number and size of many hematopoietic progenitors [269]. Dose-related increases in mobilization of progenitor cells of myeloid, erythroid, and megakaryocyte lineages were noted in breast cancer patients who were given SCF and G-CSF for mobilization [269]. To date, SCF has not been fully tested in the clinical bone marrow transplant setting, but it is likely that it will undergo extensive evaluation in the next few years because of its great potential.

Interleukin-11 (IL-11)

IL-11 is a stromal-derived cytokine that appears to be similar in functional activity to IL-6 [272–274]. In in vitro studies, IL-11 alone and in conjunction with other cytokines stimulates megakaryocyte, erythroid, and myeloid colony growth and stimulates the number of immunoglobulin-secreting B lymphocytes in vitro [272,273,275–277]. In addition, this agent is synergistic with many other cytokines, including G-CSF, IL-3, IL-6, and SCF to produce multilineage colonies [278]. Preclinical animal trials have shown significant activity in increasing the platelet count in mice and nonhuman primates, as well as enhancing platelet recovery in experimental bone marrow transplant systems [279–283]. Furthermore, IL-11 was demonstrated to have effects on both bone marrow stromal elements and the gastrointestinal tract [284,285]. In a study by Du et al. [285], IL-11 treatment led to increased survival of treated animals after cytotoxic drug exposure compared to control animals. IL-11 appeared to provide protection to the small bowel mucosa by promoting rapid recovery of intestinal villi length and increased proliferative activity in the intestinal crypt cells [285].

Although several clinical trials have been initiated to examine the utility of recombinant human IL-11 in bone marrow transplantation, few results are available at this time. Champlin et al. [286] presented preliminary data on platelet recovery in patients who received G-CSF 5 µg/kg per day plus escalating doses of IL-11 beginning after infusion of bone marrow (table 11). Dose-limiting atrial arrhythmias and fluid retention occured at 75 µg/kg/day, leading this group to conclude that in combination with G-CSF the maximum tolerated dose of IL-11 was 50 µg/kg/day. Median day to platelet recovery ≥20,000/µL was 21 days after bone marrow infusion. These results are promising, especially in view of the dual benefit of enhancing platelet count recovery as well as the potential protective effects on the gastrointestinal tract.

Table 11. Representative trials illustrating the influence of recombinant hematopoietic growth factors alone and in combination on recovery of peripheral blood counts in patients undergoing autologous bone marrow transplantation for breast cancer

Cytokine therapy	Number of patients	Median day neutrophils ≥1000/µL	Median day platelets ≥20,000/µL
None	50	36	40
GM-CSF	75	33	32
G-CSF	80	18	30
Concurrent IL-6/GM-CSF (337)	26	16	20
Concurrent IL-11/G-CSF (286)	15	13	21

Interleukin-2 (IL-2)

Interleukin-2 (IL-2) is a prime activator of both T-cell and natural killer-(NK-) cell-based antitumor mechanisms and has been shown to exhibit anti-cancer properties in a variety of human malignancies [287–290]. This cytokine possesses significant toxicities, including fever, chills, rash, diarrhea, nausea, vomiting, hypotension, capillary leak syndrome, and renal, pulmonary, and hepatic dysfunction; these toxic effects resolve with discontinuation of the drug or can be attenuated or prevented by the use of high-dose corticosteroid therapy [290–294].

IL-2 production appears to be deficient after autologous bone marrow transplantation, but exogenous administration can activate the host immune system, facilitating hematopoietic recovery and providing antitumor benefit [295,296]. A number of phase I–II single-institution clinical trials have examined the use of recombinant human IL-2 administered after bone marrow infusion, i.e., 'posttransplantation immunotherapy.' These studies have demonstrated that such treatment is tolerable, appears to enhance immune recovery, and provides antitumor effects in some patients, including those who received T-cell-depleted allogeneic bone marrow [294,297–306]. No phase III trials testing the utility of IL-2 in this setting have been completed, however, and the role of this agent as 'post-transplantation immunotherapy' remains speculative. Since IL-2 appears to be most effective in the setting of minimal residual disease rather than overt disease, and since this agent has significant toxicity when used systemically, a number of trials have used IL-2 as an in vitro purging agent [307–311]. Activated killer cells can be generated by incubating bone marrow with IL-2 prior to marrow infusion, potentially without affecting engraftment [311]. This approach appears to hold promise not only as an antitumor modality but also as a means of eliminating cytomegalovirus (CMV) infection in marrow [312].

Thrombopoietin

After a lengthy search, thrombopoietin, the cytokine predominantly responsible for megakaryocytopoiesis, was identified and cloned [110–113,172–173,313–316]. Initially known as c-mpl ligand, this agent has just entered clinical trials. It is anticipated that recombinant thrombopoietin will dramatically speed platelet recovery and lessen (or possibly eliminate) platelet transfusion requirements. Such an effect will add significantly to supportive care improvements in bone marrow transplantation in a manner analogous to those contributions made by GM-CSF and G-CSF.

Combination cytokine trials

A number of in vitro as well as preclinical animal studies have demonstrated the synergistic effects of various cytokines, such as G-CSF and GM-CSF

[214,317–322]. It has been theorized that in a clinical application, the combination of agents in vivo may be more effective in promoting hematopoietic recovery than either agent alone [323,324]. Hence, a number of combination cytokine trials were undertaken. Table 11 compares several representative trials illustrating the positive influence of using recombinant hematopoietic growth factors in combination to stimulate recovery of peripheral blood counts in patients undergoing autologous bone marrow transplantation for breast cancer.

Erythropoietin in combination with other agents

Erythropoietin and GM-CSF may act synergistically in vitro, with enhancement of megakaryocyte colony formation [325,326]. Rabinowitz and colleagues [327] also demonstrated in vivo that autologous bone marrow transplant patients receiving recombinant GM-CSF therapy had significantly higher endogenous erythropoietin serum concentrations than a comparable control group that did not receive GM-CSF therapy. As a result, Pene et al. [328] conducted a prospective, randomized trial to evaluate the effect of the addition of exogenous recombinant erythropoietin therapy to GM-CSF treatment. Eighteen autologous marrow transplant patients were given both erythropoietin and GM-CSF and were compared to six concurrent controls and 65 historic controls, each given GM-CSF. Although neutrophil recovery (>500/ μL) appeared to occur earlier in the erythropoietin plus GM-CSF group (median 12.5 days after marrow reinfusion versus 18 days for concurrent and 19 days for historic control patients), there was no apparent impact on red cell transfusion requirements, platelet recovery, or duration of hospitalization. Similarly, Chao et al. [329] showed in a prospective, randomized study that the combination of erythropoietin and G-CSF did not influence the total number of red blood cell or platelet units transfused, or the time to recovery of peripheral blood counts. These autotransplant studies, conducted primarily in adults, are at odds with a pediatric allogeneic bone marrow transplant trial conducted by Locatelli and coworkers [330]. In children given G-CSF and erythropoietin after allografting, they noted a significantly shorter neutrophil recovery, fewer infections, fewer febrile days, and more rapid platelet reconstitution and number of platelet transfusions. Thus, as was the case for single-agent erythropoietin therapy, the G-CSF-erythropoietin combination may be effective only in the allogeneic bone marrow transplant setting.

G-CSF and GM-CSF

Since endogenous G-CSF was elevated in the plasma of neutropenic bone marrow transplant patients, Weisdorf et al. [34] postulated that the addition of GM-CSF to G-CSF would provide superior recovery and reduce the morbidity and mortality of delayed engraftment. In a prospective, randomized phase III trial, they treated 47 engraftment failure allogeneic and autologous transplant patients; GM-CSF was given to 23 patients for 14 days versus the sequence of seven days GM-CSF followed by seven days of G-CSF ($N = 24$ patients). Time to neutrophil recovery and erythrocyte transfusion- and platelet transfusion-independence were not statistically different in both groups. Although the 100-day survival was superior in the single-agent GM-CSF group compared to the sequential combination ($p = 0.026$), there does not appear to be an obvious benefit to the sequential combination of G-CSF and GM-CSF in the engraftment failure setting.

IL-3 and GM-CSF

Donohue and coworkers [218] demonstrated in vivo synergism of these cytokines by treating cynomolgus monkeys (who were not given cytotoxic therapy) using the sequence of single-agent IL-3 followed by single-agent GM-CSF. Albin and associates [331] studied progenitor cell recovery after IL-3 or GM-CSF treatment given after infusion of mafosfamide-purged autologous bone marrow. Their data prompted them to postulate that IL-3 and GM-CSF have different mechanisms of action on hematopoietic recovery, and suggested a potential synergistic effect that favored sequential administration of these cytokines after autologous bone marrow transplantation. These data formed the basis for sequential cytokine clinical trials in patients with engraftment failure.

Suttorp et al. [332] reported the case of a boy with chronic myeloid leukemia who developed graft failure after a matched, unrelated allogeneic bone marrow transplant. He recovered autologous marrow function after receiving GM-CSF followed later by two courses of IL-3 therapy. Similarly, Nagler and associates [333] reported the use of continuous infusion IL-3 and GM-CSF $250\,\mu g/m^2$/day in a radiation accident victim given T-depleted sibling mismatched allogeneic bone marrow. Neutrophil engraftment was documented nine days after marrow infusion, and diagnostic marrow examination suggested rapid engraftment. The patient expired, however, 36 days after transplant, due apparently to lung injury from the 1000–2000 cGy total body irradiation, cytomegalovirus pneumonitis, hepatic veno-occlusive disease, and acute graft-versus-host-disease.

A clinical trial was completed by Crump et al. [334] in seven autologous bone marrow transplant patients who had delayed engraftment and were severely pancytopenic despite GM-CSF therapy for 28 days after marrow infusion. Seven hematologic malignancy patients received the combination of IL-3 2–5 μg/kg/day for 21 days followed immediately by GM-CSF 10 μg/kg/day for 7–10 days. This approach produced transient increases in circulating neutrophils and eosinophils, but no effect on platelet or red cell production.

As a result of these sequential study design protocols, Fay and colleagues [335] completed a complex, phase I–II combination study in relapsed lymphoma and Hodgkin's disease patients using IL-3 (2.5–5.0 $\mu g/m^2$/day for 5 to 10 days) followed by recombinant GM-CSF 250 µg/m^2/day commencing immediately after infusion of autologous bone marrow. Compared to historic controls, there was enhanced recovery of both neutrophils >1000/µL (median 16 days) as well as platelets >20,000/µL (median 15 days) (table 10). Several prospective, randomized comparison trials to address this concept in phase III fashion recently have been completed but are not yet analyzed.

IL-6 and GM-CSF

Gonter and colleagues [336] used a nonhuman primate model to demonstrate enhanced marrow recovery after chemotherapy with the combination of IL-6 and either GM-CSF or G-CSF. Given this background, Fay et al. [337] reported in preliminary fashion the results of a phase I–II study involving concurrent use of IL-6 (0.5–2.5 µg/kg/day) and GM-CSF (2.5–5.0 µg/kg/day) in 26 breast cancer patients undergoing autologous bone marrow transplantation. At the higher cytokine doses, toxic effects were significant and included fever, fluid retention, rash, pericardial effusion, and capillary leak syndrome. Median times to neutrophil and platelet recovery were 12 and 20 days, respectively. A phase II trial using this combination recently has been completed, but the results are not yet available.

SCF and G-CSF

SCF has marked in vitro and in vivo synergism with other cytokines [267,268,338–342]. The combination of recombinant rat SCF and recombinant human G-CSF given to normal mice induced a greater than additive increase in blood neutrophil numbers and colony-forming units-spleen (CFU-S) than when either was given as a single agent [340]. Recombinant rat SCF and G-CSF in normal rats resulted in an increase in bone marrow neutrophils yet significantly decreased erythroid and lymphoid elements [338,339]. Finally, not only did the combination of SCF and G-CSF mobilize peripheral blood progenitor cells at a markedly higher rate than G-CSF alone but also engraftment of these cells was faster than G-CSF-mobilized cells [341,343]. Similar intriguing data have been generated in vivo in nonhuman primates fostering new clinical trials [344,345]. In preliminary studies, SCF plus G-CSF increased the yield of peripheral blood progenitor cell collections and decreased the time, by up to four days after transplant, to in vivo platelet recovery to 50,000/µL [270]. It is unclear at present, however, what role this combination of cytokines will play when given in conjunction with bone marrow infusions.

Delayed use of cytokines after transplant

In almost all published trials, recombinant hematopoietic growth factors were initiated immediately after or within one day after the infusion of hematopoietic cells. Several studies, however, systematically examined the effect of delaying administration of recombinant cytokines after bone marrow transplantation. Clark and colleagues [346] evaluated the effects of withholding G-CSF until 7 to 10 days after marrow reinfusion in 19 patients undergoing autologous bone marrow transplantation for Hodgkin's disease, non-Hodgkin's lymphoma, multiple myeloma, acute lymphoblastic leukemia, and several solid tumor types. Time to recovery of neutrophils was faster and duration of hospitalization was shorter than in 18 historic subjects who underwent transplant without the use of G-CSF; there were no differences in febrile days and duration of antibiotic therapy. The overall costs of the procedure were a median £750 less per transplant even if the expense of G-CSF therapy was included. Vey et al. [347] compared 49 Hodgkin's disease, non-Hodgkin's lymphoma, breast cancer, and ovarian cancer patients given G-CSF either one or six days after marrow reinfusion with 29 historic controls who underwent transplant without the use of hematopoietic growth factors. Granulocyte recovery >500/μL occured significantly faster in both G-CSF-treated groups (median 12 days in both groups) compared to the historic controls (median 16 days). The number of red cell and platelet transfusions, platelet recovery, infectious complications, and duration of hospitalization, however, did not differ in both G-CSF groups and the controls. Of note, the group in which G-CSF therapy was delayed received a median of 9 (range: 6–17) days of G-CSF therapy compared to a median of 16 (range: 9–22) days in the patients given cytokine early after transplant. Both these authors concluded that a delay in G-CSF therapy gives the same clinical benefit, which can result in significant cost savings. Similar results using G-CSF in a delayed manner were presented in preliminary fashion by Khwaja and associates [348]. These studies justify undertaking randomized, phase III trials testing the concept of delaying the use of late-acting cytokines; such a practice cannot yet be recommended on the basis of phase II studies, which contain inherent patient selection biases.

Cost issues of recombinant hematopoietic growth factors

Bone marrow transplantation is recognized to be an extremely costly therapeutic modality, although it can be quite cost-effective (per year of life saved) when compared to other medical therapies [349,350]. While hematopoietic growth factors themselves are expensive agents, use of these new technologic advances could offset their own cost and reduce the cost of the procedure. Such therapy, by enhancing recovery of bone marrow function, may reduce the need for antibiotics, red blood cell and platelet transfusions, and additional diagnostic testing and may permit earlier hospital discharge. Not all the phase III studies that involve colony-stimulating factors discussed herein demonstrate a consistent positive effect on these variables. As yet, no phase III trials have demonstrated that these agents lower the mortality due to visceral organ damage or infection, or enhance tumor response or patient survival. In part, failure to demonstrate a positive benefit relates to inadequacies in those study endpoints, usually objectives secondary to the primary aim of establishing other benefits of the cytokine(s) in question [351].

Several authors have outlined methods for analyzing the potential benefits [352–354]. In one small, randomized trial, Gulati and Bennett [84] determined that despite the cost of the cytokine therapy, treatment of Hodgkin's disease patients with colony-stimulating factors after marrow reinfusion was associated with a substantial reduction in patient care costs ($40,000 versus $63,000) [84]. Similar results were noted by Clark et al. [346] as discussed above. Future investigations of bone marrow transplantation and colony-stimulating factors should include cost-effectiveness analyses.

Table 12. Additional uses of cytokines during bone marrow transplantation

Potential cytokine uses	Cytokine(s)	Clinical situations and citation(s)
Anticancer agents	GM-CSF, G-CSF, IL-2, IL-4	Therapy for relapse after allogeneic bone marrow transplant [355–358]
Increase tumor cell sensitivity to cytotoxic agents	GM-CSF, G-CSF	Stimulate host leukemia cells before initiating transplant conditioning regimen [359]
Antimicrobial agents	GM-CSF, M-CSF	Adjunct to amphotericin B for invasive aspergillosis [165–167,360]
Immunomodulatory substances	IL-2	Induce autologous graft-versus-host disease and graft-versus-tumor effect [296,361]
Normal cell protectors	IL-1, TGF-β, TNF-α	Prevent cytotoxic damage to bone marrow cells [246,251,254,361–363]
Effectors in wound healing and repair	IL-11	Protection of gastrointestinal tract damage due to cytotoxic therapy [285,361]
Immunization enhancers	GM-CSF	Augment response to immunogens after vaccination, i.e., vaccine adjuvants [364]
Mobilize hematopoietic progenitor cells for collection and transplant	G-CSF, GM-CSF, IL-3, EPO, SCF	Mobilize hematopoietic progenitors from peripheral blood for transplantation [365,366]
Expand autologous and allogeneic hematopoietic progenitors ex vivo before infusion	IL-1, IL-3, IL-6, EPO, SCF, GM-CSF	Culture-expansion ex vivo of hematopoietic progenitor cells for transplant [367–370]
Facilitate gene insertion	IL-1, IL-3, IL-6, SCF	Stimulate earliest progenitors to enhance gene transfer for transplant [371–379][a]

[a] Most clinical genetic marking studies to date do not use hematopoietic growth factors, but it is anticipated in future studies that use of these agents will enhance the frequency and efficiency of transfection.
Abbreviations: TGF-β, transforming growth factor-β; TNF-α, tumor necrosis factor-α; EPO, erythropoietin.

280

Other cytokines uses during bone marrow transplantation

Recombinant cytokines have numerous potential applications in the bone marrow transplant setting in addition to enhancing recovery of marrow function. Several of these applications, including some of those already in practice, are shown in table 12.

Summary

Use of recombinant hematopoietic growth factors in the course of bone marrow transplantation has revolutionized this modality by significantly improving the safety of the procedure. It is anticipated that use of cytokines in combination and the introduction of newer agents will further reduce costs and improve antitumor responses as well.

References

1. Metcalf D. The Molecular Control of Blood Cells. Boston: Harvard University Press, 1988.
2. Clark SC, Kamen R. The human hematopoietic colony-stimulating factors. Science 236:1229–1237, 1987.
3. Metcalf D. The colony-stimulating factors: discovery, development and clinical application. Cancer 65:2185–2195, 1990.
4. Lieschke GJ, Burgess AW. Granulocyte colony-stimulating factor and granulocyte-macrophage colony-stimulating factor. N Engl J Med 327:28–35, 99–106, 1992.
5. Rapoport AP, Abboud CN, DiPersio JF. Granulocyte-macrophage colony-stimulating factor (GM-CSF) and granulocyte colony-stimulating factor (G-CSF): receptor biology, signal transduction and neutrophil activation. Blood Rev 6:43–57, 1992.
6. Weisbart RH. Colony-stimulating factors and host defense. Ann Intern Med 110:297–303, 1989.
7. Bortin MM, Horowitz MM, Rimm AA. Increasing utilization of allogeneic bone marrow transplantation: results of the 1988–1990 survey. Ann Intern Med 116:505–512, 1992.
8. Armitage JO. Bone marrow transplantation. N Engl J Med 330:827–838, 1994.
9. Lazarus HM. Hematopoietic growth factors in bone marrow transplantation for hematologic malignancies. In Dainiak N, Cronkite EP, McCaffrey R, Shadduck RK (eds), Biology of Hematopoiesis. Proceedings of the 15th Annual Frederick Stohlman Jr., M.D. Memorial Symposium: An International Symposium. Cambridge, Massachusetts, October 15–20, 1989. Wiley-Liss, New York: 1990, pp. 531–538.
10. Metcalf D. Hematopoietic growth factors and marrow transplantation: an overview. Transplant Proc 21:2932–2933, 1989.
11. Yamasaki K, Solberg LA, Jamal N, et al. Hemopoietic colony growth-promoting activities in the plasma of bone marrow transplant recipients. J Clin Invest 82:255–261, 1988.
12. Mangan KF, Mullaney MT, Barrientos TD, Kernan NA. Serum interleukin-3 levels following autologous or allogeneic bone marrow transplantation: effects of T-cell depletion, blood stem cell infusion, and hematopoietic growth factor treatment. Blood 81:1915–1922, 1993.
13. Cairo MS, Suen Y, Sender L, Gillan ER, Ho W, Plunkett JM, van de Ven C. Circulating granulocyte colony-stimulating factor (G-CSF) levels after allogeneic and autologous bone marrow transplantation: endogenous G-CSF production correlates with myeloid engraftment. Blood 79:1869–1873, 1992.

14. Cairo MS, Gillan ER, Weinthal J, Yancik S, van de Ven C, Ho W, Shen V, Buzby JS, Suen Y. Decreased endogenous circulating steel factor (SLF) levels following allogeneic and autologous BMT: lack of an inverse correlation with post-BMT myeloid engraftment. Bone Marrow Transplant 11:155–161, 1993.

15. Rabinowitz J, Petros WP, Stuart AR, Peters WP. Characterization of endogenous cytokine concentrations after high-dose chemotherapy with autologous bone marrow support. Blood 81:2452–2459, 1993.

16. Miksits K, Beyer J, Siegert W. Serum concentrations of G-CSF during high-dose chemotherapy with autologous stem cell rescue. Bone Marrow Transplant 11:375–377, 1993.

17. Sallerfors B, Olofsson T, Lenhoff S. Granulocyte-macrophage colony-stimulating factor (GM-CSF) and granulocyte colony-stimulating factor (G-CSF) in serum in bone marrow transplanted patients. Bone Marrow Transplant 8:191–195, 1991.

18. Haas R, Gericke G, Witt B, Cayeux S, Hunstein W. Increased serum levels of granulocyte colony-stimulating factor after autologous bone marrow or blood stem cell transplantation. Exp Hematol 21:109–113, 1993.

19. Iacone A, Pierelli L, Quaglietta AM, et al. Survival after PBSC transplantation and comparison of engraftment speed with autologous and allogeneic marrow transplantation: results of multicenter study. Int J Artif Organs 16(S-5):45–50, 1993.

20. Cassileth PA, Andersen J, Lazarus HM, Colvin OM, Bennett JM, Stadtmauer EA, Kaizer H, Weiner RS, Edelstein M, Oken MM. Autologous bone marrow transplant in acute myeloid leukemia in first remission. J Clin Oncol 11:314–319, 1993.

21. Körbling M, Fliedner TM, Holle R, Magrin S, Baumann M, Holdermann E, Eberhardt K. Autologous blood stem cell (ABSCT) versus purged bone marrow transplantation (pABMT) in standard risk AML: influence of source and cell composition of the autograft on hemopoietic reconstitution and disease-free survival. Bone Marrow Transplant 7:343–349, 1991.

22. Wang JM, Chen ZG, Golella S, et al. Chemotactic activity of recombinant G-CSF. Blood 72:1456–1460, 1988.

23. Fibbe WE, Damme JV, Biolliau A, et al. Human fibroblasts produce granulocyte-CSF, macrophage-CSF, and granulocyte-macrophage-CSF following stimulation by interleukin-1 and poly(rl). poly(rC). Blood 72:860–866, 1988.

24. Motoyoshi K, Yoshida K, Hatake K. Recombinant and native human urinary colony-stimulating factor directly augments granulocytic and granulocyte-macrophage colony-stimulating factor production of human peripheral blood monocytes. Exp Hematol 17:68–71, 1989.

25. Wieser M, Bonifer R, Oster W. Interleukin-4 induces secretion of CSF for granulocytes and CSF for macrophages by peripheral blood monocytes. Blood 73:1105–1108, 1989.

26. Macey MG, Sangster J, Kelsey SM, Newland AG. Pilot study: effects of G-CSF on neutrophil ex-vivo function post bone marrow transplantation. Clin Lab Haematol 15:79–85, 1993.

27. Bleiberg I, Riklis I, Fabian I. Enhanced resistance of bone marrow transplanted mice to bacterial infection induced by recombinant granulocyte-macrophage colony-stimulating factor. Blood 75:1262–1266, 1990.

28. Frenck RW, Sarman G, Harper TE, Buescher ES. The ability of recombinant murine granulocyte-macrophage colony-stimulating factor to protect neonatal rats from septic death due to Staphylococcus aureus. J Infect Dis 162:109–114, 1990.

29. Smith PD, Lamerson CL, Banks SM, et al. Granulocyte-macrophage colony-stimulating factor augments human monocyte fungicidal activity for Candida albicans. J Infect Dis 161:999–1005, 1989.

30. Nienhaus AW, Donohue RE, Karlsson S, et al. Recombinant human granulocyte macrophage colony-stimulating factor (GM-CSF) shortens the period of neutropenia after autologous bone marrow transplantation in a primate model. J Clin Invest 80:573–577, 1987.

31. Monroy RL, Skelly RR, Mac Vittie TJ, et al. The effect of recombinant GM-CSF on the recovery of monkeys transplanted with autologous bone marrow. Blood 70:1696–1699, 1987.

32. Kernan NA, Bartsch G, Ash RC, et al. Analysis of 462 transplantations from unrelated donors facilitated by the National Marrow Donor Program. N Engl J Med 328:593–602, 1993.

33. Nemunaitis J. The role of hematopoietic growth factor in the treatment of graft failure. Bone Marrow Transplant 12(Suppl 3):S50–S52, 1993.

34. Weisdorf DJ, Verfaillie CM, Davies SM, Filipovich AH, Wagner JE Jr, Miller JS, et al. Hematopoietic growth factors for graft failure after bone marrow transplantation: a randomized trial of granulocyte-macrophage colony-stimulating factor (GM-CSF) versus sequential GM-CSF plus granulocyte-CSF. Blood 85:3452–3456, 1995.

35. Nemunaitis J, Singer JW, Buckner CD, Durnam D, Epstein C, Hill R, et al. Use of recombinant granulocyte-macrophage colony-stimulating factor in graft failure after bone marrow transplantation. Blood 76:245–253, 1990.

36. Brandwein JM, Nayar R, Baker MA, Sutton DMC, Scott JG, Sutcliffe SB, Keating A. GM-CSF therapy for delayed engraftment after autologous bone marrow transplantation. Exp Hematol 19:191–195, 1991.

37. Sierra J, Terol MJ, Urbano-Ispizua A, Rovira M, Marin P, Carreras E, Batlle M, Rozman C. Different response to recombinant human granulocyte-macrophage colony-stimulating factor in primary and secondary graft failure after bone marrow transplantation. Exp Hematol 22:566–572, 1994.

38. Ippoliti C, Przepiorka D, Giralt S, Andersson BS, Wallerstein RO, Gutterman J, Deisseroth AB, Champlin RE. Low-dose non-glycosylated rhGM-CSF is effective for the treatment of delayed hematopoietic recovery after autologous marrow or peripheral blood stem cell transplantation. Bone Marrow Transplant 11:55–59, 1993.

39. Vose JM, Bierman PJ, Kessinger A, Coccia PF, Anderson J, Oldham FB, Epstein C, Armitage JO. The use of recombinant human granulocyte-macrophage colony stimulating factor for the treatment of delayed engraftment following high dose therapy and autologous hematopoietic stem cell transplantation for lymphoid malignancies. Bone Marrow Transplant 7:139–143, 1991.

40. Klingemann H-G, Eaves AC, Barnett MJ, Reece DE, Shepherd JD, Belch AR, Brandwein JM, Langleben A, Koch PA, Phillips GL. Recombinant GM-CSF in patients with poor graft function after bone marrow transplantation. Clin Invest Med 13:77–81, 1990.

41. Kanamaru A, Hara H. Hematopoietic factors in graft-versus-host reaction. Int J Cell Cloning 5:450–462, 1987.

42. Lazarus HM, Rowe JM, Clinical use of hematopoietic growth factors in allogeneic bone marrow transplantation. Blood Rev 8:169–178, 1994.

43. Lazarus HM, Rowe JM. New and experimental therapies for treating graft-versus-host disease. Blood Rev, 9:117–133, 1995.

44. Holler E, Kolb HJ, Moeller A, et al. Increased serum levels of tumor necrosis factor alpha precede major complications of bone marrow transplantation. Blood 75:1011–1016, 1990.

45. Piguet P-F, Grau GE, Allet B, Vassalli P. Tumor necrosis factor/cachesin is an effector of skin and gut lesions of the acute phase of graft versus host disease. J Exp Med 166:1280–1289, 1987.

46. Moore RN, Oppenheim JJ, Farrar JJ, Carter CS Jr, Waheed A, Shadduck RK. Production of lymphocyte-activating factor (interleukin 1) by macrophages activated with colony-stimulating factors. J Immunol 125:1302–1305, 1980.

47. Shalaby MR, Fendly B, Sheehan KC, Schreiber RD, Ammann AJ. Prevention of the graft-versus-host reaction in newborn mice by antibodies to tumor necrosis factor-alpha. Transplantation 47:1057–1061, 1989.

48. Farrar WL, Mizel SB, Farrar JJ. Participation of lymphocyte activating factor (interleukin-1) in the induction of cytotoxic T cell responses. J Immunol 124:1371–1377, 1980.

49. Nemunaitis J. Growth factors in allogeneic transplantation. Semin Oncol 20(Suppl 6):96–101, 1993.

50. Masaoka T, Motoyoshi K, Takaku F, Kato S, Harada M, Kodera Y, Kanamaru A, Moriyama

Y, Ohno R, Ohira M, et al. Administration of human urinary colony stimulating factor after bone marrow transplantation. Bone Marrow Transplant 3:121–127, 1988.

51. Motoyoshi K, Takaku F, Mizoguti H, Miura Y. Purification and some properties of colony stimulating factor from normal human urine. Blood 52:1012–1020, 1978.

52. Wong GG, Temple PA, Leary AC, Witek-Giannoti JS, Yang YC, Ciarletta AB, et al. Human CSF-1: molecular cloning and expression of 4-kb cDNA encoding the human urinary protein. Science 235:1504–1508, 1987.

53. Denzlinger C, Tetzloff W, Gerhartz HH, et al. Differential activation of the endogenous leukotriene biosynthesis by two different preparations of granulocyte-macrophage colony-stimulating factor in healthy volunteers. Blood 81:2007–2013, 1993.

54. Dorr RT. Clinical properties of yeast-derived versus Escherichia coli-derived granulocyte-macrophage colony-stimulating factor. Clin Ther 15:19–29, 1993.

55. Oheda M, Hasegawa M, Hattori K, et al. O-linked sugar chain of human granulocyte colony-stimulating factor protects it against polymerization and denaturation allowing it to retain its biological activity. J Biol Chem 265:11432–11435, 1990.

56. Brandt SJ, Peters WP, Atwater SK, Kurtzberg J, Borowitz MJ, Jones RB, et al. Effect of recombinant human granulocyte-macrophage colony-stimulating factor on hematopoietic reconstitution after high-dose chemotherapy with autologous bone marrow transplantation. N Engl J Med 318:869–876, 1988.

57. Blazar BR, Kersey JH, McGlave PB, et al. In vivo administration of recombinant human granulocyte/macrophage colony-stimulating factor in acute lymphoblastic leukemia patients receiving purged autografts. Blood 73:849–857, 1989.

58. Link H, Seidel J, Stoll M, Kirchner H, Linderkamp C, Freund M, Bucsky P, Welte K, Riehm H, Burdach S, et al. Regeneration of granulopoiesis with recombinant human granulocyte-macrophage colony-stimulating factor after bone marrow transplantation. Haematol Blood Transf 33:741–746, 1990.

59. Taylor KM, Jagannath S, Spitzer G, et al. Recombinant human granulocyte colony-stimulating factor hastens granulocyte recovery after high-dose chemotherapy and autologous bone marrow transplantation in Hodgkin's disease. J Clin Oncol 7:1791–1799, 1989.

60. Sheridan WP, Morstyn G, Wolf M, et al. Granulocyte colony-stimulating factor and neutrophil recovery after high dose chemotherapy and autologous bone marrow transplantation. Lancet 2:891–894, 1989.

61. Nemunaitis J, Singer JW, Buckner CD, et al. Use of recombinant human granulocyte-macrophage colony-stimulating factor in autologous marrow transplantation for lymphoid malignancies. Blood 72:834–836, 1988.

62. Nemunaitis J, Singer JW, Buckner CD, Epstein C, Hill R, Storb R, Thomas ED, Appelbaum FR. Long-term followup of patients who received recombinant human granulocyte-macrophage colony stimulating factor after autologous bone marrow transplantation for lymphoid malignancy. Bone Marrow Transplant 7:49–52, 1991.

63. O'Day SJ, Rabinowe SN, Neuberg D, Freedman AS, Soiffer RJ, Spector NA, et al. A phase II study of continuous infusion recombinant human granulocyte-macrophage colony-stimulating factor as an adjunct to autologous bone marrow transplantation for patients with non-Hodgkin's lymphoma in first remission. Blood 83:2707–2714, 1994.

64. Carlo-Stella C, Mangoni L, Almici C, Cottafavi L, Meloni G, Mandelli F, Rizzoli V. Use of recombinant human granulocyte-macrophage colony-stimulating factor in patients with lymphoid malignancies transplanted with purged or adjusted-dose mafosfamide-purged autologous marrow. Blood 80:2412–2418, 1992.

65. Devereaux S, Linch DC, Gribben JG, McMillan A, Patterson K, Goldstone AH. GM-CSF accelerates neutrophil recovery after autologous bone marrow transplantation for Hodgkin's disease. Bone Marrow Transplant 4:49–54, 1989.

66. Lazarus HM, Andersen J, Chen MG, Variakojis D, Mansour EG, Oette D, et al. Recombinant granulocyte-macrophage colony-stimulating factor after autologous bone marrow transplantation for relapsed non-Hodgkin's lymphoma: blood and bone marrow progenitor

growth studies. A phase II Eastern Cooperative Oncology Group Trial Blood. 78:830–837, 1991.

67. Klingemann H-G, Wilkie-Boyd K, Rubin A, Onetto N, Nantel SH, Barnett MJ, Reece DE, Shepherd JD, Phillips GL. Granulocyte-macrophage colony-stimulating factor after autologous marrow transplantation for Hodgkin's disease. Biotech Therapeut 5(1&2):1–13, 1994.

68. Asano S, Masaoka T, Takaku F. Clinical effect of recombinant human granulocyte colony-stimulating factor in bone marrow transplantation. Jpn J Cancer Chemother 17:1201–1209, 1990.

69. Biggs D, Stadtmauer E, Mangan P, Edelstein M, Powlis W, Buzby G, Magee D, Sachs B, Silberstein L: 4-Hydroperoxycyclophosphamide purged autologous bone marrow transplantation of relapsed, responding non-Hodgkin's lymphoma with granulocyte colony stimulating factor support results in reliable hematopoietic recovery. In Advances in Bone Marrow Purging and Processing: Fourth International Symposium. New York: Wiley-Liss, 1994, pp. 9–15.

70. Kennedy MJ, Davis J, Passos-Coelho J, Noga SJ, Huelskamp AM, Ohly K, Davidson NE. Administration of human recombinant granulocyte colony-stimulating factor (filgrastim) accelerates granulocyte recovery following high-dose chemotherapy and autologous marrow transplantation with 4-hydroperoxycyclophosphamide-purged marrow in women with metastatic breast cancer. Cancer Res 53:5424–5428, 1993.

71. Schriber JR, Negrin RS, Chao NJ, Long GD, Horning SJ, Blume KG. The efficacy of granulocyte colony-stimulating factor following autologous bone marrow transplantation for non-Hodgkin's lymphoma with monoclonal antibody purged bone marrow. Leukemia 7:1491–1495, 1993.

72. Nemunaitis J, Buckner CD, Appelbaum FR, et al. Phase I/II trial of recombinant human granulocyte-macrophage colony-stimulating factor following allogeneic bone marrow transplantation. Blood 77:2065–2071, 1991.

73. Masaoka T, Takaku F, Kato S, Moriyama Y, Kodera Y, Kanamaru A, Shimosaka A, Shibata H, Nakamura H. Recombinant human granulocyte colony-stimulating factor in allogeneic bone marrow transplantation. Exp Hematol 17:1047–1050, 1989.

74. Atkinson K, Bradstock K, Biggs JC, Lowenthal RM, Downs K, Dale B, Juttner C, Szer J. GM-CSF after allogeneic bone marrow transplantation: accelerated recovery of neutrophils, monocytes, and lymphocytes. Aust NZ J Med 21:686–692, 1991.

75. Nemunaitis J, Anasetti C, Storb R, et al. Phase II trial of recombinant human granulocyte-macrophage colony-stimulating factor in patients undergoing allogeneic bone marrow transplantation from unrelated donors. Blood 79:2572–2577, 1992.

76. Nemunaitis J, Anasetti C, Bianco JA, Hansen J, Singer JW. rhGM-CSF after allogeneic bone marrow transplantation from unrelated donors: a pilot study of cyclosporine and prednisone as graft-versus-host disease prophylaxis. Leuk Lymphoma 10:177–181, 1993.

77. Nemunaitis J, Anasetti C, Buckner CD, Appelbaum FR, Shannon-Dorcy K, Hansen J, Singer JW. Long-term follow-up of 103 patients who received recombinant human granulocyte-macrophage colony-stimulating factor after unrelated donor bone marrow transplantation (letter). Blood 81:865, 1993.

78. Schriber JR, Chao NJ, Long GD, Negrin RS, Tierney DK, et al. Granulocyte colony-stimulating factor after allogeneic bone marrow transplantation. Blood 84:1680–1684, 1994.

79. Lickliter JD, Roberts AW, Grigg AP. Phase II study of glycosylated recombinant human granulocyte colony-stimulating factor after HLA-identical sibling bone marrow transplantation. Aust NZ J Med 24:541–546, 1994.

80. Kodo H, Tajika K, Takanhashi S, Ozawa K, Asano S, Takaku F. Acceleration of neutrophilic granulocyte recovery after bone-marrow transplantation by administration of recombinant human granulocyte colony-stimulating factor (letter). Lancet 2:38–39, 1988.

81. Rabinowe SN, Neuberg D, Bierman PJ, et al. Long-term follow-up of a phase III study of recombinant human granulocyte-macrophage colony-stimulating factor after autologus bone marrow transplantation for lymphoid malignancies. Blood 81:1903–1908, 1993.

82. Nemunaitis J, Rabinowe SN, Singer JW, et al. Recombinant granulocyte-macrophage colony-stimulating factor after autologous bone marrow transplantation for lymphoid malignancies. N Engl J Med 324:1773–1778, 1991.

83. Advani R, Chao NJ, Horning SJ, et al. Granulocyte-macrophage colony-stimulating factor (GM-CSF) as an adjunct to autologous hemopoietic stem cell transplantation for lymphoma. Ann Intern Med 116:183–189, 1992.

84. Gulati S, Bennett C. Granulocyte-macrophage colony-stimulating factor (GM-CSF) as adjunct therapy in relapsed Hodgkin's disease. Ann Intern Med 116:177–182, 1992.

85. Gorin NC, Coiffier B, Hayat M, et al. Recombinant human granulocyte-macrophage colony-stimulating factor after high-dose chemotherapy and autologous bone marrow transplantation with unpurged marrow in non-Hodgkin's lymphoma: a double-blind placebo-controlled trial. Blood 80:1149–1157, 1992.

86. Link H, Boogaerts MA, Carella AM, et al. A controlled trial of recombinant human granulocyte-macrophage colony-stimulating factor after total body irradiation, high-dose chemotherapy, and autologous bone marrow transplantation for acute lymphoblastic leukemia or malignant lymphoma. Blood 80:2188–2195, 1992.

87. Visani G, Gamberi B, Greenberg P, Advani R, Gulati S, Champlin R, Hoglund M, Karanes C, Williams S, Keating A, et al. The use of GM-CSF as an adjunct to autologous/syngeneic bone marrow transplantation: a prospective randomized controlled trial (abstract). Bone Marrow Transplant 7(Suppl 2):81, 1991.

88. Khwaja A, Linch DC, Goldstone AH, et al. Recombinant human granulocyte-macrophage colony-stimulating factor after autologous bone marrow transplantation for malignant lymphoma: a British National Lymphoma Investigation double-blind, placebo-controlled trial. Br J Haematol 82:317–323, 1992.

89. Hiraoka A, Masaoka T, Mizoguchi H, Asano S, Kodera Y, Kitamura K, Takaku F, Komenushi S. Recombinant human non-glycosylated granulocyte-macrophage colony-stimulating factor in allogeneic bone marrow transplantation: double-blind placebo-controlled phase III clinical trial. Jpn J Clin Oncol 24:205–211, 1994.

90. Schmitz N, Dreger P, Zander A, et al. Recombinant human granulocyte colony stimulating factor (filgrastim) after autologous bone marrow transplantation for lymphoma: an open label randomized trial in Germany (abstract). Blood 80 (Suppl):292a, 1992.

91. Gisselbrecht C, Prentice HG, Bacigalupo A, Biron P, Milpied N, Rubie H, et al. Placebo-controlled phase III trial of lenograstim in bone-marrow transplantation. Lancet 343:696–700, 1994.

92. Stahel RA, Jost LM, Cerny T, Pichert G, Honegger H, Tobler A, Jacky E, Fey M, Platzer E. Randomized study of recombinant human granulocyte colony-stimulating factor after high-dose chemotherapy and autologous bone marrow transplantation for high-risk lymphoid malignancies. J Clin Oncol 12:1931–1938, 1994.

93. Blaise D, Vernant JP, Fiere D, et al. A randomised, controlled, multicenter trial of recombinant human granulocyte colony stimulating factor (filgrastim) in patients treated by bone marrow transplantation (BMT) with total body irradiation (TBI) for acute lymphoblastic leukemia (ALL) or lymphoblastic lymphoma (LL) (abstract). Blood 80(Suppl):982a, 1992.

94. Michon J, Bouffet E, Bernard JL, Lopez M, Philip I, Gentet JC, Zucker JM, Philip T. Administration of recombinant human GM-CSF (rHuGM-CSF) after autologous bone marrow transplantation (ABMT). A study of 21 stage IV neuroblastoma patients undergoing a double intensification regimen (abstract 712). Proc Am Soc Clin Oncol 9:184, 1990.

95. Linch DC, Scarffe H, Proctor S, Chopra R, Taylor PRA, Morgenstern G, Cunningham D, Burnett AK, Cawley JC, Franklin IM, Bell AJ, Lister TA, Marcus RE, Newland AC, Parker AC, Yver A. Randomised vehicle-controlled dose-finding study of glycosylated recombinant human granulocyte colony-stimulating factor after marrow transplantation. Bone Marrow Transplant 11:307–311, 1993.

96. De Witte T, Gratwohl A, Van Der Lely N, Bacigalupo A, Stern AC, Speck B, et al. Recombinant human granulocyte-macrophage colony-stimulating factor accelerates neutro-

phil and monocyte recovery after allogeneic T-cell-depleted bone marrow transplantation. Blood 79:1359–1365, 1992.

97. Powles R, Treleaven J, Millar J, et al. Human recombinant GM-CSF in allogeneic bone marrow transplantation for leukemia: double-blind placebo control trial. Bone Marrow Transplant 7(Suppl 2):85–86, 1991.

98. Powles R, Smith C, Milan S, et al. Human recombinant GM-CSF in allogeneic bone-marrow transplantation for leukemia: double-blind, placebo-controlled trial. Lancet 336:1417–1420, 1990.

99. Gupta P, Tiley C, Powles R, Treleaven J, Millar J, Catalano J. No increase in relapse in patients with myeloid leukaemias receiving rhGM-CSF after allogeneic bone marrow transplantation. Bone Marrow Transplant 9:491–493, 1992.

100. Nemunaitis J, Rosenfeld C, Ash R, et al. Phase III double-blind trial of rhGM-CSF (sargramostin) following allogeneic bone marrow transplant (BMT) (abstract 1128). Blood 82(Suppl 1):286a, 1993.

101. Masaoka T, Moriyama Y, Kato S, et al. A randomized, placebo-controlled study of KRN8601 (recombinant human granulocyte colony-stimulating factor) in patients receiving allogeneic bone marrow transplantation. Jpn J Med 3:233–239, 1990.

102. Reissmann KR. Studies on the mechanism of erythropoietic stimulation in parabiotic rats during hypoxia. Blood 5:372–380, 1950.

103. Krantz SB, Goldwasser E. Specific binding of erythropoietin to spleen cells infected with the anemia strian of Friend virus. Proc Natl Acad Sci USA 81:7574–7578, 1984.

104. Graber SE, Krantz SB. Erythropoietin and the control of red blood cell production. Annu Rev Med 29:51–66, 1978.

105. Spivak J. The mechanism of action of erythropoietin. Int J Cell Cloning 4:139–166, 1986.

106. Dessypris EN, Krantz SB. Effects of pure erythropoietin on DNA-synthesis by human marrow day 15 erythroid burst forming units in short term liquid culture. Br J Haematol 56:295–306, 1984.

107. Dessypris EN, Graber SE, Krantz SB, et al. Effects of recombinant erythropoietin on the concentration any cycling status of human marrow hematopoietic progenitor cells in vivo. Blood 72:2060–2062, 1988.

108. Goldwasser E. Erythropoietin and its mode of action. Blood Cells 4:89–103, 1984.

109. Spivak JL. Erythropoietin: a brief review. Nephron 52:289–294, 1989.

110. Bartley TD, Bogenberger J, Hunt P, et al. Indentification and cloning of a megakaryocyte growth and development factor (MGDF) which is a ligand for Mpl. Cell 77:1117–1124, 1994.

111. de Sauvage FJ, Haas PE, Spencer SD, et al. Stimulation of megakaryocytopoiesis and thrombopoiesis by the c-Mpl ligand. Nature 369:533–538, 1994.

112. Metcalf D. Thrombopoietin — at last. Nature 369:519–520, 1994.

113. Vigon I, Mornon JP, Cocault L, et al. Molecular cloning and characterization of Mpl, the human homolog of the v-mpl oncogene: identification of a member of the hematopoietic growth factor receptor superfamily. Proce Natl Acad Sci USA 89:5640–5644, 1992.

114. Ishibashi T, Koziol JA, Burstein SA. Human recombinant erythropoietin promotes differentiation of murine megakaryocytes in vitro. J Clin Invest 79:286–289, 1987.

115. Mazur EM, South K. Human megakaryocyte colony-stimulating factor in sera from aplastic dogs: partial purification, characterization, and determination of hematopoietic cell lineage specificity. Exp Hematol 13:1164–1172, 1985.

116. Lazarus HM, Rowe JM. Erythropoietin therapy after bone marrow transplantation. Erythropoiesis 5:9–15, 1994.

117. Atkinson K, Norrie S, Chan P, et al. Hemopoietic progenitor cell function after HLA-indentical sibling bone marrow transplantation: influence of chronic graft-versus-host disease. Intl J Cell Cloning 4:203–220, 1986.

118. Beguin Y, Oris R, Fillet G. Dynamics of erythropoietic recovery following bone marrow transplantation: role of marrow proliferative capacity and erythropoietin production in autologous versus allogeneic transplants. Bone Marrow Transplant 11:285–292, 1993.

287

119. Ma DDF, Varga DE, Biggs JC. Haemopoietic reconstitution after allogeneic bone marrow transplantation in man: recovery of haemopoietic progenitors (CFU-Mix, BFU-E and CFU-GM). Br J Haematol 65:5–10, 1987.
120. Prioso E, Erslev AJ, Caro J. Inappropriate increase in erythropoietin titers during chemotherapy. Am J Haematol 32:248–254, 1989.
121. Hellebostad M, Marstrander J, Slordahl SH, et al. Serum immunoreactive erythropoietin in children with acute leukemia at various stages of disease and the effects of treatment. Eur J Haematol 44:159–164, 1990.
122. Bowen DT, Janowska-Wieczorek A. Serum erythropoietin following cytostatic therapy (letter). Br J Haematol 74:372–373, 1990.
123. Birgegård G, Wide L, Simonsson B. Marked erythropoietin increase before fall in haemoglobin after treatment with cytostatic drugs suggests a mechanism other than anaemia for stimulation. Br J Haematol 72:462–466, 1989.
124. Grace RJ, Kendall RG, Chapman C, et al. Changes in serum erythropoietin levels during allogeneic bone marrow transplantation. Eur J Haematol 47:81–85, 1991.
125. Abdei MR, Bäckman L, Boström L, et al. Markedly increased serum erythropoietin levels following conditioning for allogeneic bone marrow transplantation. Bone Marrow Transplant 6:121–126, 1990.
126. Ireland RM, Atkinson K, Concannon A, et al. Serum erythropoietin changes in autologous and allogeneic bone marrow transplant patients. Br J Haematol 76:128–134, 1990.
127. Lazarus HM, Goodnough LT, Goldwasser E, et al. Serum erythropoietin levels and blood component therapy after autologous bone marrow transplantation: implications for erythropoietin therapy in this setting. Bone Marrow Transplant 10:71–75, 1992.
128. Miller CB, Jones RJ, Zahurak ML, et al. Impaired erythropoietin response to anemia after bone marrow transplantation. Blood 80:2677–2682, 1992.
129. Schapira, L, Antin JH, Ransil BJ, et al. Serum erythropoietin levels in patients receiving intensive chemotherapy and radiotherapy. Blood 76:2354–2359, 1990.
130. Bosi A, Vannucchi AM, Grossi A, et al. Serum erythropoietin levels in patients undergoing autologous bone marrow transplantation. Bone Marrow Transplant 7:421–425, 1991.
131. Beguin Y, Clemons GK, Oris R, et al. Circulating erythropoietin levels after bone marrow transplantations: inappropriate response to anemia in allogeneic transplants. Blood 77:868–873, 1991.
132. Schuster SJ, Wilson HJ, Erslev AJ, et al. Physiologic regulation and tissue localization of renal erythropoietin messenger RNA. Blood 70:316–318, 1987.
133. Holler E, Kolb HJ, Moeller A, et al. Increased serum levels of tumor necrosis factor alpha precede major complications of bone marrow transplantation. Blood 75:1011–1016, 1990.
134. Piguet PF, Grau GE, Allet B, et al. Tumor necrosis factor/cachesin is an effector of skin and gut lesions of the acute phase of graft versus host disease. J Exp Med 166:1280, 1987.
135. Faquin WC, Schneider TJ, Goldberg MA. Effects of inflammatory cytokines on erythropoietin production in Hep3B cells (abstract 560). Blood 6:142a, 1990.
136. Abboud SL, Gerson SL, Berger NA. The effect of tumor necrosis factor on normal human hematopoietic progenitors. Cancer 60:2965–2970, 1987.
137. Locatelli F, Pedrazzoli P, Barosi G, et al. Recombinant human erythropoietin is effective in correcting erythropoietin-deficient anaemia after allogeneic bone marrow transplantation. Br J Haematol 80:545–549, 1992.
138. Link H, Diedrich H, Ebell W, et al. Recombinant human erythropoietin after allogeneic bone marrow transplantation (abstract). Bone Marrow Transplant 5:219, 1990.
139. Miller CB, Huelskamp AM, Mills SR, et al. A pilot trial of recombinant human erythropoietin (rhEPO) after allogeneic bone marrow transplantation (alloBMT) (abstract). Exp Hematol 19:577, 1991.
140. Ayash L, Elias A, Demetri G, et al. Recombinant human erythropoietin (EPO) in anemia associated with autologous bone marrow transplantation (ABMT) (abstract 513). Blood 76:131a, 1990.

141. Vannucchi AM, Bosi A, Grossi A, et al. Stimulation of erythroid engraftment by recombinant human erythropoietin in ABO-compatible, HLA-identical, allogeneic bone marrow transplant patients. Leukemia 6:215–219, 1992.

142. Steegmann JL, López J, Otero MJ, et al. Erythropoietin treatment in allogeneic BMT accelerates erythroid reconstitution: results of a prospective controlled randomized trial. Bone Marrow Transplant 10:541–546, 1992.

143. Bishop MR, Stiff PJ, McKenzie RS, et al. Recombinant human erythropoietin (rHuEPO) administration does not affect peripheral leukocyte counts in patients with delayed erythropoietin after marrow transplantation (abstract D201). J Cell Biochem 16A:189, 1992.

144. Paltiel O, Cournoyer D, Rybka W. Pure red cell aplasia following ABO-incompatible bone marrow transplantation: response to erythropoietin. Transfusion 33:418–421, 1993.

145. Heyll A, Aul C, Runde V, et al. Treatment of pure red cell aplasia after major ABO-incompatible bone marrow transplantation with recombinant erythropoietin (letter). Blood 77:906, 1991.

146. Peliska J, Miller C, Bishop M, Mills S, Sosman J, Bayer R, et al. Recombinant human erythropoietin therapy for patients with delayed erythropoiesis after bone marrow transplantation (abstract 2541). Blood 82(Suppl):639a, 1993.

147. Link H, Boogaerts MA, Fauser AA, et al. A controlled trial of recombinant human erythropoietin after bone marrow transplantation. Blood 84:3327–3335, 1994.

148. York A, Clift RA, Sanders JE, Buckner CD. Recombinant human erythropoietin (rh-Epo) administration to normal marrow donors. Bone Marrow Transplant 10:415–417, 1992.

149. Masaoka T, Shibata H, Ohno R, Katoh S, Harada M, Motoyoshi K, Takaku F, Sakuma A. Double-blind test of human urinary macrophage colony-stimulating factor for allogeneic and syngeneic bone marrow transplantation: effectiveness of treatment and 2-year follow-up for relapse of leukaemia. Br J Haematol 76:501–505, 1990.

150. Beckers S, Warren MK, Haskill S. Colony-stimulating factor-induced monocyte survival and differentiation into macrophages in serum-free cultures. J Immunol 139:3703–3708, 1987.

151. Ralph PW. Biological properties and molecular biology of the human macrophage growth factor, CSF-1. Immunobiology 172:194–204, 1986.

152. Sternberg S. The emerging fungal threat. Science 266:1632–1634, 1994.

153. Meyers JD. Fungal infection in bone marrow transplant patiens. Semin Oncol 17:10–13, 1990.

154. Wingard JR, Advances in the management of infectious complications after bone marrow transplantation. Bone Marrow Transplant 6:371–383, 1990.

155. Watson JG. Problems of infection after bone marrow transplantation. J Clin Pathol 36:683–686, 1986.

156. Zimmerli W, Zarth A, Gratwohl A, Nissen C, Speck B. Granulocyte-macrophage colony-stimulating factor for granulocyte defects of bone marrow transplant patients (letter). Lancet 1:494, 1989.

157. Fabian I, Kletter Y, Bleiberg I, Gadish M, Naparsteck E, Slavin S. Effect of exogenous recombinant human granulocyte and granulocyte-macrophage colony-stimulating factor on neutrophil function following allogeneic bone marrow transplantation. Exp Hematol 19:868–873, 1991.

158. Petros WP, Rabinowitz J, Stuart AR, Gupton C, Alderman EM, Peters WP. Elevated endogenous serum macrophage colony-stimulating factor in the early stage of fungemia following bone marrow transplantation. Exp Hematol 22:582–586, 1994.

159. Gale RP, Sparkes LS, Golde DW. Bone marrow origin of hepatic macrophages (Kupffer cells) in humans. Science 201:937–938, 1978.

160. Nemunaitis J, Singer JW. Macrophage colony-stimulating factor (M-CSF). Biology and clinical applications. In Armitage JO, Antman K (eds), High-dose Cancer Therapy. Pharmacology, Hematopoietins, and Stem Cells. Baltimore, MD: Williams & Willkins, 1992, pp. 344–361.

161. Smith PD, Lamerson CL, Banks SM, et al. Granulocyte-macrophage colony-stimulating

factor augments human monocyte fungicidal activity for Candida albicans. J Infect Dis 161:999–1005, 1990.

162. Mufson RA, Aghajanian J, Wong G, et al. Macrophage colony-stimulating factor enhances monocyte and macrophage antibody-dependent cell-mediated cytotoxicity. Cell Immunol 119:182–192, 1989.

163. Sampson-Johannes A, Carlino JA. Enhancement of human monocyte tumoricidal activity by recombinant M-CSF. J Immunol 141:3680–3686, 1988.

164. Fabian I, Shapira E, Gadish M, et al. Effects of human interleukin 3, macrophage and granulocyte-macrophage colony-stimulating factor on monocyte function following autologous bone marrow transplantation. Leuk Res 16:703–709, 1992.

165. Nemunaitis J, Meyers JD, Buckner CD, et al. Phase I trial of recombinant human macrophage colony-stimulating factor in patients with invasive fungal infections. Blood 78:907–913, 1991.

166. Nemunatits J, Shannon-Dorcy K, Appelbaum FR, et al. Long-term follow-up of patients with invasive fungal disease who received adjunctive therapy with recombinant human macrophage colony-stimulating factor. Blood 82:1422–1427, 1993.

167. Schiller G, O'Neill C, Lee M, Nemunaitis J, Ando D, O'Byrne J, Lazarus H. A phase II study of placebo versus recombinant human macrophage colony-stimulating factor to augment antifungal therapy in patients with invasive candida or aspergillus fungal infection (abstract 2002). Blood 82:504a, 1993.

168. Morrow JF, Braine HG, Kickler TS, Ness PM, Dick JD, Fuller AK. Septic reactions to platelet transfusions. A persistent problem. JAMA 266:555–558, 1991.

169. Yomtovian R, Lazarus HM, Goodnough LT, Hirschler NV, Morrissey AM, Jacobs MR. A prospective microbiologic surveillance program to detect and prevent the transfusion of bacterially contaminated platelets. Transfusion 33:902–909, 1993.

170. Stack G, Snyder EL. Cytokine generation in stored platelet concentrates. Transfusion 34:20–25, 1994.

171. Muylle L, Joos M, Wouters E, De Bock R, Peetermans ME. Increased tumor necrosis factor α (TNFα), interleukin 1, and interleukin 6 (IL-6) levels in the plasma of stored platelet concentrates: relationship between TNFα and IL-6 levels and febrile transfusion reactions. Transfusion 33:195–199, 1993.

172. Gordon MS, Hoffman R. Growth factors affecting human thrombocytopoiesis: potential agents for the treatment of thrombocytopenia. Blood 80:302–307, 1992.

173. Hoffman R. Regulation of megakaryocytopoiesis. Blood 74:1196–1212, 1989.

174. Chambers LA, Garcia LW. Lack of effect on platelet increments of granulocyte-macrophage-colony-stimulating factor following autologous bone marrow transplantation for malignant lymphoma. Transfusion 34:221–225, 1994.

175. Morstyn G, Foote M, Perkins D, Vincent M. The clinical utility of granulocyte colony-stimulating factor: early achievements and future promise. Stem Cells 12(Suppl 1):213–227, 1994.

176. Bishop JF. Platelet support and the use of cytokines. Stem Cells 12:370–377, 1994.

177. Kimura H, Ishibashi T, Uchida T, Maruyama Y, Friese P, Burstein SA. Interleukin 6 is a differentiation factor for human megakaryocytes in vitro. Eur J Immunol 20:1927–1931, 1990.

178. Ishibashi T, Kimura H, Uchida T, Kariyone S, Friese P, Burstein SA. Human interleukin 6 is a direct promoter of maturation of megakaryocytes in vitro. Proc Natl Acad Sci USA 86:5953–5957, 1989.

179. Patchen ML, MacVittie TJ, Williams JL, Schwartz GN, Souza LM. Administration of interleukin-6 stimulates multilineage hematopoiesis and accelerated recovery from radiation-induced hematopoietic depression. Blood 77:472–480, 1991.

180. Burstein SA, Downs T, Friese P, et al. Thrombocytopoiesis in normal and subethally irradiated dogs: response to human interleukin-6. Blood 80:420–428, 1992.

181. Asano S, Okano A, Ozawa K, et al. In vivo effects of recombinan human interleukin-6 in primates: stimulated production of platelets. Blood 75:1602–1605, 1990.

290

182. Stahl CP, Zucker-Franklin D, Evatt BL, Winton EF. Effects of human interleukin-6 on megakaryocyte development and thrombocytopoiesis in primates. Blood 78:1467–1475, 1991.
183. Herodin F, Mesries J-C, Janodet D, et al. Recombinant glycosylated human interleukin-6 accelerates peripheral blood platelet count recovery in radiation-induced bone marrow depression in baboons. Blood 80:688–695, 1992.
184. Van Snick J. Interleukin-6: an overview. Annu Rev Immunol 8:253–278, 1990.
185. Kishimoto T. The biology of interleukin-6. Blood 74:1–10, 1989.
186. Ogawa M. IL-6 and hematopoietic stem cells. Res Immunol 143:749–751, 1992.
187. Peng J, Friese P, George JN, Dale GL, Burstein SA. Alteration of platelet function in dogs mdiated by interleukin-6. Blood 83:398–403, 1994.
188. Slavin S, Kedar E. Current problems and future goals in clinical bone marrow transplantation. Blood Rev 2:259–269, 1988.
189. Aronson FR, Sznol M, Mier JW, et al. Interleukin 6: phase I trials of 1 and 120 hour intravenous infusions (abstract 952). Proc Am Soc Clin Oncol 12:292, 1993.
190. Weber J, Yang JC, Topalian SL, et al. Phase I trial of subcutaneous interleukin-6 in patients with advanced malignancies. J Clin Oncol 11:499–506, 1993.
191. Colwill R, Crump M, Stewart AK, et al. Phase I trial of interleukin-6 (IL-6) after autologous bone marrow transplantation (ABMT) for patients with poor prognosis Hodgkin's disease (abstract 2569). Blood 82(Suppl 1):646a, 1993.
192. Lazarus HM, Winton EF, Williams SF, Grinblatt D, Campion M, Cooper BW, Gunn H, Manfreda S, Isaacs RE. A phase I multicenter trial of interleukin 6 therapy after autologous bone marrow transplantation in advanced breast cancer. Bone Marrow Transplant 15:935–942, 1995.
193. Wing EJ, Magee DM, Whiteside TL, Kaplan SS, Shadduck RK. Recombinant human granulocyte/macrophage colony-stimulating factor enhances monocyte cytotoxicity and secretion of tumor necrosis factor-α and interferon in cancer patients. Blood 73:643–646, 1989.
194. Moore RN, Oppenheim JJ, Farrar JJ, Carter CS Jr, Waheed A, Shadduck RK. Production of lymphocyte-activating factor (interleukin 1) by macrophages activated with colony-stimulating factors. J Immunol 125:1302–1305, 1980.
195. Halaby MR, Fendly B, Sheehan KC, Schreiber RD, Ammann AJ. Prevention of the graft-versus-host reaction in newborn mice by antibodies to tumor necrosis factor-alpha. Transplantation 47:1057–1061, 1989.
196. Holler E, Kolb HJ, Moeller A, et al. Increased serum levels of tumor necrosis factor alpha precede major complications of bone marrow transplantation. Blood 75:1011–1016, 1990.
197. Neta R, Vogel SN, Sipe JD, Wong GG, Nordan RP. Comparison of in vivo effects of human recombinant IL 1 and human recombinant IL 6 in mice. Lymphokine Res 7:403–412, 1988.
198. Neta R, Perlstein R, Vogel SN, Ledney GD, Abrams J. Role of interleukin 6 (IL-6) in protection from lethal irradiation and in endocrine responses to IL-1 and tumor necrosis factor. J Exp Med 175:689–694, 1992.
199. Ogawa M. IL-6 and hematopoietic stem cells. Res Immunol 143:749, 1992.
200. Givon T, Revel M, Slavin S. Potential use of interleukin-6 in bone marrow transplantation: effects of recombinant human interleukin-6 after syngeneic and semiallogeneic bone marrow transplantation in mice. Blood 83:1690–1697, 1994.
201. Ihle JN, Keller J, Oroszlan S, Hendersohn LE, Copeland TD, Fitch F, et al. Biologic properties of homogeneous interleukin-3. I. Demonstration of WEHI-3 growth factor activity, mast cell growth factor activity, p cell-stimulating factor activity, colony-stimulating factor activity, and histamine-producing cell-stimulating factor activity. J Immunol 131:282–287, 1983.
202. Platzer E, Welte K, Gabrilove JL, Lu L, Harris P, Mertelsmann R, Moore MA. Biological activities of a human pluripotent hemopoietic colony stimulating factor on normal leukemic cells. J Exp Med 162:1788–1801, 1985.
203. Ishibashi T, Bursten SA. Interleukin 3 promotes the differentiation of isolated single megakaryocytes. Blood 67:1512–1514, 1986.

204. Takaue Y, Kawano Y, Reading CL, Watanbe T, Abe T, Ninomiya T, et al. Effects of recombinant human G-CSF, GM-CSF, IL-3, and IL-lα on the growth of purified human peripheral blood progenitors. Blood 76:330–335, 1990.
205. Saeland S, Caux C, Favre C, Aubry JP, Mannoni P, Pebusque MJ, et al. Effects of recombinant human interleukin-3 on CD34-enriched hematopoietic progenitors and on myeloblastic leukemia cells. Blood 72:1580–1588, 1988.
206. Sorensen P, Farber NM, Krystal G. Identification of the interleukin-3 receptor using an iodinatable, cleavable, photoreactive cross-linking agent. J Biol Chem 261:9094–9097, 1986.
207. Wang M, Friedman H, Djeu JY. Enhancement of human monocyte function against Candida albicans by the colony-stimulating factors (CSF): IL-3, granulocyte-macrophage-CSF, and macrophage-CSF. J Immunol 143:671-677, 1989.
208. Leary AG, Yang YC, Clark SC, et al. Recombinant gibbon interleukin-3 supports human multi-lineage colonies and blast cell colonies in culture: comparison with recombinant human granulocyte-macrophage colony-stimulating factor. Blood 70:1343–1348, 1987.
209. Young DA, Lowe LD, Clark SC. Comparison of the effects of IL-3, granulocyte-macrophage colony-stimulating factor, and macrophage colony-stimulating factor in supporting monocyte differentiation in culture. Analysis of macrophage antibody-dependent cellular cytotoxicity. J Immunol 145:607–615, 1990.
210. Elliott MJ, Vadas MA, Eglinton JM, Park LS, To LB, Cleland LG, Clark SC, Lopez AF. Recombinant human interleukin-3 and granulocyte-macrophage clolny-stimulating factor show common biological effects and binding characteristics on human monocytes. Blood 74:2349–2359, 1989.
211. Kindler V, Thorens B, DeKossodo S, Allet B, Eliason JF, Thatcher D, Farber N, Vassalli P. Stimulation of hematopoiesis in vivo by recombinant bacterial murine interleukin 3. Proc Natl Acad Sci USA 83:1001–1005, 1986.
212. Bruno E, Cooper RJ, Briddel RA, Hoffman R. Further examination of the effects of recombinant cytokines on the proliferation of human megakaryocyte progenitor cells. Blood 77:2339–2346, 1991.
213. Sieff CA, Niemeyer CM, Nathan DG, Ekern SC, Bieber FR, Yang YC, Wong G, Clark SC. Stimulation of human hematopoietic colony formation by recombinant gibbon multi-colony-stimulating factor of interleukin 3. J Clin Invest 80:818–823, 1987.
214. Paquette RL, Zhou J-Y, Yang Y-C, Clark SC, Koeffler HP. Recombinant gibbon interleukin-3 acts synergistically with recombinant human G-CSF and GM-CSF in vitro. Blood 71:1596–1600, 1988.
215. Gillio AP, Gasparetto C, Laver J, Abboud M, Bonilla MA, Garnick MB, O'Reilly RJ. Effects of interleukin-3 on hematopoietic recovery after 5-fluorouracil or cyclophosphamide treatment of cynomolgus primates. J Clin Invest 85:1560–1565, 1990.
216. Krumwieh D, Seiler FR. In vivo effects of recombinant colony stimulating factors on hematopoiesis in cynomolgus monkeys. Transplant Proc 21:2964–2967, 1989.
217. Geissler K, Valent P, Mayer P, Liehl E, Hinterberger W, Lechner K, Bettelheim P. Recombinant human interleukin-3 expands the pool of circulating hematopoietic progenitor cells in primates — synergism with recombinant human granulocyte-macrophage colony-stimulating factor. Blood 75:2305–2310, 1990.
218. Donahue RE, Seehra J, Metzger M, Lefebvre D, Rock B, Carbone S, Nathan DG, Garnick M, et al. Human IL-3 and GM-CSF act synergistically in stimulating hematopoiesis in primates. Science 241:1820–1823, 1988.
219. Mayer P, Valent P, Schmidt G, Liehl E, Bettelheim P. The in vivo effects of recombinant human interleukin-3: demonstration of basophil differentiation factor, histamine-producing activity, and priming of GM-CSF-responsive progenitors in nonhuman primates. Blood 74:613–621, 1989.
220. Vose JM, Kessinger A, Bierman PJ, et al. The use of rhIL-3 for mobilization of peripheral blood stem cells in previously treated patients with lymphoid malignancies. Int J Cell Cloning (Suppl 1) 10:62–64, 1992.

292

differentiation and IL-1 receptor induction on BM cells in vivo. Exp Hematol 21:303–310, 1993.

259. McConkey DJ, Hartzell P, Chow SC, Orrenius S, Jondal M. Interleukin 1 inhibits T cell receptor-mediated apoptosis in immature thymocytes. J Biol Chem 265:3009–3011, 1990.

260. Nemunaitis J, Appelbaum FR, Lilleby K, Buhles WC, Rosenfeld C, Zeigler ZR, Shadduck RK, Singer JW, Meyer W, Buckner CD. Phase I study of recombinant interleukin-1β in patients undergoing autologous bone marrow transplant for acute myelogenous leukemia. Blood 83:3474–3479, 1994.

261. Weisdorf D, Katsanis E, Verfaillie C, Ramsay NKC, Haake R, Garrison L, Blazar BR. Interleukin-1α administered after autologous transplantation: a phase I/II clinical trial. Blood 84:2044–2049, 1994.

262. Katsanis E, Weisdorf DJ, Xu Z, Dancisak BB, Halet ML, Blazar BR. Infusions of interleukin-1α after autologous transplantation for Hodgkin's disease and non-Hodgkin's lymphoma induce effector cells with antilymphoma cytolytic activity. J Clin Immunol 14:205–211, 1994.

263. De Vries P, Brasel KA, Eisenman JR, Alpert AR, Williams DE. The effect of recombinant mast cell growth factor on purified murine hematopoietic stem cells. J Exp Med 173:1205–1211, 1991.

264. Broxmeyer HE, Cooper S, Lu L, Hangoc G, Anderson D, Cosman D, Lyman SD, Williams DS. Effects of murine mast cell growth factor (c-kit proto-concogene ligand) on colony formation by human marrow hematopoietic progenitor cells. Blood 77:2142–2149, 1991.

265. Briddell RA, Bruno E, Cooper RJ, Brandt JE, Hoffman R. Effect of c-kit ligand on in vitro human megakaryocytopoiesis. Blood 78:2854–2859, 1991.

266. Du XX, Keller D, Maze R, Williams DA. Comparative effects of in vivo treatment using interleukin-11 and stem cell factor on reconstitution in mice after bone marrow transplantation. Blood 82:1016–1022, 1993.

267. Hoffman R, Tong J, Brandt J, Traycoff C, Bruno E, McGuire BW, Gordon MS, McNiece I, Srour EF. The in vitro and in vivo effects of stem cell factor on human hematopoiesis. Stem Cells 11(Suppl 2):76–82, 1993.

268. Metcalf D, Nicola NA. Direct proliferative actions of stem cell factor on murine bone marrow cells in vitro: effects of combination with colony-stimulating factors. Proc Natl Acad Sci USA 88:6239–6243, 1991.

269. Briddell R, Glaspy J, Shpall EJ, LeMaistre F, Menchaca D, McNicec I. Mobilization of myeloid, erythroid and megakaryocyte progenitors by recombinant human stem cell factor (rhSCF) plus filgrastim (rhG-CSF) in patients with breast cancer (abstract 109). Proc Am Soc Clin Oncol 13:77, 1994.

270. Glaspy J, McNiece I, LeMaistre F, Menchaca D, Briddell R, Lill M, Jones R, Tami J, Morstyn G, Brown S, Shpall EJ. Effects of stem cell factor (rh-SCF) and filgrastim (rhG-CSF) on mobilization of peripheral blood progenitor cells (PBPC) and on hematological recovery post-transplant: early results from a phase I/II study (abstract 76). Proc Am Soc Clin Oncol 13:68, 1994.

271. Crawford J, Lau D, Erwin R, Rich W, McGuire B, Meyers, F. A Phase I trial of recombinant methionyl human stem cell factor (SCF) in patients with advanced non-small cell lung carcinoma (NSCLC) (abstract 338). Proc Am Soc Clin Oncol 12:135, 1993.

272. Paul SR, Bennett F, Calvetti JA, Kelleher K, Wood CR, O'Hara RM Jr, Leary AC, Sibley B, Clark SC, Williams DA, Yang Y-C. Molecular cloning of a cDNA encoding interleukin 11, a stromal cell-derived lymphopoietic and hematopoietic cytokine. Proc Natl Acad Sci USA 87:7512–7516, 1990.

273. Du XX, Williams DA. Interleukin-11: a multifunctional growth factor derived from the hematopoietic microenvironment. Blood 83:2023–2030, 1994.

274. Paul SR, Yang Y-C, Donahue RE, Goldring S, Williams DA. Stromal cell-associated hematopoiesis: immortalization and characterization of a primate bone marrow-derived stromal cell line. Blood 77:1723–1733, 1991.

275. Schibler KR, Yang Y-C, Christensen RD. Effect of interleukin-11 on cycling status and clonogenic maturation of fetal and adult hematopoietic protentiators. Blood 80:900–903, 1992.

276. Bruno E, Briddell RA, Cooper RJ, Hoffman R. Effects of recombinant interleukin 11 on human megakaryocyte progenitor cells. Exp Hematol 19:378–381, 1991.

277. Quesniaux VF, Clark SC, Turner K, Fagg B. Interleukin-11 stimulates multiple phases of erythropoietin in vitro. Blood 80:1218–1223, 1992.

278. Tsuji K, Lyman DS, Sudo T, Clark SC, Ogawa M. Enhancement of murine hematopoiesis by synergistic interactions between steel factor (ligand for c-kit), interleukin-11, and other early acting factors in culture. Blood 79:2855–2860, 1992.

279. Du X, Neben T, Goldman S, Williams DA. Effects of recombinant human interleukin-11 on hematopoietic reconstitution in transplant mice: acceleration of recovery of peripheral blood neutrophils and platelets. Blood 81:27–34, 1993.

280. Neben TY, Loebelenz J, Hayes L, McCarty K, Stoudemire J, Schaub R, Goldman SJ. Recombinant human interleukin-11 stimulates megakaryocytopoiesis and increases peripheral platelets in normal and splenectomized mice. Blood 81:901–908, 1993.

281. Bree A, Schlerman F, Timony G, McCarthy K, Stoudemire J. Pharmacokinetics and thrombopoietic effects of recombinant human interleukin-11 (rhIL-11) in nonhuman primates and rodents (abstract). Blood 78(Suppl 1):132, 1991.

282. Hangoc G, Yin T, Cooper S, Schendel P, Yang Y-C, Broxmeyer HE. In vivo effects of recombinant interleukin-11 on myelopoiesis in mice. Blood 81:965–972, 1993.

283. Nash RA, Seidel K, Storb R, Slichter S, Schuening FG, Appelbaum FR, Becker AB, Bolles L, et al. Effects of rhIL-11 on normal dogs and after sublethal radiation. Exp Hematol 23:389–396, 1995.

284. Orazi A, Cooper R, Tong J, Gordon MS, Battiato L, Sledge GW Jr, Kaye J, Hoffman R. Recombinant human interleukin-11 (Neumega™, rhIL-11 growth factor; rhIL-11) has multiple profound effects of human hematopoiesis (abstract). Blood 82:1460a, 1993.

285. Du XX, Doerschuk CM, Orazi A, Williams DA. A bone marrow stromal-derived growth factor, interleukin-11, stimulates recovery of small intestinal mucosal cells after cytoablative therapy. Blood 83:33–37, 1994.

286. Champlin RE, Mehra R, Kaye JA, Woodin MB, Geisler D, Davis M, et al. Recombinant human interleukin eleven (rhIL-11) following autologous BMT for breast cancer (abstract 1567). Blood 84(Suppl):395a, 1994.

287. Dutcher JP, Gaynor ER, Boldt DH, Doroshow JH, Bar MH, Sznol M, et al. A phase II study of high-dose continuous infusion interleukin-2 with lymphokine-activated killer cells in patients with metastatic melanoma. J Clin Oncol 9:641–648, 1991.

288. Sosman JA, Kohler PC, Hank J, Moore KH, Bechhofer R, Storer B, Sondel PM. Repetitive weekly cycles of recombinant human interleukin-2: rsponses of renal carcinoma with acceptable toxicity. J Natl Cancer Inst 80:60–63, 1988.

289. Rosenberg SA, Lotze MT, Yang JC, Aebersold PM, Linehan WM, Seipp CA, White DE. Experience with the use of high dose interleukin-2 in the treatment of 652 patients with cancer. Ann Surg 210:474–484, 1989.

290. Rosenberg SA, Lotze MT, Muul LM, Chang AE, Avis FP, Leitman S, Linehan WM, et al. A progress report on the treatment of 157 patients with advanced cancer suing lymphokine-activated killer cells and interleukin-2 or high-dose interleukin-2 alone. N Engl J Med 316:889–897, 1987.

291. Rosenstein M, Ettinghausen SE, Rosenberg SA. Extravasation of intravascular fluid mediated by the systemic administration of recombinant interleukin-2. J Immunol 137:1735–1742, 1986.

292. Vetto JT, Papa MZ, Lotze MT, Chang AE, Rosenberg SA. Reduction of toxicity of interleukin-2 and lymphokine-activated killer cells in humans by the adminisration of corticosteroids. J Clin Oncol 5:496–503, 1987.

293. Funke I, Prummer O, Schrezenmeier H, et al. Capillary leak syndrome associated with

296

elevated IL-2 serum levels after allogeneic bone marrow transplantation. Ann Hematol 68:49–52, 1994.

294. Michon J, Négrier S, Coze C, Mathiot C, Frappaz D, Oskam R, et al. Administration of high-dose recombinant interleukin 2 after autologous bone marrow transplantation in patients with neuroblastoma: toxicity, efficacy, and survial. A Lyon-Marseille-Curie-East of France Group Study. In Advances in Neuroblastoma Research 4. New York: Wiley-Liss, 1994, pp. 293–300, 1994.

295. Bosly A, Price P, Humblet Y, Doyen C, Faille A, Chatelain B, Franks C, Gisselbrecht C, Symann M. Interleukin-2 after autologous bone marrow transplantation as consolidation immunotherapy against minimal residual disease. Nouv Revue Franc Hematol 32:13–16, 1990.

296. Bilgrami S, Silva M, Cardoso A, Miller KB, Ascensao JL. Immunotherapy with autologous bone-marrow transplantation: rationale and results. Exp Hematol 22:1039–1050, 1994.

297. Gottlieb DJ, Prentice HG, Heslop HE, Bello-Fernandez C, Bianchi AC, Galazka AR, Brenner MK. Effects of recombinant interleukin-2 administration on cytotoxic function following high-dose chemo-radiotherapy for hematological malignancy. Blood 74:2335–2342, 1989.

298. Gottlieb DJ, Brenner MK, Heslop HE, Bianchi AC, Bello-Fernandez C, Mehta AB, et al. A phase I clinical trial of recombinant interleukin-2 following high dose chemo-radiotherapy for haematological malignancy: applicability to the elimination of minimal residual disease. Br J Cancer 60:610–615, 1989.

299. Blaise D, Olive D, Stoppa AM, Viens P, Pourreau C, Lopez M, Attal M, et al. Hematologic and immunologic effects of the systemic administration of recombinant interleukin-2 after atuologous bone marrow transplantation. Blood 76:1092–1097, 1990.

300. Weisdorf DJ, Anderson PM, Blazar BR, Uckun FM, Kersey JH, Ramsay NK. Interleukin 2 immediately after autologous bone marrow transplantation for acute lymphoblastic leukemia — a phase I study. Transplant 55:61–66, 1993.

301. Higuchi CM, Thompson JA, Petersen FB, Buckner DC, Fefer A. Toxicity and immunomodulatory effects of interleukin-2 after autologous bone marrow transplantation for hematologic malignancies. Blood 77:2561–2568, 1991.

302. Fefer A, Benyunes MC, Massumoto C, et al. Interleukin-2 therapy after autologous bone marrow transplantation for hematologic malignancies. Semin Oncol 20(Suppl 9):41–45, 1993.

303. Prentice HG, MacDonald ID, Hamon MD. Understanding the mechanism of cure of acute myeloid leukemia by allogeneic bone marrow transplantation: toward the application of interleukin-2 in autologous bone marrow transplantation. J Hematother 3:47–50, 1994.

304. Klingemann H-G, Eaves C, Eaves AC, Nantel SH, Barnett MJ, Reece DE, et al. Transplantation of autologous bone marrow cultured in interleukin-2 to support myeloablative chemotherapy in poor prognosis acute myeloid leukemia (AML) (abstract). Blood 78(Suppl 1):246a, 1991.

305. Soiffer RJ, Murray C, Cochran K, Cameron C, Want E, Schow PW, Daley JF, Ritz J. Clinical and immunologic effects of prolonged infusion of low-dose recombinant interleukin-2 after autologous and T-cell-depleted allogeneic bone marrow transplantation. Blood 79:517–526, 1992.

306. Soiffer RJ, Murray C, Gonin R, Ritz J. Effect of low-dose interleukin-2 on disease relapse after T-cell-depleted allogeneic bone marrow transplantation. Blood 84:964–971, 1994.

307. Agah R, Malloy B, Kerner M, Mazumder A. Generation and characterization of IL-2-activated bone marrow cells as potent graft vs tumor effector in transplantation. J Immunol 143:3093–3099, 1989.

308. Agah R, Malloy B, Kerner M, Girgis E, Bean P, Twomey P, Mazumder A. Potent graft antitumor effect in natural killer-resistant disseminated tumors by transplantation of interleukin 2-activated syngeneic bone marrow in mice. Cancer Res 49:5959–5963, 1989.

309. Ades EW, Peacocke N, Sabio H. Lymphokine-activated killer cell lysis of human neuroblas-

toma cells: a model for purging tumor cells from bone marrow. Clin Immunol Immunopathol 46:150–156, 1988.

310. Charak BS, Malloy B, Agah R, Mazumder A. A novel approach to purging of leukemia by activation of bone marrow with interleukin 2. Bone Marrow Transplant 6:193–198, 1990.

311. Gambacorti-Passerini C, Rivoltini L, Fizzotti M, Rodolfo M, Sensi MI, Castelli C, et al. Selective purging by human interleukin-2 activated lymphocytes of bone marrows contaminated with a lymphoma line or autologous leukemic cells. Br J Haematol 78:197–205, 1991.

312. Agah R, Mazumder A. The potential usefulness of interleukin-2 activated bone marrow cells as an active therapeutic tool against cytomegalovirus infection in a bone marrow transplantation setting. J Clin Immunol 9:223–228, 1989.

313. Straneva JE, van Besien KW, Derigs G, Hoffman R. Is interleukin 6 the physiologic regulator of thrombopoiesis? Exp Hematol 20:47–50, 1992.

314. Lok S, Kaushansky K, Holly RD, et al. Cloning and expression of murine thrombopoietin cDNA and stimulation of platelet prodcution in vivo. Nature 369:565–568, 1994.

315. Miyasaki H, Kato T, Ogami K, et al. Isolation and cloning of a novel human thrombopoietin factor (abstract). Exp Hematol 22:838a, 1994.

316. Kaushansky K, Lok S, Holly RD, et al. Promotion of megakaryocyte progenitor expansion progenitor expansion and differentiation by the c-Mpl ligand thrombopoietin. Nature 369:568–571, 1994.

317. Hogge DE, Cashman JD, Humphires RK, Eaves CJ. Differential and synergistic effects of human granulocyte-macrophage colony-stimulating factor and human granulocyte colony-stimulating factor on hematopoiesis in human long-term marrow cultures. Blood 77:493–499, 1991.

318. McNiece I, Andrews R, Stewart M, et al. Action of interleukin-3, G-CSF, and GM-CSF on highly enriched human hemaptopoietic progenitor progenitor cells: synergistic interaction of GM-CSF plus G-CSF. Blood 74:110–114, 1989.

319. McNicec IK, Robinson BE, Quesenberry PJ. Stimulation of murine colony-forming cells with high proliferative potential by the combination of GM-CSF and CSF-1. Blood 72:191–195, 1988.

320. Krumwieh D, Siebold B, Weinmann E, Seiler FR. Combined effects of granulocyte-macrophage colony-stimulating factor with erythropietin in subhuman primates. Am J Clin Oncol 14(Suppl 1):S1–S4, 1991.

321. Krumwieh D, Weinmann E, Sieblod B, Seiler FR. Preclinical studies on synergistic effects of IL-1, IL-3, G-CSF, and GM-CSF in cynomolgus monkeys. Int J Cell Cloning 8(Suppl 1):229–248, 1990.

322. Musashi M, Yang YC, Paul SR, Clark SC, Sudo T, Ogawa M. Direct and synergistic effects of interleukin 11 on murine hemopoiesis in culture. Cell 88:765–769, 1991.

323. Moore MA. The future of cytokine combination therapy. Cancer 67(10, Suppl):2718–2726, 1991.

324. Kanz L, Brugger W, Bross K, Mertelsmann R. Combination of cytokines: current status and future prospects. Br J Haematol 79:96–104, 1991.

325. Bruno E, Miller ME, Hoffman R. Interacting cytokines regulate in vitro human megakaryopoiesis. Blood 73:671–677, 1989.

326. Groopman JE, Molina J-M, Scadden DT. Hematopoietic growth factors. Biology and clinical applications. N Engl J Med 321:1449–1459, 1989.

327. Rabinowitz I, Stuart A, Petros W, et al. Endogenous cytokine secretion after high-dose chemotherapy with autologous bone marrow support (abstract). Blood 76:162a, 1990.

328. Pene R, Appelbaum FR, Fisher L, et al. Use of granulocyte-macrophage colony-stimulating factor and erythropoietin in combination after autologous marrow transplantation. Bone Marrow Transplant 11:219–222, 1993.

329. Chao NJ, Schriber JR, Long GD, Negrin RS, Catolico M, Brown BW, Miller LL, Blume KG. A randomized study of erythropoietin and granulocyte colony-stimulating factor (G-CSF) versus placebo and G-CSF for patients with Hodgkin's and non-Hodgkin's lymphoma undergoing autologous bone marrow transplantation. Blood 83:2823–2828, 1994.

330. Locatelli F, Zecca M, Ponchio L, Beguin Y, Giorgiani G, Maccario R, Bonetti F, De Stefano P, Cazzola M. Pilot trial of combined administration of eryhtropoietin and granulocyte colony-stimulation factor to children undergoing allogeneic bone marrow transplantation. Bone Marrow Transplant 14:929–935, 1994.

331. Albin N, Douay L, Fouillard L, Laporte JP, Isnard F, Lesage S, et al. In vivo effects of GM-CSF and IL-3 on hematopoietic cell recovery in bone marrow and blood after autologous transplantation with mafosfamide-purged marrow in lymphoid malignancies. Bone Marrow Transplant 14:253–259, 1994.

332. Suttorp M, Schmitz N, Prange E, Ganser A, Löffler H, Schaub J, et al. Successful stimulation of autologous bone marrow recovery by GM-CSF and IL-3 after an unrelated donor BMT for juvenile CML complicated by graft failure (abstract). Bone Marrow Transplant 7(Suppl 2):84, 1991.

333. Nagler A, Naparstek E, Drakos P, Brautbar C, Goldman M, Kaplan O, Fridman A, Slavin S. Interleukin-3 in combination with granulocyte-macrophage-colony-stimulating factor following bone marrow transplantation in a radiation accident victim (letter). Med Oncol 11:27–28, 1994.

334. Crump M, Couture F, Kovacs M, Saragosa R. McGrae J, Brandwein J, Huebsch L, Beauregard-Zollinger L, Keating A. Interleukin-3 followed by GM-CSF for delayed engraftment after autologous bone marrow transplantation. Exp Hematol 21:405–410, 1993.

335. Fay JW, Lazarus H, Herzig R, Saez R, Stevens DA, Collins RH Jr, et al. Sequential administration of recombinant human interleukin-3 and granulocyte-macrophage colony-stimulating factor after autologous bone marrow transplantation for malignant lymphoma: a phase I/II multicenter study. Blood 84:2151–2157, 1994.

336. Gonter PW, Hillyer CD, Strobert EA, et al. Enhanced post-chemotherapy platelet and neutrophil recovery using combination rhIL-6 and rhGM-CSF or rhG-CSF in a nonhuman primate model (abstract 1444). Blood 82:365a, 1993.

337. Fay JW, Stein B, Collins R, Piñeiro L, Dutcher J. Gucalp R, et al. Concomitant administration of interleukin-6 (rhIL-6) and rhGM-CSF following autologous bone marrow transplantation — a phase I trial update (abstract 247). Proc Am Soc Clin Oncol 13:111, 1994.

338. Ulich TR, del Castillo J, Yi ES, Yin S, McNiece I. Yung YP, Zsebo KM. Hematologic effects of stem cell factor in vivo and in vitro in rodents. Blood 78:645–650, 1991.

339. Ulich TR, del Castillo J, McNiece IK, Yi ES. Alzona CP, Yin SM, Zsebo KM. Stem cell factor in combination with granulocyte colony-stimulating factor (CSF) or granulocyte-macrophage CSF synergistically increases granulopoiesis in vivo. Blood 78:1954–1962, 1991.

340. Molineux G, Migdalska A, Szmitkowski M, Zsebo K, Dexter TM. The effects on hematopoiesis of recombinant stem cell factor (ligand for c-kit) administered to mice either alone or in combination with granulocyte colony-stimulating factor. Blood 78:961–966, 1991.

341. Briddell RA, Hartley CA, Smith KA, McNiece IK. Recombinant rat stem cell factor synergizes with human granulocyte colony-stimulating factor in vivo in mice to mobilize peripheral blood progenitor cells that have enhanced repopulating potential. Blood 82:1720–1723, 1993.

342. Morstyn G, Glaspy J, Shpall EJ, LeMaistre F. Briddell R, Menchaca D, Lill M, Jones RB, Tami J, Brown S, et al. Clinical applications of filgrastim and stem cell factor in vivo and in vitro. J Hematother 3:353–355, 1994.

343. Yan XQ, Briddell R, Hartley C, Stoney G, Samal B, McNiece I. Mobilization of long-term hematopoietic reconstituting cells in mice by the combination of stem cell factor plus granulocyte colony-stimulating factor. Blood 84:795–799, 1994.

344. Andrews RG, Briddell RA, Knitter GH, Rowley SD, Appelbaum FR, McNiece IK. Rapid engraftment by peripheral blood progenitor cells mobilized by recombinant human stem cell factor and recombinant human granulocyte colony-stimulating factor in nonhuman primates. Blood 85:15–20, 1995.

345. Andrews RG, Briddell RA, Knitter GH, Opie T, Bronsden M, Myerson D, Appelbaum FR, McNiece IK. In vivo synergism between recombinant human stem cell factor and recombi-

nant human granulocyte colony-stimulating factor in baboons enhanced circulation of progenitor cells. Blood 84:800–810, 1994.

346. Clark RE, Shlebak AA, Creagh MD. Delayed commencement of granulocyte colony-stimulating factor following autologous bone marrow transplantation accelerates neutrophil recovery and is cost effective. Leuk Lymphoma 16:141–146, 1994.

347. Vey N, Molnar S, Faucher C, Le Corroller AG, Stoppa AM, Viens P, et al. Delayed administration of granulocyte colony-stimulating factor after autologous bone marrow transplantation: effect on granulocyte recovery. Bone Marrow Transplant 14:779–782, 1994.

348. Khwaja A, Mills W, Leveridge K, Goldstone AH, Linch DC. Efficacy of delayed granulocyte colony-stimulating factor (G-CSF) after autologous bone marrow transplantation (ABMT) (abstract). Br J Haematol 84(Suppl 1):12, 1993.

349. Hillner BE, Smith TJ, Desch CE. Efficacy and cost-effectiveness of autologous bone marrow transplantaion in metastatic breast cancer. Estimates using decision analysis while awaiting clinical trial results. JAMA 267:2055–2061, 1992.

350. Welch HG, Larson EB. Cost effectiveness of bone marrow transplantaion in acute nonlymphocytic leukemia. N Engl J Med 321:807–812, 1989.

351. Vose JM, Armitage JO. Clinical applications of hematopoietic growth factors. J Clin Oncol 13:1023–1035, 1995.

352. Petros WP, Peters WP. Cost implications of haematopoietic growth factors in the BMT setting. Bone Marrow Transplant 11(Suppl 2):36–38, 1993.

353. Finley RS. Measuring the cost-effectiveness of hematopoietic growth factor therapy. Cancer 67:2727–2730, 1991.

354. Lyman GH, Lyman CG, Sanderson RA, et al. Decision analysis of hematopoietic growth factor use in patients receiving cancer chemotherapy. J Natl Cancer Inst 85:1935–1936, 1993.

355. Charack BS, Sadowski RM, Mazunder A. Granulocyte-macrophage colony stimulating factor in autologous bone marrow transplantation: augmentation of graft versus tumor effect via antibody dependent cellular cytotoxicity. Leuk Lymphoma 9:453–457, 1993.

356. Giralt S, Escudier S, Kantarjian H, Deisseroth A, Freireich EJ, Andersson BS, et al. Preliminary results of treatment with filgrastim for relapse of leukemia and myelodysplasia after allogeneic bone marrow transplantation. N Engl J Med 329:757–761, 1993.

357. Richard C, Baro J, Bello-Fernandez C, Hermida G, Calavia J, Olalla I, et al. Recombinant human granulocyte-macrophage colony stimulating factor (rhGM-CSF) administration after autologous bone marrow transplantation for acute myeloblastic leukemia enhances activated killer cell function and may diminish leukemic relapse. Bone Marrow Transplant 15:721–726, 1995.

358. Nemunaitis J. Biological activities of hematopoietic growth factors that lead to future clincial application. Cancer Invest 12:516–529, 1994.

359. Takahashi S, Okamoto S-I, Shirafuji N, Ikebuchi K, Tani K, Shimane M, et al. Recombinant human glycosylated granulocyte colony-stimulating factor (rhG-CSF)-combined regimen for allogeneic bone marrow transplantation in refractory acute myeloid leukemia. Bone Marrow Transplant 13:239–245, 1994.

360. Bodey GP, Anaissie E, Gutterman J, Vadhan-Raj S. Role of granulocyte-macrophage colony-stimulating factor as adjuvant therapy for fungal infection in patients with cancer. Clin Infect Dis 17:705–707, 1993.

361. Peschel C, Huber C, Aulitzky WE. Clinical applications of cytokines. Presse Med 23:1083–1091, 1994.

362. Bonewald LF. Can transforming growth factor beta be useful as a protective agent for pluripotent hematopoietic progenitor cells? Exp Hematol 20:1249–1251, 1992.

363. Moore MAS. Clinical implications of positive and begative hematopoietic stem cell regulators. Blood 78:1–19, 1991.

364. Jones TC. Future uses of granulocyte-macrophage colony-stimulating factor (GM-CSF). Stem Cells 12(Suppl 1):229–240, 1994.

365. Lowry PA, Tabbara IA. Mini review. Peripheral blood hematopoietic stem cell transplantation: current concepts. Exp Hematol 20:937–942, 1992.

366. Kessinger A, Bishop M, Jackson J, Anderson J, O'Kane Murphy B, Vose J, et al. Erythropoietin (EPO) for mobilization of circulating progenitor cells in patients with previously treated malignancies (abstract 892). Blood 82(Suppl):227a, 1993.

367. Naparstek E, Hardan Y, Ben-Shaher M, Nagler A. Or R, Mumcuoglu M, Weiss L, Samuel S, Slavin S. Enhanced marrow recovery by short preincubation of marrow allografts with human recombinant interleukin 3 and granulocyte-macrophage colony stimulating factor. Blood 80:1673–1678, 1992.

368. Atkinson K, Bartlett A, Dodds A, Rallings M. Lack of efficacy of a short ex vivo incubation of human allogeneic donor marrow with recombinant human GM-CSF prior to its infusion into the recipient. Bone Marrow Transplant 14:573–577, 1994.

369. Kooler MR, Emerson SG, Palsson BO. Large-scale exansion of human stem and progenitor cells from bone marrow mononuclear cells in continuous perfusion cultures. Blood 82:378–384, 1993.

370. Brugger W, Heimfeld S, Berenson RJ, Mertelsmann R, Kanz L. Reconstitution of hematopoiesis after high-dose chemotherapy by autologous progenitor cells generated ex vivo. N Engl J Med 333:283–287, 1995.

371. Barge AJ. A review of the efficacy and tolerability of recombinant haematopoietic growth factors in bone marrow transplantation. Bone Marrow Transplant 11(Suppl 2):1–11, 1993.

372. Ward M, Richardson C, Pioli P, et al. Transfer and expression of the human multiple drug resistance gene in human CD34+ cells. Blood 84:1408–1414, 1994.

373. Brenner MK, Rill DR, Moen RC, Krance RA. Miro J Jr, Anderson WF, Ihle JN. Gene-marking to trace origin of relapse after autologous bone-marrow transplantatin. Lancet 341:85–87, 1993.

374. Brenner MK, Rill DR, Holladay MS, Heslop HE. Moen RC, Buschle M, et al. Gene marking to determine whether autologous marrow infusion restores long-term haemopoiesis in cancer patients. Lancet 342:1134–1137, 1993.

375. Deisseroth A, Zu Z, Claxton D, Hanania EG, Fu S. Ellerson D, et al. Genetic marking shows tat Ph+ cells present in autologous transplants of chronic myelogenous leukemia (CML) contribute to relapse after autologous bone marrow in CML. Blood 83:3068–3076, 1994.

376. Dunbar CE, Cottler-Fox M, O'Shaughnessy JA. et al. Retrovirally marked CD34-enriched peripheral blood and bone marrow cells contribute to long term engraftment after autologous transplantation. Blood 85:3048–3057, 1995.

377. Hughes PFD, Eaves CJ, Hogge DE, Humphries RK. High-efficiency gene transfer to human hematopoietic cells maintained in long-term marrow culture. Blood 74:1915–1922, 1989.

378. Nolta JA, Smogorzewska EM, Kohn DB. Analysis of optimal conditions for retroviral-mediated transduction of primitive human hematopoietic cells. Blood 86:101–110, 1995.

379. Bodine DM, Seidel NE, Gale MS, Nienhuis AW. Orlic D. Efficient retrovirus transduction of mouse pluripotent hematopoietnc stem cells mobilized into the peripheral blood by treatment with granulocyte colony-stimulating factor and stem cell factor. Blood 84:1482–1491, 1994.

IV

Clinical Applications: Continued Progress and New Frontiers

13. Bone marrow transplantation in thalassemia

Guido Lucarelli, Claudio Giardini, and Emanuele Angelucci

Thalassemia refers to various types of hereditary anemias identified by a reduced production of one of the globin chains that form the hemoglobin molecule [1]. In β-thalassemia, there is a deficient or absent synthesis of β-globin chains that constitute the adult hemoglobin molecule, which causes several deleterious effects on erythrocyte production and survival. Hemolysis and ineffective erythropoiesis lead to a chronic anemia with erythroid marrow hyperplasia; this determines an increase in the plasma iron turnover and, consequently, increased iron absorption. A progressive iron overload is associated with the above mechanism and is the consequence of the red cell transfusional regimen adopted to correct the anemia. Transfusions and regular iron chelation with deferoxamine constitute the conventional treatment for severe β-thalassemia. Homozygous thalassemia, which once resulted in early death, has become a chronic disease compatible with prolonged survival [2,3], although it remains a progressive disease.

Bone marrow transplantation

The first successful transplant in β-thalassemia was performed in Seattle on December 5, 1981, in an untransfused 14-month-old child [4]. At the same time, a 14-year-old thalassemic patient who had received 150 red cell transfusions was transplanted in Pesaro on December 17, 1981, but he had recurrence of thalassemia after rejection of the graft [5]. The experiences that followed, which were promptly reported in the literature by the Group of Pesaro, were disappointing, with the first series of patients transplanted using high doses of cyclophosphamide and total body irradiation (TBI) showing a high percentage of failures related to marrow rejection and early toxicity [5,6]. From 1983, a modification of the conditioning regimen originally proposed by Santos for leukemia [7] was adopted. This included a combination of busulfan (BU) and cyclophosphamide (CY) without use of radiation [8,9]. In 1990, a retrospective evaluation made in 222 consecutively transplanted patients led us to categorize patients under 16 years of age into three prognostically different classes of patients [10,11]. The risk factors considered included the presence of

Jane N. Winter (ed.) BLOOD STEM CELL TRANSPLANTATION. 1997. Kluwer Academic Publishers. ISBN 0-7923-4260-7. All rights reserved.

hepatomegaly (enlargement of more than 2 cm below the costal margin), the presence of liver fibrosis in the pretransplant liver biopsy, and the quality of iron chelation received before transplantation. The quality of chelation was considered adequate when deferoxamine therapy was initiated within 18 months after the first transfusion and administered subcutaneously for 8 to 10 hours for at least five days each week. Chelation was defined as inadequate if there was any deviation from this requirement. As of September 1995, 761 transplants in thalassemic patients have been performed in Pesaro, 714 from HLA-identical siblings, 22 from phenotypically identical parents, 24 from partially matched family members, and one from an HLA-identical unrelated donor. In this review, we update our experience in bone marrow transplantation in thalassemia from HLA-identical donors in 697 patients, with the last patient transplanted on December 29, 1994, and the analyses performed on September 30, 1995.

Bone marrow transplantation in class I patients

Class I patients are identified by absence of hepatomegaly, regular iron chelation therapy performed before transplant, and absence of fibrosis at the pretransplant liver biopsy [10–12].

Between June 1983 and December 31, 1994, 111 class I patients under the age of 16 years were transplanted using a conditioning protocol consisting of BU 14 mg/kg and CY 200 mg/kg. The graft-versus-host disease (GVHD) prophylaxis consisted of weekly methotrexate (MTX) before December 1985 and cyclosporine A alone from this date onwards. The median age of this group of patients was four years (range: 1–16 years); the median number of transfusions received pretransplant was 40 (range: 4–304; the median serum ferritin level was 1171 ng/ml (83–5200)). Patterns of liver function are shown in table 1. Thirty percent of patients had serological markers of hepatitis B (HBV) infection, and 31% (10 out of 32 patients tested) had evidence of hepatitis C (HCV) (table 1).

In patients receiving marrow transplants for thalassemia, liver fibrosis has never been observed before the age of three years [13]. In view of the known hazards of the liver biopsy procedure in very young children, patients under the age of three years did not undergo liver biopsy unless hepatomegaly was present; such infants were considered not to have liver fibrosis. In the remaining 79 patients, a pretransplant liver biopsy was performed (table 2). Liver iron overload was graded with semiquantitative estimation according to previously published criteria [14]. Using this procedure, 42 patients (53%) had a mild, 35 (44%) a moderate, and two patients (3%) a severe liver iron overload. A quantitative estimation of the liver iron content has been obtained for 28 patients: the median liver iron concentration was 7.0 mg/gram of dry tissue (range 1–24) (table 2).

In a Kaplan–Meier analysis, the probabilities of survival, event-free sur-

Table 1. Pretransplant characteristics of patients

	Children			Adults
	Class 1	Class 2	Class 3	
Patients	$n = 111$	$n = 294$	$n = 165$	$n = 86$
Age (years)				
Median	4	9	11	19
Range	1–16	1–16	3–16	17–32
No. transfusions				
Median	40	116	150	310
Range	4–304	2–430	4–435	130–600
Ferritin (ng/ml)				
Median	1171	1913	3187	1888
Range	83–5207	33–8547	604–17,450	322–9071
Bilirubin (mg/dl)				
Median	0.8	1.0	1.1	1.2
Range	0.2–3.8	0.2–4.4	0.1–7.0	0.1–5.9
AST (IU/l)				
Median	28	33	54	41
Range	9–123	6–166	5–415	13–419
ALT (IU/l)				
Median	27	57	104	73
Range	7–840	3–371	9–742	12–520
HBV Ab — Pos/Neg	34/77	116/178	94/71	62/24
HCV Ab— Pos/Neg	10/22	24/36	38/44	59/9

Table 2. Pretransplant liver histology and liver iron concentration

	Children			Adults
	Class 1	Class 2	Class 3	
Liver iron	$n = 79$	$n = 273$	$n = 165$	$n = 86$
Mild	42 (53%)	64 (23%)	16 (10%)	18 (21%)
Moderate	35 (44%)	162 (59%)	60 (35%)	41 (47%)
Severe	2 (3%)	47 (17%)	89 (55%)	27 (31%)
Liver fibrosis	$n = 79$	$n = 265$	$n = 165$	$n = 86$
Absent	79 (100%)	69 (26%)	0	0
Mild	0	98 (37%)	41 (24%)	26 (30%)
Moderate	0	75 (29%)	54 (32%)	20 (23%)
Severe	0	23 (9%)	70 (44%)	40 (46%)
Liver iron concentration[a]	$n = 28$	$n = 51$	$n = 35$	$n = 34$
25 percentile	5.0[a]	6.7	10.3	6.2
Median	7.0	10.0	15.1	12.7
75 percentile	10.0	18.0	30.0	22.3
Standard dev.	4.53	9.78	12.8	10.8
Range	1.0–24	0.8–43.0	3.0–47.0	1.4–46.7

[a] mg/gram dry tissue.

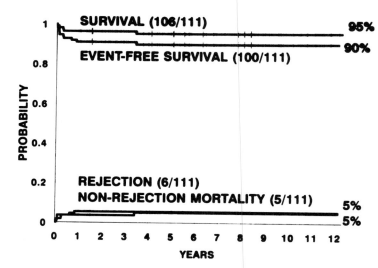

Figure 1. Kaplan–Meier probability statistics on survival, event-free survival, rejection, and nonrejection mortality for 111 class I patients less than 16 years old transplanted from HLA-identical family members.

vival, rejection, and nonrejection mortality are respectively 95%, 90%, 5%, and 5%, with a maximum follow-up of about 12 years (figure 1). Five patients died from causes related to the transplant. Six patients experienced rejection of the graft and all reconstituted autologous marrow. The last death occurred on day 1244, and the last episode of rejection on day 365. Two additional patients died from causes unrelated to the transplant procedure and the disease itself (car accidents) at day +993 and +3190; these patients have been censored from the Kaplan–Meier analysis at the day of the event.

Thirty patients (27%) presented with acute graft-versus-host disease (AGVHD), grade II to IV, and 12 patients (12%) developed a clinical form of chronic GVHD. From January 1986, all class I patients had received AGVHD prophylaxis consisting of cyclosporine A, 5 mg per kilogram intravenously daily from day −2 through day 5, followed by 3 mg per kilogram daily until the patient was able to tolerate oral administration at a daily dose of 12.5 mg per kilogram. The dose of cyclosporine was then tapered from day 60 until the drug was discontinued after one year (protocol 6).

Bone marrow transplantation in class II patients

Between June 1983 and December 1994, bone marrow transplants were performed in 293 class II patients. These patients are identified by the presence of either hepatomegaly, a history of irregular chelation performed before transplant, or histological evidence of liver fibrosis, or various combinations of two

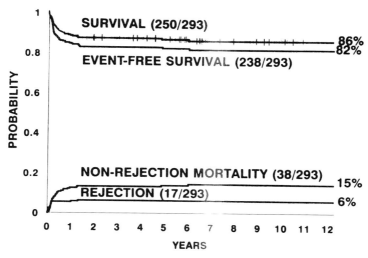

Figure 2. Kaplan–Meier probability statistics on survival, event-free survival, rejection, and nonrejection mortality for 293 class II patients less than 16 years old transplanted from HLA-identical family members.

of the above risk factors. The mean age was nine years (range: 1–16), the approximate total number of transfusions was 116 (range: 2–430), and the mean serum ferritin level was 1913 ng/ml (33–8547). One hundred and sixteen patients (39%) had serological markers of hepatitis B infection, and 40% (24 of 60 patients tested) of hepatitis C (table 1). The pretransplant liver biopsy (total number of biopsies performed and evaluable: 273) showed in 64 patients (23%) a mild, in 162 (59%) a moderate, and in 47 (17%) a severe iron overload. Liver fibrotic damage was absent in 69 patients (26%), mild in 98 (37%), moderate in 75 (29%), and severe in 23 (9%) (table 2). Quantitative estimation of the liver iron content has been obtained for 51 patients; liver iron concentration ranged from 0.8 to 43 mg/gram, with a median of 10.0 (table 2). This group includes three patients who, although affected by a genetically different disease (double heterozygotes, sickle-cell/β-thalassemia), were all regularly transfused and chelated from a young age; these patients have been evaluated and conditioned for transplant following the same strict schedule already in use for thalassemia.

The probabilities of survival, event-free survival, rejection, and nonrejection mortality are respectively 86%, 82%, 6%, and 15%, with a maximum follow-up of 12 years (figure 2). Forty-three patients died from transplant-related causes: 22 patients died within the first 100 days (most of them during the aplastic phase and, during the early engraftment, from septic-hemorrhagic causes and acute GVHD); and 21 patients died after the first 100 days, 17 of them during the first year while on immunosuppressive therapy with cyclosporine A. Four patients died after the first year posttransplant: two of them from complications of a severe form of chronic GVHD, and two from

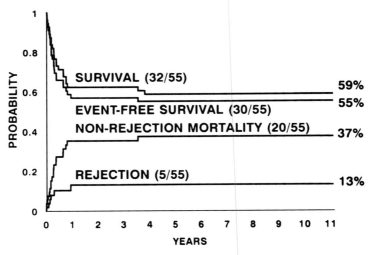

Figure 3. Kaplan–Meier probability statistics on survival, event-free survival, rejection, and nonrejection mortality for 55 class III patients less than 16 years old transplanted from HLA-identical family members before March 1989.

septic shock that suddenly caused death in a 24-hour period after the first symptoms began, most likely related to the splenectomized state. An additional patient died from accidental causes at day +1700, and he has also been censored from the analysis at the time of death. Seventeen patients rejected the graft; 12 of them have survived with autologous reconstitution, under transfusional support. Seventy-seven patients (28%) presented with acute GVHD, grade II to IV; 44 patients (17%) developed chronic GVHD.

Bone marrow transplantation in class III patients

Between June 1983 and March 1989, 55 patients were included in class III, since they presented all the aforementioned risk factors and had been transplanted after a total dose of BU 14 mg/kg and CY 200 mg/kg. The results of this clinical experience, when analyzed in 1990 [10,11] (updated in figure 3), were considered unsatisfactory because of a high incidence of early mortality due to toxicity and infections. It was thought that this toxicity was a consequence of high-dose CY in patients with preexisting liver damage, and admission of class III patients to protocol 6 was interrupted.

Beginning in March 1989, new conditioning protocols with a reduced dose of cyclophosphamide were introduced in search of less toxic adverse effects and according to the experiences in malignancies [15]. Between March 1989 and December 31, 1994, 110 patients were included in class III. The median age of the overall group, historical and post-March 1989 (165 patients), is 11 years (range 3–16), the median number of pretransplant transfusions 150

310

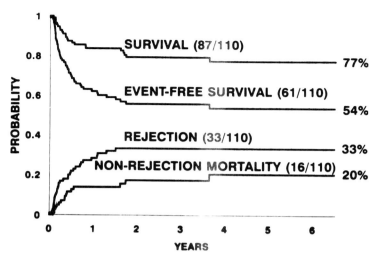

Figure 4. Kaplan–Meier probability statistics on survival, event-free survival, rejection, and nonrejection mortality for 110 class III patients less than 16 years old transplanted from HLA-identical family members from March 1989 through December 1994.

(range 4–435), the median serum ferritin level 3, 187 ng/ml (range 604–17,450). Ninety-four patients (57%) had serological markers of hepatitis B infection and 46% (38 out of 82 patients tested) of hepatitis C (table 1). The pre-transplant liver biopsy showed a mild iron overload in 16 patients (10%), a moderate form in 60 patients (35%), and a severe iron overload in 89 patients (55%); 41 patients (24%) had mild fibrosis, 54 (32%) moderate, and 70 (44%) a severe fibrotic liver damage. Quantitative estimation of the liver iron content has been obtained for 35 patients; liver iron concentration ranged from 3.0 to 47.0, with a median of 15.1 mg/gram (table 2).

The conditioning regimens studied since March 1989 included BU 14–16 mg/kg, a dose of CY variable from 120–160 mg/kg and, in some protocols, the use of antilymphocytic globuline (ALG). In a Kaplan–Meier curve, the probabilities of survival, event-free survival, rejection, and nonrejection mortality for this group of 110 patients are 77%, 54%, 33%, and 20%, respectively, with a maximum follow-up of six years (figure 4). Twenty-three patients died from causes related to the transplant. Thirty-three patients rejected the graft; 25 of them are alive with return of the thalassemia, and one patient has been successfully retransplanted. Fifteen patients (16%) developed grade II to IV acute GVHD, and seven (10%) developed chronic GVHD. The most recent analysis of a Kaplan–Meier curve including the subgroup of the 48 most recent class III patients, transplanted since June 1992 after busulfan 14 mg/kg and a total dose of 160 mg/kg of cyclophosphamide and with a maximum follow up of 37 months, shows 85% survival, 68% event-free survival, 25% rejection, and 15% nonrejection mortality. From the data presented here, the introduction of new protocols with a reduced dose of CY represents a promising step in the attempt to reduce the transplant-related mortality in this patient population. In fact, mortality is reduced from 37% to 20% (15% with the last modification of the conditioning regimen), although the rejection rate at the same time varied from 13% to 33%.

Bone marrow transplant in adult thalassemic patients

The early experience with transplantation for patients over 16 years was disappointing, with 4 of 6 patients dying of AGVHD and 2 patients dying 9 months and 6 years, respectively, after recurrence of the thalassemia [16]. In October 1988, bone marrow transplantation in patients older than 16 years was restarted after categorization of the patients into class II or class III and the adoption of the protocols used for these classes in younger patients. Through December 31, 1994, 86 adult thalassemic patients have been transplanted. The age ranged from 17 to 32 years (median 19). The median serum ferritin level was 1888 ng/ml (range: 322–9071). Sixty-two patients (73%) had serological makers of hepatitis B infection and 87% (59 out of 68 patients tested) of hepatitis C. Liver biopsy was performed before transplant in all 86 patients. Eighteen patients (21%) had mild, 41 (47%) moderate, and 27 (31%) severe iron overload; with regard to fibrosis, 26 patients (30%) had mild, 20 (23%) moderate, and 40 patients (46%) severe liver fibrosis. In some of these patients, the histological documentation was liver cirrhosis. All patients had a history of irregular iron chelation at the time of the pretransplant evaluation. This group also includes two patients affected by double heterozygous sickle-cell/β-thalassemia. By a Kaplan–Meier analysis, the probabilities of survival,

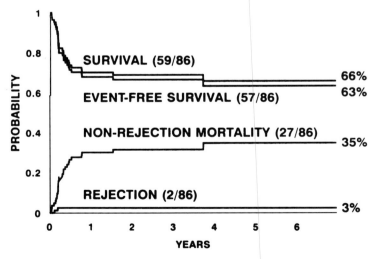

Figure 5. Kaplan–Meier probability statistics on survival, event-free survival, rejection, and nonrejection mortality for 86 patients 17 years of age or older transplanted from HLA-identical family members from October 1988 through December 1994.

event-free survival, rejection, and nonrejection mortality are 66%, 63%, 3%, and 35%, respectively (figure 5). Twenty-seven patients (32%) died from causes directly related to the transplant, mainly of sepsis or hemorrhage within the first 100 days. One patient, who was splenectomized before transplant, died from septic shock on day +1363. Two patients experienced rejection of the allogeneic marrow and are alive with complete autologous reconstitution. Twenty-three patients (27%) presented with acute GVHD, grade II to IV, and 10 patients (16%) developed chronic GVHD.

Mortality and causes of death

Table 3 summarizes the causes of death in the examined population. A total of 145 patients (21%) died. The incidence of infections was 37% (54 patients), with a prevalence of fungal (23 patients) and viral (18 patients) infections. The large majority of these lethal infections occurred during the period of bone marrow aplasia. Thirteen patients did not recover autologous hemopoeitic reconstitution after rejection of the allograft and died of causes directly related to the prolonged marrow aplasia. Acute and chronic GVHD have been direct or indirect causes of death in 34 patients (23%). An unusual cause of death, observed only after bone marrow transplantation in thalassemia, has been sudden cardiac tamponade, which occurred in six cases (4%) [17]. The mortality for veno-occlusive disease in this patient population has been lower than

Table 3. Causes of death

Cause	No.of patients (% of deaths)
Infections	54 (37%)
Bacterial	8 (6%)
Fungal	23 (16%)
Viral	18 (13%)
Protozoal	5 (3%)
Graft-versus-host disease	34 (23%)
Graft failure or rejection	13 (9%)
Cardiac	8 (6%)
Hemorrhage	6 (4%)
Adult respiratory distress syndrome	3 (2%)
B-cell lymphoma	2 (1%)
Idiopathic interstitial pneumonia	4 (3%)
Veno-occlusive disease of the liver	3 (2%)
Acute liver failure	3 (3%)
Thalassemia (late deaths after graft) rejection and autologous reconstitution	4 (3%)
Late septic shocks in splenectomized patients	3 (2%)
Died at home (cause uncertain)	4 (3%)
Car accident	4 (3%)
TOTAL	145 (100%)

expected in transplants done in patients with a high rate of liver damage and with BU as part of the preparative regimen. Three patients had late fulminant infections with fatal sudden shock. This complication has been attributed to the fact that these patients had been splenectomized years before the transplant and therefore could have had a higher susceptibility to encapsulated bacterial infections. For this reason, immunization against encapsulated bacteria such as pneumoncoccus, haemophilus, and meningococcus, and/or long-term antibiotic prophylaxis is highly recommended in these patients. Four patients who experienced rejection of the allograft and had complete autologous reconstitution died from causes related to progression of the disease itself (cardiac and infectious causes) between day +2213 and day +3180 posttransplant. Four patients died from causes unrelated to the transplant and the original disease (car accidents); these patients, as already mentioned, have been censored from the Kaplan–Meier analysis at the time of the event.

Conclusions

Today, allogeneic bone marrow transplantation represents the only therapeutic modality for the eradication of β-thalassemia major [18]. Several bone marrow transplant centers have ongoing clinical experience in this setting [19,25]. The first thalassemic patient was transplanted more than 13 years ago. Since then, the results of marrow transplantation have improved steadily, with major progress in the management of transplant-related complications. This is due to the use of cyclosporine, more effective treatment for cytomegalovirus infection, improvement of aseptic techniques, and evolution of systemic antibiotic therapy. At the moment, a patient in class I has a 5% probability of mortality, 4% probability of rejection, and 91% probability of disease-free survival posttransplant. In patients in classes II and III, the organ damage related to iron overload and to acquired blood-borne viral infections, is more advanced, and therefore transplant-related mortality is higher. However, these are patients who have developed progressive and significant organ damage while receiving conventional treatment. The survival expectations of such patients are poor in the absence of intervention by marrow transplantation [26,27]. Hopefully, in the future the improved management of graft-versus-host disease and the development of technologies for bone marrow transplantation from unrelated donors may expand the pool of potential candidates.

References

1. Weatherall DJ, Clegg JG. The Thalassemia Syndromes. Oxford: Blackwell Scientific Publications, 1981, pp. 744–782.
2. Piomelli S, Loew T. Management of thalassemia major (Cooley's anemia). Hematol Oncol Clin North Am 5:557–560, 1991.

3. Modell B, Letsky EA, Flynn DM, et al. Survival and desferrioxamine in thalassemia major. Br Med J 284:1081–1084, 1982.
4. Thomas ED, Buckner CD, Sanders JE, et al. Marrow transplantation for thalassemia. Lancet 2:227–229, 1982.
5. Lucarelli G, Izzi T, Polchi P, et al. Bone marrow transplantation in thalassemia. J Exp Clin Cancer Res 3:313–315, 1983.
6. Lucarelli G, Polchi P, Izzi T, et al. Allogeneic marrow transplantation for thalassemia. Exp Hematol 12:676–681, 1984.
7. Santos GW, Tutschka PJ, Brookmeyer R, et al. Marrow transplantation for acute nonlymphocytic leukemia after treatment with busulfan and cyclophosphamide. N Engl J Med 309:1347–1353, 1983.
8. Lucarelli G, Polchi P, Galimberti M, et al. Marrow transplantation for thalassemia following busulfan and cyclophosphamide. Lancet 1:1355–1357, 1985.
9. Lucarelli G, Galimberti M, Polchi P, et al. Bone marrow transplantation in advanced thalassemia. N Engl J Med 316:1050–1055, 1987.
10. Lucarelli G, Galimberti M, Polchi P, et al. Bone marrow transplantation in patients with thalassemia. N Engl J Med 322:417–421, 1990.
11. Lucarelli G, Galimberti M, Polchi P, et al. Bone marrow transplantation in thalassemia. Hematol Oncol Clin North Am 5:549–556, 1991.
12. Lucarelli G, Galimberti M, Polchi P, et al. Marrow transplantation in patients with thalassemia responsive to iron chelation therapy. N Engl J Med 329:840–844, 1993.
13. Muretto P, Angelucci E, Del Fiasco S, et al. Reversal feature of hepatic haemodisderosis and aemochromatiosis in thalassemia after bone marrow transplantation. In Buckner CD, Gale RP, Lucarelli G (eds), Advances and Controversies in Thalassemia Therapy: Bone Marrow Transplantation and Other Approaches. Prog Clin Biol Res 309:299–314, 1989.
14. Muretto P, Del Fiasco S, Angelucci E, et al. Bone marrow transplantation in thalassemia: modifications of hepatic iron overload and associated lesions after long-term engrafting. Liver 14:14–24, 1994.
15. Tutschka PJ, Copelan EA, Kapoor N. Bone marrow transplantation for leukemia following a new busulfan and cyclophosphamide regimen. Blood 70:1382–1388, 1987.
16. Lucarelli G, Galimberti M, Polchi P, et al. Bone marrow transplantation in adult thalassemia. Blood 80:1603–1607, 1992.
17. Angelucci E, Mariotti E, Lucarelli G, et al. Sudden cardiac tamponade after chemotherapy for marrow transplantation in thalassemia. Lancet 339:287–289, 1992.
18. Weatherall DJ. Bone marrow transplantation for thalassemia and other inherited disorders of hemogloin (editorial). Blood 80:1379–1381, 1992.
19. Di Bartolomeo P, Di Girolamo G, Agrilli F. et al. Treatment of thalassemia by allogeneic bone marrow transplantation. Bone Marrow Transplant 12(Suppl 1):37–41, 1993.
20. Lin KH, Linn KS. Allogeneic bone marrow transplantation for thalassemia in Taiwan: factors associated with graft failure. Am J Pediatr Hematol Oncol 11:417–420, 1989.
21. Frappaz D. Allogeneic bone marrow graft in thalassemia major. The French Experience. Arch Fra Pediatr 47:97–100, 1990.
22. Issagrilis S, Visudhisakchai S, Suvatte V, et al. Bone marrow transplantation for thalassemia in Thailand. Bone Marrow Transplant 12(Suppl 1):42–44, 1993.
23. Contu L, La Nasa G, Pizzati A, et al. Bone marrow transplantation in thalassemia. The Cagliari team experience. Bone Marrow Transplant 12(Suppl 1):45–46, 1993.
24. Walters MC, Thomas ED. Bone marrow transplantation for thalassemia: the United States experience. Am J Pediatr Hematol Oncol 16:11–17, 1994.
25. Vellodi A, Picton S, Downie CJC, et al. Bone marrow transplantation for thalassemia: experience of two British centers. Bone Marrow Transplant 13:559–562, 1994.
26. Nathan DG, Oski FA. Hematology of infancy and childhood, vol. 1, 4th ed. Philadelphia: WB Saunders, 1993, p. 845.
27. Ehlers KH, Giardina PJ, Lesser ML, et al. Prolonged survival in patients with beta-thalassemia major treated with deferoxamine. Pediatr 118:540–545, 1991.

14. Immune ablation and hematopoietic stem cell rescue for severe autoimmune diseases (SADS)

Richard K. Burt

Patients afflicted by an autoimmune disorder have generally been considered to have a normal life expectancy complicated by a relapsing/remitting or chronic disease. However, depending upon the disease, there may exist a subset of affected individuals who have a shorter survival than the general population. It is this high-risk group with early mortality for whom Marmont coined the term *SADS*, *severe autoimmune diseases* [1].

These disorders are believed to arise from an immune system that has lost tolerance to tissue-specific self epitopes. Treatment of SADS by broad spectrum immunosuppression is complicated by long-term toxicities and infections, and in most instances is not curative. Specific immunotherapy could be targeted to regulate an autoreactive subset of lymphocytes while leaving the overall immune system intact to avoid the infectious risks of broad-spectrum immunosuppression. However, animal studies suggest that once inflammation is initiated against an immunodominant epitope, T-cell clones are recruited against other subdominant or cryptic epitopes [2]. This phenomenon of epitope spreading would argue against any long-lasting effectiveness of specific immunotherapy. Consequently, it has recently been suggested that patients with SADS be considered candidates for complete immune ablation and autologous or allogeneic hematopoietic stem cell (HSC) reconstitution [3–6].

Rationale

High-dose chemoradiotherapy can ablate an aberrant immune system, and following either autologous or allogeneic HSC reconstitution, the immune system appears to be skewed towards suppression. The CD4 count is depressed, and the CD4/CD8 ratio is inverted for 12 to 18 months despite an otherwise healthy graft [7,8]. Memory for prior immunity to childhood vaccines is lost, and patients generally need to be reimmunized. Theoretically, lasting remission of an autoimmune disease may occur by 1) recapitulation of a naive immune system that may remain unresponsive to 'self' until reexposure to the original disease-initiating agent, 2) generation or infusion of suppressor cells, 3) infusion of genetically distinct allogeneic stem cells giving

Jane N. Winter (ed.) BLOOD STEM CELL TRANSPLANTATION. 1997. Kluwer Academic Publishers. ISBN 0-7923-4260-7. All rights reserved.

rise to T cells and antigen-presenting cells with different major and/or minor histocompatiblity-complex surface molecules, and/or 4) generation of tolerance through exposure of lymphocyte precursors to self epitopes early in development, possibly resulting in anergy and/or deletion of autoreactive repertoires.

Animal models of autoimmune disease

Autoimmune diseases in animals may arise spontaneously or after immunization. In general, those that occur spontaneously are restricted to inbred strains and arise from genetic defects in the hematopoietic stem cell compartment. Those that arise after immunization may occur in a variety of outbred species and are due to priming (i.e., activation) of normal, previously naive (i.e., unresponsive) lymphocytes.

Examples of spontaneously occurring autoimmune diseases are a systemic lupus erythematosus-like syndrome in New Zealand black (NZB)/New Zealand white (NZW) F1 (B/W) and MRL/lpr mice [9–11]; a scleroderma-like illness in Tsk mice [12,13] and UCD L200 chickens [14,15]; an inflammatory bowel disease in cotton top tamarin monkeys [16]; and an islet cell inflammatory disease similar to type I diabetes mellitus in NOD mice [17,18] (table 1). With exception of the MRL/lpr mouse, the exact genetic defect(s) remains enigmatic.

MRL/lpr mice develop a massive lymphoproliferative disease characterized by arthritis, glomerulonephritis, vasculitis, and anti-ds DNA antibody. These mice have a single gene defect that prevents high-level expression of the Fas receptor, a surface receptor that signals for apoptosis [20,21]. Normal mice express high levels of the Fas receptor protein on CD4/CD8 double-positive thymocytes, inducing apoptosis of potentially autoreactive T-cell clones. T cells normally upregulate Fas-receptor surface protein when activated, which by inducing cell death serves to control a lymphoproliferative response. In MRL/lpr mice, autoimmunity results from a lack of normal lymphocyte programmed cell death. Transplant of HSCs from MRL/lpr mice into an unaffected strain of mice results in the lpr phenotype and early death.

The NZB mouse develops spontaneous hemolytic anemia and high-titer antierythrocyte antibodies [9,10]. When the NZB mouse is bred with the phenotypically normal NZW mouse, the offspring (F1 hybrid, B/W) develop a fatal immune glomerulonephritis and high-titer anti-ds DNA antibody but low-titer antierythrocyte antibodies. Although hemolysis may occur, it is not prominent. The genetic defect in B/W mice is unknown, but transplantation of lymphocyte-depleted marrow to a normal mouse from another strain causes fatal immune glomerulonephritis [11]. Similarly, transplantation of lymphocyte-depleted marrow from Tsk [22] or NOD mice [23] to a genetically nonsusceptible strain results in disease.

Animal autoimmune diseases that arise after immunization with the appro-

318

priate self epitope include adjuvant-induced arthritis (AIA) [24], collagen-induced arthritis (CIA) [24,25], experimental autoimmune myasthenia gravis (EAMG) [26,27], experimental allergic encephalomyelitis (EAE) [28,29], experimental autoimmune myositis [30], and allergen-induced asthma [31] (table 1). Injection of tissue-specific protein in complete Freund's adjuvant initiates disease in susceptible species. Adoptive transfer of lymphocytes from affected animals to a naive syngeneic recipient can also induce disease through transfer of effector lymphocytes. Discussion will be limited to EAE, although the same principles apply to other models of autoimmune disease that arise by immunization with target-organ homogenate or immunodominant peptide(s).

EAE was first discovered as a disease in humans following immunization with the Pasteur vaccine for prevention of rabies [32]. Patients developed an ascending paralysis due to contamination of the vaccine by rabbit central nervous system antigens. Subsequently, it was found that injection of spinal cord homogenate with adjuvant causes neurologic deficits in a wide variety of species including mice, rats, rabbits, guinea pigs, and monkeys. Disease manifestations vary by species. Lewis rats develop a monophasic ascending paralysis with a transient inflammatory spinal cord infiltrate. Complete recovery without relapse or demyelination is the rule. In the Buffalo rat, EAE presents as an acute hemorrhage encephalomyelitis.

In the SJL/J mouse, EAE manifests as an inflammatory, demyelinating, relapsing remitting disease similar to relapsing remitting multiple sclerosis. Although EAE was initially induced with spinal cord homogenate, it was subsequently realized that small (10–14) amino acid sequences of myelin have the capacity to initiate disease. These specific immunogenic myelin peptide sequences include proteolipid protein (PLP) peptide sequence 139–151 or 178–191 and myelin basic protein (MBP) peptide sequence 169–181. If the animal is immunized with PLP 139–151, peripheral lymphocytes during the first relapse proliferate to 139–151. During subsequent relapses, epitope spreading occurs with lymphocytes proliferating to both PLP 139–151 and other immunogenic myelin peptides such as PLP 178–191 [2].

Viruses also offer models for autoimmune diseases. For example, Theiler's murine encephalomyelitis virus (TMEV) is a picornavirus that causes a chronic progressive neurologic disease clinically similar to primary progressive multiple sclerosis [33]. Histologically, the disease is marked by an inflammatory demyelination. Susceptible strains of mice are unable to clear the virus from the CNS, while strains resistant to TMEV resolve symptoms at the time of disappearance of the virus from the CNS [34]. Human autoimmune diseases, such as multiple sclerosis, have intermittently been associated with viral agents for which the TMEV model offers an experimental parallel [35].

Bone marrow transplant in animal models of autoimmune disease

Immune ablation and hematopoietic rescue has been attempted in several animal autoimmune disorders (table 2). Those that arise spontaneously and

Table 1. Animal models of human autoimmune diseases

Autoimmune disease [ref]	Animal model	Comment
Asthma [31]	Airborne allergen sensitization — various species — mouse, rat, guinea pig, rabbit, dog, horse, sheep	Inhalation of aerosolized protein, e.g., ovalbumin, ten minutes daily for five days, three weeks later breathing pattern in a whole-body plethysmograph recorded after reexposure to the aerosolized protein
Diabetes [17,18]	Nonobese animal — type I diabetes (NOD) mouse, BB rat, etc.	Spontaneous T-cell-mediated inflammation and destruction of islet cells causing hypoinsulinemia and hyperglycemia
[17,19]	Obese animals — type II diabetes KK mice, etc.	Spontaneous onset of peripheral insulin resistance with hyperinsulinemia and hyperglycemia
Inflammatory bowel disease [16]	Cotton top tamarin	A new world monkey on the endangered species list; develops spontaneous colitis resembling ulcerative colitis
Multiple sclerosis [28,29]	Experimental allergic encephalomyelitis (EAE) — SJL/J mice, Lewis rat, Buffalo rat, primates, etc.	Immunization with spinal cord homogenate or specific encephalogeneic myelin peptides causes ascending paralysis. Disease may be adoptively transferred by T cells
[33]	Theiler's murine encephalomyelitis (TMEV) — SJL/L mice	Oral ingestion or intracerebral injection of TMEV, a picornavirus, results in ascending paralysis and demyelination
Myasthenia gravis [27,26]	Experimental autoimmune myasthenia gravis (EAMG) — mice, rats, guinea pigs, rabbits, primates	Immunization by injection of acetycholine receptor in complete Freund's adjuvant. Animals develop anti-acetylcholine receptor antibody and paralysis that improves after injection of tensilon

Disease	Model	Description
Myositis [30]	Experimental autoimmune myositis (EAM) — SJL/L mice, guinea pig, rat	Immunization by injection of xenogeneic muscle homogenates in complete Freund's adjuvant
	Familial canine dermatomyositis (FCD)	Autosomal-dominant disease of purebred collies: spontaneous onset 7–11 weeks old
Rheumatoid arthritis [24]	Adjuvant-induced arthritis (AIA) —rat	Injection of complete Freund's adjuvant intradermal
[25]	Collagen-induced arthritis (CIA) — rat	Injection of type II collagen in complete Freund's adjuvant intradermal
Scleroderma [13]	Tight skin mouse (Tsk)	Autosomal-dominant spontaneous disease, thickened skin with inflammatory infiltrate, antitopo I, and anti-RNA pol I antibodies
[14]	Avian scleroderma University of California Davis line 200 chicken (UCD L200)	Spontaneous scleroderma-like changes with inflammatory mononuclear infiltrate, antibodies to topoisomerase I (Scl-70)
Systemic lupus erythematosus (SLE) [9–11]	New Zealand Bielschowsky Black mated with New Zealand Whiteb mouse (NZB/NZW F1)	Spontaneous lethal immune complex glomerulonephritis, anti-ds DNA and anti-ss DNA antibody, anti-histone antibodies
	Murphy and Roth Lab/lymphoproliferation mouse (MRL/1pr)	Spontaneous massive lymphoproliferation, polyarthritis, high titer rheumatoid factor, anti-Sm, anti-ds DNA, anti-ss DNA antibody, immune complex glomerulonephritis. Arises from stem cell defect in Fas induced apoptosis

321

Table 2. Results of bone marrow transplant in animal models of autoimmune disease

Human disease [ref]	Animal model	Type of marrow transplant	Conditioning regimen	Result
Diabetes [23]	NOD mouse	Allogeneic	TBI	Reconstitution of marrow from a resistant strain prevents disease
Multiple sclerosis [42–45]	Experimental allergic encephalomyelitis (EAE) — Lewis rat, Buffalo rat, SJL/J mouse	Syngeneic	TBI or cyclophosphamide	BMT before onset of disease prevents disease; after onset of disease, BMT arrests disease but may not reverse neurologic deficits
Myasthenia gravis [41]	Experimental autoimmune myasthenia gravis (EAMG)	Syngeneic	Cyclophosphamide and TBI	BMT abolishes immune response to acetylcholine receptor
Rheumatoid arthritis [40]	Adjuvant-induced arthritis (AIA)	Syngeneic, allogeneic, or autologous	TBI	Syngeneic, allogeneic, and autologous BMT equally effective in curing AIA after onset of disease
[39]	Collagen-induced arthritis (CIA)	Syngeneic or allogeneic	TBI	BMT before onset of CIA prevented disease; after onset of CIA decreased progression
Systemic lupus erythematosus [36–38]	(NZB/NZW)F1, BXSB, MRL/lpr	Allogeneic	TBI	Allogeneic BMT from nonautoimmune-prone strain cures or prevents glomerulonephritis and immune and serologic abnormalities

are thought to be secondary to a stem cell defect have been cured by allogeneic BMT from a strain resistant to disease. For example, diabetes in the NOD mouse may be prevented by HSC transplant from a nonsusceptible strain [23]. Immune glomerulonephritis, anti-ds DNA antibody, and lymphocytic infiltration of the liver and kidneys disappear in lupus-prone mice after allogeneic BMT from a nonsusceptible strain [36–38].

In contrast to stem-cell-mediated autoimmunity, immunization-induced autoimmune disease has been reported to be arrested not only by allogeneic but also syngeneic and autologous BMT (table 2). Following autologous BMT, the inflammatory synovitis of AIA resolves [39,40]. After syngeneic BMT in animals with EAMG, anti-acetylcholine-receptor antibodies disappear and weakness reverses [41], while in EAE, neurologic progression is stopped [42–45]. Syngeneic BMT from an unimmunized animal prevents EAE if done before onset of disease. After onset of neurologic disease, syngeneic BMT prevents clinical progression, and peripheral lymphocytes no longer proliferate to myelin epitopes. However, depending on the animal and stage of disease, neurologic deficits may not completely resolve. Although the immunologic attack may be arrested, remyelination and/or axonal repair is necessary to reverse established neurologic damage.

The results of BMT in animal autoimmune disorders suggest that diseases that arise due to a stem cell defect require an allogeneic donor from an unaffected strain to be cured. In contrast, autoimmune diseases that arise from environmental stimuli (i.e., immunization) may be cured by a syngeneic or autologous graft. The contribution of genes versus environment in human autoimmune disease is poorly understood, but the implication is that some human autoimmune diseases may be cured by an autologous graft; others may require an allogeneic donor. For an autologous graft, the role of purging lymphocytes from the graft has not yet been addressed in animal models. Finally, results of BMT in EAE suggest that cure of an autoimmune disease may not cure the patient, since repair of the affected target organ may not occur.

Results of BMT in patients with autoimmune disorders

Allogeneic bone marrow transplant for leukemia or aplastic anemia has been performed in patients with a coincidental autoimmune disease (table 3). Most of these patients had rheumatoid arthritis because they developed aplastic anemia from gold or D-penicillamine therapy [46]. A total of nine patients with rheumatoid arthritis have undergone allogeneic matched sibling BMT. Eight patients had a complete clinical remission with disappearance of active disease including rheumatoid factor for several years after discontinuing all immunosuppressive medications. Similarly, one patient each with ulcerative colitis [47] and psoriasis [47] entered sustained remissions following allogeneic

Table 3. Results of BMT in humans with coincidental autoimmune disease

Type of BMT	Disease [ref]	Comment
Allogeneic	Multiple sclerosis [48]	Subjective neurologic symptoms (pain, fatique) improved; some objective neurologic signs improved, others worsened; early death from leukemia relapse
	Psoriasis [47]	1 case; no symptoms off all medications
	Rheumatoid arthritis [46]	9 reported cases; 1 relapsed, 8 without evidence of disease off all immunosuppressive medications
	Ulcerative colitis [47]	1 case; no symptoms off all medications
Autologous (unpurged)	Systemic lupus erythematosus [50]	Disappearance of symptoms but recurrence of anti-ds DNA antibody
	Myasthenia gravis [49]	Disappearance of anticholinergic receptor antibody, early death from lymphoma relapse

genotypically matched BMT for leukemia. A patient with myelodysplastic syndrome and multiple sclerosis died six months after transplant from relapsed leukemia [48]. Neurologic symptoms of pain and fatigue resolved and visual acuity improved, but new tremor, weakness, and cerebellar signs developed at the time of leukemia relapse. These symptoms could have been attributed to cyclosporine (e.g., tremors), disuse atrophy, infection, meningeal carcinomatosis, or progression of multiple sclerosis with reemergence of host hematopoiesis.

An autologous unpurged BMT performed in a patient with lymphoma and myasthenia gravis was complicated by early death from relapsed lymphoma [49]. However, following transplant, anti-acetylcholine-receptor antibody titers disappeared. Unpurged autologous transplant has also been reported in a patient with lymphoma and systemic lupus erythematosus with subsequent resolution of clinical disease but recurrence of disease specific anti-ds DNA antibody [50].

These case reports suffer from publication bias, since it is unlikely that an autoimmune process that fails to improve after BMT would be reported. To overcome this bias, the International Bone Marrow Transplant Registry has included a questionnaire on autoimmune disorders for all patients enrolled in the registry. Finally, several centers are activating protocols to transplant patients with SADS. To date, an otherwise normal patient with severe CREST syndrome was treated with high-dose cyclophosphamide and autologous marrow rescue in Genoa, Italy, resulting in a complete but transient remission [51]. Therefore, preliminary data suggest that if autologous marrow is to be used for hematopoietic rescue, the hematopoeitic stem cell product should be purged of lymphocytes before reinfusion.

Table 4. Severe autoimmune diseases/potential for BMT

Disease	Potential candidate	Monitoring disease
Crohn's disease	All or most of the following: young age at onset, multiple surgical procedures, short bowel/malabsorption, chronic steroid therapy, narcotic addiction, history of sepsis	Crohn's disease activity index (CDAI)
Multiple sclerosis	Primary or secondary progressive MS with rapid deterioration, e.g., greater than 1–2 Kurtzke EDSS points within 12 months	MRI, Kurtzke extended status disability scale, Scripps neurology rating scale
Myasthenia gravis	Respiratory involvement within 8 months of onset; rapid bulbar involvement	EMG, anticholinergic receptor antibody
Rheumatoid arthritis	Extra-articular disease, vasculitis; greater than 30 involved joints and poor functional status (e.g., >120 seconds to button and unbutton five buttons, or >21 seconds to walk 25 feet)	Rheumatoid factor, C3, C4, CH50, X-rays and/or MRI of involved joints, swollen joint count, arthritis impact measurement scales (AIMS), patient assessment of pain, erythrocyte sedimentation rate (ESR)
Scleroderma	Cardiopulmonary involvement; renal involvement	Scl-70 titer, end organ function, skin elasticity measurement, i.e., Rodnan score
Systemic lupus erythematosus (SLE)	Vasculitis; catastrophic antiphospholipid syndrome: cytopenias refractory to steroids, splenectomy, and alkylating agent; WHO class III, IV glomerulonephritis failing NIH short-course cyclophosphamide	ANA, anti-ds and anti-ss DNA antibody, anti-Sm, C3, C4, CH50 creatinine, creatinine clearance, proteinuria, SLE disease activity index

Patient selection for bone marrow transplant

In general, the expected mortality is less than 5% for autologous and 20% to 30% for allogeneic hematopoietic stem cell transplants. Therefore, despite the morbidity associated with autoimmune diseases, immune ablation and HSC rescue as a treatment alternative should be offered only to those individuals with a life expectancy shorter than the general age-matched population. Indeed, we have used the term *severe autoimmune diseases* (SADS), to define those with a shortened survival (Table 4).

Multiple sclerosis

Multiple sclerosis (MS) generally affects young individuals (age 20–40) and has a variable natural history: relapsing/remitting, primary progressive, secondary progressive, etc. [52]. Most patients have relapsing/remitting disease (70%) with the same life expectancy as the general population. However, the majority with progressive MS are wheelchair bound, bedridden, or dead within ten years of onset of progressive disease. Survival correlates best with the level of disability. Less than 6% of patients with an unrestricted activity level are dead within ten years, compared to a 70% mortality within ten years for patients confined to a wheelchair. The cause of death is generally infection, pulmonary embolus, arrhthymia, or suicide. BMT candidates should have high risk features for early mortality, i.e., relatively advanced disease (e.g., unable to walk more than 600 yards), with a rapid chronic progressive course (decline of 1 or more Kurtzke disability scales over one year).

The clinical course of MS may be followed by neurologic function disability scales such as the Kurtzke extended status disability scale or the Scripps neurology rating scale [53,54]. Changes in CNS inflammatory plaques may be monitored by gadolinium enhancement on MRI [55]. However, the correlation between the MRI findings and clinical disability is poor. Severe neurologic deficits may be present with minimal MRI activity. Conversely, a large number of plaques may be detected in patients with minimal clinical disability. The β-interferon trial demonstrated a reduction in MRI lesions in patients on interferon compared to placebo. Therefore, MRI imaging data may be useful as an outcome measure in identifying subclinical disease burden and possibly in predicting future disability.

Rheumatoid arthritis

Rheumatoid arthritis affects 0.5% to 1% of the U.S. population. Most patients have a normal life expectancy. Consequently, therapy has traditionally been based on an incremental pyramid scheme of nonsteroidal anti-inflammatory agents (NSAIA) and physical therapy, advancing to steroids if NSAIAs fail, and finally disease-modifying antirheumatic drugs (DMARDS) such as

326

methotrexate, gold, hydroxychloroquine, or D-penacillamine if steroids alone fail. Patients referred to in university medical centers tend to fare worse, with a progressive chronic course, radiologic joint distruction, and extraarticular disease. Poor prognostic indicators are more than 30 abnormal joints (50% survival at five years), time of more than 21 seconds required to walk 25 feet (60% survival at five years), and time of more than 120 seconds necessary to unbutton and button five buttons (50% survival at five years) [56,57]. Therefore, a questionnaire on activities of daily living, joint count, and simple functional tests can identify patients at high risk for early mortality who could be potential BMT candidates.

Systemic scleroderma

Patients with systemic scleroderma, characterized by fibrosis and vasculopathy, have a survival significantly shorter than the general population. Those patients with renal, cardiac, or pulmonary involvement have the worst prognostic variables [58–60]. Patients with renal disease, defined as rapid progressive insufficiency or proteinuria greater than 3.5 g/day, have a 40% three-year survival. Cardiac involvement (pericarditis, CHF, or arrthymias) has a 50% three-year survival. Patients with pulmonary scleroderma diagnosed by an interstitial disease on chest roentograph, carbon monoxide diffusing capacity (DLCO) less than 13 ml/min/mm Hg, or pulmonary hypertension on cardiac catheterization or Doppler echocardiogram have a survival of 60% at five years. Therefore, patients with early vital organ involvement may be considered potential BMT candidates. Disease may be followed by monitoring affected organ function and serology, e.g., Scl-70 titer.

Myasthenia gravis

Myasthenia gravis (MG) manifests as generalized weakness, fatigability, ophthalmoplegia, dysarthria, or dysphagia due to antibodies directed against the postsynaptic acetylcholine receptor [61]. These antibodies reduce the number of acetylcholine receptors by increasing endocytosis, complement-mediated damage, or blockade of the neurotransmitter binding site. MG has a prevalence of 5 to 12.5 per 100,000 and a bimodal incidence, with one peak at age 20 to 30 and another at age 60. Today most patients with MG have a normal life expectancy, and survival is 80% at ten years. Patients may be categorized by Osserman group into group I — ocular MG; group IIA — mild generalized MG; group IIB — moderate generalized MG; group III — acute fulminating, MG; and group IV — late severe MG. Patients in Osserman group III or IV with respiratory or bulbar muscle involvement, especially if onset was rapid, i.e., within eight months of diagnosis, have high risk features [62,63] and could be considered candidates for BMT. Disease may be followed by clinical muscle strength, antibody titer, and electromyography (EMG).

Systemic lupus erythematosus (SLE)

SLE is a multisystem, inflammatory disorder characterized by a variable presentation and clinical course that generally affects young women 20 to 40 years old. Diagnosis depends on fulfilling at least 4 of 11 American Rheumatism Association (ARA) criteria, which are antinuclear antibody, malar rash, discoid rash, photosensitivity, oral ulcers, arthritis, serositis, and a renal, neurologic, hematologic, or immunologic disorder(s) [64]. Anti-ds DNA and anti-Sm antibodies in high titer are specific for SLE. Five-year survival estimates vary widely and range from 68% to 98% [65–68]. The usual cause of death is sepsis, renal failure, vasculitis, or cytopenias. For patients with renal failure, survival is 80% at five years. BMT may, therefore, be considered for patients with cytopenias unresponsive to steroids, splenectomy, and an alkylating agent; vasculitis, e.g., cerebritis; or progressive renal failure, defined as WHO class III or IV glomerulonephritis that has failed NIH short-course cyclophosphamide ($500–1000 \, mg/m^2$ IV monthly for six months and then quarterly for two years) [69–72]. The renal status should be documented by biopsy and have a low chronicity (fibrosis, scarring) score and high activity (acute inflammation) index. A rare presentation of SLE is the catastrophic antiphospholipid syndrome, which gives rise to acute devastating multiple organ failure from occlusion of large and small arterial and venous vessels in a patient with antiphospholipid antibody [73]. If the patient survives the acute event, BMT may be considered to prevent recurrence.

Inflammatory bowel disease

Ulcerative colitis may be cured by resection of the colon. Crohn's disease may involve any part of the alimentary canal from mouth to anus. Although most patients with Crohn's disease have a normal life expectancy, for some patients mortality is slightly increased over the general population, with a ten-year overall survival of 85% [74,75]. The risk of early death is increased in those patients with most or all of the following: young age at onset, multiple surgical procedures, short bowel/malabsorption, chronic steroid therapy, narcotic addiction, and a history of sepsis [75].

Summary

In addition to our center (Northwestern University, Chicago), several institutions in the United States (Fred Hutchinson Cancer Center, University of California at Los Angeles, and Medical College of Wisconsin) and Europe are activating protocols to transplant patients with SADS. In this age of cost-effectiveness, it will be difficult to arrange third-party reimbursement for a hematopoietic stem cell transplant that may lead to medical charges of between $100,000 and $200,000. However, the cost of standard medical care for patients with SADS is not trivial. Dialysis for an SLE patient with renal failure costs $40,000 per year, while the medical resources required to care for a patient with progressive multiple sclerosis may exceed $35,000 per year.

Unique BMT regimen-related toxicities may occur, including intracranial hemorrhage in the SLE or rheumatoid arthritis patient who has vasculitis; acute neurologic decompensation in patients with multiple sclerosis, especially if the conditioning regimen contains neurotoxic agents that cross a compromised blood–brain barrier; respiratory failure in patients with myasthenia gravis; and increased renal or pulmonary toxicity in patients with scleroderma and parenchymal fibrosis. Scleroderma-associated gastrointestinal dysmotility and bacterial overgrowth may also lead to greater fungal and bacterial infections [76].

BMT is currently considered appropriate therapy for patients with chronic-phase Chronic myelogenous leukemia (CML) and indolent lymphomas who otherwise have a relatively long life expectancy of 5 and 10 years, respectively. The roughly similar long survival but greater functional impairment of patients with SADS may justify consideration of immune ablation and hematopoietic stem cell rescue.

Acknowledgment

I wish to acknowledge those physicians who have gone before me: Professor Marmont (Genoa), Professor van Bekkum (Netherlands), and Professor Robert Good (Moffit Cancer Center, Florida).

References

1. Marmont A. Personal comunication. Genoa. Italy.
2. McRae BL, Vanderlugt CL, Dal Canto MC. Miller SD. Functional evidence for epitope spreading in the relapsing pathology of experimental autoimmune encephalomyelitis: J Exp Med 182:75–85, 1995.
3. Marmont AM, van Bekkum DW. Stem cell transplantation for severe autoimmune diseases: new proposals but still unanswered questions. Bone Marrow Transplantation 16:497–498, 1995.
4. Burt RK, Burns W, Hess A. Bone marrow transplantation for multiple sclerosis. Bone Marrow Transplant 16:1–6, 1995.
5. Marmont A, Tyndall A, Gratwohl A, et al. Haemopoietic precursor-cell transplants for autoimmune diseases. Lancet 345(8955):978. 1995.
6. Marmont AM. Perspective immune ablation with stem-cell rescue: a possible cure for systemic lupus erythematosus? Lupus 2:151–156, 1993.
7. Forman SJ, Nocker P, Gallagher M. Pattern of T cell reconstitution following allogeneic bone marrow transplantation for acute hematologic malignancy. Transplantation 34:96–98, 1982.
8. Olsen GA, Gockerman JP, Bast RC, et al. Altered immunologic reconstitution after standard dose chemotherapy or high dose chemotherapy with autologous bone marrow support. Transplantation 46:57–60, 1988.
9. Heyler BJ, Howie JB. Renal disease associated with positive lupus erythematosus tests in a cross bred strain of mice. Nature 197:197. 1963.

10. Putterman C, Naparstek Y. Murine models of spontaneous systemic lupus erythematosus. In Cohen IR, Miller A (eds) Autoimmune Disease Models: A Guidebook. San Diego, CA: Academic Press 1994, pp. 217–243.
11. Akizuki M, Reeves JP, Steinberg AD. Expression of autoimmunity by NZB/NZW marrow. Clin Immunol Immunopathol 10:247–250, 1978.
12. Jimenez SA, Christner P. Animal models of systemic sclerosis. Clin Dermatol 12:425–436, 1994.
13. Kasturi KN, Shibata S, Muryoi T, et al. Tight-skin mouse an experimental model for scleroderma. Intern Rev Immunol 11:253–271, 1994.
14. van de Water J, Boyd R, Wick G, et al. The immunologic and genetic basis of avian scleroderma, an inherited fibrotic disease of line 200 chickens. Intern Rev Immunol 11:273–282, 1994.
15. Rose NR. Avian models of automimmune disease: lessons from the birds. Poultry Science 73:984–990, 1994.
16. Warren BF, Watkins PE. Animal models of inflammatory bowel disease. J Pathol 172:313–316, 1994.
17. Mendez JD, Ramos HG. Animal models in diabetes research. Arch Med Res 25(4):367–375, 1994.
18. Hanafusa T, Miyagawa J, Nakajima H, et al. The NOD mouse. Diabetes Res Clin Pract 24(Suppl):S307–S311, 1994.
19. Ikeha H. KK mouse. Diabetes Res Clin Pract 24(Suppl):S313–S316, 1994.
20. Cohen PL, Eisenberg RA. The lpr and gld genes in systemic autoimmunity: life and death in the Fas lane. Immunol Today 13(11):427–428, 1992.
21. Drappa J, Brot N, Elkon KB. The Fas protein is expressed at high levels on double positive thymocytes and activated mature T cells in normal but not MRL/lpr mice. Proc Natl Acad Sci U S A 90:10340–10344, 1993.
22. Walker MA, Harley RA, Delustro FA, et al. Adoptive transfer of tight-skin fibrosis to +/+ recipients by tsk bone marrow and spleen cells. Proc Soc Exp Biol Med 192:196–200, 1989.
23. LaFace DM, Peck AB. Reciprocal allogeneic bone marrow transplantation between NOD mice and diabetes-nonsusceptible mice associated with transfer and prevention of autoimmune diabetes. Diabetes 38:894–901, 1989.
24. Hayashida K, Ochi T, Fujimoto M, et al. Bone marrow changes in adjuvant-induced and collagen-induced arthritis. Arthritis Rheum 35(2):241–245, 1992.
25. Durie FH, Fava RA, Noelle RJ. Collagen-induced arthritis as a model of rheumatoid arthritis. Clin Immunol Immunopathol 73(1):11–18, 1994.
26. Patrick J, Lindstrom J. Autoimmune response to acetylcholine receptor. Science 180:871–872, 1973.
27. Vincent A. Experimental autoimmune myasthenia gravis. In Cohen IR, Miller A (eds) Autoimmune Disease Models: A Guidebook. San Diego, CA: Academic Press 1994, pp. 83–106.
28. Brocke S, Gijbels K, Steinman L. Experimental autoimmune encephalomyelitis in the mouse. In Cohen IR, Miller A (eds) Autoimmune Disease Models: A Guidebook. San Diego, CAL Academic Press 1994, pp. 1–14.
29. Steinman L, Schwartz G, Waldor M, et al. 1984. In Alvord EC Jr, Kies MW, Suckling AJ EAE: A Good Model for MS. New York, NY, A R Liss 1984, pp. 393–397.
30. Rosenberg N. Experimental models of inflammatory myopathies. Bailliere's Clin Neurol 2(3):693–703, 1993.
31. Karol MH. Animal models of occupational asthma. Eur Respir J 7:555–568, 1994.
32. Remlinger J. Accidents paralytiques au cours du traitment antirabique. Ann Inst Pasteur 19:625–646, 1905.
33. Miller SD, Karpus WJ, Pope JG, et al. Theiler's virus-induced demyelinating disease. In Cohen IR, Miller A (eds) Autoimmune Disease Models: A Guidebook. San Diego, CA: Academic Press 1994, p. 23.
34. Chamorro M, Aubert C, Brohic M. Demyelinating lesions due to Theiler's virus are associated with ongoing central nervous system infection. J Virol 57:992–997, 1986.

35. Johnson RT. The virology of demyelinating diseases. Ann Neurol 36 (Suppl):S54–60, 1994.
36. Ikehara S, Good RA, Nakamura T, et al. Rationale for bone marrow transplantation in the treatment of autoimmune diseases. Proc Natl Acad Sci U S A 82:2483–2487, 1985.
37. Himeno K, Good RA. Marrow transplantation from tolerant donors to treat and prevent autoimmune diseases in BXSB mice. Immunology. Proc Natl Acad Sci U S A 85:2235–2239, 1988.
38. Ikehara S, Yasumizu R, Inaba M, et al. Long-term observations of autoimmune-prone mice treated for autoimmune disease by allogeneic bone marrow transplantation. Immunology. Proc Natl Acad Sci U S A 86:3306–3310, 1989.
39. Kamiya M, Sohen S, Yamane T, et al. Effective treatment of mice with type II collagen induced arthritis with lethal radiation and bone marrow transplantation. J Rheumatol 20:225–230, 1993.
40. Knaan-Shanzer S, Houben P, Kinwel-Bohre EPM, et al. Remission induction of adjuvant arthritis in rats by total body irradiation and autologous bone marrow transplantation. Bone Marrow Transplant 8:333–338, 1991.
41. Pestronk A, Drachman DB, Teoh R, et al. Combined short-term immunotherapy cures experimental autoimmune myasthenia gravis. Ann Neurol 14:235–241, 1983.
42. Karussis DM, Vourka-Karussis U, Lehmann D, et al. Prevention and reversal of adoptively transferred, chronic relapsing experimental autoimmune encephalomyelitis with a single high dose cytoreductive treatment followed by syngeneic bone marrow transplantation. J Clin Invest 92:765–772, 1993.
43. van Gelder M, Kinwel-Bohre EPM, van Bekkum DW. Treatment of experimental allergic encephalomyelitis in rats with total body irradiation and syngeneic BMT. Bone Marrow Transplant 11:233–241, 1993.
44. van Gelder M, van Bekkum DW. Treatment of relapsing experimental autoimmune encephalomyelitis in rats with allogeneic bone marrow transplantation from a resistant strain. Bone Marrow Transplant 16:343–351, 1995.
45. Burt RK, Hess A, Burns W, et al. Syngeneic bone marrow transplantation eliminates V$_\beta$8.2T lymphocytes from the spinal cord of lewis rats with experimental allergic encephalomyelitis. J Neurosci Res 41:526–531, 1995.
46. Lowenthal RM, Cohen ML, Atkinson K, et al. Apparent cure of rheumatoid arthritis by bone marrow transplantation. J Rheumatol 20(1):137–140, 1993.
47. Yin JA, Jowitt SN. Resolution of immune-mediated diseases following allogeneic bone marrow transplantation for leukaemia. Bone Marrow Transplant 9:31–33, 1992.
48. Burt RK, Meehan K, Richert J, et al. Genotypically matched allogeneic bone marrow transplantation for myelodysplastic syndrome in a patient with coincidental multiple sclerosis. Submitted.
49. Salzman P, Tami J, Jackson C, et al. Clinical remission of myasthenia gravis after high dose chemotherapy and autologous transplantation with CD34+ stem cells (abstract 808). Blood 84 (10, Suppl 1):206a, 1994.
50. Fastenrath S, Dreger P, Schmitz N. Autologous unpurged bone marrow transplantation in a patient with lymphoma and SLE: short-term recurrence of antinuclear antibioties. Arthritis Rheumatol 38(9):S303, 1995.
51. Marmont AM. Immune ablation followed by stem cell transplantation for SLE and other severe autoimmune diseases: an overview. Lupus 4(Suppl 1):97, 1995.
52. Weinshenker BG. The natural history of multiple sclerosis. Multiple Sclerosis 13(1):119–146, 1995.
53. Kurtzke, JF. Rating neurologic impairment in multiple sclerosis: an expanded disability status scale (EDSS). Neurlogy 33:1444–1452, 1983.
54. Sipe JC, Knobler RL, Braheny SL, et al. A neurologic rating scale (NRS) for use in multiple sclerosis. Neurology 34:1368–1372, 1984.
55. Francis GS, Evans AC, Arnold DL. Neuroimaging in multiple sclerosis. Multiple Sclerosis 13(1):147–171, 1995.
56. Pincus T, Brooks RH, Callahan LF. Prediction of long-term mortality in patients with rheu-

331

matoid arthritis according to simple questionnaire and joint count measures. Ann Intern Med 120:26–34, 1994.

57. Pincus T, Callahan LF. Rheumatology function tests: grip strength, walking time, button test and questionnaires document and predict longterm morbidity and mortality in rheumatoid arthritis. J Rheumatol 19(7):1051–1057, 1992.

58. Bulpitt KJ, Clements PJ, Lachenbruch PA, et al. Early undifferentiated connective tissue disease. III. Outcome and prognostic indicators in early scleroderma (Systemic Sclerosis). Ann Intern Med 118:602–609, 1993.

59. Langevitz LP, Alderdice CA, Aubrey M, et al. Mortality in systemic sclerosis (scleroderma). J Med New Series 82(298):139–148, 1992.

60. Altman RD, Medsger TA Jr, Bloch DA, et al. Predictors of survival in systemic sclerosis (scleroderma). Arithritis Rheum 34(4):403–413, 1991.

61. Drachman DB. Myasthenia Gravis. Engl J Med 330(25):1797–1810, 1994.

62. Sanders DB, Scoppetta C. The treatment of patients with myasthenia gravis. Neurol Chin North Am 12(2):343–368, 1994.

63. Somnier FE, Keiding N, Paulson OB. Epidemiology of myasthenia gravis in Denmark. Arch Neurol 48:733–739, 1991.

64. Tan EM, Cohen AS, Fries JF, et al. The revised criteria for the classification of systemic lupus erythematosus. Arthritis and Rheum 25(11):1271–1277, 1982.

65. Cheigh JS, Kim H, Stenzel KH, et al. Systemic lupus erythematousus in patients with end-stage renal disease: long-term follow-up on the prognosis of patients and the evolution of lupus activity. Am J Kidney Dis 16(3):189–195, 1990.

66. Seleznick MJ, Fries JF. Variables associated with decreased survival in systemic lupus erythematosus. Semin Arthritis Rheum 21(2):73–80, 1991.

67. Gladman DD. Prognosis of systemic lupus erythematosus and factors that affect it. Rheumatology 4:681–687, 1992.

68. Cohen MG, Li EK. Mortality in systemic lupus erythematosus: active disease is the most important factor. NZ J Med 22:5–8, 1992.

69. Appel GB, Valeri A. The course and treatment of lupus nephritis. Annu Rev Med 45:525–537, 1994.

70. Bates WD, Halland AM, Tribe RD, et al. Lupus nephritis: Part I. Histopathological classification, activity and chronicity scores. S Afr Med J 79:256–259, 1991.

71. Golbus J, McCune WJ. Lupus nephritis: classification, prognosis, immunopathogenesis, and treatment. Syst Lupus Erythematosus 20(1):213–226, 1994.

72. Boumpas DT, Austin HA III, Vaughn EM, et al. Controlled trial of pulse methylprednisolone versus two regimens of pulse cyclophosphamide in severe lupus nephritis. Lancet 340(8822):741–745, 1992.

73. Asherson RA. The catastrophic antiphospholipid syndrome (editoral). J Rheumatol 19(4):508–512, 1992.

74. Probert CS, Jayanthi V, Wicks AC, et al. Mortality from Crohn's disease in Leicestershire, 1972–1989: an epidemiological community based study. Gut 33:1226–1228, 1992.

75. Mendelsohn RR, Korelitz BI, Gleim GW. Death from Crohn's disease and lessons from a personal experience. J Clin Gastroenterol 20(1):22–26, 1995.

76. Sjogren RW. Gastrointestinal motility disorders in scleroderma. Arthritis Rheum 37(9):1265–1282, 1994.

15. Autologous bone marrow transplantation in pediatric solid tumors

Morris Kletzel and Ae Rang Kim

Cancer is one of the major causes of death in children ages 1 to 14 years. Although solid tumors represent only 40% of all pediatric cancers, they result in a high mortality rate due to their biologic behavior and stage. Therefore, it is imperative that all possible therapeutic approaches be carefully studied.

Autologous bone marrow transplantation (ABMT) is a method for delivering high doses of cytoreductive therapy to cancer patients that is based on the existence of a steep dose–response curve for many tumors [1]. Whereas hematopoietic toxicity limits the intensity of many of the chemotherapeutic regimens available for the treatment of children with malignant disease, autologous bone marrow rescue has eliminated the primary dose-limiting toxicity of intensive cytoreductive regimens, namely, myelosuppression [2]. This has permitted drug doses to be increased three- to fivefold above those used without marrow rescue [3].

The first description of ABMT in pediatrics was by Clifford et al. in 1961, who infused autologous marrow into children with advanced lymphoreticular tumors following treatment with high-dose nitrogen mustard [4]. Subsequent studies in patients with malignant lymphoma were quite successful. Unfortunately, the initial studies in solid tumors were characterized by a high degree of morbidity and mortality [1]. New treatment regimens and improvements in supportive care, however, have increased the efficacy of ABMT for children with solid tumors over the last few years. Consequently, ABMT is playing an increasingly important role in the treatment of pediatric patients with solid tumors. Although response rates appear to be improved with the use of dose-intensive therapy, disease recurrence is the most common cause of treatment failure [5]. Neoplastic cells contaminating the autologous marrow may contribute to relapse rates, but incomplete eradication of the tumor by ineffective chemotherapeutic regimens is the primary cause of treatment failure. Techniques have been developed to purge the autologous marrow of neoplastic cells, but the effectiveness of these methods and their relative contribution towards cure rates remains to be determined.

Since each specific solid tumor has its own prognosis and biologic characteristics, the effect of ABMT on each disease also varies. This chapter will review the rationale, effectiveness, and future directions of ABMT in the following

Jane N. Winter (ed.) BLOOD STEM CELL TRANSPLANTATION. 1997. Kluwer Academic Publishers. ISBN 0-7923-4260-7. All rights reserved.

solid tumors: neuroblastoma, Ewing's Sarcoma, rhabdomyosarcoma, brain tumor, and Wilms' tumor.

Neuroblastoma

Introduction

Neuroblastoma (NBL), a tumor of the neural crest cells from which the sympathetic nervous systems develops, is the most common childhood solid tumor occurring outside the central nervous system, with an annual incidence of approximately eight per million children in the U.S. [6]. Children with completely localized tumor or those with only local spread to adjacent tissues or lymph nodes have an excellent prognosis when treated by surgical resection, with or without chemotherapy [7,8]. This includes children with stage I and stage II disease according to the Evan's classification. Infants diagnosed at less than one year of age and children with stage IVS also have an excellent prognosis. Forty percent to 70% of patients with stage III disease who have favorable prognostic markers, such as a single copy of N-myc or hyperdiploid tumors, can also be cured by conventional therapy, depending in part on the feasibility of surgical excision [9]. Unfortunately, between one third and one half of NBLs in children older than one year of age are stage IV [10]. These children present with advanced disease and dissemination to distant sites such as the liver, bone marrow, and skeleton, or other unfavorable features such as amplified expression of the N-myc oncogene [11].

Stage IV NBL is the most common childhood malignancy between the ages of one and five [12]. Although new treatments and therapy regimens have increased the chances of initial survival for children with stage IV NBL, the long-term disease-free survival still remains quite poor. In the 1950s and early 1960s, when the only available chemotherapy was vincristine and cyclophosphamide, the long-term disease-free survival was only 5%. In the late 1960s and 1970s, after the introduction of multiagent chemotherapy in addition to debulking surgery and radiotherapy, the cure rate increased to approximately 10% to 20% [10]. Since the mid-1980s, however, more aggressive multimodality therapy, including extensive surgery to remove the primary tumor and sites of bulk disease, irradiation to localized tumor masses, and increasingly, intensive combinations of chemotherapy, has produced significant response rates in up to 80% of afflicted children and has prolonged overall survival from a few months to several years in many patients [13–15]. Nonetheless, long-term survival remains poor. Among the new strategies investigated in the last decade, high-dose therapy has emerged as a promising approach with the demonstration that both rate and quality of response may be improved by increasing the dosage of some anticancer compounds, administered alone or in combination [16]. Supportive care with autologous bone marrow or peripheral blood stem cell rescue has enabled further significant dose escalation of cytotoxic agents active against neuroblastoma, resulting in disease-free survival for 25% to 50% of patients at two years, an improvement over all historical experience with conventional chemotherapy [17].

For children with disseminated poor-risk NBL who respond to first-line therapy and then receive consolidation with megatherapy (MGT) and bone marrow transplantation, survival rates are 40% to 45% at two years and 20% at five yearsl [18]. Intensive myeloablative consolidation therapy followed by ABMT has resulted in estimated disease-free survival rates of up to 44% at three years [19]. A recent update on results in stage IV patients over one year of age confirmed that high-dose melphalan and bone marrow transplantation prolong the duration of remission (23 months versus 6 months with no further treatment after induction), but only marginally alters long-term survival [17]. Reasons for the poor long-term survival rates may include inadequate chmotherapy delivery, development of drug resistance, and toxicity [20].

Although results are not yet conclusive, it can be concluded that some patients benefit from AMBT in terms of prolonged life. The results for long-term disease-free survival, however, currently remain quite dim. Yet, with the new approaches there is hope for an increased survival rate and possibly a cure for what once seemed to be a hopeless disease.

Results

In this section, the results of different approaches and treatments for combating NBL will be compared and reviewed (see table 1).

The role of tumor burden and pretransplant cytoreduction is underscored by the series reported by Hartmann et al. [21] in which 15 patients with advanced NBL (one with stage III and 14 with stage IV) were treated with high-dose melphalan (HDM) followed by ABMT. All patients had been extensively treated with multimodality therapy including surgical excision, and four were in complete remission at the time of transplant. One of the 15 patients died of early toxicity, but five were free of disease at 29+ to 54+ months after ABMT. These five patients had minimal residual disease or were in a complete remission (CR) before HDM. These results suggest that chemotherapy including high-does melphalan followed by ABMT is tolerable in children with advanced NBL, and effective when used as consolidation therapy in patients who have attained CR or significant cytoreduction with conventional therapy.

A study by Kushner et al. [22] presents a long-term study of 28 patients who were diagnosed with poor risk NBL at more than 12 months of age and who received high-dose melphalan (HDM) as consolidation therapy followed by ABMT. The majority of patients also received dianhydrogalactitol, and some also received total body irradiation (TBI). Bone marrow was purged in all but two cases. Of the 17 patients in first remission, one is relapse free more than 6.5 years post-ABMT, three died of ABMT-related toxicity, and 13 had progressive disease at 2 to 23 months. Among the patients with progressive disease, 11

Table 1. Current results of myeloablative treatments followed by ABMT for children with NBL

Investigators	Patients	Disease-free survival	Therapy regimen	Information/conclusions
Hartmann et al. [21]	15 patients	33% at 29–54 months after ABMT	High-dose melphalan followed by ABMT	All patients with DFS had minimal or o residual disease before MGT
Kushner et al. [22]	28 patients	29% at 12 months; 18% at 18 months; 6% at 24 months post ABMT	High-dose melphalan followed by ABMT; 11/28 also received TBI	Marrow was purged with 6-hydroxydopamine/all patients with refractory disease or in second remission died
LCME1 [23]	72 patients (62 underwent MGT with ABMT)	40% at 2 years; 20% at 4 years; 13% at 7 years	Vincristine, high-dose melphalan, and fractionated TBI followed by BMT (57 Auto and 5 allo).	Patients not grafted had 0% survival rate at 4yr; subgroup of patients with normalization of bone metastasis before AMBT had 30% DFS at 5yrs.
LCME2 [12]	33 patients with refractory disease or relapse	36% at 2 years and 32% at 5 years	Double megatherapy and ABMT — MGT1-teniposide, carmustine, and cisplatinum; MGT2 vincristine, Melphalan, TBI followed ABMT1 at 4 weeks; and ABMT2 at 60–90 days+.	Toxic rate high at 24% and delayed double harvest engraftment may support single graft even with the encouraging results
Corbett R et al. OMEC pilot [24]	20 patients	10% 24–35 months after OMEC	Multiagent regimen consisting of vincristine, melphalan, etoposide, and carboplatin (OMEC, followed by ABMT)	High toxicity; mortality at 20%; 65% of patients relapsed 10 months after OMEC; concluded that OMEC is no more effective than HDM alone

Study	Patients	Results	Treatment	Conclusion
Italian Cooperative Group for NBL [28]	181 patients (75 patients in group NB82; 106 patients in ND85)	9% for NB82 and 18% for NB85 at five years	NB82 standard treatment and NB85 high-dose chemotherpy. Chemotherapy involved peptichemio and cisplatin at SD of HD, respectively, following BMT.	Intensified treatment for NBL improves response rates and increase survival.
Kletzel et al. [29]	7 patients with VGPR	57% in CR at 23–48+ months	High-dose cyclophosphamide, continuous infusion of vincristine, escalating doses of VP-16-213, TBI, unpurged ABMT	Regimen is tolerated and beneficial. Unpurged marrow did not contribute to relapse. Small smaple of patients warrant further tests.
Lam-Po-Tang et al. [30]	12 patients	100% at 42 months from time of ABMT	VAM-TBI regimen (teniposide, doxorubicin, melphalan, cisplatin, and total body irradiation) followed by ABMT	Very encouraging results for the VAM-TBI treatment, but small sample number requires further tests be done
Matthay et al. [31]	56 patients	25% for allogeneic patients and 49% for autologous patients at 4 years	Myeloablative therapy consisting of etoposide, melphalan, cisplatin, and TBI followed by allogeneic (20 patients) or autologous (36 patients) BMT.	Overall outcome same for allogenic versus autologous BMT in treating high-risk NBL

of 13 had disease involving bone and/or bone marrow. Event-free survival was 29% at 12 months, 18% at 18 months, and 6% at 24 months post-ABMT. All of the patients with refractory disease or in second remission died; one patient in second partial remission relapsed 32 months post-ABMT; eight patients had progressive disease within five months of ABMT, and two patients died of toxicity. These results suggest that high-dose melphalan is relatively ineffective in patients with residual disease or refractory tumors. Also, the pattern of relapse in several patients suggests that 6-hydroxydopamine may not be completely efficient at eliminating contaminating malignant cells from the autograft.

The LCME1 study by Philip et al. [23] is unique because it included unselected patients, and because the strategy for megatherapy and ABMT purging was constant over a six-year period. Seventy-two patients entered the LMCE1 study between 1982 and 1987. In response to the induction regimen, 18 achieved CRs, eight attained very good partial remissions (VGPR), 42 achieved partial remissions (PRs), and four experienced disease progression. Sixty-two out of the 72 patients were then treated with consolidation therapy consisting of vincristine (total $4\,mg/m^2$), high-dose melphalan ($180\,mg/m^2$), and fractionated TBI followed by bone marrow transplantation (57 had ABMT and five had allogeneic BMT). The progression-free survival (PFS) for the ten patients not treated with high-dose therapy and transplantation is 20% at two years and 0% four years. The PFS for the 62 grafted patients is 40% at two years, 20% at four years, and 13% at seven years. Comparing the survival without progression, there is no significant difference in CR vs. PR/VGPR or CR/VGPR vs. PR. However, there is a subgroup defined by healing of bone metastases before ABMT in which long-term PFS could be obtained. This group had a 30% PFS at five years. This study showed definitive improvement in the management of stage IV disease. It identifies a group of patients that is potentially curable.

In a follow-up study, the LCME2 [12] study uses a double harvest/ double graft approach with two different megatherapy regimens. Since most relapses in the LCME1 trial occurred during the first two years after ABMT 1, this new investigation is designed to test the role of increased dose intensity on response rates, relapse patterns, and overall survival. Thirty-three patients with refractory disease in partial remission after second-line treatment for stage IV NBL or at the time of relapse from stage IV or III disease enrolled in this study. The first megatherapy regimen consisted of a combination of teniposide, carmustine, and cisplatin, whereas the second contained vincristine, melphalan, and TBI. The first harvest was four weeks after the last chemotherapy, and the second occurred 60 to 90 days after megatherapy. Response rates were 65% (16% CR) for MGT 1 and 60% (25% CR) for MGT 2. The overall survival rate was 36% at two years and 32% at five years. Although these results are hopeful for patients with refractory or relapsed disease, the degree of toxicity is high (24%), and the delayed engraftment associated with the double transplant may give support to the the use of a single harvest approach. This study does, however, show that increased dose intensity may improve the outlook for some patients. Other high-dose procedures should be investigated.

A pilot study by Corbett et al. [24], investigated the efficacy and toxicity of a high-dose multiagent consolidation regimen. OMEC (vincristine, 4 mg/m^2; melphalan, 180 mg/m^2; etoposide, 1 g/m^2; and carboplatin 1.0–1.75 g/m^2) followed by ABMT was studied in 20 patients with poor-prognosis NBL. Eighteen patients received OMEC after induction chemotherapy and two following relapse. Four patients died of treatment-related toxicity. Sixty-five percent (13 of 20) have relapsed a median of ten months after receiving OMEC. Overall, four patients are alive 24 to 35 months after receiving OMEC; two of these patients have disease. These results are extremely disappointing, in view of the fact that this regimen was especially designed to include agents that are individually active against NBL, exhibit a steep dose–response curve, are noncross-resistant and preferably synergistic, and produce tolerable, yet different nonmyelotoxic side effects at the administered dose. Melphalan has been shown to maintain a fractional tumor cell kill with increasing dose in vitro [25]. Etoposide, in combination with cisplatin, produced a 55% response rate in patients with NBL [26]. A five-day continuous infusion of vincristine has documented efficacy in patients with solid tumors, and in combination with high-dose melphalan and total body irradiation was well tolerated [27]. Unfortunately, although the rationale for this sort of multiagent regimen is logical, the results are very disappointing. The OMEC regimen is no more effective than HDM alone, and the level of toxicity is much higher.

The Italian Cooperative Group for Neuroblastoma (ICGNB) published a paper in 1992 [28] comparing two studies on 181 children age one year or older with newly diagnosed disseminated NBL from January 1982 to November 1989. Seventy-five patients (group NB82), enrolled from 1982 to 1984, were treated with standard-dose chemotherapy (SD). One hundred six patients (group NB85), enrolled from 1985 to 1989, received high-dose (HD) chemotherapy. In both groups, induction therapy included peptichemio (a mixture of six oligopeptides of m-l-phenylalanine mustard thought to act by both alkylating and antimetabolic mechanisms) and cisplatin at SD or HD, respectively. In NB82, children who achieved complete or partial tumor regression received SD consolidation therapy; in contrast, patients enrolled on study NB85 received three cycles of HD chemotherapy or one cycle of myeloablative therapy followed by ABMT. Comparing the two protocols, the NB85 group had significantly fewer failures (no tumor response or disease progression) than NB82 after administration of peptichemio (9% vs. 32%) and had greater percentages of CRs and PRs both after treatment with cisplatin (60% vs. 43%) and after surgery (76% vs. 46%). The overall survival and progression-free survival at five years were respectively 11% and 9% for NB82 and 27% and 18% for NB85. Patients in the NB85 group who after achievement of CR were consolidated with three cycles of HD chemotherapy versus those consolidated with myeloablative therapy followed by ABMT was 24% to 32%. These results show that intensified treatment for NBL — either multiple cycles of HD chemotherapy or myeloablative treatment with ABMT — improves response rates and increases survival.

A single-institution experience studying the toxicity and efficacy of multiagent chemotherapy plus TBI in children with NBL was reported by Kletzel et al. [29]. Seven children with NBL with very good partial remissions underwent a multiagent ablative regimen including high-dose cyclophosphamide, continuous infusion vincristine, escalating doses of VP-16-213, and TBI followed by unpurged ABMT. The dose-limiting toxicity was mucositis observed when the dose of VP-16-213 was escalated to 2400 mg/m^2 total dose. Four of seven patients achieved CRs lasting 23 to 48+ months. The use of unpurged marrow did not appear to contribute to relapse in that patients relapsed at their primary site of disease and the bone marrow remained disease free at relapse. This finding is of particular interest because at the time of diagnosis, 6 of 7 of these patients did in fact have bone marrow metastasis. However, due to the small sample of patients, further tests will have to be performed to determine the therapeutic value of this regimen. The results demonstrate that this regimen is well tolerated and effective.

Lam-Po-Tang et al. [30] reported their experience with ABMT using a modified version of the VAM-TBI regimen (teniposide, doxorubicin, melphalan, cisplatin, and total body irradiation) in a group of 12 patients treated between 1985 and 1992. All 12 are alive and are in clinical remission at a median follow-up of 42 months from the time of ABMT. These data confirm that ABMT using modified VAMP-TBI conditioning treatment is safe, prolongs survival, and appears to increase cure rates. This study was done with a small sample number; larger numbers of patients must be studied in order to confirm these results.

Questions concerning the advantages and disadvantages of autologous over allogeneic bone marrow transplant were investigated by Matthay et al. [31] in their study of 56 patients with high-risk NBL. The concept of allogeneic bone marrow transplantation presents the problems of graft-versus-host disease and lack of donor availability; however, it avoids the possibility of tumor-cell reinfusion associated with ABMT. In the comparison study by Matthay et al., two groups of patients received identical induction chemotherapy, surgery, and local radiation. Patients who remained progression free at the end of induction received myeloablative chemotherapy consisting of etoposide, melphalan, cisplatin, and TBI followed by allogeneic (20 patients) or autologous (36 patients) bone marrow transplantation. Time for both neutrophil and platelet engraftment was significantly shorter after allogeneic than autologous BMT. The relapse rate among allogeneic BMT patients was 69% compared with 46% for autologous. The estimated progression-free survival rates four years after BMT were 25% for allogeneic and 49% for autologous. Although these rates appear to be different, they are not significantly so. In this comparison, allogeneic and autologous transplantation were equivalent,

340

although caution must be used in interpreting a nonrandomized comparative study.

In conclusion, the most intensively studied therapeutic approach for advanced-stage NBL has been chemotherapy with or without total body irradiation or local irradiation, followed by stem cell rescue. The approaches and methods or study are different, but the objective is to determine whether an increase in the intensity of therapy improves outcome for children with NBL. The prognosis of children with disseminated NBL still remains poor. However, intensified therapy followed by ABMT may provide higher survival rates and eventual cure for some children with NBL.

Controversies

Purging. The role of purging autologous bone marrow in NBL remains controversial. Despite the intensification of cytotoxic therapy facilitated by autotransplantation, relapse or refractory disease still remains a major source of failure. Thirty-fifty percent of patients with stage IV NBL have metastatic disease detectable in marrow prior to auto transplantation [32]. Gene-marking of human bone marrow cells provides a more sensitive and efficient method of directly addressing the issue of whether malignant cells in an autograft contribute to relapse because a transferred gene is present in equal concentration in all progeny of a marked cell for every generation [33]. By use of a neomycin-resistance (NeoR) marker gene, Brenner et al. showed that bone marrow cells marked in remission and their progeny contributed to relapse. In all relapsed patients, resurgent cells contained the NeoR marker. Therefore, there would seem to be a need for eliminating malignant cells from the autograft. However, the controversy lies in whether relapse is caused by other factors, such as failure to eradicate the primary tumor, and whether current purging methods, while successful in removing neoplastic cells efficiently in vitro, perform the same in vivo. In considering the number of cells required for reconstitution and a marrow contaminated with 1% tumor cells, 2000 to 20,000 tumor cells could remain and be infused into a 20-kg patient [34] (see table 2).

Table 2. Potential number of tumor cells infused with autologous bone marrow [38]

Total cells[a]	×	Tumor cells	=	Total tumor cells
2×10^9		10^{-3}		2×10^6
2×10^9		10^{-4}		2×10^5
2×10^9		10^{-5}		2×10^4
2×10^9		10^{-6}		2×10^3
2×10^9		10^{-7}		2×10^2

[a] For hematologic and immunologic reconstitution, assume that $10^8 \times 20\,kg$ equal 2×10^9 total cells.

There are a number of methods that may be useful for removing NBL cells from marrow, such as pharmacological, physical separation, and immunological techniques. The use of toxins for killing NBL cells in bone marrow has not been extensively studies. The drug 4-hydroperoxycyclophosphamide (4-HC) has been shown to kill human NBL cell lines in vitro, but the half-life of 4-HC is very short, and cells not in cycle may not be killed [35]. The pattern of relapse following purging with the drug 6-hydroxydopamine mentioned above in the Kushner et al. results [22] suggests that this agent may be ineffective at purging malignant NBL cells from the bone marrow. Density gradients have been used to separate malignant cells from stem cells. Centrifugation methods using an elutriation rotor for the removal of neuroblastoma cells from bone marrow have been developed, but they are relatively ineffective. Only 95% of neuroblasts can be removed from artificially contaminated bone marrow [36].

Immunological methods for purging involving the use of monoclonal antibodies and immunomagnetic microspheres have been most widely used. Single monoclonal antibody methods have been performed with success [37,38]. However, in a recent paper by Moss et al. [39], the authors stated that their antibodies bound no more than 87% of the cultured cells. The magnetic separation device removes NBL cells coated with magnetic microspheres by using high-field-strength permanent magnets. Tumor cells in the marrow cannot be detected at sensitivity levels of less than 1/10,000. These problems provoked investigators to research techniques combining methods for detecting small numbers of malignant cells. Recently, Moss et al. [39] developed a multiassay system consisting of fluorescence microscopy, immunocytology, and tumor colony assay. Eight experiments were performed on two different NBL cell lines with 2% to 5% contamination. Moss et al. demonstrated greater than 3 log removal with one cycle of antibody/bead treatment and greater than 1 log further reduction with a second cycle. The sensitivity of this method can detect 1/30,000 to 1/100,000 malignant cells over 4 logs of tumor cell removal.

Although purging techniques have been greatly improved, their usefulness in vivo and their effects on normal healthy stem cells remain a major concern. There seems to be a significant loss of mononuclear cells associated with immunomagnetic purging, with an average mononuclear recovery of 35%. In addition, some investigators have expressed concern about slow engraftment or failure to engraft when marrow has been purged with monoclonal antibody or pharmacologic agents [40]. The occurrence of early marrow relapse, despite purging, might be taken as an indication that purging is not fully effective [41]. Most purging techniques can be demonstrated to have activity in vitro, although the limitations of assays for occult NBL pose problems. The major difficulty is demonstrating effectiveness in vivo. At present, it is likely that the main obstacle to disease-free survival is the ineffectiveness of our therapeutic regimens [42], not the reinfusion of small numbers of malignant cells.

342

Some patients who have received unpurged or inadequately purged marrow are reported to have developed metastatic disease in a pattern suggestive of tumor embolization, such as lung metastases [43,44]. However, in general, the patterns of recurrence in purged and nonpurged marrow transplant have been similar, usually at the site of primary tumor, residual gross disease, bone, or bone marrow, suggesting that the major cause of relapse is ineffective cytotoxic therapy which fails to eradicate the tumor [20]. Also, when the results of allogeneic and autologous bone marrow transplant are compared, the relapse rates do not appear to be significantly different [32].

Although increased sensitivity and specificity has improved the efficiency of purging techniques, its role in transplantation remains controversial. Research now must take on the task of demonstrating the efficacy of purging in vivo through clinical trials.

TBI. The benefits of TBI must be weighed against its toxicity. NBL is a very radiosensitive cancer, such that radiation therapy to residual disease sites may be quite valuable [45,46]. However, since most NBL patients are young, the role of TBI remains controversial. There is an understandable reluctance to use such therapy in young children because of the considerable and as yet ill-defined long-term toxicity [3].

Some researchers suggest that until targeted radiotherapy using radiolabeled metaiodobenzylguanadine (MIBG) has been shown to be effective, they would be reluctant to omit external irradiation from the overall treatment plan in NBL. Although like chemotherapy, radiation therapy has its own undesirable side effects, it is an effective treatment for NBL, and its inclusion may be responsible for the absence of late relapses in some studies [47]. In a study by Philip et al., who were the first group to use fractionated TBI associated with HDM regimen, the relapse rates in patients who received HDM with TBI were lower than those treated with HDM alone or in combination with other drugs [44].

However, other reviews demonstrate opposing results. A review of more than 300 ABMTs from Europe showed a constant 15% toxic death rate with no difference between patient status at graft, conditioning regimen, and even single- or double-graft programs [48]. A TBI-containing regimen is not statistically more toxic, and the long-term progression-free survival is not better. Therefore, a TBI regimen should be used sparingly and cautiously, especially in young children. Although it would appear to make sense to use TBI against radiosensitive and disseminated tumors such as NBL, a clear survival advantage of TBI- containing regimens versus non-TBI-containing regimens has not been demonstrated [49].

The arguments for or against TBI are both convincing. Since children have rapidly developing normal tissues, the long-term toxicity associated with any high-dose regimen — particularly TBI, which could limit growth and development and possibly lead to secondary malignancies — is of concern [50]. Although each patient must be carefully considered with regard to his or her prognosis, the more recent reviews suggest that TBI may not be that effective and that other methods such as local irradiation and targeted radio-isotope therapy such as ^{131}I-mIBG (metaiodobenzylguanidine) should be investigated.

Recommendation/future directions

Autotransplantation is most effective in children with advanced-stage NBL who have obtained a significant response to combination chemotherapy, together with surgery and localized radiation therapy when indicated, and before disease progression [34]. Intensive therapy followed by ABMT has shown itself to be effective in increasing survival rates. Unfortunately, the absence of a plateau in the survival curves and recent reports on very late relapses warn us against drawing premature conclusions about eventual cure rates [17].

Allogeneic transplantation is also a viable option for children with NBL. However, the availability of HLA and DR-matched allografts is very limited, restricting this type of marrow transplant to fewer than 1 in 5 children [3]. The existence of an immunologic antitumor effect has been established as a therapeutic tool in allogeneic BMT [51]. However, this benefit does not translate into an improved overall survival because of a higher transplant-related mortality, largely due to graft-versus-host disease [19].

A newer alternative is the use of peripheral blood stem cells (PBSCs). The first studies describing the successful use of autologous PBSC transplantation (PBSCT) were reported in 1985 and 1986. These patients underwent PBSCT instead of ABMT because of residual marrow disease of fibrotic marrow collection sites resulting in inadequate yields of harvested cells [52]. PBSCT is gaining support because of its numerous advantages over ABMT, e.g., general anesthesia is not required, there is less discomfort for the patient, rapid hematopoietic recovery occurs, and there is the potential for a reduced risk of tumor cell contamination [53]. Unfortunately, experiments do show that PBSC harvests may be contaminated with significant numbers of tumor cells. In a study by Moss et al. [54], 75% of PBSC harvests obtained from 31 patients with disseminated NBL contained neoplastic cells at diagnosis, 36% during therapy, and 14% at harvest. Six of 13 patients with minimal or no bone marrow disease had positive blood specimens. In another experience reported by Di Caro et al. [55], nine patients with NBL were treated with high-dose chemotherapy and autologous PBSC transplantation. Immunocytological analysis of the PBSC harvests showed the presence of circulating neoplastic cells in 3 of 9 patients. One child is still alive with no evidence of disease at five years. The others died at a median of 14 months after transplantation. In this study, there was no conclusive evidence that PBSCs gave way to a more rapid stem cell recovery. In contrast, a report by Kletzel et al. [56] demonstrated very positive results using PBSC rescue in six patients with advanced-stage NBL. All samples from bone marrow and PBSCs tested negative for the presence of NBL cells, leading the investigators to conclude that the risk of tumor contamination in peripheral blood seems to decrease with therapy. Only one patient has relapsed, while the remaining five remain disease free at 150 to 450+ days posttransplant. In this evaluation, the PBSCs engrafted more rapidly than bone marrow in comparable patients.

Allogeneic bone marrow or PBSC rescue following myeloablative therapy is a definite alternative to ABMT. Like autologous bone marrow rescue, these approaches are used to overcome the toxic effects of megatherapy regimens. These approaches have resulted in higher response rates in NBL patients, but the problems of toxicity and relapse still remain. In advanced NBL, multiagent regimens with overlapping toxicities appear inadvisable with regard to high toxic death rates [25]. Most studies document relapse in approximately 45% to 60% of patients, usually within the first year following infusion [57]. Children with NBL have a low long-term disease-free survival rate. Despite this fact, one cannot dispute the definite progress that has occurred with the intensive chemotherapy regimens made feasible by ABMT.

For the future, new therapeutic approaches such as immunotherapy [58] should be further investigated. In order for new curative approaches to be discovered and for future breakthroughs to occur, a better understanding of the biology underlying the proliferative and metastatic characteristics of NBL must be obtained.

Ewing's sarcoma (see table 3)

Ewing's sarcoma (ES) is a primary malignant tumor of the bone, which occurs is children and adolescents. The prognosis for children with peripheral small-volume ES is generally good [9], whereas the prognosis for patients with multifocal primary bone disease or those who have experienced early or multiple relapses is dismal with conventional chemoradiotherapy and surgery

Table 3. Current results of myeloablative treatments followed by ABMT for children with Ewing's sarcoma

Investigators	Patients	Survival rate	Therapy regimen
Burdach et al. [59]	17 patients with previous remission induction chemotherapy	47% alive in CR at 49 months	12 Gy of hyperfractionated TBI, fractionated HDM, high-dose etoposide, stem cell rescue (auto, allo, peripheral)
Miser et al. [66]	68 patients (30 with Ewing's)	Overall disease-free survival is 40%	VCR, adriamycin, cyclophosphamide, TBI, unpurged marrow
Horowitz et al. [67]	90 patients (44 with Ewing's)	14% survival in Ewing's patients, 30% overall	8 Gy of fractionated TBI and ABMT

[59]. Introduction of multimodality therapy in the late 1960s and its refinement in the 1970s steadily improved the prognosis [60,61]. However, by 1980, a group of patients at high risk for treatment failure could be readily identified [62]. Few of those with overt metastatic disease at diagnosis or those with localized but extensive unresectable primary lesions of the trunk were curable [63]. The majority responded initially to treatment, but eventually suffered recurrences in the lung, bone, or bone marrow, and died of disseminated disease [64]. Myeloablative approaches with bone marrow rescue have been used by various investigators to improve the poor prognosis of ES.

Results

Initially promising results were achieved by Cornbleet et al. in 1981 using high-dose melphalan with ABMT. The patients had a high initial response rate, but generally relapsed when treated in PR [1]. In 1984, the European Bone Marrow Transplant (EBMT) group reviewed 35 cases and similarly demonstrated a response rate of 66% in evaluable patients [65].

The 1992 analysis of the EBMT solid tumor registry showed a two-year survival rate of 31% for 14 patients with metastatic ES grafted in first CR and a two-year survival rate of 37% for patients grafted in second CR. For 28 patients grafted with measurable disease for intensification of primary therapy, the survival rate at two years was 25%. In relapsed patients, the two-year survival rate was 33% for 19 patients with sensitive relapse and 10% for patients with resistant relapse [29].

Burdach et al. [59] investigated the efficacy and feasibility of myeloablative regimens administered as consolidation therapy. The study included 17 patients who underwent remission-induction chemotherapy and local treatment before myeloablative therapy. Seven had multifocal primary ES, and ten had early or multiple relapses. The regimen consisted of 12 Gy hyperfractionated TBI (two doses of 1.5 Gy for four days) plus fractionated HDM (30–45 mg/m^2 for four days) followed by high-dose etoposide (40–60 mg/kg) and hemopoietic stem cell rescue (either allo, auto, or peripheral). The results were an improvement from a 2% to 45% event-free survival rate in comparison to historical controls. Eight of 17 patients are alive in CR at median observation time of 49 months.

Similarly, Miser et al. [66] have used ABMT in high-risk sarcoma as consolidation therapy. Sixty-eight patients diagnosed with high-risk sarcomas underwent ABMT after their first remission was obtained. The patients' diagnoses included 30 ES, 18 rhabdomyosarcomas, 10 primitive sarcomas, 9 peripheral neuroepithelioma, and 1 NBL. The cytoreductive therapy included VCR, adriamycin, cyclophosphamide, and TBI followed by infusion of frozen unpurged bone marrow. Five of 68 patients had treatment-related deaths, and 32 of 68 relapsed. Overall disease-free survival at 24 months is 40%.

Horowitz et al. [67] also explored the use of TBI plus ABMT as consolidation therapy. High-risk patients (25 with rhabdomyosarcoma, 44 with ES, 17

346

with peripheral neuroepithelioma, 4 with primitive sarcoma of bone, and 1 with ectomesenchymoma) who responded completely to induction chemotherapy and local irradiation proceeded with the consolidation therapy, which consisted of fractionated TBI of 8 Gy and ABMT. Nineteen of 91 failed to achieve CR at induction therapy, and seven elected to forgo consolidation. Twenty of the transplant patients are long-term disease-free survivors. There was a 14% survival rate of the ES patients. This regimen had minimal to no impact on the outcome of patients with either localized or metastatic ES when compared with patients enrolled on a conventional chemotherapy protocol.

The role of TBI is still questionable in ES. In vitro studies using Ewing's cell lines show TBI to be effective therapy. In vivo, this is not always the case. In vitro, two 4 Gy TBI fractions result in a maximum tumor cell kill of 3 to 4 logs. However, since patients who achieve CR to combined modality induction therapy may have up to 10^8 to 10^9 tumor cells (down from 10^{11} to 10^{12} at presentation), it is not surprising that TBI might not benefit high-risk patients [64] with ES, despite the fact that their tumors are known to be radiosensitive.

In review of these studies, it appears that myeloablative therapy with ABMT benefits patients with poor-prognosis ES. The role of ABMT must still, however, be researched more thoroughly in this disease. Although initial responses seem to be promising, long-term disease-free survival still is in question.

Rhabdomyosarcoma

Rhabdomyosarcoma (RMS), tumor of the striated muscle, is the most common soft tissue sarcoma and represents between 5% and 15% of all malignant solid tumors in children [4]. Most children with RMS are cured by conventional therapy, while a small group of patients with metastatic disease or unfavorable histology have a poor outcome [9]. The role of ABMT in this disease is unknown due to the small number of patients transplanted.

Results

In 1985, Houghton et al. demonstrated melphalan's activity against a series of seven childhood rhabdomyosarcomas, each derived from a different patient and maintained in vivo as xenografts in immune-deprived mice. A single administration of melphalan caused complete regressions of advanced tumor in 6 of 7 lines [68]. Melphalan was more cytotoxic than vincristine, cyclophosphamide, doxorubicin, or dactinomycin in this model. Phase II studies in children with relapsed or resistant rhabdomyosarcoma have demonstrated a high response rate to high-dose melphalan with ABMT, confirming the data obtained in the xenograft model. The duration of response was almost invariably brief, with few long-term survivors [3].

347

Building on the HDM regimen, Pinkerton et al. [3] added TBI. Because the long-term survival of children with stage IV disease remains poor, myeloablative therapy could be considered as consolidation treatment once CR had been achieved. Seven patients (four received myeloablative therapy in first CR having presented with advanced disease involving metastasis to bone in one case; one was in second CR after relapsing in lymph nodes; and two had residual disease after a partial response to salvage therapy) underwent treatment composed of vincristine infusion of $4\,mg/m^2$ over five days, melphalan $140\,mg/m^2$, and TBI 12 Gy in six fractions followed by ABMT purged with Asta-Z or melphalan 120 to $140\,mg/m^2$ and TBI with unpurged marrow. In the two that underwent ABMT with disease, one died with candida septicemia, and one died relapsing on day 75 after achieving CR. Five patients remain disease free, all of whom were in CR at the time of high-dose therapy; however, follow-up in these cases is short, with a median of 8 months.

In a report from the EBMT solid tumor registry, 7 of 20 children with metastatic RMS are alive in CR post-BMT, 12 to 100 months from diagnosis. This heterogenous group received a variety of induction and transplant regimens. No advantage could be attributed to TBI or to tandem transplant programs at this time. However, a disease-free survival of 40% at two years compares very favorably with the best available conventional chemotherapy regimen [9,69].

The role of ABMT in RMS is not clear at this point. Results are positive, but long-term success has yet to be documented. Preclinical and clinical studies revealing the benefits of myeloablative therapy show the potential need for more studies with high-dose chemoradiotherapy with stem cell rescue.

Brain tumor

Central nervous system tumors are a diverse group of neoplasms that account for 16% to 20% of all pediatric neoplasms and are exceeded only by leukemia as a malignancy occurring in children less than 15 years of age [70]. The five-year survival rate associated with all childhood CNS tumors is approximately 50% [71]. Most common childhood CNS tumors are either low-grade astrocytomas or embryonic neoplasms such as medulloblastomas and ependymonas. Malignant brain tumors in children are known to have a poor outcome. Disease-free survival for the most common tumors — medulloblastomas and ependymomas — is not more than 40% to 60% [72]. High-grade malignant glial tumors are usually fatal when treated with conventional therapy. Although the addition of radiation and chemotherapy extends survival, fewer than 10% of patients live beyond three years [73]. Surgery and radiation therapy have been used to treat malignant CNS tumors for many years. Whereas cure rates with conventional therapy have been stagnant, new approaches such as aggressive chemotherapy have been utilized in treating brain tumors. To prevent the characteristic myelopsuppression involved with high-dose chemotherapy, ABMT has been used. The results of clinical investigations using high-dose chemotherapy followed by stem cell rescue are presented below.

Patients with gliomas that progress following initial therapy have a very poor prognosis, with a median survival of seven months. Giannone and Wolff [74] conducted a study with 16 patients with progressive CNS gliomas previously treated with maximal radiation therapy and chemotherapy. The patients entered a phase II study with high-dose etoposide followed by ABMT. Nineteen percent (3 of 16) experienced a tumor response. The responding patients were then treated with two more cycles of high-dose etoposide. The median survival for all 16 patients was four months, with the three responders alive at 9, 10, and 54+ months. These results seem to correlate with the results using standard-dose etoposide [75]. The severe myelosuppression involved with this regimen and its modest activity suggests that this regimen is not efficient. Further tests are warranted with etoposide alone or in conjunction with other cytotoxic agents.

No phase III randomized trials have demonstrated an obvious advantage of chemotherapy in addition to radiotherapy. However, the efficacy of single agents or combinations of drugs have clearly been observed [76,77]. A reason for failure of chemotherapy could be in part due to the poor penetration of chemotherapeutic agents into the CNS tumors [70,78]. Alkylating agents such as busulfan and thiotepa are expected to exhibit a steep dose effect with no overlapping extramedullary toxicity. Therefore, Kalifa et al. [79] designed a study treating children with measurable recurrent brain tumors with busulfan and thiotepa, two drugs know to have an excellent distribution into the CNS system in humans. Twenty children were treated with $150 \, mg/m^2/day \times 4$ of busulfan and $350 \, mg/m^2/day \times 3$ of thiotepa followed by ABMT. The overall response rate was 26%. One patient died of early toxicity. Out of the 19 evaluable patients, five partial responses, three objective responses, ten with stable disease, and one with progressive disease were observed. These results are encouraging because this high-dose regimen seems to be effective in some pediatric brain tumors refractory to all conventional therapies.

Kedar et al. [73] evaluated high-dose chemotherapy with marrow reinfusion for patients with newly diagnosed brain tumors having a high risk of failure with standard treatment. Nine patients (six with brain stem glioma, one with high-grade oligodendroglioma-astrocyoma, one with thalamic anaplastic astrocytoma, and one with high-grade parietal glioma) were treated with high-dose thiotepa/cyclophosphamide chemotherapy followed by ABMT. Five patients died, two due to toxicity and three due to disease. Two patients are in CR at 22+ and 24+ months after diagnosis, and two patients are alive with disease. The overall response rate is not any better than that observed with conventional chemotherapy. However, the results and response of the two CR patients are encouraging, suggesting that there is a select group of patients who may benefit from this type of regimen. Additional studies are needed to test this concept.

Although transient, responses have been reported in several trials of high-dose chemotherapy with stem cell support in children with recurrent CNS malignancies [79–81]. Classical bifunctional alkylators in combination appear to be beneficial, but only temporarily. The use of high-dose chemoradiotherapy to extended fields involving the CNS in young children should be weighed very carefully due to long-term consequences such as compromised growth and mental development. This type of high-dose chemotherapy seems to be a valid alternative, especially for those with refractory unresectable brain tumors. Most of the studies on high-dose treatment with stem cell rescue in patients with brain tumors have small sample numbers without extensive follow-up. More studies are warranted to provide a conclusive argument for the use of myeloablative therapy followed by ABMT in treating children with brain tumors.

Wilms' tumor

Wilms' tumor represents approximately 6% of childhood malignancies [2]. This tumor is among the most curable neoplasms in childhood, with more than 80% in continuous CR. Due to its high cure rate, high-dose therapy with stem cell rescue is rarely considered; however, new approaches and strategies must be undertaken to cure those children who fail first-line and salvage therapy and to reduce treatment toxicity [9,82].

Early results from the Royal Marsden group, using high-dose melphalan alone for patients with high-risk Wilms', demonstrated 6 of 6 responses in patients with relapsed disease and two long-term survivors [3]. In a recent report by the EBMT solid tumor registry [82], 25 children with relapsing or resistant Wilms' tumor underwent high-dose chemotherapy associated with ABMT in the period June 1984 to December 1991. Seventeen children were in CR and eight had measurable disease at the time of high-dose chemotherapy. Three children died of early pneumonitis; two developed acute transient renal failure, and one developed chronic renal failure. Out of the eight with measurable disease, two died of toxicity, five achieved CR, one obtained PR, and only one is presently alive in continuous CR at 39 months after ABMT. Of the 17 children grafted in CR, eight are alive event-free at 14 to 90 months from ABMT. Seven relapsed at 3 to 23 months; one died of toxicity; one was lost to follow-up in CR at 12 months. Although pulmonary and renal toxicities seem to be high, the results from patients who received consolidation salvage therapy in CR is quite positive. High-dose chemotherapy with ABMT in patients with measurable disease can induce a tumor response, but long-term results are poor. This study reveals that high-dose chemotherapy with ABMT in children with resistant or relapsed poor prognosis Wilms' tumor is beneficial and of interest. Since this study is small and selective, additional large randomized trials need to be performed. Currently, the National Wilms' Tumor Study Group #5 has proposed a study in which patients with Wilms' tumors will be

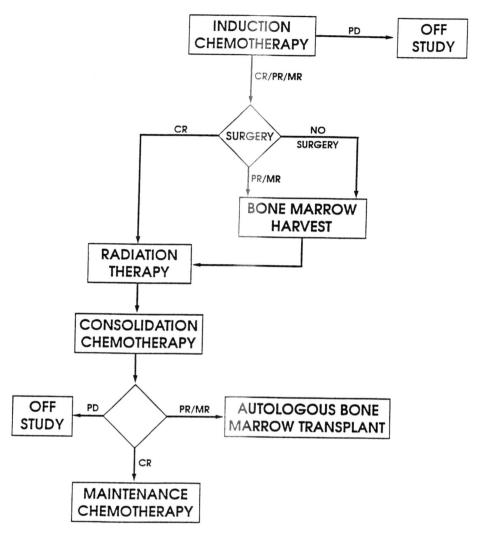

Figure 1. National Wilms' Tumor Study-5 regimen flow chart.

treated similarly at time of relapse. The high-risk patients will be treated with ABMT after high-dose drug therapy consisting of Thiotepa and VP-16 (see figure 1). Comprehensive studies such as these are necessary to determine the definitive role of ABMT in treating Wilms' tumor.

Other tumors

Small studies on other solid tumors have been performed using ABMT. In a study of 24 relapsed osteosarcoma patients, Miser used a massive cytoreductive regimen consisting of high-dose methotrexate, VCR, cyclophosphamide, doxorubicin, dicarbazine, melphalan, and high-dose cisplatin followed by ABMT. Twelve patients responded and were disease free 6.5 months post-ABMT [1].

ABMT has also been reported in malignant germ-cell tumors. In a melphalan and etoposide regimen with ABMT, the EBMT solid tumor registry confirmed that patients with refractory disease did not benefit from ABMT, whereas the role of ABMT as consolidation in first CR or PR was questionable [9].

The studies on these tumors are small, and more research with myeloablative regimens and ABMT must be performed before the role of ABMT in these tumors can be deciphered.

Conclusion

Autologous bone marrow is a valuable source of hemopoietic recovery when used in conjunction with nyeloablative regimens for treating pediatric solid tumors. The results using this type of regimen seem to benefit patients, and are in general an improvement over conventional historical treatments. However, hopeful enthusiasm resulting from these initial responses has been tempered in view of the disappointing long-term results. To achieve greater success using ABMT in pediatric tumors, it is unlikely that further increments in dose will be helpful. More clinical research must be conducted using myeloablative chemotherapy with stem cell rescue to clearly define its role in curing pediatric solid tumors. Yet at the same time, there exists a need to research new insights into the biology of these diseases, to improve the preparative regimens, to design innovative therapies such as combinations of chemotherapeutic drugs and immunotherapies, and to improve patient selection in studies. Hopefully, these tactics will lead to promising results such as reducing toxicity, lowering the percentage of relapse, achieving more complete remissions, and eventually reaching a time where more patients can be cured.

References

1. Pick TE. Autologous bone marrow transplant in children. CRC Crit Rev Oncol Hematol 8:311–337, 1988.
2. Kingston J, Malpas S, Stiller CA, et al. Autologous bone Marrow transplant contributes to haemopoietic recovery in children with solid tumors treated with high-does melphalan. Engl J of Haematol 58:589–595, 1984.
3. Pinkerton R, Philip, T, Bouffet E, et al. Autologous bone marrow transplantation in paediatric solid tumors. Clin Hematol 15:187–203, 1986.
4. Clifford P, Clift RA, Duff JK. Nitrogen mustard therapy combined with autologous marrow infusion. Lancet i:687–690, 1961.
5. Rill RD, Santana VM, Roberts WM, et al. Direct demonstration that autologous bone

marrow transplant for solid tumors can return a multiplicity of tumorigenic cells. Blood 84:380–383, 1994.

6. Kemshead JT, Heath L, Gibson FM, et al. Magnetic microspheres and monoclonal antibodies for the depletion of neuroblastoma cells from bone marrow: experiments, improvements, and observations. Br J Cancer 54:771–78 1986.

7. Evans EE, D'Angio GJ, Koup CE. The role of multimodal therapy in patients with local and regional NBL. J Pediatr Surg 19:77–80 1984.

8. Matthay KK, Sather HN, Seeger RC, et al. Excellent outcome for stage II neuroblastoma is independent of residual disease and radiation therapy. J Clin Oncol 7:236–44 1989.

9. Yaniv I, Bouffet E, Irle C, et al. Autologous bone marrow transplant in pediatric solid tumors. Pediatr Hematol Oncol 7:35–46, 1990.

10. Vossen JM. Autologous bone marrow rescue as part of a curative approach for pediatric solid tumors (editorial). Pediatr Hematol Oncol 7:iii–vii. 1990.

11. Seeger RC, Villablanca JG, Matthay KK, et al. Chemoradiotherapy and autologous bone marrow transplant for poor prognosis neuroblastoma. In Evans AE, D'Angio G, Knudson A, Seeger RC (eds), Advances in Neuroblastoma Research 3. New York: Wiley-Liss, 1991, p. 52.

12. Philip T, Ladenstein R, Zucker JM, et al. Double megatherapy and autologous bone marrow transplant for advanced neuroblastoma: The LCME2 study. Br J Cancer 67:119–127, 1993.

13. Haase GM, O'Leary MC, Ramsay NKC, et al. Aggressive surgery combined with intensive chemotherapy improves survival in poor risk neuroblastoma. J Pediatr Surg 26:1119–23, 1991.

14. Hayes FA, Smith EI. Neuroblastoma. In Pizzo PA, Poplack DG (eds), Principles of Pediatric Oncology. Philadelphia: JB Lippincott, 1989, p. 607.

15. Graham-Pole J. The role of marrow autografting in neuroblastoma. Bone Marrow Transplant 4:3, 1989.

16. Shafford EA, Rogers DW, Pritchard J. Advanced neuroblastoma: improved response rate using a multiagent regimen (OPEC) including cis-platinum and VM-26. J Clin Oncol 2:742–747, 1984.

17. Lanino E, Boni L, Corcuslo R, DeBernardi B. Did bone marrow transplant change the clinical course of neuroblastoma? Bone Marrow Transplant 7(Suppl 3):114–7, 1991.

18. Philip T, Hartmann O, Agust C, et al. Stage IV neuroblastoma alive progression-free 17 months post BMT are not cured. Bone Marrow Transplant 3(Suppl 1), 1988.

19. Ladenstein R, Lasset C, Hartmann O, et al. 1994. Comparison of auto vs. allografting as consolidation of primary treatments in advanced neuroblastoma over one year of age at diagnosis: report from the European Group for Bone Marrow Transplant. Bone Marrow Transplant 14:37–46, 1994.

20. Matthay KK, Atkinson JB, Stram DO, et al. Patterns of relapse after autologous purged bone marrow transplant for neuroblastoma: a children's cancer group pilot study. J Clin Oncol 11:2226–2233, 1993.

21. Hartman O, Kaifa C, Benhamou E, et al. Treatment of advanced neuroblastoma with high-dose melphalan and autologous bone marrow transplant. Cancer Chemother Pharmacol 16:165–169, 1986.

22. Kushner BH, Gulati SC, Kwon JH, et al. High dose melphalan with 6-hydroxy-dopamine-purged autologous marrow transplant for poor risk neuroblastoma. Cancer 68:242–247, 1991.

23. Philip T, Zucker JM, Bernard JL, et al. Improved survival at 2 and 5 years in the LMCE 1 unselected group of 72 Children with stage IV neuroblastoma older than 1 year of age at diagnosis: is a cure possible in a small subgroup. J Clin Oncol 9:1037–1044, 1991.

24. Corbett R, Pinderton R, Pritchard J, et al. Pilot study of high-dose vincristine, etoposide, carboplatin, and melphalan with autologous bone marrow rescue in advanced neuroblastoma. Eur J Cancer 28A:1324–1328, 1992.

25. Frei E, Antman K, Teicher B, et al. Bone marrow autotransplantation for solid tumors — prospects. J Clin Oncol 7:511–526, 1989.

26. Philip T, Ghalie R, Pinkerton R, et al. A phase II study of high dose cisplatin and VP16 in neuroblastoma: a report from the Societe Francaise D'Oncologie Pediatrique. J Clin Oncol 5:941–950, 1987.

27. Pinkerton R, Philip T, Biron P, et al. Vincristine infusion with advanced relapsed tumor. J Clin Oncol 3:1437–1438, 1985.
28. DeBernardi B, Bagnulo S, Brisgotti M, et al. Standard-dose and high-dose peptichemio and cisplatin in children with disseminated poor-risk neuroblastoma: 2 studies by the Italian Cooperative Group for Neuroblastoma. J Clin Oncol 10:1860–1878, 1992.
29. Kletzel M, Becton DL, Berry DH. Single institution experience with high-dose cyclophosphamide, continuous infuson vincristine, escalating doses of VP-16-213, unpurged bone marrow rescue in children with neuroblastoma. Med Pediatr Oncol 20:64–67, 1992.
30. Lam-Po-Tang PRL, McCowage GB, Vowels MR. Teniposide, doxorubicin, melphalan, cisplatin and total body irradiation with autologous bone marrow transplantation for advanced neuroblastoma. Transplant Proc 25:2881–2, 1993.
31. Matthay KK, Seeger RC, Reynolds CP, et al. Allogeric vs. autologous purged bone marrow transplant for neurobalstoma: a report from the children's cancer group. J Clin Oncol 12:2382–2389, 1994.
32. Johnson LR, Goldman S. Role of autotransplantation in neuroblastoma. Hematol Oncol Clin North Am 7(3):647–62, 1993.
33. Brenner MK, Rill DR, Moen RC, et al. Gene marking and autologous bone marrow transplantation (review). Ann NY Acad Sci 716:204–215, 225–227, 1994.
34. Seeger RC, Reynolds CP, Dang Vo D, et al. Depletion of neuroblastoma cells from bone marrow with monoclonal antibodies and magnetic immunobeads. In Evans AE, D'Angio GJ, Seeger RC (eds), Advances in Neuroblastoma Research. New York: Alan R. Liss, 1985, pp. 443–485.
35. Hartmann O, Zucker JM, Philip T, et al. Metastatic neuroblastoma in children more than one year old at diagnosis. Treatment with intensive chemo-radiotherapy and autologous bone marrow transplantation. Nouv Rev Franc d'Hematol, in press.
36. Fidgor CG, Voute PA, DeKraker J, et al. Physical cell separation of neuroblastoma cells from bone marrow. In Evans AE, D'Angio GJ, Seeger RC (eds), Advances in Neuroblastoma Research. New York: Alan R. Liss, 1985, pp. 471–483.
37. Treleaven JG, Kemshead JT. Removal of tumor cells from bone marrow: an evaluation of the available techniques. Hematol Oncol, 3:65–75, 1985.
38. Seeger RC, Moss TJ, Feig SA, et al. Bone marrow transplantation for poor prognosis neuroblastoma. Prog Clin Biol Res 271:41–50, 1988.
39. Moss TJ, Xu ZJ, Mansour VH, et al. Quantitation of tumor cell removal for bone marrow: a preclinical model. J Hematol 1:65–73, 1992.
40. Beaujean F, Hartmann O, Pico JL, et al. Incubation of autologous bone marrow graft with Asta-Z: comparative studies of hematological reconstitution after purged or non-purged bone marrow transplantation. Pediatr Hematol Oncol 4:105–115, 1987.
41. Philip T, Brehard JL, Zucker JM, et al. High-dose chemoradiotherapy with bone marrow transplantation as a consolidation treatment in neuroblastoma: an unselected group of stage IV patients over 1 year of age. J Clin Oncol 15:266–271, 1987.
42. Pinkerton R, Philip T, Biron P, et al. High dose melphalan, vincristine, and total body irradiation with autologous bone marrow transplant in children with relapsed neuroblastoma: a phase II study. Med Pediatr Oncol 15:236–240, 1987.
43. Glorieux P, Bouffet E, Philip I, et al. Metastatic interstitial pneumonitis after autologous bone marrow transplantation: a consequence of reinjection of malignant cells. Cancer 85:2136, 1986.
44. Graeve JLA, DeAlacron PA, Sato Y, et al. Milliary pulmonary neuroblastoma. A risk of autologous bone marrow transplant. Cancer 62:2125–7, 1988.
45. Rosen EM, Cassady JR, Frantz CN, et al. Neuroblastoma: The Joint Center for Radiation Therapy/Dana-Farber Cancer Institute/Children's Hospital experience. J Clin Oncol 2:719–732, 1984.
46. Jacobson HM, Marcu RB, Thar TR, et al. Pediatric neuroblastoma: a postoperative radiation therapy using less than 2000 radiation. Int J Radiat Oncol 9:501–505, 1983.
47. Evans A, Scher C, D'Angio G. Treatment of advanced neuroblastoma. Eur J Cancer 28A:1301–1302, 1992.

354

48. Dini G, Philip T, Hartmann O, et al. Bone marrow transplantation for neuroblastoma: a review of 513 cases. In Bernasconi G, Biergio GR (eds), Bone Marrow Transplantion in Children and Adults. Pavia, Italy: Medico Scientifiche Eds, 1989, pp. 42–46.

49. Kremens B, Kingebiel T, Herrmann F, et al. High-dose consolidation with local radiation and bone marrow rescue in patients with advanced neuroblastoma. Med Pediatr Oncol 23:470–475, 1994.

50. Sander J, Sullivan K, Witherspoon K, et al. Long-term effects and quality of life in children and adults after marrow transplantation. Bone Marrow Transplant 4:27–29, 1989.

51. Jones RJ, Ambinder RE, Piantoadosi S, Santos G. Evidence of a Graft vs. leukemia lymphoma effect associated with allogeneic bone marrow transplantation. Blood 77:649–653, 1971.

52. Jottner CA, To LB, Haylock DN, et al. Autologous blood stem cell transplantation. Transplantation Proc 21:2929–31, 1989.

53. Moss TJ, Ross AA. The risk of tumor cell contamination in peripheral blood stem cell collections. J Hematother 1:225–232, 1992.

54. Moss TJ, Sander DG, Lasky LC, Bostrom B. Contamination of peripheral blood stem cell harvest by circulating neuroblastoma cells. Blood 76(9):1879–1883, 1990.

55. Dicaro A, Bostrom B, Moss T, et al. Autologous peripheral blood cell transplant in the treatment of advanced neuroblastoma. Am J Pediatr Hem Oncol 16:200–206, 1994.

56. Kletzel M, Longino R, Danner K, et al. Peripheral blood stem cell rescue in children with advanced stage IV neuroblastoma. Prog Clin Biol Res 389:513–9, 1994.

57. Graham-Pole J, Casper J, Elfenbeen G, et al. High-dose chemoradiotherapy supported by marrow infusions for advanced neuroblastoma: a pediatric oncology group study. J Clin Oncol 9:152–158, 1991.

58. Favrot MC, Mchon J, Floret D, et al. Interleukin 2 immunotherapy in children with neuroblastoma after high-dose chemotherapy and autologous bone marrow transplant. Pediatr Hematol Oncol 7:275–284, 1990.

59. Burdach S, Jurgens H, Peters C, et al. Myeloablative radiochemotherapy and hematopoietic stem-cell rescue in poor-prognosis Ewing's sarcoma. J Clin Oncol 11:1482–1488, 1993.

60. Kinsella TJ, Miser JS, Waller B, et al. Long-term follow up of Ewing's sarcoma of bone treated with combined modality therapy. Int J Radiat Oncol Biol Phys 20:389–395, 1991.

61. Maurer HM, Moon T, Donaldson M, et al. The Intergroup Rhabdomyosarcoma Study: a preliminary report. Cancer 40:2015–2026, 1977.

62. Glaubiger DL, Makuch RW, Schwarz J. Influence of prognostic factors on survival in Ewing's sarcoma. Nat Cancer Inst Monogr 56:285–288, 1981.

63. Wilkins RM, Pritchard DJ, Burgert EO, et al. Ewing's Sarcoma of Bone Experience with 140 Patients. Cancer, 58:2551–2555, 1986.

64. Horowitz ME, Kinsella TK, Wexler LH, et al. Total-body irradiation and ABMT in the treatment of high-risk Ewing's sarcoma and rhabdomyosarcoma. J Clin Oncol 11:1911–1918, 1993.

65. Pinkerton R, Philip T. Autologous bone marrow transplant in pediatric solid tumors. Hematol Blood Transfus 31:92–96, 1987.

66. Miser J. Autologous bone marrow transplant for the treatment of sarcomas. In John FL, Pocheduj C (eds), Bone Marrow Transplant in Children. New York: 1990, pp. 289–298.

67. Horowitz ME, Etcubanas E, Christensen ML, et al. Phase II testing of melphalan in children with newly diagnosed rhabdomyosarcoma: a model for anti cancer drug development. J Clin Oncol 6:308–314, 1988.

68. Houghton JA, Cook RL, Lutz PJ, Houghton PJ. Melphalan: a potential new agent in the treatment of childhood rhabddomyosarcoma. Cancer Treatment Rep 69(1):91–6, 1985.

69. Pinkerton R, Philip T, Hartmann O, et al. High-dose chemoradiotherapy with autologous bone marrow rescue in pediatric soft tissue sarcoma. In Dicke K, Spitzer G, Jagnnath S (eds), Proceedings of the 4th International Symposium on Autologous Bone Marrow Transplant. Houston: University of Texas, 1989.

70. Arenson E, Waldman JB. Central nervous system tumors of childhood. Current Concepts Oncol Spring: 15–22, 1986.
71. Shulte FJ. Intracranial tumors in childhood — concepts of treatment and prognosis. Neuropediatrics 15:3–12, 1984.
72. Evans AE, Jenkin RD, Sposto R, et al. The treatment of medulloblastoma results of a prospective randomized trial of radiation therapy with and without CCNU, vincristine, and prednisone. J Neurosurg 72:572–582, 1990.
73. Kedar A, Maria BL, Graham-Pole J, et al. High dose chemotherapy with marrow reinfusion and hyperfractionated irradiation for children with high risk brain tumors. Med Pediatr Oncol 23:428–436, 1994.
74. Giannone L, Wolff SN. Phase II treatment of CNS gliomas with high-dose etoposide and autologous bone marrow transplantation. Cancer Treatment Rep 71:7–8, 1987.
75. Tirelli U, D'Incalci M, Canetta R, et al. Etoposide (VP-15-213) in malignant brain tumors: a phase II study. J Clin Oncol 2:432–437, 1984.
76. Bertolone SJ, Baum E, Krivit W, et al. Phase II trial of cis-platinum diamino dichloride in recurrent childhood brain tumors: a CCSG trial. Proc Am Soc Clin Oncol 72, 1983.
77. Allen JC, Walker RW, Luks E, et al. Carboplatin and recurrent childhood brain tumors. J Clin J Oncol 5:459–463, 1987.
78. Cohen ME, Duffner PK. Brain tumors in children: principles of diagnoses and treatment. In International Review of Child Neurology Series. New York: Raven Press, 1984, pp. 1–7, 103–211.
79. Kalifa C, Hartmann O, Demecq, et al. High-dose busulfan and thiotepa with ABMT in childhood malignant brain tumors: a phase II study. Bone Marrow Transplant 9:237–233, 1992.
80. Finlay JL, August C, Packer R, et al. High dose multi-agent chemotherapy followed by bone marrow rescue for malignant astrocytomas of childhood and adolescence. J Neuro-Oncol 9:239–248, 1990.
81. Hochberg FH, Parker LM, Takvorian T, et al. High dose BCNU with autologous bone marrow rescue for recurrent glioblastoma multi-forme. J Neurosurg 54:455–460, 1981.
82. Garaventa A, Hartmann O, Bernard JL, et al. Autologous bone marrow transplantation for pediatric Wilms' tumor: the experience of the European Bone Marrow Transplantation Solid Tumor Registry. Med Pediatr Oncol 22:11–14, 1994.

16. Autologous stem cell transplantation for the treatment of chronic myelogenous leukemia

Ravi Bhatia and Philip B. McGlave

Chronic myleogenous leukemia (CML) is a malignant disorder arising from the hematopoietic stem cell. It is characterized by abnormal expansion of malignant hematopoietic progenitor and precursor cells with concomitant suppression of normal hematopoiesis. CML is characterized cytogenetically by the 9;22 translocation resulting in the characteristic Philadelphia chromosome (Ph) [1] and, at the molecular level, the bcr/abl fusion oncogene [2]. Several studies have demonstrated a critical role for the bcr/abl oncogene in the pathogenesis of CML [3]. In contrast to other leukemias, treatment with conventional chemotherapy usually fails to induce a persistent complete cytogenetic remission in CML, and does not alter the course of the disease or prevent progression to accelerated phase (AP) and blast crisis (BC) over a median of 3 to 5 years. Allogeneic bone marrow transplantation using HLA-matched sibling or unrelated donor marrow is at present the most effective therapy for CML and successfully eliminates the malignant clone in a large proportion of patients. However, allogeneic transplants are available to less than 50% of CML patients either because of lack of a suitable donor or because older patients are unable to tolerate the associated morbidity and mortality. In view of this, there is a clear need to develop alternative therapeutic strategies. Perhaps because of the perceived difficulty in obtaining a leukemia-free graft and the anticipated lack of benefit from a graft that is contaminated with leukemic cells, the use of autologous transplantation for the treatment of CML has been explored but not widely applied. However, evidence indicating that normal Ph-negative hematopoietic stem cells persist in CML and preliminary clinical experience with autografting suggest that this approach is feasible and may be beneficial in CML.

Evidence for the persistence of residual normal Ph-negative hematopoietic stem cells in CML

Several lines of evidence suggest that normal Ph-negative hematopoietic stem cells persist in the marrow of patients with CML. It was observed that the occasional patient recovering from busulfan-induced marrow hypoplasia had

Jane N. Winter (ed.) BLOOD STEM CELL TRANSPLANTATION. 1997. Kluwer Academic Publishers. ISBN 0-7923-4260-7. All rights reserved.

long periods of Ph-negative hematopoiesis [4]. Transient cytogenetic remissions were observed in some CML patients following treatment with intensive chemotherapy similar to that used in the treatment of acute myeleogenous leukemia [5–7]. Similarly, in early autotransplant studies, Ph-negative hematopoiesis resulted transiently in some patients when marrow was collected in chronic phase (CP), cryopreserved, and reinfused at the time of disease progression [8]. Recently, it has been demonstrated that treatment with interferon-α, besides inducing hematological responses in the majority of patients, results in complete cytogenetic remissions with restoration of Ph-negative hematopoiesis in some patients with CML [9]. Thus, different treatment modalities can result in the induction of varying degrees of Ph-negative hematopoiesis in patients with CML, indicating the persistence of normal stem cells.

A number of laboratory studies have also confirmed the presence of Ph-negative progenitors in CML. The presence of both Ph-positive and Ph-negative colonies was observed following in vitro culture of bone marrow from patients with Ph-positive CML, indicating the existence of a normal stem cell population in at least some patients with CML [10]. In other studies, a significantly increased proportion of Ph-negative colonies was observed following treatment of CML bone marrow with interferon-γ [11]. Eaves and colleagues demonstrated that ex vivo culture of CML bone marrow in Dexter-type long-term bone marrow culture resulted in selective outgrowth of Ph-negative progenitors in about 40% of patients [12]. Further studies demonstrated that these progenitors were nonclonal and therefore presumably normal [13]. In addition, other studies have suggested that normal stem cells in CML bone marrow can be differentiated from their malignant Ph-positive counterparts on the basis of phenotypic differences. CD34 + HLA-DR- primitive progenitors in CML are Ph-negative by cytogenetics and fluorescence in situ hybridization (FISH) and bcr/abl negative by the polymerase chain reaction (PCR) as opposed to the CD34 + HLA-DR+ progenitors that comprise the malignant CML cell population [14,15]. These studies confirm the presence of Ph-negative stem cells in at least some patients with CML and support the use of autologous transplantation as treatment for CML.

Clinical experience

Autologous transplantation with unmanipulated blood or marrow grafts

Early experience with autologous transplant for CML was in patients with blast crisis CML. In the early 1970s, Buckner et al. performed autologous transplantation on seven CML patients who were in BC, utilizing intensive therapy with cyclophosphamide and total body irradiation followed by infusion of cryopreserved autologous marrow collected previously while the patients were still in CP [8]. Blast cells were cleared from the marrow of all seven patients. However, complete engraftment occurred in only two patients, and the one evaluable patient relapsed with BC within four months. These studies demonstrated the feasibility of using cryopreserved marrow for autologous transplantation for CML.

These studies were extended by the Hammersmith group, which transplanted 51 patients with CML BC between 1977 and 1983 using cryopreserved peripheral blood (PB) cells obtained by leukapheresis during CP [16]. Forty-eight patients achieved a second CP after autografting; however, the duration of the remissions was short, and the median survival was only 26 weeks. Twenty-one patients with relatively long remissions from BC were treated with second transplants either as consolidation or following recurrence of BC. This group appeared to achieve a longer survival (52 weeks) compared to patients transplanted only once. In three patients, 14% to 67% Ph-negative metaphases were observed transiently following transplantation.

Similar results were subsequently reported by Reiffers et al. [17] and confirmed in several smaller studies [18]. It was observed that although CP was reestablished in most patients, it was usually short-lived, with recurrence of advanced disease and death within six months to one year. Similar results were recently reported from the Dana-Farber Cancer Institute, where 12 patients with BC CML were treated with high-dose cytarabine and melphalan followed by reinfusion of peripheral blood mononuclear cells (PBMNCs) collected during CP [19]. None of the patients returned to a Ph-negative status. Seven patients achieved complete or partial hematological remission, while five showed no response to therapy. Further, 6 of 7 patients who returned to chronic phase required treatment for acceleration within three months.

These results led to studies evaluating the efficacy of autotransplantation for patients before the onset of transformation. The Hammersmith group reported the results for transplantation for 21 CP CML patients between 1984 and 1992 with unmanipulated autologous PBMNCs [20]. Twelve patients survive at a median of 82 months from the time of autografting (range: 9–105 months). The five-year survival of the autografted patients was significantly higher compared with 636 age-matched controls treated with conventional chemotherapy (56% vs. 28%). Harvesting of peripheral blood stem cells soon after diagnosis or later in CP did not affect survival. Nine patients achieved some degree of Ph-negative hematopoiesis, including two patients who achieved completely Ph-negative hematopoiesis late (one year and three years) after transplantation.

Reiffers et al. analyzed the results of 49 patients autografted for CML in CP entered in the European Bone Marrow Transplant registry between 1989 and 1991 [21], some of whom may have been included in the above-mentioned study. Engraftment occurred in 45 patients and was significantly faster after PBMNC (30 patients) than bone marrow (19 patients) transplantation. Fifteen of 34 evaluable patients had a major cytogenetic response (>65% Ph-negative metaphases), ten of whom had complete cytogenetic responses. Eight of ten patients were still in cytogenetic remission 6 to 36 months after transplant.

Table 1. Autotransplantation for CML with unmanipulated grafts

Study	No. of patients transplanted	Stem cell source	Cytogenetic response CR	Cytogenetic response PR(%Ph-)[a]	Survival (No. months)
Blast crisis					
Haines [16] Hammersmith	51	PBMNC	0	3 (14–67)	0.5–35
Reiffers [17] Bordeaux	47	PBMNC	0	14 (>10)	4.0–49
Matulonis [19] Dana-Farber	12	PBMNC	0	0	5.5
Chronic Phase					
Hoyle [20] Hammersmith	21	PBMNC	0[b]	9 (not defined)	9–105 56% at 5 years
Reiffers [21] EBMTR	49	BM 19 PBMNC 30	10[c]	5 (>65)	17–52 81% at 3 years

[a] % Ph- metaphases.
[b] Two late (1 and 3 years) responders.
[c] Duration of cytogenetic response: 6–36 months.
Abbreviations: PBMNC, Peripheral blood mononuclear cells; BM, bone marrow

Thirty-seven patients were still alive 17 to 52 months after autotransplantation. The actuarial survival at three years was 81.5 ± 15%. No factors were identified that predicted CR or survival.

These studies, summarized in table 1, suggest that autografting with unpurged autologous marrow or PBMNCs may extend survival for CML patients, particularly those transplanted in CP, and may be an option for patients who cannot undergo allogeneic transplantation. The mechanism by which autografting extends patient survival is unclear, although it may be related to a reduction in the size of the leukemic stem cell population by the transplant conditioning regimen.

Autologous transplantation with marrow and blood purged ex vivo

Eaves et al. demonstrated that incubation of bone marrow from some CML patients for ten days in long-term bone marrow culture causes a selective loss of primitive Ph-positive progenitors and enrichment with Ph-negative progenitors [12]. A variety of studies have shown that these Ph-negative hematopoeitic cells are nonclonal and presumably normal [13]. The Vancouver group has recently reported the results of a pilot study demonstrating that ex vivo culture of bone marrow in 36 of 87 patients (41%) resulted in the selective elimination of malignant progenitors [22]. Twenty-two of these 36 patients underwent transplantation with autologous ex vivo cultured bone marrow between November 1987 and March 1992; 16 of these patients were in

360

CP and 6 had advanced disease. Hematological recovery occured in 16 of 22 patients (73%). Regenerating bone marrow cells were 100% Ph negative in 13 patients and 75% to 94% Ph negative in the other three patients. However, Ph-positive cells became detectable in 12 of 13 patients in CR 4 to 36 months following transplant, while one patient died in remission. Thirteen of 16 CP patients and 3 of 6 advanced-disease patients are alive from 1 to 5.7 years from transplant. Four of 7 patients treated with low-dose interferon-α were returned to complete cytogenetic remission. Five patients failed to engraft or experienced slow engraftment and required 'back-up' untreated cells. This raises the concern that ex vivo manipulation may damage or deplete stem cells. These results indicate that use of a Ph-negative graft, rather than an unpurged graft, may result in an increased frequency of cytogenetic remission posttransplant. Elimination of the malignant clone after ex vivo culture, attainable in only 40% of patients, may be an important factor in the induction of cytogenetic remissions posttransplant. Brion et al. autografted two patients with ex vivo cultured marrow that contained residual bcr/abl+ cells after culture in both cases. Neither patient obtained cytogenetic remission posttransplant [23].

Rizzoli and colleagues demonstrated that mafosfamide treatment of CML bone marrow selectively enriches for Ph-negative stroma-adherent progenitors in some patients with CML. They evaluated treatment of bone marrow autografts with mafosfamide prior to autotransplantation [24]. Patients were selected for this therapy on the basis of laboratory assessment of the percentage of Ph-negative stroma-adherent progenitor cells that resulted from mafosfamide treatment of the bone marrow. In 16 of 25 patients evaluated, more than 50% of stroma-adherent progenitors were Ph-negative. Using this as the criterion to select patients for transplantation, bone marrow from ten patients (five in CP, three in AP, and two in second CP) was treated with mafosfamide (100 µg/ml for 30 minutes) and used for autografting. Recovering marrow metaphases were 100% Ph negative in 6 of 9 evaluable patients for a median duration of 6.5 months. However, with a median follow-up of 16 months (range: 3–31 months), only one patient remained Ph negative; one was Ph positive in CP, while five patients evolved to BC. Two patients died of nonhematological causes.

McGlave et al. performed autotransplantation with bone marrow cultured for 36 hours ex vivo in the presence of 1000 u/ml γ-interferon in 22 CP, 20 AP, and 2 second CP CML patients from 1988 to 1994 [25]. Twenty-nine patients had initial sustained engraftment, while 15 patients had delayed engraftment requiring reinfusion of autologous PBMNCs. The regenerating marrow metaphases were 100% Ph negative in 10 of 39 (26%) evaluable patients and 11% to 95% Ph negative in 12 of 39 (31%) patients. In all but three evaluable cases, Ph-negative metaphases had dropped to less than 10% by one year after transplant. The projected three-year survival for CP patients was 71% and for AP CML patients was 15%. Fifteen patients failed to engraft or showed slow engraftment requiring 'back-up' BM/PBMNC infusion.

Table 2. Autotransplantation for CML with purged marrow grafts: ex vivo purging

Study	Purging method	No. of patients studied	No. of patients transplanted	No. with cytogenetic response		Duration of cytogenetic CR (no. months)	Survival (no. years)
				CR	PR (%Ph-)		
Barnett [22] Vancouver	LTBMC	87[a]	22 (16CP,3AP,1CP2)	13	3 (>75%)	4.0-36	1.0-5.7
McGlave [25] Minnesota	gamma-Interferon	44[b]	44 (22CP,20AP,2CP2)	10	12 (10-95%)	<12	CP 71% at 3y AP 15% at 3y
Rizzoli [24] Parma	Mafosfamide	25[a]	10 (5CP,3AP,2CP2)	6	1 (75%)	6.5	0.3-1.8

[a] Only patients achieving a significant response to ex vivo purging were transplanted.
[b] Patients underwent autotransplantation regardless of the effect of purging on the Ph status of the autograft.
Abbreviations: LTBMC, Long-term bone marrow culture; CP, chronic phase; AP, accelerated phase; CP2, second chronic phase.

These studies, summarized in table 2, demonstrate that ex vivo purging of CML marrow prior to autografting may increase the cytogenetic remission rate after transplant in those patients in whom the Ph-positive clone can be eliminated. Consideration needs to be given to the possible contribution of patient selection to the favorable outcome of this group of patients. However, even in this selected group, the leukemia usually relapses over a variable period of time posttransplant, indicating the need for improved methods for purging of the autograft and/or better therapy to maintain remissions.

Autologous transplantation with peripheral blood or marrow purged in vivo

It was demonstrated in early 1980s that treatment with intensive combination chemotherapy similar to that used for acute myeloid leukemia resulted in a significant reduction in the percentage of Ph-positive cells and allowed restoration of Ph-negative hematopoiesis in up to 50% of patients with CML. However, the cytogenetic remissions were transient, and attempts to extend the duration of Ph-negative hematopoiesis by using different chemotherapy combinations were unsuccessful [5–7]. These results, however, raised the possibility that bone marrow or peripheral blood progenitor cells (PBPCs) collected during the recovery phase following chemotherapy could provide a suitable source of leukemia-free stem cells for autografting. In an early study, Korbling et al. collected PB cells from a CML CP patient following chemotherapy at a time when the patient's marrow was 100% Ph negative and used these for autografting when the patient's disease subsequently transformed to BC. This patient had 100% Ph-negative hematopoiesis on recovery [26].

More recently, Carella et al. tried a similar approach to autotransplantation of CML patients, using intensive chemotherapy consisting of idarubicin, cytarabine, and etoposide (ICE). PBPC were collected by leukapheresis during recovery from chemotherapy-induced myelosuppression. Forty-six patients were treated in this manner [27]. Apheresis products from 12 of 24 CP (50%) and five of 22 AP (23%) patients were 100% Ph negative, and were more than 50% Ph negative in an additional three CP and three AP patients. Sixty-four percent of patients treated within the first year from diagnosis had 100% Ph-negative apheresis collections. Collections that were 100% Ph negative were used as autografts in 16 patients (11 CP, 5 AP) following intensive chemoradiotherapy. Thirteen patients have engrafted and are alive, and five of these patients are Ph negative (31%) 5 to 29 months after transplant. Hematopoiesis was polyclonal in all four female patients evaluated posttransplantation for X-chromosome inactivation patterns [28].

Simonsson et al. reported the results of 97 newly diagnosed patients treated in a study conducted by the Swedish CML group [29]. Patients without a donor for allogeneic transplant were treated initially with hydroxyurea and α-interferon for at least six months. Those who did not achieve a complete cytogenetic remission were treated with one to three courses of intensive combination chemotherapy in an attempt to induce a complete cytogenetic remission. Remissions were eventually achieved in 23 cases. Eighteen patients were autografted, 15 of them in CR and three with more than 50% Ph-positive metaphases. Seventeen patients remain alive posttransplant. Of the 16 patients analyzed, nine are Ph negative 1 to 32 months from transplant, while seven relapsed cytogenetically 3 to 22 months after transplant. Of the remaining 79 patients, 32 are in continued CP, 34 underwent allogeneic transplantation, and 13 have died, four from treatment-related causes and nine in BC. These results support the concept that intensive treatment reduces the size of the Ph-postive clone in CML and that autografting of these patients results in Ph-negative hematopoiesis posttransplant.

Talpaz et al. collected PBMNCs and marrow cells during recovery from myelosuppression from 21 CML patients treated with conventional-dose chemotherapy [30]. CD34+ cells seperated from PBMNCs and marrow cells were used for autografting following high-dose chemoradiotherapy. Nine of 10 CP patients and 7 of 8 AP patients remain alive posttransplant, while none of the three BC patients remains alive posttransplant. Following conventional-dose chemotherapy, CD34+ cells from 3 of 21 patients were completely Ph negative; positively selected CD34+ cells were partially Ph negative in 7 of 21 cases (30% to 92%). Following autografting, the regenerating marrow was 100% Ph negative in 5 of 21 patients and partially Ph negative (26% to 96%) in another five patients. A direct correlation was observed between the frequency of Ph-negative cells in the autograft and the percentage of Ph-negative marrow cells 17 to 55 weeks after transplant (figure 1). These results suggest that the

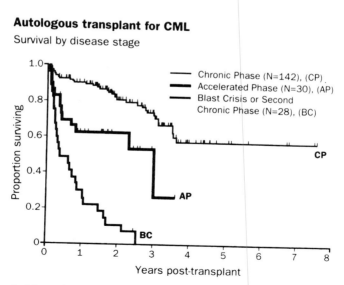

Figure 1. Survival for patients receiving autologous transplants. Chronic phase (CP), accelerated phase (AP), and blast crisis or second chronic phase (BC). Hatch marks represent surviving patients.

Table 3. In vivo purging

Study	Regimen	No. of patients studied	IN VIVO PURGING No. with cytogenetic response CR	PR(%Ph-)	Stem cell source	No. of patients transplanted	AUTOGRAFTING No. with cytogenetic response CR	PR(%Ph-)	Duration of cytogenetic CR (No. of months)	Survival (No. of months)
Carella [27] Genoa	ICE, G-CSF	46 (24CP,22AP)	17	6(>50%)	PBPC	16 (11CP,5AP)	5	NA	5.0–29	15–29
Talpaz [30] MD Anderson	DC/FMC/ICE	21 (10CP,8AP,3BC)	3	7(30–92%)	PBPC/BM CD34 selected	21	5	5(26–90%)	4.0–15	1.0–21
Simonsson [29] Sweden	Hu/Ifn, DC MI,C,CA	97 (97CP)	23	NA	BM	18 (18CP)	13	2(>65%)	3.0–32	13–32
Durrant [34] Australia	ICE, G-CSF	15 (8CP,5AP,2BC)	3	4(-65%)	PBPC	5	4	NA	NA	NA
O'Brien [32] Hammersmith	ICE, G-CSF	9 CP	NA	NA	PBPC	6 (6CP)	0	3(NA)	NA	0.6–10.9
Chalmers [33] Glasgow	I,C	25 (25CP)	11	2(>50%)	PBPC	8 (8CP)	1	1(>50%)	4	NA
Tringali [31] Palermo	Cy	6 (4CP,2AP)	0	1(NA)	PBPC4 PBPC+BM2	6 (4CP,2AP)	1	1(>60%)	NA	14–26
Sureda [35] Barcelona	ICE, G-CSF	3 (2CP,1AP)	1	1(>33%)	PBMNC	2	NA	NA	NA	NA

Abbreviations: CP, chronic phase; AP, accelerated phase; BC, blast crisis; I, idarubicin; C, ARA-C; E, etoposide; D, daunorubicin; F, fludarabine; M, mitoxantrone; Hu, hydroxyurea; Ifn, inteferon-alpha; A, amsacrine, Ara-C; Cy, high-dose cytoxan.

365

chances of obtaining cytogenetic remissions posttransplant are related to the achievement of cytogenetic responses with pretransplant treatment.

Several other centers have initiated similar trials exploring the use of chemotherapy to induce Ph-negative hematopoiesis prior to harvesting bone marrow or PBMNCs for autografting [31–35]. The results of these studies are shown in table 3. Although there is considerable variability in the results from different centers, it appears that this approach may lead to the achievement of a Ph-negative state and/or a reduction in the leukemic load in the autograft. Achievement of Ph-negative hematopoiesis posttransplant may occur. It is less clear whether this is a result of the reduced leukemic burden resulting from effective purging of the autograft or whether a good response to conventional chemotherapy preselects those patients who are likely to respond well to the more intensive chemoradiotherapy used in transplant preparative regimens.

Survival benefit from autologous stem cell transplantation

Several reports from individual centers suggest that autologous transplantation may be associated with prolongation of survival of CML patients, especially those transplanted in CP, compared with patients treated with conventional chemotherapy. McGlave et al. compiled the results for 200 patients with Ph-positive CML who underwent autologous transplantation with purged or unpurged marrow or primed peripheral blood progenitor cells or PBMNCs at eight different transplant centers in Europe and North America from June 1984 to January 1992 [36]. This was the first multicenter report on autologous transplantation for CML and included the largest number of autotransplanted CML patients studied to date. Of the 200 patients studied, 125 were alive at the end of the study (median follow-up of 42 months; range 1–91 months). The median survival time for 142 patients with CP CML had not been reached; the median survival was 35.9 months for patients with AP and 4.1 months for patients in BC. The survival probability for CP patients was 58%, with the last of 36 deaths occurring at 43.3 months (figure 2). Although relatively few patients are evaluable 43.3 months after transplant, these data suggest that autotransplantation may result in a plateau in the survival curve that is not observed with conventional chemotherapy. Furthermore, autotransplant may increase survival of AP CML patients over that seen with conventional-dose chemotherapy. Aside from the disease phase at transplant, no other patient characteristics predicted survival, including source of stem cells (bone marrow versus PBMNCs) or ex vivo purging methods. These results confirm those from several smaller studies mentioned earlier, many of which were included in this analysis. It is of note that the majority of the survivors had recurrent or persistent CML based on cytogenetic or hematological criteria. Therefore, improved survival cannot be attributed to the elimination of malignant progenitors following autografting. This suggests that the beneficial effect of autografting may be related to a reduction rather

366

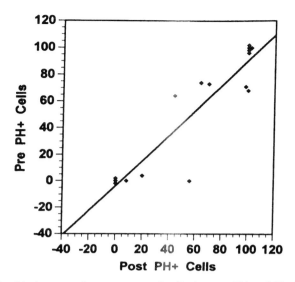

Figure 2. Relationship between the percentage of cells that are Ph⁺ and Ph⁻ before and after transplantation. Using the Spearman rank test, there is a less than 0.001% probability that the observed correlation (coefficient of correlation = 0.91) would have occurred if the null hypothesis of no correlation were true.

than elimination of the leukemic cell load following myeloablative therapy. These results should be interpreted cautiously, since patient selection may have influenced these results and the analysis included a heterogenous group of patients from eight transplant centers. Controlled clinical trials will be required to definitively demonstrate the superiority of this approach over other treatment modalities in CML.

Future approaches

Reasons for failure of autologous transplantation treatment for CML

The above results demonstrate that although autografting may result in a transient Ph-negative state, leukemia usually recurs within the first year following transplant. Relapse following autologous transplantation could result either from the transplantation of residual primitive leukemic cells in the autograft or from the persistence of leukemic cells in the host following myeloablative therapy. This issue may be resolved by retroviral marking of the autograft prior to transplantation; the contribution of transplanted malignant stem cells to posttransplant relapse could then be assessed. Etkin et al. demonstrated that the marrow from patients with CML could be marked efficiently, allowing the use of this marking technique to study the question of relapse origin [37]. To evaluate the contribution of infused Ph-positive cells to relapse posttransplant, the MD Anderson group used a safety-modified retrovirus containing the Neomycin resistance gene (NEO) to mark autologous marrow cells collected early in the recovery phase after conventional dose chemotherapy. CD34+ cells were selected from the harvested marrow. Thirty percent of these cells were marked by exposure to the retrovirus and then mixed with unmarked cells and used for autotransplantation [38]. Following transplantation, NEO-marked leukemic cells were found in blood and marrow at least 280 days after transplant in both reported patients. These studies, besides demonstrating the feasibility of this approach, demonstrate that infused malignant cells contribute to relapse after transplant and indicate the need for improved methods for purging the autograft of leukemic stem cells.

Improved methods for purging of CML blood and marrow

A number of novel approaches to the in vitro purging of CML marrow are being developed. One promising approach is the selection of benign progenitors on the basis of phenotypic characteristics. Verfaillie et al. demonstrated that the CD34+ HLA-DR- cells obtained from CML bone marrow contain primitive progenitors that generate progeny that are nonmalignant by cytogenetics and RT-PCR [14]. This was subsequently confirmed in a high proportion of patients in early CP (less than one year after diagnosis). Other investigators have verified this finding [15,39]. The recent observation that this progenitor population lacks the bcr/abl rearrangement at the genomic level [15,40] addresses the concern expressed by some investigators that primitive CML progenitors that do not express bcr/abl message and may not be detectable by RT-PCR could be present [41]. Sufficient numbers of benign progenitors for autologous transplantation appear to be present in the marrow of early CP patients. However, in late CP, AP, or BC, the CD34+ DR- population is markedly reduced in number and contaminated with malignant cells [40]. Selection of CD34+ DR- cells from the bone marrow of patients with early CP may thus offer a source of leukemia-free cells for autografting, although other approaches will be required for patients with more advanced disease.

The use of antisense oligonucleotides (ASOs) directed against either the bcr/abl oncogene or the myb gene is also being explored for ex vivo purging of CML bone marrow. ASOs complementary to the breakpoint junctions of bcr/abl mRNA inhibit the expression of the p210 bcr/abl fusion protein and prevent development of tumors in experimental animals [42,43]. ASOs directed against c-myb, a proto-oncogene important in cell proliferation, selectively inhibit growth of CML progenitors in vitro [44]. De Fabritiis et al. autografted a patient with AP CML progenitors using bone marrow treated with ASOs to bcr/abl [45]. Posttransplant marrow evaluation with FISH and cytogenetics demonstrated approximately 10% of cells to be bcr/abl or Ph negative for up to nine months post-transplant. Luger et al. treated CD34+ marrow cells from five CML patients with c-myb ASOs prior to autografting

368

[46]. Bone marrow from two patients evaluated soon after transplant had approximately 15% Ph-negative metaphases. Although these results are encouraging and indicate that this approach is likely to be feasible, additional studies will be needed to determine the benefit of this approach. Recently, ribozyme RNA sequences capable of cleaving other RNA molecules in a catalytic manner have been adapted to create targeted antisense molecules that specifically bind a target sequence and cleave adjacent sites. Leopold et al. constructed a multiunit ribozyme that binds the b3a2 bcr-abl junction and cleaves three sites close to the breakpoint [47]. Transfection of the ribozyme into bcr/abl transformed cells reduced bcr/abl mRNA levels by a thousandfold, suggesting that this approach could be useful for ex vivo purging autografts in CML.

Several studies have demonstrated that Ph-positive CML hematopoietic progenitors, in contrast to normal Ph-negative cells, are deficient in their ability to adhere to the marrow stromal microenvironment [48,49]. It may be possible to employ differences in adhesion to stroma and fibronection between CML and normal marrow progenitors to select for Ph-negative progenitors. In contrast to normal Ph-negative progenitors, Ph-positive CML progenitors do not respond to normal inhibitory signals and continue to proliferate even when in contact with stroma or fibronectin; treatment of CML bone marrow with cell-cycle-specific chemotherapeutic agents following culture in the presence of these ligands may result in selective elimination of the Ph-positive population [50]. Eaves et al. reported that the chemokine macrophage inflammatory protein-1α (MIP-1α) inhibits the proliferation of primitive normal progenitors, but does not inhibit the proliferation of CML progenitors. Treatment of marrow cultures with MIP-1α may therefore accentuate differences in proliferation between CML and normal progenitors [51]. This differential response following MIP-1α exposure could be exploited in therapeutic interventions with cell-cycle-specific chemotherapeutic agents directed against cycling malignant CML progenitors. Another possible approach being evaluated is based on the observation that malignant CML progenitors have significantly reduced survival on stroma deficient in SCF (stem cell factor) compared with normal progenitors. This results in the generation of an increased proportion of Ph-negative colonies when CML marrow is cultured on such stromal layers [52]. It may be possible to purge CML marrow or peripheral blood progenitors by culture on SCF-deficient feeders, leading to selective depletion of Ph-positive progenitors.

Another approach to ex vivo purging of CML bone marrow currently being evaluated is the use of immune effector cells to selectively target leukemic cells. Verma et al. reported that culture of CML marrow with rIL-2 for 1 to 2 weeks resulted in the generation of cells cytotoxic for the A375 melanoma cell line and K562 cells of CML origin [53]. This technique resulted in the elimination of Ph-positive cells from the bone marrow of four patients with CML. Miller et al. have developed techniques for large-scale ex vivo cultivation of activated NK cells that can be applied to immunotherapy protocols [54].

Cervantes et al. demonstrated that activated NK cells generated from CML peripheral blood cells selectively suppress autologous primitive CML but not normal bone marrow progenitors [55]. Likewise, autologous T lymphocytes cultured from CML bone marrow were demonstrated to suppress autologous hematopoietic progenitors, whereas T lymphocytes similarly generated from normal bone marrow failed to suppress autologous progenitors [56]. These studies suggest that ex vivo culture of CML bone marrow with rIL-2 or with autologous rIL-2-activated NK or T cells may constitute a useful purging approach.

Therapies to maintain remissions following autologous transplantation

It is likely that resistant leukemic cells that survive myeloablative chemo-radiotherapy contribute to the leukemic relapses observed after autologous transplantation. Allogeneic transplants with bone marrow from normal individuals that has been T depleted, or syngeneic transplants using bone marrow from identical twins, result in relapse in more than 50% of patients two years following transplant [57]. Therefore, in addition to improved purging methods, treatment directed against leukemic cells that survive myeloablative therapy will also be required.

In several of the clinical studies discussed above, α-interferon treatment following relapse posttransplant has resulted in restoration of a Ph-negative state. This occurs in some patients who failed to achieve cytogenetic responses to α-interferon treatment pretransplant. However, the use of α-interferon is limited by side effects that may be more pronounced in patients post-transplant, and its effectiveness may be limited to a small proportion of patients. Therefore, there is a need for the development of other effective posttransplant treatments.

The above-mentioned studies demonstrating the utility of interleukin-2 in ex vivo purging of CML marrow also suggest that it may be of use as systemic therapy following autotransplantation for CML. In fact, systemic interleukin-2 is being studied as posttransplant immunotherapy for acute myelogenous leukemia and lymphomas [58]. Similarly, studies are underway to determine the effect of the immunomodulator Linomide (roquinimex) following autologous marrow for CML [59]. Another potentially useful approach is the use of cellular therapy with activated NK- and T-cell populations, discussed above with reference to ex vivo purging, for systemic antileukemia therapy in the posttransplant setting.

Another potentially useful approach to posttransplant therapy following CML autotransplantation is the introduction of drug resistance genes into Ph-negative autologous hematopoietic cells prior to transplant. Following transplantation, systemic chemotherapy may be employed to selectively target nontransduced cells, including residual malignant cells that may have persisted in the host. This approach is currently being used in patients undergoing autografting for breast cancer, in whom the multidrug resistance

(MDR) gene is introduced into autologous marrow stem cells [60]. A similar approach may be possible in CML in combination with selection of Ph-negative progenitors.

Conclusions

Autologous transplantation, even with an unpurged graft, can result in a transient Ph-negative state in CML patients. Ex vivo and in vivo purging methodologies can be employed to obtain a completely or partially Ph-negative autograft and appear to be associated with improved chances of achieving Ph-negative hematopoiesis following transplant. Although most patients will relapse within a year of transplantation, autografting of CML patients, especially in CP, may result in improved survival compared to conventional treatment in spite of disease relapse posttransplant. Autologous transplantation using either marrow or blood as a source of progenitors offers an alternative treatment option for patients without a suitable allogeneic donor. It may eventually be possible to achieve long-term restoration of Ph-negative hematopoiesis once improved methods for marrow purging are available and better antileukemia treatments for use after transplant have been developed.

References

1. Rowley JD. A new consistent chromosome abnormality in chronic myelogenous leukemia. Nature 243:209, 1973.
2. DeKlein A, Van Kessel AG, Grosveld G, Bartram CR, Hagemeijer A, Bostooma D, Spurr NK, Heisterkamp N, Groffen J, Stephenson JR. A cellular oncogene is translocated to the Philadelphia chromosome in chronic myelocytic leukemia. Nature 300:765, 1982.
3. Daley GQ, Van Etten RA, Baltimore D. Induction of chronic myelogenous leukaemia in mice by the p210 bcr/abl gene of the Philadelphia chromosome. Science 247:824–829, 1990.
4. Finney R, McDonald A, Baikie AG, Douglas AS. Chronic granulocytic leukaemia with Ph[1] negative cells in bone marrow and a ten year remission after Busulphan hypoplasia. Br J Haematol 23:283–288, 1972.
5. Cunningham I, Gee T, Dowling M. Results of treatment of Ph[1] positive chronic myeloid leukemia with an intensive treatment regimen (L-5 protocol). Blood 53:375–395, 1979.
6. Goto T, Nishikori M, Arlin Z, Gee T, Kempin S, Burchenal J, Strife A, Wisniewski D, Lambek C, Little C, Jhanwar S, Chaganti R. Clarkson B. Growth characteristics of leukemia and normal hematopoietic cells in Ph1+ chronic myelogenous leukemia in vivo and in vitro and effects of intensive treatment with the L15 protocol. Blood 59:793–808, 1982.
7. Smalley RV, Vogel J, Huguley CM Jr, Miller D. Chronic granulocytic leukemia: cytogenetic conversion of the bone marrow with cycle-specific chemotherapy. Blood 50:107–113, 1977.
8. Buckner CD, Stewart P, Clift RA, Fefer A. Neiman PE, Singer J, Storb R, Thomas ED. Treatment of blastic transformation of chronic granulocytic leukemia by chemotherapy, total body irradiation and infusion of cryopreserved autologous marrow. Exp Hematol 6:96–109, 1978.
9. Talpaz M, Kantarjian HM, Kurzrock R, Trujillo JM, Gutterman JU. Interferon-alpha produces sustained cytogenetic responses in chronic myelogenous leukemia Philadelphia chromosome positive patentis. Ann Intern Med 114:532–538, 1991.

10. Chervenick PA, Ellis LD, Pan SF, Lawson AL. Human leukemic cells: in vitro growth of colonies containing the Philadelphia (Ph) chromosome. Science 174:1134–1136, 1971.
11. McGlave P, Mamus S, Vilen B, Dewald G. Effect of recombinant gamma interferon on chronic myelogenous leukemia bone marrow progenitors. Exp Hematol 15:331–335, 1987.
12. Coulombel L, Kalousek DK, Eaves CJ, Gupta CM, Eaves AC. Long term marrow culture reveals chromosomally normal hematopoietic progenitor cells in patients with Philadelphia chromosome-positive chronic myelogenous leukemia. N Engl J Med 306:1493–1498, 1983.
13. Hogge DE, Coulombel L, Kalousek DK, Eaves CJ, Eaves AC. Nonclonal hematopoietic progenitors in a G6PD hetrerozygote with chronic myelogenous leukemia revealed after long-term marrow culture. Am J Hematol 24:389–394, 1987.
14. Verfaillie CM, Miller WJ, Boylan K, McGlave PB. Selection of benign primitive hematopoietic progenitors in chronic myelogenous leukemia on the basis of HLA-DR antigen expression. Blood 79:1003–1010, 1992.
15. Kirk JA, Reems JA, Roecklein BA, Van Devanter DR, Bryant EM, Radich J, Edmands S, Lee A, Torok-Storb B. Benign marrow progenitors are enriched in the CD34+/HLA-DRlo population but not in the CD34+/CD38lo population in chronic myelogenous leukemia: an analysis using interphase fluorescence in situ hybridization. Blood 86:737–743, 1995.
16. Haines ME, Goldman JM, Worsely AM, McCarthy DM, Wyatt SE, Dowding C, Kearney L, Th'ng KH, Wareham NJ, Pollock A, Galvin MC, Samson D, Geary CG, Catovsky D, Galton DAG. Chemotherapy and autografting for chronic granulocytic leukaemia in transformation: probable prolongation of survival for some patients. Br J Haematol 58:711–721, 1984.
17. Reiffers J, Troutte R, Marit G, Montastruc M, Faberes C, Cony-Makhoul P, David B, Bordeau MJ, Bilhou-Nabera C, Lacombe F, Feuillatre-Fabre F, Vezon G, Bernard PH, Broustet A. Autologous blood stem cell transplantaion for chronic granulocytic leukaemia in transformation: a report of 47 cases. Br J Haematol 77:339–345, 1991.
18. Butturini A, Keating A, Goldman J, Gale RP. Autotransplants in chronic myelogenous leukemia: strategies and results. Lancet 335:1255–1258, 1990.
19. Matulonis UA, Griffin JD, Canellos GP. Autologous peripheral blood stem cell transplantation of the blastic phase of chronic myelogenous leukemia following sequential high-dose cytosine arabinoside and melphalan. Am J Hematol 45:283–287, 1994.
20. Hoyle C, Gray R, Goldman J. Autografting for patients with CML in chronic phase: an update. Br J Hematol 86:76–81, 1994.
21. Reiffers J, Goldman J, Meloni G, Cahn JY, Gratwohl A. Autologous stem cell transplantaion in chronic myelogenous leukemia: a retrospective analysis of the European Group for Bone Marrow Transplantation. Bone Marrow Transplant 14:407–410, 1994.
22. Barnett MJ, Eaves CJ, Phillips GL, et al. Autografting with cultured marrow in chronic myelogenous leukemia: results of a pilot study. Blood 84:724–732, 1994.
23. Brion A, Charbord P, Flesch M, Deconinck E, Deschaseux M, Racadot EW, Cahn JY. Autografting with cultured marrow in CML: problem of hematopoietic reconstitution. Bone Marrow Transplant 15:S22, 1995.
24. Carlo-Stella C, Mangoni L, Almici C, Caramatti C, Cottafavi L, Dotti GP, Rizzoli V. Autologous transplant for chronic myelogenous leukemia using marrow treated ex vivo with mafosfamide. Bone Marrow Transplant 14:425–432, 1994.
25. McGlave P, Miller J, Miller W, Perry E, Fautsch S, Ramsay NKC, Verfailie CM, Weisdorf DW. Autologous marrow transplant therapy for CML using marrow treated ex vivo with human recombinant interferon gamma. Blood 84(10, Suppl 1):537A, 1994.
26. Korbling M, Burke P, Braine H, Elfenbien G, Santos G, Kaizer H. Successful engraftment of blood derived stem cells in chronic myelogenous leukemia. Exp Hematol 9:684–690, 1981.
27. Carella AM, Frassoni F, Podesta M, Pungolino E, Pollicardo N, Ferrero R, Soracco M. Idarubicin containing regimen and G-CSF are able to recruit a high rate of normal progenitor cells during early hematopoietic recovery in patients with CML. J Hematother 3:199–202, 1994.
28. Carella AM, Frassoni F, Negrin RS. Autografting in chronic myelogenous leukemia: new questions. Leukemia 9:365–369, 1995.

29. Simonsson B, Oberg G, Killander A, et al. Intensive treatment in order to minimize the Ph-positive clone in chronic myelogenous leukemia. Stem Cells 111(Suppl 3):73–76, 1993.
30. Talpaz M, Kantarjian H, Liang J, Calvert L, Hamer J, Tibbits P, Durett A, Claxton D, Giralt S, Khouri I, Przepiorka D, Van Besien K, Andersson B, Mehra R, Gajewski J, Seong D, Hester J, Estey E, Korbling M, Pollicardo N. Berenson R, Heimfeld S, Champlin R, Deisseroth AB. Percentage of Philadelphia chromosome (Ph)-negative and Ph positive cells found after autologous transplantation for chronic myelogenous leukemia depends on percentage of diploid cells induced by conventional-dose chemotherapy before collection of autologous cells. Blood 85:3257–3263, 1995.
31. Tringali S, Santoto A, Scimi R, Vasta S, Pampinella M, Marino MA, Majolino I. High-dose cyclophosphamide for mobilization of circulating stem cells in chronic myelogenous leukemia. Eur J Haematol 53:1–5, 1994.
32. O'Brien SG, Rule S, Spencer A, Savage D, Apperly J, Chase AJ, Mconald C, Davidson RJ, Goldman JM. Autografting in chronic phase CML using PBPCs mobilized by intermediate-dose chemotherapy. Bone Marrow Transplant 15:S11, 1995.
33. Chalmers EA, Franklin IM, Kelsey S, Clarke R. Sproul AM, Goldstone AH, Hepplestone A, Watson W, Sharp S, Tansey P. Mobilization of Ph negative progenitors into peripheral blood in chronic myelogenous leukemia (CML) using Idarubicin and Cytarabine. Blood 84(10, Suppl 1):400A, 1994.
34. Durrant S, Taylor K, Moore D, Hutchins C, Eliadis P, Grigg A, Atkinson K. Bone marrow transplant following intensive chemotherapy with filgrastim support and progenitor cell collection in advanced chronic myelogenous leukemia. Bone Marrow Transplant 15:S19, 1995.
35. Sureda A, Brunet S, Amill B, Aventin A, Sanchez JA, Mateu R, Portos JM, Madoz P, Gomez de Segura G, Garcia Lopez J, Domingo-Albos A. Peripheral blood stem cell mobilization in patients with chronic myelogenous leukemia. Bone Marrow Transplant 15:S20, 1995.
36. McGlave PB, De Fabritiis P, Deisseroth A, Goldman J, Barnett M, Reiffers J, Siminsson B, Carella A, Aeppli D. Autologous transplants for chronic myelogenous leukemia: results from eight transplant groups. Lancet 343:1486–1488, 1994.
37. Etkin M, Filaccio M, Ellerson D, Suh S-P. Claxton D, Gaozza E, Brenner M, Moen R, Belmont J, Moore KA, Moseley AM, Reading C, Khouri I, Talpaz M, Kantarjian H, Deisseroth A. Use of cell-free retroviral vector preparations for transduction of cells from the marrow of chronic phase and blast crisis chronic myelogenous leukemia patients and from normal individuals. Human Gene Ther 3:137–145, 1992.
38. Deisseroth AB, Zhifei Zu, Claxton D, Hanania EG, Fu S, Ellerson D, Goldberg L, Thomas M, Janicek K, French Anderson W, Hester J, Korbling M, Durett A, Moen R, Berenson R, Heimfeld S, Hamer J, Calvert L, Tibbits P. Talpaz M, Kantarjian H, Champlin R, Reading C. Genetic marking shows that Ph positive cells present in autologous transplants of chronic myelogenous leukemia (CML) contribute to relapse after autologous bone marrow in CML. Blood 83:3068–3076, 1994.
39. Leemhuis T, Leibowitz D, Cox G, Silver R. Srour EF, Tricot G, Hoffman R. Identification of BCR/ABL-negative primitive hematopoietic progenitor cells within chronic myelogenous leukemia marrow. Blood 81:801–807, 1993.
40. Verfaillie CM, Miller W, Miller JS, Bhatia R. McGlave PB. Benign primitive progenitors can be selected on the basis of the CD34 + HLA-DR- phenotype in early chronic phase (ECP) but not advanced phase (AP) CML. Blood 84(10, Suppl 1):382A, 1994.
41. Keating A, Wang XN, Laraya P. Variable transcription of bcr-abl by Ph positive cells arising from hematopoietic progenitors in chronic myelogenous leukemia. Blood 83:1744–1751, 1994.
42. Szczylik C, Skorski T, Nicolaides NC, Manzella L, Malaguernara L, Venturelli D, Gewirtz AM, Calabretta B. Selective inhibition of leukemia cell proliferation by BCR-ABL antisense oligodeoxynucleotides. Science 253:562–565, 1991.
43. Skorski T, Nieborowska-Skowrska M, Nicolaides NC, Szczylik C, Iversen P, Iozzo RV, Zon G, Calabretta B. Suppression of Philadelphia leukemia growth in mice by bcr-abl antisense oligonucleotides. Proc Natl Acad Sci U S A 91:4504–4508, 1994.
44. Calabretta B, Sims PB, Valiteri M, Caracciolo D, Szczylik C, Venturelli D, Rtajczak M, Beran

M, Gewirtz AM. Normal and leukemic hematopoietic cells manifest differential sensitivity to inhibitory effects of c-myb antisense oligonucleotides: an in vitro study relevant to bone marrow purging. Proc Natl Acad Sci U S A 88:2351–2315, 1991.

45. de Fabritiis P, Amadori S, Petti MC, Mancini M, Montefusco E, Picardi A, Geiser T, Campbell K, Calabretta B. In vitro purging with BCR-ABL antisense oligodeoxynucleotides does not prevent haematological reconstitution after autologous bone marrow transplantation. Leukemia 9:662–664, 1995.

46. Luger SM, Ratjczak MZ, Stadtmauer EA, Mangan P, Magee D, Silberstein L, Edelstein M, Nowell P, Gewirtz AM. Autografting for chronic myelogenous leukemia with c-myb antisense oligonucleotide purged bone marrow: a preliminary report. Blood 84(10, Suppl 1):151A, 1994.

47. Leopold LH, Shore SK, Newkirk TA, Reddy RMV, Reddy EP. Multi-unit ribozyme-mediated cleavage of bcr-abl mRNA in myeloid leukemias. Blood 85:2162–2170, 1995. 48.

48. Gordon MY, Dowding CR, Riley GP, Goldman JM, Greaves MF. Altered interactions with marrow stroma of haematopoietic progenitor cells in chronic myelogenous leukemia. Nature 328:342–344, 1987.

49. Verfaillie CM, McCarthy JB, McGlave PB. Mechanisms underlying abnormal trafficking of malignant progenitors in chronic myelogenous leukemia: decreased adhesion to stroma and fibronectin but increased adhesion to the basement membrane components laminin and collagen type IV. J Clin Invest 90:1232–1241, 1992.

50. Eaves CJ, Cashman JD, Gaboury LA, Kalousek DK, Eaves AC. Unregulated proliferation of primitive chronic myelogenous leukemia progenitors in the presence of normal marrow adherent cells. Proc Natl Acad Sci U S A 83:5306–5310, 1986.

51. Eaves CJ, Cashman JD, Wolpe SD, Eaves AC. Unresponsiveness of primitive chronic myelogenous leukemia cells to macrophage inflammatory protein 1α, an inhibitor of primitive normal cells. Proc Natl Acad Sci U S A 90:12015–12019, 1993.

52. Agarwal R, Doren S, Hicks B, Dunbar CE. Long-term culture of chronic myelogenous leukemia marrow cells on stem cell factor-deficient stroma favours benign progenitors. Blood 85:1306–1312, 1995.

53. Verma UN, Bagg A, Brown E, Mazumder A. Interleukin-2 activation of human bone marrow in long-term cultures: an effective strategy for purging and generation of antitumor cytotoxic effectors. Bone Marrow Transplant 13:115–123, 1994.

54. Miller JS, Verfaillie C, McGlave PB. Expansion and activation of human natural killer cells as therapy for autologous transplantation. Prog Clin Biol Res 389:39–45, 1994.

55. Cervantes F, McGlave PB, Miller JS. Autologous activated natural killer cells (ANK) suppress CML progenitors but spare normal hematopoiesis in long term bone marrow cultures (LTC). Blood 84(10, Suppl 1):150A, 1994.

56. Bhatia R, McGlave PB. T lymphocytes cultured from chronic myelogenous leukemia bone marrow suppress autologous hematopoietic progenitors. Leukemia 9:1006–1012, 1995.

57. Gale RP, Champlin R. How does bone marrow transplantation cure leukemia? Lancet ii:28–29, 1984.

58. Weisdorf DJ, Anderson PM, Blazar BR, Uckun FM, Kersey JH, Ramsay NKC. Interleukin-2 immediately after autologous bone marrow transplantation for acute lymphoblastic leukemia — a phase I study. Transplantation 55:61–66, 1993.

59. Rowe J, Ryan D, Dipersio J, Nilsson B, Larsson L, Liesveld J, Kouides P, Simonsson B. Autografting in chronic myelogenous leukemia followed by immunotherapy. Stem Cells 11(Suppl 3):34–42, 1993.

60. O'Shaughnessy JA, Cowan KH, Nienhuis AW, McDonagh KT, Sorrentino BP, Dunbar CE, Chiang Y, Wilson W, Goldspiel B, Kohler D, Cottler-Fox M, Leitman S, Gottesman M, Pastan I, Denicoff A, Noone M, Gress R. Retroviral mediated transfer of the human multidrug resistance gene (MDR-1) into hematopoietic stem cells during autologous transplantation after intensive chemotherapy for metastatic breast cancer. Human Gene Ther 5:891–911, 1994.

A New Challenge for the Field of Stem Cell Transplantation: Financial Constraints

17. Health care economics and bone marrow transplantation

Ilana Westerman, Teresa Waters and Charles Bennett

Cancer care is expensive, and Americans paid over $35 billion for cancer related treatment in 1990. One of the most costly cancer treatments is bone marrow transplantation (BMT) for malignant diseases which, in 1989, cost approximately $193,000 per patient [1.2]. In an era of health care reform, increasing importance is placed on costs and cost-effectiveness estimates of expensive therapies. These factors are taking on a larger role in the decision to use such expensive therapies. However, American efforts for quickly evaluating new or expensive therapies on an economic basis lag behind the progress in other countries that have government-subsidized health care systems, such as Canada and Australia. In these countries, evidence of both clinical effectiveness and cost-effectiveness is required before allowing new drugs to be marketed [3]. In the past five years, medical research journals have begun to publish articles on the costs of care of many therapies. Without this information, insurers, formulary committees, physicians, and health maintenance organizations must make policy decisions hindered by the absence of objective data on cost-effectiveness.

The cost-effectiveness of a therapy is only one of the concerns that need to be addressed when evaluating medical technologies. A therapy such as BMT that is very effective and that provides a higher quality of life or long-term survival requires more than a cost-effectiveness analysis. Alternative therapies, especially standard therapies, must be studied as well. While studies on costs of care are appropriate to guide the development of more cost-effective therapies and supportive care agents, such considerations should not diminish enthusiasm for investigation of new therapies that may be expected to be very expensive and possibly not cost-effective.

As physicians and health policy makers, we must be able to evaluate the cost-effectiveness of medical therapies. To address these questions, it is important to analyze the following issues: costs; benefits; cost-effectiveness; cost-reduction methods; and health care decision making, which compares alternatives in therapies based on cost-effectiveness. In this chapter, we will outline these terms frequently used by policy analysts to evaluate medical technologies. Then we will illustrate how these measures can be applied to evaluate costs and cost-effectiveness for bone marrow transplantation.

Jane N. Winter (ed.) BLOOD STEM CELL TRANSPLANTATION. 1997. Kluwer Academic Publishers. ISBN 0-7923-4260-7. All rights reserved.

Defining cost, effectiveness, and cost-effectiveness

While there are many important economic terms being applied to health care policy, the concepts of costs, effectiveness, and cost-effectiveness are central ingredients in most health policy assessments. We will define each of these terms below.

Costs of therapy

The cost of therapy is defined in terms of the associated economic burden it creates, measured in monetary terms [4–11]. The perspective from which the evaluation is undertaken is crucial to the cost of therapy. If the perspective is that of the patient, then costs can be measured in terms of out-of-pocket expenditures as well as indirect costs related to lost wages (morbidity costs) and lost income from premature death (mortality costs). However, if the perspective is that of a third-party insurance payer, the cost of therapy will be measured in terms of the dollar volume of claims that must be paid for patients who are treated with the particular form of therapy, with the incorporation of some return on investment for the stockholders. Finally, many studies evaluate costs from a societal perspective. This strategy requires that we attempt to measure the actual economic value of all resources that are used in therapy. The societal cost is therefore measured as the value of these resources in terms of their next best alternative use, and is determined by what is paid for these resources in viable economic markets. As an example, if the going rate for a physician assistant is assumed to be $40/per hour, the social opportunity cost of an hour of the physician assistant's time is typically assumed to be $40/per hour — a number that is substantially different in various countries, since that is the fee that someone else would be willing to pay for that hour in another situation. The social opportunity cost of all other inputs for a therapy can be considered in a similar fashion.

The costs of therapy are generally divided into direct and indirect costs. Direct costs reflect medical care given during the episode of illness and include physician fees, hospital charges, medications, blood products, etc. [12]. Direct medical costs may account for as little as 10% of all transplantation-related expenses. Indirect costs include morbidity costs and mortality costs. Morbidity costs are expenses incurred due to illness, such as travel, lodging, and food, which may amount to 30% to 40% of family income and be as high as 60% of the indirect costs. Mortality costs are usually calculated as the value of forgone earnings or the value of life calculated by a willingness to trade perfect health for days of life. In this chapter, we will concentrate on direct costs, since this is the standard practice in most cost-effectiveness analyses [13–21]. The rationale for use of these costs is that indirect costs are markedly variable (e.g., they differ based on geographic location) and are linked closely with most measures of effectiveness.

378

Cost measurement

In the health care arena, medical charges are a poor measure of the costs of therapy [22]. Internal accounting systems often allocate overhead costs to various centers and departments in a manner that may not closely resemble cost consumption. In addition, charges are also determined by market demand forces, which have little to do with underlying cost. Thus, internal and external forces often distort the relationship between medical charges and medical resource consumption, making charges less useful in cost analyses.

The full cost of therapy will include all treatment and follow-up costs, and should also take into consideration the costs of diagnosis and terminal care costs. The usual scenarios presented are in the acute care setting and are carried out for short periods of time. These studies frequently show very high costs for BMT: costs of managing leukemic patients for the first year after bone marrow transplantation were almost 30 times greater than those for standard maintenance chemotherapy [23]. However, if the patients treated with standard chemotherapy relapse and require induction chemotherapy or BMT, costs were only 1.7 times greater. Relapse and supportive terminal care is expensive, and costs continue to accrue as long as the patient lives. Leukemia BMT/HDC patients live longer than standard chemotherapy patients, and this longer follow-up time is needed to offset the higher early costs.

The costs of therapy assessments must also include those incurred from expensive supportive and terminal care [24,25]. Almost one third of one's total lifetime medical expenditures are spent in the last six months of life on average, with mean medical expenditures for cancer patients being reported as over $21,000 (in 1980) for the last 12 months of life and over $16,000 for the last six months of life. These costs do not vary markedly across different cancer diagnoses and are not decreased markedly by hospice or home care. Terminal care costs for persons with cancer are high, with little opportunity to decrease costs unless services are withheld. A few patients do voluntarily do this by writing living wills.

The investigators must decide at a very early stage what categories of cost items they wish to include in the analysis and the level of detail at which they will focus. The choice of the proper cost items to include is closely linked to the questions or hypotheses that are being evaluated. For example, if one wanted to know the cost savings available from using PBPCTs rather than ABMT, then one would include only the costs incurred after induction. However, if one wanted to know what costs would be saved if one shifted from the inpatient to the outpatient setting (i.e., the incremental cost difference between the two settings), one would again include all costs in both settings, including costs such as personnel, if this shift in practice settings would be likely to have an impact on the type and number of staff personnel that are involved. If the perspective of the analysis were long term, then it would also be necessary to include the effects on fixed costs of the medical center, such as the cost of maintaining the treatment center building.

In practice, the types of data required for cost analyses are difficult to obtain unless the medical system involved has a very sophisticated billing/utilization database and cost-accounting system [24,25]. It is often difficult to obtain data on all resources in the typical multicenter trial. This approach requires the identification of all the inputs associated with a health care service and the assignment of an appropriate cost to each. This task is very easy for simple services such as antibiotic administration, radiograph performance, or laboratory tests. However, a more complex therapy, such as BMT, is a considerably greater challenge because of the variability of inputs from one patient to the next. Most complicated of all is the entire episode of care from diagnosis to death, because this requires detailed cost and resource-use data from many medical providers over an extended period of time. Very few medical systems have an accounting system detailed enough to support this type of complete analysis, referred to as 'microcosting,' and even fewer systems have performed the necessary time-motion studies required to identify the inputs used in the microcosting system.

However, with the advent of managed care and large integrated medical systems, a few providers have developed sophisticated microcosting management systems that allow for estimation of patient-specific cost. The labor inputs in these systems are usually based on estimates by laboratory and department supervisors rather than by direct measurements, and a variety of assumptions are built into these systems. It is likely that as the number and size of managed care systems increases, many more providers will adopt these information systems. While management systems have not received a large amount of attention in medical research, they will be increasingly used in multicenter trials.

Costs have been measured by direct accounting of all services used by HDC patients in the study of Gulati and Bennett [26,27]. An alternative accounting method estimates the consumption of resources and costs in a multivariate prediction model in which predicted charges serve as a proxy for costs and are estimated for room and board, radiographs, laboratories, and the operating room. This model has been used to estimate charges for leukemia patients and general medical patients [28].

Another strategy that has been used for estimating costs is based on converting hospital charges from medical bills into costs using the ratio of cost to charges (RCCs) included in each medical system's annual report to Medicare. Medicare RCCs are mostly a holdover from the era before DRGs (diagnosis-related groups), when Medicare reimbursed hospitals on the basis of incurred costs. Medicare developed a system for estimating the reasonable and necessary costs of providing medical care rather than paying the full hospital charges. This system involved a detailed report from each hospital that was filed yearly with the Health Care Financing Agency (HCFA). Each hospital included in this report a set of ratios, the RCCs. The Medicare RCCs and per diem costs (for the lodging part of the hospital bill) are a moderately standardized means of estimating costs across medical systems in the United States in

380

which a Medicare Cost Report is filed. Although the Medicare Cost Report is no longer used to determine reimbursement, it still serves as the primary source of government data on hospital costs.

There are several limitations to the RCC method of cost estimation. First, this system does not separate out overhead and other fixed costs and therefore provides an estimate of average rather than marginal costs. It may overstate potential cost savings as a result. Second, Medicare Cost Reports are based on complex, detailed instructions that may be interpreted differently by individual hospital systems. Finally, RCCs are averages of all the cost/charge ratios within a large medical system's revenue center, such as radiology, pharmacy, or pathology. If an individual patient's use of resources is far from average, the Medicare RCCs are not likely to be an accurate reflection of true costs for a given revenue center.

Departmental RCCs can be determined from the detailed budget data from a medical system. Conversion of charges to costs using these ratios more closely approximates the marginal cost than do the Medicare RCCs, but they still represent average rather than marginal costs and may still be imprecise if individual patients have cost/charge relationships that differ significantly from the average of the department. In addition, researchers require access to detailed financial records if they are to use these data sources in multicenter cost research.

Rather than adding up a complete laundry list of the individual resources being consumed, most cost studies start with an aggregated measure of costs, such as hospital or physician bills, and attempt to count 'big-ticket' items. The prices assigned to each big-ticket item are usually charges derived from a single institution or an estimate based on expert opinion. While this approach is practical for many cost studies, it does limit the ability to control the factors that are included as a 'cost' in the analysis. This approach has several other limitations as well. First, it has never been empirically validated within a given institution or across institutions. Second, the appropriate set of big-ticket items necessary to estimate costs has never been agreed upon. Third, the method usually treats big-ticket items such as leukapheresis as if they are homogenous, while they may differ in terms of duration, frequency, and post-harvest manipulations.

In addition to 'costing out' hospital services, one must also consider how to estimate the cost of physician services. Most commonly, physician fees, based on actual charges, have been used. Unfortunately, physician charges may vary widely, especially in the fee-for-service setting. Based on these issues, the new Medicare Fee Schedule based on the Resource-Based Relative Value Scale (RBRVS) developed by Hsiao and colleagues is likely to be more appropriate for assigning costs to physician services [29]. The basic principle of the RBRVS is that the price of a service is a reflection of the long-term cost of providing that service. Hsiao et al. used three cost components to calculate the RBRVS: (1) the work input required to provide a service; (2) the opportunity cost of specialty training; and (3) the practice overhead expenses, such as office staff and malpractice coverage. The first component of the RBRVS reflects the time spent and the intensity or difficulty of the service provided. Most of the RBRVS system has been incorporated into the Medicare Fee Schedule. Medicare fees under RBRVS are linked to the Physician's Current Procedural Terminology (CPT) classification system, so that in order to model physician costs in a cost-analysis project, some map must be created between CPT codes and the data on physician services.

Cost analyses are usually classified into one of three types: randomized controlled trials, nonrandomized or observation studies, and cost-effectiveness models [30–32]. A proper cost study in a randomized clinical trial is most often associated with secondary objectives of the trial. We have now completed several cost substudies involving oncology therapies. In each case, cost or resource consumption patterns were not a primary endpoint. Some have argued that since randomized clinical trials do not include cost as a primary endpoint, the trials are therefore not designed to answer most economic questions of interest. In addition, requirements for monitoring phase III trials may distort the true economic implications of the study.

While the conflicting demands of economic and clinical trials are apparent, and not all clinical trials are suitable for an economic substudy, we feel that many randomized trials are suitable for an economic analysis. The ability to analyze the data by an 'intention to treat' offers good protection against biases that may affect other types of analyses. Also, some of the distortions that randomized clinical trials create for economic analyses apply equally well to analyses of clinical outcomes.

Observational cost studies include both nonrandomized treatment comparisons and descriptive studies that lack a comparison group. These cost studies are often carried out in areas where there is still very little published empirical cost data. The data can be used to make sample size projections for randomized controlled trials or to provide estimates for cost-effectiveness and other health policy studies, but they require careful attention to sensitivity analyses and are subject to the bias of the investigator; thus, these studies are the least reliable. Large pharmaceutical benefit managers (PBMs) have detailed medical and claims information on millions of persons and are being used by large medical system providers and insurers to generate cost-effectiveness profiles. However, very little attention has been given to statistical adjustment techniques to control for bias of the investigators nonrandom patient selection variations over time, and differences in practice settings.

Time effects are an important consideration in medical cost analyses [33]. First, the value of money diminishes over time because of inflation, so that cost studies from different years are not directly comparable unless adjustments for inflation are made. The most common way is to use the medical care component of the Consumer Price Index (CPI) or its subcomponents. The costs of therapy may also decrease over time as more procedures are performed [34,35]. The marginal cost (cost of treating one more patient) may decrease as more patients are treated at an individual institution. For example, once dedicated space and staff time are allocated to BMT, the cost of treating one more patient should be lower. Integrated health systems in the managed care environment seek to provide comprehensive inpatient and outpatient services and attempt to minimize the financial impact of BMT by referring patients to specially designated 'centers of excellence' whose volume of procedures help to control costs.

Also, time effects are important because future medical expenditures are considered less costly than current ones, due to the fact that current expenditures remove money today, while future expenditures allow one to invest money at the market rate of return until it is needed. For this reason, cost studies use a technique called 'discounting' to account for the difference between the present and future value of money.

Geographic and market economic factors also affect health care costs, although these effects have not been well studied. Different practice settings (e.g., fee-for-service or capitated medical care plans) can affect the cost of providing a given type of care due to variations in organizational structures and incentives, different practice patterns, and different levels of efficiency. Care in an academic tertiary care center may differ markedly from care in a community hospital and may have different costs. Cost differences result from different staffing patterns, use of intensive care beds, and availability of post-discharge facilities. In a study evaluating the clinical and economic effects of GM-CSF as adjunct therapy for ABMT for lymphoid malignancies at six medical centers, clinical differences between GM-CSF and placebo were similar at all six hospitals. GM-CSF was consistently associated with a marked decrease in the duration of severe neutropenia, generally the limiting factor for hospital discharge. Economic results, as measured by duration of hospitalization, were more variable. Two of the six hospitals actually had a slightly higher mean hospitalizations for the GM-CSF group than the placebo group. However, the overall estimated mean benefit for the GM-CSF group was 3.4 days.

Material and labor costs for medical care can vary according to the type and location of the medical system and can create differences in the cost of providing a medical service. Labor costs are the most variable according to geographic location. However, large managed care systems have also lowered pharmaceutical costs dramatically through negotiated discounts from pharmaceutical companies. Therefore, comparison of cost studies from different health care systems should not be done without some adjustment for these differences.

In addition, the perspective of the investigators needs to be considered because of concerns about potential bias. In unblinded studies, the investigator or the pharmaceutical firm may minimize side effects or toxicities attributed to a new agent. In many phase III double-blind studies, pharmaceutical companies are involved in trials designed to help with FDA approval of new agents. However, as noted by Hillman et al., discussions and agreements about what to do with the economic results of the study must be considered prior to initiating the research project [19]. Guidelines have been proposed to help investigators who are involved with economic evaluations of new pharmaceuticals [19].

Effectiveness of therapy

Most studies seek to identify whether a medical intervention results in a statistically demonstrable improvement over established therapies. When this impact is limited to only a few important outcomes of BMT such as mortality or is under tightly controlled clinical situations, this is an evaluation of *efficacy*. The *effectiveness* of a therapy is more broadly defined to include its impact on all outcomes of importance to the patient and in situations consistent with everyday medical practice. There are several broad categories of effectiveness measures [36,37].

The simplest and most common measures of effectiveness are unidimensional indicators of outcome, e.g., life-years saved. Next, for a more detailed measure of effectiveness, one can choose to consider the impact of a therapy on a number of outcome dimensions (e.g., physical, social, and mental functioning). Instruments such as the SF-36 and the FLIC are used in these assessments [38–41]. The patient usually receives an overall score based on the responses to questions about functional ability or capacity; typically, the scoring algorithm reflects the instrument developer's judgments about the relative importance of the individual items, rather than the respondent's own preferences. Unidimensional or multidimensional measures may be disease specific (e.g., for breast cancer) or else generic (e.g., the SF-36) in which case comparisons can be made across diseases.

Another measure of effectiveness incorporates the decision maker's own *preferences* for the alternative outcomes of the therapy [42,43]. Decision analysis is a technique that allows for comparison of therapies for clinical and cost-effectiveness. It evaluates alternative therapies by estimating the probability of all relevant events or outcomes in the future. In a decision analysis pertaining to the individual patient, it is that patient's preferences that are used to value-weight the outcomes associated with alternative therapies. In these cases, a value-weighted measure of therapy effectiveness, the Quality Adjusted Life Year (QALY), is used [44].

The QALY is based on two important aspects of outcomes generally perceived by patients as important: quantity of life and quality of life. If an individual could live one's entire life in excellent health, the QALY score would be the same as one's life expectancy. If the individual experiences toxicities, such as overwhelming sepsis or respiratory failure, the QALY score is basically life expectancy reduced by the value-weighted amount of time the individual suffers the effects of the sepsis or respiratory failure. The value associated with being in respiratory failure (per unit of time) — often called the 'disutility' of the respiratory failure state — should reflect individual preferences. In most studies, if the health state being evaluated is deemed to be as good as excellent health state, it is assigned a value of 1.0. If it is felt to be as undesirable as the worst state (typically assumed to be death), it is assigned a value of zero. States that are intermediate in preference to the best and worst are assigned a number along the interval from 0 to 1 accordingly [44].

There is no consensus as to the best way for making adjustments for quality of life. Clearly, quality of life is subjective. In one randomized trial comparing continuous versus intermittent therapy, prolongation of life was valued more than life with recurrent cancer, despite the side effects of chemotherapy [43]. While little is known about quality of life for patients undergoing BMT, pilot studies suggest that quality of life estimates are similar to those for patients who receive standard chemotherapy.

General strategies for measuring cost-effectiveness

The term *cost-effectiveness* is often applied to many aspects of medical therapies [45]. However, its meaning is very specific. Cost-effectiveness analysis involves the explicit comparison of one option or program with one or more alternatives. When one of two therapies is more effective and is more expensive than the other, it is cost-effective if the additional effectiveness is worth the additional cost. Similarly, if one intervention is less effective and less costly than a second, it is cost-effective if the loss in effectiveness is judged to be more than offset by the reduction in cost. Therefore, cost-effectiveness analysis cannot address whether a specific therapy is worthwhile by itself, but rather how it compares to other potential alternatives. The main objective of cost-effectiveness analyses is to evaluate multiple options so that policy makers can choose among the alternatives. With health care expenditures being the major concern of policy makers, legislators, patients, providers, and insurers, cost-effectiveness analyses are an objective method of deciding, for example, to spend more money on preventive services, screening, or therapies. However, cost-effectiveness analyses are not meant to limit the total health care expenditures.

Under the category of cost-effectiveness analyses, there are several different methods of economic analysis. In each method, the final measure is given as a ratio, with incremental costs in the numerator and incremental health care benefits/outcomes in the denominator. One popular measure of incremental health benefit is the difference in life expectancy between alternative treatments. This is the most common type of health care analysis. In cost utility analysis, remaining survival is adjusted for less than full quality with QALYs. Cost-effectiveness analysis may also focus on 'nonsurvival' outcomes, such as complication avoided.

The basic assumption for all forms of economic analyses is that one is trying to find the most efficient means of maximizing the net health benefits of a particular group of people given a constraint of limited financial resources.

These analyses are neutral to the group of patients and therapies being studied, and only the net health benefits are taken into consideration.

Cost–benefit analysis

Cost–benefit analysis allows for comparison of medical expenditures with other types of expenditures — such as education, defense, transportation, and public health. Benefits are expressed in units of dollars. The two most common methods for evaluating the financial benefits of a therapy are the human-capital approach and the willingness-to-pay approach. Both have significant limitations. In the human-capital approach, survival is valued in terms of how much an individual could produce for society, usually measured by lost wages. One objection is that it does not seem appropriate to value people solely by their economic contributions. Second, it is not clear how to estimate the benefits of individuals who do not work or who are retired.

The other approach is to measure benefit by using the willingness-to-pay method. This approach requires that patients estimate how much they would be willing to pay to obtain a certain health benefit or to avoid a bad outcome. However, individuals with fewer resources are willing to pay significantly less than wealthier individuals.

Costs and effectiveness of allogeneic bone marrow transplants

A limited number of studies have been conducted on the costs and cost-effectiveness of allogeneic bone marrow transplantation. A review of three signature papers will follow, each of which includes a distinct analytic framework. Since there have been numerous medical advances in transplantation and supportive care, the findings of these studies must be viewed in a dynamic fashion. The literature review will provide both a methodological background and estimates of the cost and cost-effectiveness of bone marrow transplantations.

Since the 1970s, allogeneic organ transplantation has greatly proliferated, primarily because of technological advances in minimizing rejection of donor organs. While studies in the 1970s and 1980s reported the costs of liver, heart, and kidney transplantations, the first study of bone marrow transplantation for a hematologic malignancy, acute nonlymphocytic leukemia, was conducted by Welch et al. in 1989 [46]. This study evaluated 41 patients who participated in a prospective trial of allogeneic bone marrow transplantation versus intensive chemotherapy at the Fred Hutchinson Cancer Center in Seattle. Seventeen patients had a HLA-matched donor and therefore received an allogeneic bone marrow transplant, while 19 patients did not have a suitable donor and received two courses of consolidation chemotherapy followed by monthly maintenance chemotherapy.

386

Resource-based measures of costs were collected for five areas: number of nonintensive care unit days spent in hospital, number of days spent in the intensive care unit, number of lab tests performed, number of X-rays, and the number of operating room procedures. Because of the large discrepancy between charges and costs, hospital charges were not directly included in cost estimates. A charge estimate equation was derived to serve as a proxy for the costs of each procedure. All the resource data were collected by one observer to diminish variability. Because patients were divided into study arms solely on the basis of donor availability, bias was minimized for accrual into the different arms.

Clinical results of the study showed that the overall survival rate of bone marrow transplant patients was much higher than that of chemotherapy patients: 10 of 17 versus 5 of 19 were alive at five years. Differences in resource intensity of bone marrow transplant patients versus chemotherapy patients were observed. Patients treated with chemotherapy alone averaged seven hospitalizations, while bone marrow transplant patients had 4.6 hospitalizations. However, although chemotherapy patients spent 10% more time in the hospital, bone marrow transplant patients spent most of their hospital time in ICU centers (57% for bone marrow transplant patients versus 5% for chemotherapy patients). Over a five-year period, patients who survived had lower costs than patients who did not. For example, the average cost of a chemotherapy survivor was $79,000 versus $157,000 for a nonsurvivor, and the average cost of a bone marrow transplant survivor was $166,000 versus $232,000 for a nonsurvivor.

Although chemotherapy costs were lower than bone marrow transplantation costs, bone marrow transplantation for acute nonlymphocytic leukemia had a favorable incremental cost-effectiveness (ICE) ratio relative to standard chemotherapy:

$$ICE = \frac{\text{Cost}\left(BMT-\text{Chemotherapy}\right)}{\text{\# of years of survival after therapy}\left(BMT-\text{Chemotherapy}\right)}$$

The bone marrow transplant procedure cost only $10,000 more than chemotherapy per life year gained, which is even lower than the incremental costs of treatment of moderate hypertension in middle-aged men ($13,500 per life year gained).

Allogeneic bone marrow transplants became less cost effective as the practice of mismatched donors proliferated, which creates a lower survival rate, and as the age of recipients increased. For example, if the upper age limit were increased to 55 years, a 125% rise in bone marrow transplant dollars results. Concerns of age discrimination are also raised in this type of study. Finally, the amount of time bone marrow transplant patients spend in intensive care units may be shortened as changes in practice patterns occur. The use of step-down units will greatly increase the cost-effectiveness estimates of bone marrow transplants.

387

As the clinical efficacy of a medical treatment improves and treatment protocols become standardized, many hospitals and managed care organizations require detailed data on the costs of transplantation and the extent of resources utilized. A 1989 paper entitled, 'Cost of allogeneic bone marrow transplants in four diseases' analyzed the costs of allogeneic bone marrow transplants for several different pathologies and aided physicians and health care managers in planning and designing new treatment programs [47]. The four diseases studied were acute myelogenous leukemia (AML), severe combined immunodeficiency (not considered here), severe aplastic anemia, and chronic granulocytic leukemia.

Data were collected for 12 months after the initial diagnosis because most acute clinical complications occur within six months to one year of transplantation. The study was conducted in three Parisian hospitals where the same treatment protocol for allogeneic HLA-identical BMT was administered for each disease. Cost components included pharmaceuticals and blood products, disposable medical supplies, laboratory tests, radiological imaging, medical and nursing care, HLA typing and donor costs, and outpatient care. A very comprehensive data set was created through collection of data on medical resource use and the inclusion of indirect and personnel costs into cost estimates.

Patients with acute nonlymphocytic leukemia were admitted to the hospital at least twice. The first admission prior to transplantation was for chemotherapy (vincristine, daunorubicine, cytarabine, lomestine) and supportive care (with antibiotics for febrile episodes, transfusions of irradiated blood and platelets, and oral decontamination). Patients then were readmitted for the bone marrow transplantation. After preparation with total body irradiation and cyclophosphamide, methotrexate was given to prevent GVHD, and other medications were used as necessary. Costs associated with the most common posttransplant complications were calculated: severe thrombocytopenia lasting three months, interstitial pneumonia, and localized zoster infection. The standard costs of bone marrow transplantation and the costs with complications for bone marrow transplantation for patients with acute myelogenous leukemia are listed in table 1. Uncomplicated cases cost an estimated $40,923, and complicated cases cost an estimated $55,839.

A second series of estimates were derived for transplantations for patients with severe aplastic anemia. Patients with severe aplastic anemia were admitted to the hospital on average 40 days prior to transplantation. They were treated with chemotherapy (cyclophosphamide), radiation therapy (6 Gy thoraco-abdominal irradiation), ketaconzole, and antibiotics. Cyclosporin A and methotrexate were administered to prevent GVHD. Patients remained in the hospital for 35 days on average after transplantation. Complications secondary to GVHD almost tripled the cost of the procedure. All costs are listed in table 2, including costs for complications (primarily representing the costs for GVHD treatment). Uncomplicated cases cost an estimated $84,537, and complicated cases cost an estimated $232,007.

Table 1. Allogeneic bone marrow transplantation cost in adult acute myelogenous leukemia (in U.S. dollars)[b]

Cost components	Direct standard cost[a,c]		Cost with complications[a,c]	
Medical supplies	2,188	5.4%	2,569	4.6%
Pharmaceutical products	6,841	16.7%	9,027	16.2%
Blood products	6,467	15.8%	11,514	20.6%
Laboratory tests and X-ray	12,002	29.3%	13,803	24.7%
Nursing care	11,266	27.5%	15,327	27.5%
Physicians' time	2,159	5.3%	3,599	6.4%
Total	40,923	100%	55,839	100%

[a] Note: table lists costs, not patient charges
[b] From Viens-Bitker C, Fery-Lemonnier E, Blum-Boisgard C, et al. Cost of allogeneic bone marrow transplantation in four diseases. Health Policy 12:309–317, 1989.
[c] French Francs converted to U.S. dollars at the 1989 rate of 0.16339 $/FF (an average of January, June, and December rates).

Table 2. Allogeneic bone marrow transplantation cost in severe aplastic anemia (in U.S. dollars)[b]

Cost components	Direct standard cost[a,c]		Cost with complications[a,c]	
Medical supplies	6,189	7.3%	11,786	5.1%
Pharmaceutical products	18,982	22.5%	69,587	30.0%
Blood products	17,184	20.3%	81,835	35.3%
Laboratory tests and X-ray procedures	26,267	31.1%	42,150	18.1%
Nursing care	14,149	16.7%	22,702	9.8%
Physicians' time	1,766	2.1%	3,947	1.7%
Total	84,537	100%	232,007	100%

[a] Note: table lists costs, not patient charges
[b] From Viens-Bitker C, Fery-Lemonnier E, Blum-Boisgard C, et al. Cost of allogeneic bone marrow transplantation in four diseases. Health Policy 12:309–317, 1989.
[c] French Francs converted to U.S. dollars at the 1989 rate of 0.16339 $/FF (an average of January, June, and December rates).

Patients with chronic granulocytic leukemia had treatment very similar to patients with severe aplastic anemia, with the major differences being that patients were admitted to the hospital only ten days prior to transplantation when immunotoxins could be used for T-cell depletion of the bone marrow. Costs for this procedure are reported in table 3. Uncomplicated cases cost an estimated $64,937.

The cost for a bone marrow transplantation for hematologic malignancies appears to vary depending on the underlying pathology and the extent of complications. The cost of an uncomplicated bone marrow transplant for acute myelogenous leukemia was $40,923, for severe aplastic anemia $84,538, and for chronic granulocytic leukemia $64,938. This study did not include the costs of hospitalization/housing (beyond nursing/physician care); therefore, blood products were the largest factor in the difference in costs. However, other studies that consider hospitalization costs have concluded that days in the

389

Table 3. Allogeneic bone marrow transplantation cost in chronic granulocytic leukemia (in U.S. dollars)[b]

Cost components	Direct standard cost[a,c]	
Medical supplies	3,351	5.1%
Pharmaceutical products	16,751	25.8%
Blood products	9,984	15.4%
Laboratory tests and X-ray procedures	23,842	36.7%
Nursing care	9,787	15.1%
Physicians' time	1,222	1.9%
Total	64,937	100%

[a] Note: table lists costs not patient charges
[b] From Viens-Bitker C, Fery-Lemonnier E, Blum-Boisgard C, et al. Cost of allogeneic bone marrow transplantation in four diseases. Health Policy 12:309–317, 1989.
[c] French Francs converted to U.S. dollars at the 1989 rate of 0.16339 $/FF (an average of January, June, and December rates).

hospital account for the largest percent of total costs and largest differences in cost estimates [48].

Data have not been collected for all diseases associated with transplantation, and cost data for a particular pathology are generally not applicable to other pathologies. As the concern over health care dollars increase, more studies will be conducted. One pitfall that health care providers will encounter is the use of old data. When a treatment regimen for a disease changes, due to new surgical procedures, new pharmaceuticals, or improvements in supportive care, the costs for treating that disease must be reanalyzed.

Professionals in the health care industry who are familiar with the treatment protocols are vital to cost analysis studies. For example, if a study does not include the clinically relevant time frame, important cost data could be lost. An example would be collecting cost data for bone marrow transplantation from the time of the transplant onward in which all the costs of the initial chemotherapy, hospitalization time, and pretransplant pharmaceuticals would not be included in the analysis.

These three studies provide a good introduction to the costs of allogeneic bone marrow transplants. However, these estimates quickly become outdated as protocols and therapies change. The addition of new, more costly chemotherapuetic agents or supportive care agents can even lower the overall costs of a transplant. Additional studies will be needed as new technologies in transplantation develop and investigators gain experience with allogeneic transplants.

Costs of autologous bone marrow transplant

Like allogeneic bone marrow transplant (AlBMT), the cost of autologous bone marrow transplant (AuBMT) is quite high. Current estimates of AuBMT costs in U.S. hospitals range from $50,000 to $200,000 per patient [49]. Variations in costs result from both patient heterogeneity and institutional differences. Given this wide range of costs, it is arguable that AuBMT may be cost-effective for some types of patients and institutions and not others. Detailed research determining the costs of AuBMT for specific types of patients using specific clinical practices is necessary.

Sources of cost variation

Patient heterogeneity. AuBMT is currently being used for treatment in a wide variety of cancers, including, but not limited to, breast cancer, Hodgkin's disease, non-Hodgkin's lymphoma, and acute myeloblastic lymphoma. This range of diseases alone creates wide variation in patient characteristics and their responses to therapy. Additional sources of variation among patients are early versus late disease, age, and complete versus partial versus nonresponses to initial therapy.

Institutional differences. Costs of AuBMT differ widely among institutions. There are several potential explanations for these discrepancies. Differences may simply be the result of difficulties in determining costs as opposed to charges. This issue has been addressed earlier. If this is the primary driver of cost differences, more sophisticated and compatible cost accounting systems will relieve this problem. It is also possible, however, that true differences in efficiency exist between hospitals. For example, some hospitals are exploring the substitution of outpatient care for inpatient stays at the beginning and ending portions of a patient's AuBMT treatment. Such substitutions significantly reduce costs. The ability to make this change, however, depends crucially on the proximity of the patient's residence or the presence of nearby facilities to handle this subacute patient. Evidence that facilities can develop more efficient delivery of AuBMT over time is presented by Bennett et al. [48]. Costs of AuBMT for non-Hodgkin's lymphoma at the University of Nebraska Medical Center decreased at a rate of 10% per year from 1987 to 1991 ($p = 0.001$).

Preliminary studies

AuBMT in New Zealand. Beard et al. [50] present one of the first papers to include AuBMTs in a BMT cost analyses. The New Zealand study is unique for a number of reasons. First of all, since the authors were able to follow some of their 41 patients for a relatively long period of time, they were better able to capture the long-term benefits of BMT. Specifically, although the costs of BMT are initially quite large, when these costs can be 'spread out' over longer life years gained, the cost-effectiveness of BMT is quite remarkable. The authors were also able to construct a classification scheme for the quality of life of their patients. This classification scheme was used to weight the life years gained from the treatment and to derive a somewhat more realistic view of the value of BMT.

Beard et al. [50] find that BMT is highly cost-effective, estimating that cost of each quality adjusted life year (QALY) gained by BMT is NZ\$13,272 (after two years of follow-up) and NZ\$3868 (for the 18 patients who could be followed for ten years). This compares extremely favorably with other cost studies using the life year or quality-adjusted life year framework (e.g., renal dialysis US\$40,000 per life year [1]). The drawback to this study is, of course, that it is based on costs in a New Zealand hospital. Given the strong differences between the New Zealand and U.S. health care systems, one must be extremely careful in interpreting these results. The authors do make a number of important methodological points that should be kept in mind when conducting a cost-effectiveness of BMT study: 1) length of follow-up is critically important in determining cost-effectiveness, since the long-term benefits of BMT may be spread out over longer periods of time; 2) calculating a quality-of-life weighting scheme for BMT patients is a viable method for adjusting for complications and is especially important for AlBMT patients who may suffer significant graft versus-host disease; and 3) considerations of the age of patients (average age in sample = 23) further reinforce the cost-effectiveness of BMT from the point of view of society as life years saved represent significant earnings.

AuBMT in France. Dufoir et al. [51] reported on a study of 40 patients, comparing the costs of AuBMT ($n = 11$), AlBMT ($n = 14$), and chemotherapy ($n = 15$) for patients with acute myeloid leukemia (AML). All patients were a subset of patients from two cooperative trials (BGM 84 and BGMT 87; total $n = 196$) who were treated in a single center (Centre Hospitalier Regional de Bordeaux) and achieved complete response after induction chemotherapy. Dufoir et al. [51] found that the cost per additional year of life saved was similar for the AlBMT and chemotherapy groups (US\$20,646 versus US\$19,990, $p = $ NS), while AuBMT was significantly less cost-effective at US\$26,667. Again, we would recommend caution in extrapolating these results to the U.S. health care system. First, it is likely that some significant differences exist between the clinical practices and cost structures of CHR Bordeaux and U.S. hospitals. In addition, at least some of the difference in cost per life year between AlBMT and AuBMT may be attributable to differences in quality of life; as pointed out by Beard et al. [50], AlBMT patients are susceptible to graft-versus-host disease. Nonetheless, this study is useful because it is the first study to attempt to compare the costs of three alternatives (AlBMT, AuBMT, and chemotherapy). In addition, the study provides a nice identification of major cost drivers in the treatment of AML: pharmaceuticals, single-use materials (syringes, gloves, etc.), blood products, laboratory tests, radiographic procedures, surgical procedures, medical and paramedical staff time, and accommodations.

AuBMT versus peripheral blood stem cell transplant (PBSCT) in Europe. A presentation at the American Society of Clinical Oncology [52] by Smith et al. included estimates of the costs of PBSCT and AuBMT for recurrent Hodgkin's disease or lymphoma. Using utilization data on 58 patients treated at six hospitals in Germany, Belgium, and the U.K. and using cost data from their own Massey Cancer Center, Smith et al. estimate the cost of AuBMT at $58,281 and the cost of PBSCT at $39,960, a difference of 31%. While the long-term survival questions concerning the efficacy of AuBMT versus PBSCT have still not been answered for these patients, based on these striking economic results, the authors find strong support for PBSCT.

AuBMT in the U.S. Published studies examining the costs and cost-effectiveness of AuBMT in the U.S. are rare. Hillner et al. [49] estimate the cost-effectiveness of AuBMT for metastatic breast cancer using a hypothetical cohort of 45-year-old women, various probabilities of recurrence, complication, death, etc. from the published data, and cost data based on a small sample of patients at their medical center. The authors find that the estimate for costs per year of life saved is most sensitive to whether the risk of recurrence is constant over a patient's lifetime or decreases after some finite period. The assumption of normal survival after five years of disease-free survival reduces the cost per year of life saved associated with AuBMT from $115,800 to $28,600 and cost per quality-adjusted life year saved from $96,600 to $27,300. This result once again reinforces the need to follow AuBMT patients for long periods of time in order to accurately assess the cost-effectiveness of this procedure.

There is some evidence that the potential for institutions and/or professions to improve outcomes and lower costs for a given intervention is significant. Bennett et al. [48] investigate this 'learning curve' phenomenon in the case of high-dose chemotherapy and autologous transplant at the University of Nebraska Medical Center. Clinical and financial data were combined to develop cost measures. Medicare cost-to-charge ratios were used to convert hospital charges to costs. All patients were seen at the University of Nebraska Medical Center between 1987 and 1991 and received high-dose chemotherapy in conjunction with either autologous bone marrow or peripheral stem cell transplantation. Patients who died in the hospital were excluded from cost calculations because their costs differed markedly from those of survivors.

One hundred and seventy-eight autotransplants were performed for patients with Hodgkin's disease. The mortality rate decreased steadily over the five year period (see figure 1). The costs of autotransplants also decreased significantly between 1987 and 1991 (see figure 2). The most significant reduction in costs was due to the decrease in hospital days per patient. In 1987 a patient stayed in the hospital an average of 51 days; in 1991, this figure was only 32 days. Changes in cost per day, medications, etc. changed very little over time.

In Hospital Mortality Rate (%)

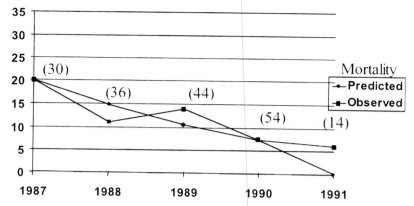

Figure 1. Bennett CL, Armitage JL, Armitage GO. Costs of care and outcomes for high-dose therapy and autologous transplantation for lymphoid malignancies: results from the University of Nebraska 1987 through 1991. JCO 13(4):969–973, 1995.

Costs/hospitalization (in thousands $)

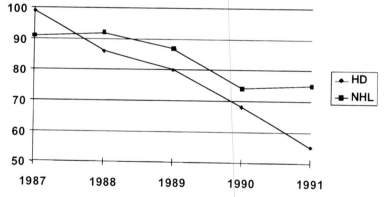

Figure 2. Bennett CL, Armitage JL, Armitage GO. Costs of care and outcomes for high-dose therapy and autologous transplantation for lymphoid malignancies: results from the University of Nebraska 1987 through 1991. JCO 13(4):969–973, 1995.

One hundred and forty-nine autotransplants were performed for patients with non-Hodgkin's lymphoma. In-hospital mortality decreased markedly over time (see figure 3). Average costs for treatment of non-Hodgkin's lymphoma also decreased from $91,000 in 1987 to $74,000 in 1991. Again, hospitalization days were important for these cost reductions: length of stay averaged 45 in 1987 and 38 days in 1991.

Factors associated with decreasing costs were hospital staff improvements, improvements in technology, and patient selection. For example, over time the

In Hospital Mortality Rate (%)

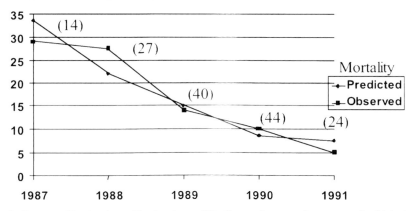

Figure 3. Bennett CL, Armitage JL, Armitage GO. Costs of care and outcomes for high-dose therapy and autologous transplantation for lymphoid malignancies: results from the University of Nebraska 1987 through 1991. JCO 13(4):969–973. 1995.

transplant team learned how to better use antibiotics by adding a specialist in infectious diseases and oncology to the transplant team. The introduction of hematopoietic growth factors also represented a significant improvement in technology, improving outcomes and decreasing costs [48].

The learning curve phenomenon is not merely an interesting note to cost and outcomes research. Careful attention must be paid to the point in the learning curve that has been reached by an institution. Figures 1 and 2 present an example of a possible learning curve. It is highly important to conduct evaluations when a technology, or the institution performing the technology, has reached part C of the curve. Only in this time frame can one be reasonably certain that differences in outcomes or costs between two technologies are not due solely to differences in where the individual institutions are in their learning curves.

An ongoing study being led by Julie M. Vose, M.D. (P.I.) at the University of Nebraska and a number of cooperative sites across the U.S. promises to provide a rich data set to examine the cost-effectiveness of AuBMT for non-Hodgkin's lymphoma, the second largest category of patients to receive AuBMT (after breast cancer). In addition, this trial will also provide critical information on the effectiveness and cost-effectiveness of AuBMT versus PBSCT. Although definitive clinical trials comparing AuBMT and PBSCT have not been conducted in U.S. hospitals, based on anecdotal evidence and experience, support for PBSCT as an effective and cost-effective alternative for many AuBMT patients is growing. Bennett and colleagues have begun to conduct cost analyses on the first patients in this trial. Using detailed patient billing information, professional practice, laboratory, and pharmacy records, and department-specific ratios of costs to charges (RCCs), the research team has the following objectives: 1) to document the costs associated with AuBMT and PBSCT in U.S. hospitals and to identify major cost drivers; and 2) to compare the costs and costs per life year associated with the two procedures and determine the relative cost-effectiveness of each.

What do we know?

Estimates of the costs and cost-effectiveness of AuBMT in the U.S. are still quite sketchy. Preliminary studies from the U.S. and abroad provide some reason to believe that AuBMT compares favorably with the cost per life year/ quality-adjusted life year of other medical procedures such as CABG and renal dialysis. We still have much to learn, however.

The good news is that we have good ideas about how to go about answering the question of the costs and cost-effectiveness of AuBMT, and we have already done a lot of leg work. We know that patients need to be followed for more than a few months to capture the long-term benefits of BMT. We are also exploring the hypothesis that certain major categories of costs drive the costs of BMT. If we can determine the major cost drivers, we will not need to collect as much detailed utilization data, and can reduce data collection costs for future analyses. Finally, it is likely that any cost-effectiveness study will have a limited shelf life. Methods of treatment and institutional patterns of care will continue to evolve as we try to treat these diseases more effectively and cost-effectively. As these changes occur, older studies of older methods will become obsolete. We must continually expand our knowledge to keep abreast of changes and improvements.

Health care policy alternatives based on cost-effectiveness

Health care costs are the major concern of policy makers, regardless of efficacy [53–55]. Decisions about care are being made on the basis of cost and many insurance plans exclude patients from BMT. Three fifths of leukemia patients who were eligible for human leukocyte antigen typing were excluded from consideration for bone marrow transplantation because of financial issues, and of those typed, 14% did not receive the transplant for the same reason.

The technology assessment of BMT has been clouded by the lack of data on outcomes, the difficulty in choosing appropriate controls, and reimbursement issues [56]. Historical control groups are frequently used, which may not have the same survival curves as concurrent controls, since patients are now diagnosed early and medical support systems have improved. Furthermore, accrual to clinical trials has been difficult, with many patients opting for BMT outside of the clinical trial setting. General strategic concerns for evaluating costs and cost-effectiveness include the following:

1. How can estimates of efficacy and cost-effectiveness be derived when the clinical trial results are not available, so as to establish thresholds for specific decisions?
2. What is the optimal strategy for maximizing life-years at minimum cost? Should all eligible patients receive BMT, or those at greatest risk of relapse, or only those with 'sensitive' relapse?
3. What is the cost per life-year gained of alternative strategies, e.g., two differing costs and toxicities?
4. How can quality-of-life values be factored into the analysis, especially when two strategies have very different risks and benefits?

Patient care decisions should be made in a rational fashion and should include data about patient preferences, efficacy, quality of life, and cost. These data will be available in the years to come, and sensitivity analyses allow for the testing of all reasonable clinical assumptions. However, caution is needed when comparing cancer therapy cost-effectiveness estimates with other medical therapies because of marked variation in methodologies and assumptions.

Rational decisions for cancer care will be based on cost-effectiveness analyses in many managed care systems. However, this process is not an easy one because of four methodological concerns:
1. Definitional problems concerning an understandable benefit, such as life-years saved.
2. Inadequate information about clinical efficacy. (sensitivity analyses are useful here when data are uncertain)
3. Conceptual and measurement issues about costs of care. (however, with large integrated health systems, this limitation should decrease)
4. Estimating the treatment effectiveness in the routine practice setting.

Despite these concerns, data can be collected for evaluation of cost-effectiveness. Rationing of health care occurs; however, it is hoped that factors other than dollars per life year saved will be used. Compassion, social equity, and justice are other important factors. Bedside rationing is not appropriate; rather, policy decisions must be made at the population or group level.

The usefulness of cost-effectiveness analyses is not limited to policy makers. It is a method that explicitly defines the risks, benefits, and outcomes of alternative therapies. Patients who are undergoing expensive therapies such as BMT — many of whom are committing a large amount of financial and emotional resources — need to evaluate the same issues.

References

1. Smith TJ, Hillner BE, Desch CE. Efficacy and cost-effectiveness of cancer treatment rational allocation of resources based on decision analysis. J Natl Cancer Inst 85:1460–1474, 1993.
2. Welch HG, Larson EB. Cost effectiveness or bone marrow transplantation in acute nonlymphocytic leukemia. N Engl J Med 321:807–812, 1989.

3. Detsky AS. Guidelines for economic analysis of pharmaceutical products: a draft document for Ontario and Canada. Pharmoecon Comics 3:354–361, 1993.
4. McVie J. Counting costs of care. J Clin Oncol: 6:1529–1531, 1988.
5. Eisenberg J. Clinical economics. Ag guide to the economic analysis of clinical practice. JAMA 262:2879–2886, 1969.
6. Drummond M, Stoddart G, LaBelle R. Health economics an introduction for clinicians. Ann Intern Med 107:88–92, 1987.
7. Smith T, Desch C, Hillner B. Analysis of economic issues. In Antman K Armitage JO (eds), High Dose Cancer Therapy: Pharmacology, Hematopoietins, and Stem Cells Philadelphia: Williams and Wilkins, 1992.
8. Goddard M, Hutton J. Economic evaluation of trends in cancer therapy: marginal or average costs. Int J Technol Assess Health Care 7:594–603, 1991.
9. Wodisnky H. The costs of caring for cancer patients. J Palliat Care 8:24–27, 1992.
10. Robinson R. Economic evaluation and heath care: costs and cost-minimization analyses. Br Med J 307:726–728, 1993.
11. Bennett C, Armitage J, Buchner D, Gulati S. Economic analysis in phase III clinical cancer trials. Cancer Invest 12:336–342, 1994.
12. Hodgson T, Meiners M. Cost-of-illness methodology: a guide to current practices and procedures. Milbank Mem Fund Q 60:429–462, 1982.
13. Weinstein M, Stason W. Foundations of cost-effectiveness analysis for health and medical practices. N Engl J Med 296:716–721, 1977.
14. Drummond M, Stoddart G, Torrance G. Methods for the Economic Evaluation of Health Care Programmes. New York: Oxford University Press, 1987
15. Lipscomb J. Time preference for health in cost-effectiveness analysis. Med Care 27:S233–S253, 1989.
16. Eddy D. Cost-effectiveness analysis. Will it be accepted? JAMA 268:132–136, 1992.
17. Detsky A, Naglie I. A clinician's guide to cost-effectiveness analysis. Ann Intern Med 113:147–154, 1990.
18. Eddy D. Cost-effectiveness analysis. Is it up to the task? JAMA 267:3342–3348, 1992.
19. Mason J, Drummond M, Torrance G. Some guidelines on the use of cost-effectiveness league tables. 306:570–572, 1993.
20. Robinson R. Economic evaluation and health care Cost-effectiveness analysis. Br Med J 307:793–795, 1993.
21. Eisenberg J. Economics. JAMA 271:1663–1666, 1994.
22. Finkler S. The distinction between cost and charges. Ann Intern Med 96:102–109, 1982.
23. Appelbaum F, Fisher L, Thomas E. Chemotherapy versus marrow transplantation for adults with acute nonlymphocytic leukemia: a five year followup. The Seattle Marrow Transplant Team. Blood 72:179–184, 1988.
24. Schapira D, Studnicki J, Bradham D, Wolff P, Jarrett A. Intensive care survival and expense of treating critically ill cancer patients. JAMA 269:783–786, 1993.
25. Robinson R. Economic evaluation and health care: The policy question. Br Med J 307:994–996, 1993.
26. Bennett C, Armitage J, LeSage S, Gulati S, Armitage J, Gorin C. Economic analyses of clinical trials in cancer: are they helpful to policy makers? Stem Cells 12:424–429, 1994.
27. Gulati S, Bennett C. Granulocyte- macrophage colony stimulating factor as adjunct therapy in relapsed Hodgkin disease. Ann Intern Med 116:177–182, 1992.
28. Kukull W, Koepsell T, Conrad D. Rapid estimation of hospitalization charges from a brief medical record review. Med Care 24:961–966, 1986.
29. Hsaio W, Braun P, Dunn D, Becker E, DeNicola M, Ketcham T. Results and policy implications of the resurce based relative value scale. N Engl J Med 319:881–888, 1988.
30. Adams M, McCall N, Gray D, Orza M, Chalmers T. Economic analysis in randomized control trials. Med Care 30:231–243, 1992.
31. Fuchs V, Garber A. The new technology assessment. N Engl J Med 323:673–677, 1992.

32. Ellwood P. Shattuck lecture — outcomes management. A technology of patient experience. N Engl J Med 318:1549–1556, 1988.
33. Discounting health care only a matter of time. Lancet 340:148–149, 1992.
34. Smith T, Buonaiuto D, Hillner B. The learning curve for cost in autologous bone marrow transplantation for breast cancer. Proc ASCO 12:63, 1993.
35. Bennett C, Armitage J, Armitage G, Schwartz C. Bierman P, Vose J, Armitage J, Anderson J. A 'learning curve' exists in autologous transplantation for Hodgkin's disease and non-Hodgkin's lymphoma as evidenced by improvements in cost in-hospital mortality. Proc Am Soci Hematol 571a, 1993.
36. Doubilet P, Weinstein M, McNeil B. Use and misuse of the term cost-effective in medicine. N Engl J Med 314:253–255, 1986.
37. Udvarhelyi I, Colditz G, Rai A. Cost-effectiveness and cost-benefit analysis in the medical literature: are the methods being used correctly. Ann Intern Med 116:238–244, 1992.
38. Skeel R. Quality of life assessments in cancer clinical trials — it's time to catch up. J Natl Cancer Inst 81:472–473, 1989.
39. Fitzpatrick R, Fletcher A, Gore S. Quality of life measures in health care. 1. Application and issues of measurement. Br Med J 305:1205–1209, 1992.
40. Fletcher A, Gore S, Spiegelhalter R. Quality of life measures in health care. Design analysis and interpretation. Br Med J 303:1561–1562, 1991.
41. Spiegelhalter D, Gore S, Fitzpatrick R. Quality of life measures in health care. 3. Resource allocation. Br Med J 305:1205–1209, 1992.
42. Pauker S, Kassierer J. Decision analyses. N Engl J Med 316:250–258, 1987.
43. Smith T, Hillner B, Desch C. Efficacy and cost-effectiveness of cancer treatment: rational allocation of resources based on decision analysis. J Natl Cancer Inst 85:1460–1474, 1993.
44. Robinson R. Economic evaluation and health care: cost-benefit analysis. Br Med J 307:924–926, 1993.
45. Rees G. Cost-effectiveness in oncology. Lancet 2:1405–1408, 1985.
46. Welch G, Larson E. Cost effectiveness of bone marrow transplantation in acute nonlymphocytic leukemia. N Engl J Med 32:807–812, 1989.
47. Viens-Bitker C, Rery-Lemonnier E, Blum-Boisgard C. Cost of allogeneic bone marrow transplantation in four diseases. Health Policy 12:309–317, 1989.
48. Bennett C, Armitage J, Armitage G. Costs of care and outcomes for high-dose therapy and autologous transplantation for lymphoid malignancies: results from the University of Nebraska 1987 through 1991. J Clin Oncol 13:969–973, 1995.
49. Hillner BE, Smith TH, Desch CE. Efficacy and cost-effectiveness of autologous bone marrow transplantation in metastitic breast cancer — estimates using decision analysis while awaiting clinical trial results. JAMA 267:2055–2062, 1992.
50. Beard M, Inder A, Allen J, Hart D. The costs and benefits of bone marrow transplantation. N Z Med J 104:303–305, 1991.
51. Dufoir T, Saux M, Terraza B. Comparative cost of allogenic or autologous bone marrow transplantation and chemotherapy in patients with acute myeloid leukaemia in first remission. Bone Marrow Transplant 10:323–329, 1992.
52. Economic analysis of a randomized clinical trial comparing peripheral blood progenitor cells or autologous bone marrow after high dose chemotherapy for recurrent Hodgkin's disease or lymphoma. Richmond, VA: American Society of Clinical Oncologists, 1995.
53. Rice D, Hodgson T, Capell F. The economic burden of cancer, 1985; United States and California. In Scheffler RM, Andrews NC (eds). Cancer Care and Cost. DRGs and Beyond. Ann Arbor: Health Admin Press, 1989.
54. Yarbro J. Changing cancer care in the 1990s and the cost. Cancer 67:1718–1727, 1991.
55. Aaron J, Schwarz W. Rationing health care: the choice before us. Science 247:418–422, 1990.
56. Gulati S. Did we focus on the most important issue in the use of growth factors and stem cell tranplantation? J Clin Oncol 12:650–652, 1994.

Index

Acute graft-vs.-host disease (GVHD), 90
    allogeneic umbilical cord blood transplants and, 188, 192
    erythropoietin and, 267
    leukemia relapse protective effects of, 61–62
    pulmonary complications and, 232
    thalassemia and, 308, 309–310, 311, 312–313
    unrelated donor transplants and, 222–223, 224, 225
Acute lymphoblastic leukemia (ALL)
    cytokines and, 258, 260, 261, 264, 265, 279
    gene therapy and, 14
    minimal residual disease and, 100, 102, 104, 105, 107–109
    radiolabeled antibodies and, 131–134
    unrelated donor transplants for, 219
Acute lymphocytic leukemia (ALL)
    allogeneic umbilical cord blood transplants for, 194, 195, 199
    donor mononuclear cells for relapse, 73
    gene therapy and, 15
    graft-vs.-host disease relapse protection, 62
    post-transplant immunotherapy and, 29, 30, 35, 43
    syngeneic bone marrow transplants and, 60, 61
Acute myeloblastic leukemia (AML), 13, 14, 391
Acute myelocytic leukemia, 199
Acute myelogenous leukemia (AML)
    allogeneic bone marrow transplants for, 388
    allogeneic umbilical cord blood

transplants for, 195, 198
    donor mononuclear cells for relapse, 73
    gene therapy and, 15
    graft-vs.-host disease relapse protection, 62
    radiolabeled antibodies in treatment of, 130–134, 135
    syngeneic bone marrow transplants and, 61
Acute myeloid leukemia (AML), 121, 363
    autologous bone marrow transplants for, 392
    cytokines and, 258, 260, 261, 265
    interleukin-1 and, 272–273
    post-transplant immunotherapy and, 29, 31, 32, 43
    unrelated donor transplants for, 219
Acute nonlymphocytic leukemia (ANLL), 35, 60, 388
Acyclovir, 18
Adeno-associated viral vectors, 10–11
Adenosine deaminase gene, 4
Adenoviral vectors, 7–10
Adjuvant-induced arthritis, 319
Adoptive immunotherapy, 65–69
    ineffectiveness in disease relapse, 72–73
    minimal residual disease and, 109
    for nonrelapse complications, 76–77
Adrenoleukodystrophy, 199
Adriamycin, see Doxorubicin
Adult respiratory distress syndrome (ARDS), 232, 245
Airflow obstruction, 245–247
Allergen-induced asthma, 319
Allogeneic bone marrow transplants
    adoptive immunotherapy and, 76–77

autologous graft-vs.-host disease
  and, 90
for chronic myelogenous leukemia,
  357
costs and effectiveness of, 386–390
cytokines and, 75–76, 255–281
graft-vs.-host disease and, 87
graft-vs.-leukemia effect of, 57–58,
  60–61, 62–72, 73–75
growth factors and, 255–281
immunotherapy following, 27, 28,
  31–32, 35–36, 43, 46–47
leukemia relapse and, 60–61, 62–72
for neuroblastoma, 340–341, 345
peripheral blood progenitor cell
  transplants vs., 146
pulmonary complications and, 232,
  244, 245
radiolabeled antibodies and, 130,
  131, 132
for severe autoimmune diseases,
  323–324
Allogeneic umbilical cord blood
  transplants, 187–212
autologous blood banking for,
  209–210
blood collection, separation and
  cryopreservation in, 200–202
ethical considerations, 210
historical background to, 188–190
immunological properties of
  lymphocytes, 205–208
progenitor cell characterization,
  202–204
regulatory issues, 211
sibling donor, 190–194
survival in, 193–194, 198
unrelated donor, 194–200
unrelated donor blood banking for,
  208–209
Amegakaryocytic thrombocytopenia,
  199
Amphotericin B, 224
Amsacrine, 365
Anemia
  aplastic, see Aplastic anemia
  Fanconi, 190, 199, 219, 220
  hemolytic, 318
Angioimmunoblastic
  lymphadenopathy, 101
Animal models
  graft-vs.-leukemia effect in, 57–59
  of severe autoimmune diseases,
    318–323

Anti-CD3 antibodies, 206
Anti-CD7 antibodies, 112
Anti-CD10 antibodies, 113
Anti-CD15 antibodies, 111
Anti-CD20 antibodies, 113, 125, 128,
  135
Anti-CD33 antibodies, 130–131, 136
Anti-CD34 antibodies, 150, 151, 163
Anti-CD37 antibodies, 125, 126
Anti-CD45 antibodies, 131–134, 135
Antigen receptor gene rearrangements,
  103–106
Antilymphocyte globulin (ALG), 311
Antisense oligonucleotides, 20–21,
  368–369
Antithymocyte globulin (ATGAM),
  88, 195, 196, 222, 226
Aplastic anemia, 219, 323
  allogeneic bone marrow transplants
    for, 388, 389
  cytokines and, 258, 260, 261, 265
  idioplastic, 199
Ara-C, 365
Arthritis
  adjuvant-induced, 319
  collagen-induced, 319
  rheumatoid, 321, 322, 323, 324, 325,
    326–327
Aspergillus, 223, 224
Asta-Z, 348
Asthma, 319, 320
Autologous bone marrow purging
  for chronic myelogenous leukemia,
    360–366, 368–370
  controversies over, 341–343
  ex vivo expansion and, 160, 163,
    360–363
  improved methods of, 368–370
  in vivo, 363–366
  for neuroblastoma treatment,
    341–343
  polymerase chain reaction
    assessment of, 110–114
Autologous bone marrow transplants,
  90, 194
  for brain tumors, 348–350
  for chronic myelogenous leukemia,
    357–371
  costs of, 379, 383, 390–396
  cytokines and, 75–76, 255–281
  in Europe, 393
  for Ewing's sarcoma, 345–347
  in France, 392
  gene therapy and, 13

growth factors and, 255–281
immunotherapy following, 27, 28,
    29–31, 34–36, 45
minimal residual disease following,
    109–110
for neuroblastoma, 334–345
in New Zealand, 391–392
for pediatric solid tumors, 333–352
peripheral blood progenitor cell
    transplants vs., 146
peripheral blood stem cell
    transplants vs., 393
pulmonary complications and, 232,
    233, 244
purging prior to, see Autologous
    bone marrow purging
radiolabeled antibodies and,
    126–127, 129, 132
for rhabdomyosarcoma, 347–348
in the United States, 393–396
for Wilms' tumor, 350–351
Autologous graft-vs.-host disease
    (GVHD), 35, 42–43, 88, 91
Autologous stem cell transplants,
    357–371
maintaining remission following, 370
reasons for failure of, 367–368
survival benefits from, 366–367
Azathioprine, 247

Bacterial pneumonia, 231
B-1 antibodies, 126, 127, 128
B-cell lymphoproliferative disorders
    (BLPD), 76
B cells, 44, 45, 274
bcl-2 gene, 20, 103, 106, 109, 113
bcr-abl fusion, 20, 73
    chronic myelogenous leukemia and,
        357, 368, 369
    minimal residual disease and, 108,
        109
    polymerase chain reaction detection
        of, 102
Blackfan-Diamond syndrome, 199
Blood banking
    autologous, 209–210
    unrelated donor, 208–209
Bone marrow aplasia, 65–67
Bone marrow transplants, 187
    allogeneic, see Allogeneic bone
        marrow transplants
    autologous, see Autologous bone
        marrow transplants

economics of, 377–397
ex vivo expansion in, 159–160, 162,
    168, 169–171, 172–173, 174, 176,
    178–179
gene therapy and, 14
graft-vs.-leukemia effect in clinical,
    59–62
immunotherapy following, see Post-
    bone marrow transplant
    immunotherapy
minimal residual disease following,
    107–109
pediatric, 240, 245
pulmonary complications and, see
    Pulmonary complications
radiolabeled antibodies and, see
    Radiolabeled antibodies
for severe autoimmune diseases, see
    Severe autoimmune diseases
syngeneic, 57, 60–61, 87, 88
for thalassemia, see Thalassemia
unrelated donors used for, 217–226
Brain tumors, 17, 18, 19, 348–350
Breast cancer
    autologous bone marrow purging
        and, 111–112
    autologous bone marrow transplants
        for, 391, 395
    CD34 cell selection in treatment of,
        152–154
    cytokines and, 258, 260, 279
    gene therapy and, 13, 14, 15, 17, 19,
        20, 22
    minimal residual disease and, 100
    post-transplant immunotherapy and,
        29, 30, 35, 41
    stem cell factor and, 273
Bronchiolitis, 231, 237, 245–247
Bronchoalveolar lavage (BAL), 244–
    245, 247–248
Bronchoscopy, 247–249
Burkitt's lymphoma, 100
Burst-forming units-erythroid (BFU-E)
    allogeneic umbilical cord blood
        transplants and, 203, 204, 205
    ex vivo expansion and, 161, 162, 171,
        173
    interleukin-2 and, 40
Busulfan
    allogeneic umbilical cord blood
        transplants and, 196
    for brain tumors, 349
    engraftment and, 222
    radiolabeled antibodies and, 131, 134

thalassemia and, 305, 306, 310, 311, 314

unrelated donor transplants and, 222

Bystander effect, 19

CAP gene, 10

Capillary leak syndrome, 259, 262, 275, 278

Carboplatin, in OMEC, 336, 339

Carcinoembryonic antigen (CEA), 16, 17

Carmustine, 129, 336, 338

CD4:CD8 cell ratio, 206, 317, 318

CD3 cells, 33, 44, 206

CD4 cells

    in allogeneic umbilical cord blood, 206

    autologous graft-vs.-host disease and, 89

    graft-vs.-host disease and, 93

    graft-vs.-leukemia effect and, 58–59, 74

    post-transplant immunotherapy and, 33, 45

    severe autoimmune diseases and, 317

CD8 cells

    in allogeneic umbilical cord blood, 206

    autologous graft-vs.-host disease and, 89

    graft-vs.-host disease and, 71, 93

    graft-vs.-leukemia effect and, 58–59, 74, 75

    post-transplant immunotherapy and, 33

CD10 cells, 202

CD11b cells, 161

CD15 cells, 161

CD28 cells, 15

CD33 cells, 202

CD34 cells

    in allogeneic umbilical cord blood, 202–205

    autologous bone marrow purging and, 114

    chronic myelogenous leukemia and, 358, 364, 368–369

    ex vivo expansion and, 161, 162, 163, 165, 168–169, 171–173, 179

    gene therapy and, 14, 21, 22

    immunoadherent selection of, 151

    immunomagnetic selection of, 150–151

    positive selection of, 144, 149–154

CD38 cells, 203, 204

CD41a cells, 161

CD45RA cells, 203, 206

CD56 cells, 207

CD71 cells, 203

c-fos gene, 21

Chediak-Higashi syndrome, 219, 220

Chemotherapy, see also specific agents

    for brain tumors, 348–350

    for chronic myelogenous leukemia, 363–366

    cost measurement of, 379

    for Ewing's sarcoma, 346–347

    hematopoietic protection from, 21–22

    interleukin-1 and, 272

    for neuroblastoma, 334–341

    peripheral blood progenitor cell mobilization with, 145–146

    pulmonary complications and, 232

    for Wilms' tumor, 350–351

Chemotherapy sensitization genes, 16–18

Children, see entries under Pediatric

Chronic graft-vs.-host disease (GVHD), 90

    leukemia relapse protective effects of, 61–62

    pulmonary complications and, 231, 232, 237, 245, 246, 247

    thalassemia and, 308, 309–310, 311, 312–313

    unrelated donor transplants and, 223

Chronic granulocytic leukemia, 388, 389

Chronic lymphocytic leukemia (CLL)

    cytokines and, 260, 261, 265

    donor mononuclear cells for relapse, 73

    gene therapy and, 15

    minimal residual disease and, 104

Chronic myelogenous leukemia (CML), 121

    adoptive immunotherapy toxicity for relapsed, 65–69

    allogeneic umbilical cord blood transplants for, 194, 195, 199

    autologous stem cell transplants for, 357–371

    CD34 cell selection in treatment of, 153

cytokines and, 75
donor mononuclear cells for
  relapsed, 63–69, 70, 75
gene therapy and, 13, 14, 15, 20
graft-vs.-host disease relapse
  protection, 62, 63–64, 67–69, 70,
  74
juvenile, 194, 195, 199
minimal residual disease and, 102
syngeneic bone marrow transplants
  and, 61
unrelated donor transplants for, 219,
  225
Chronic myeloid leukemia (CML), 160
cytokines and, 258, 260, 261, 265
GM-CSF and interleukin-3 for, 277
minimal residual disease and, 102,
  114
post-transplant immunotherapy and,
  32, 34, 35, 36, 39, 43, 46
Chronic myelomonocytic leukemia, 131
Cisplatin, 336, 337, 338, 339, 340, 352
  in VAM-TBI, 337, 340
c-kit ligand, see Stem cell factor
Clonogenic assays, 100–101
c-mpl ligand, see Thrombopoietin
c-myb gene, 369
c-myc gene, 20
Collagen-induced arthritis, 319
Colon cancer, 17, 19, 20, 44
Colony-forming units-blast (CFU-Bl),
  161
Colony-forming units-erythroid (CFU-
  E), 171
Colony-forming units-granulocyte,
  erythroid, monocyte,
  megakaryocyte (CFU-GEMM),
  40, 161, 162
Colony-forming units-granulocyte-
  macrophage (CFU-GM), 144
allogeneic umbilical cord blood
  transplants and, 191, 200, 203, 204,
  205
chemotherapy mobilization and, 145
ex vivo expansion and, 161, 162, 163,
  165–168, 171, 172, 173, 174, 176
interleukin-2 and, 36, 40
Colony-forming units-spleen (CFU-S),
  278
Competitive (quantitative) polymerase
  chain reaction (PCR), 106
Computerized tomography (CT) scans,
  239, 246
Congestive heart failure, 232

Consumer Price Index (CPI), 382
Corticosteroids, 245
Cost-benefit analysis, 386
Cost-effectiveness, 382
of allogeneic bone marrow
  transplants, 386–390
general strategies for measuring,
  385–386
health care policy alternatives based
  on, 396–397
Cost measurement, 379–384
Costs, 378
of allogeneic bone marrow
  transplants, 386–390
of autologous bone marrow
  transplants, 379, 383, 390–396
c-raf gene, 21
CREST syndrome, 324
Crohn's disease, 325, 328
c-src gene, 21
c-vas gene, 21
Cyclophosphamide, 121, 388
allogeneic umbilical cord blood
  transplants and, 195, 196
for chronic myelogenous leukemia,
  358
engraftment and, 221, 222
for Ewing's sarcoma, 345
graft-vs.-host disease and, 88
interleukin-2 and, 40–42
for neuroblastoma, 334, 337, 340
for osteosarcoma, 352
peripheral blood progenitor cell
  mobilization with, 145–146
radiolabeled antibodies and, 129,
  131, 132, 133–134
for rhabdomyosarcoma, 347
thalassemia and, 305, 306, 310, 311
unrelated donor transplants and, 222
Cyclosporine, 89, 90, 91, 92, 190, 196,
  388
graft-vs.-host disease induced by, 35
pulmonary complications and, 247
radiolabeled antibodies and, 131
severe autoimmune diseases and,
  324
thalassemia and, 308
unrelated donor transplants and,
  222, 223
Cytarabine, 359, 388
  in ICE, 363, 365
Cytokines, 255–281, see also specific
  types
combination trials with, 275–278

405

delayed use after transplant, 278–279
in engraftment failure, 257–259
gene therapy and, 161
graft enhancement and, 259–262
graft-vs.-host disease and, 75, 90–94,
259, 262, 268
graft-vs.-leukemia effect and, 75–76
pulmonary complications and, 233
rationale for administration of,
255–257
Cytomegalovirus (CMV)
allogeneic umbilical cord blood
transplants and, 195
graft-vs.-host disease mimicked by,
88
interleukin-2 and, 275
pulmonary complications and, 231,
232, 242
unrelated donor transplants and,
223, 224, 226
Cytopenia, 159–160
Cytosine deaminase gene, 17–18, 19
Cytotoxic T lymphocytes (CTLs), 31
in allogeneic umbilical cord blood,
206–207
gene therapy and, 15, 16
graft-vs.-host disease and, 88
graft-vs.-leukemia effect and, 75
pulmonary complications and, 232,
246
Cytoxan, 365

Dactinomycin, 347
Dana-Farber Cancer Institute, 113, 359
Daunorubicin, 365, 388
Deoxyadenosine, 112
2′-Deoxycoformycin, 112
Diabetes mellitus, 318, 320, 322
Diagnosis-related groups, 380
Dianhydrogalactitol, 335
Dicarbazine, 352
Diffuse alveolar hemorrhage (DAH),
244–245
Diffuse lymphoma, 103
Donor leukocyte infusions (DLI),
43–44, 46
Donor mononuclear cells (MNCs)
for chronic myelogenous leukemia
relapse, 63–69, 70, 75
graft-vs.-leukemia effect of, 63–71,
74–75
ineffectiveness in relapse of some
diseases, 72–73

for nonrelapse complications, 76–77
pancytopenia with bone marrow
aplasia and, 65–67
Doxorubicin (Adriamycin), 345, 347,
352
in VAM-TBI, 337, 340

Ectomesenchymoma, 347
Effectiveness of therapy, 384–385
Encephalomyelitis, 319, 323
Engraftment
allogeneic umbilical cord blood
transplants and, 191, 197–198
unrelated donor transplants and,
221–222
Engraftment failure, see Graft failure
env protein, 4–5, 6
Epstein-Barr virus, 76, 100, 195
Erythropoietin, 256, 263–267
allogeneic umbilical cord blood cell
transplants and, 203, 204
clinical applications of, 280
in combination with other agents,
276
endogenous, 266
exogenous administration of,
266–267
ex vivo expansion and, 165, 168, 171,
172, 179
Etoposide (VP-16-213), 269
for brain tumors, 349
for chronic myelogenous leukemia,
365
for Ewing's sarcoma, 345, 346
for germ-cell tumors, 352
in ICE, 363, 365
for neuroblastoma, 337, 340
in OMEC, 336, 339
radiolabeled antibodies and, 129
for Wilms' tumor, 351
Europe, 393
European Bone Marrow Transplant
(EBMT) registry, 65, 73, 346, 359
Ewing's sarcoma, 345–347
Ex vivo expansion, 159–179, 360–363
of allogeneic umbilical cord blood
cells, 204–205
cell characterization in, 161–162
cell processing in, 162–163
cell sources in, 162
cell types and numbers required in,
173–174
clinical trials with, 178–179
culture conditions affecting, 164–173

potential applications of, 159–161
regulatory considerations in, 177–178
systems for, 174–177

Familial erythrophagocytotic
    lymphohistiocytosis, 219
Fanconi anemia, 190, 199, 219, 220
Feeding/perfusion, in ex vivo
    expansion, 169, 170
Filgrastim, 255, see also Granulocyte
    colony-stimulating factor
Flow cytometry
    of CD34 cells, 151–152
    in ex vivo expansion, 161
flt-ligand, 165
Fludarabine, 365
Fluorescence in situ hybridization
    (FISH), 358, 368
5-Fluorocytosine (5-FC), 19
5-Fluorouracil (5-FU), 19, 179
Follicular lymphoma, 13, 103
Food and Drug Administration
    (FDA), 177, 211, 255, 383
France, 392
Fred Hutchinson Cancer Research
    Center, 240, 241, 243, 386
Fungal infections, 268

gag protein, 4–5, 6
Ganciclovir, 18, 224
Gaucher's disease, 220
Gene therapy, 3–23
    antisense, see Antisense
        oligonucleotides
    chemotherapy sensitization genes in,
        16–18
    ex vivo expansion in, 160–161
    gene marking trials in, 13–14
    viral vector systems in, 3–12
Germ-cell tumors, 352
Globoid cell leukodystrophy, 199
Glomerulonephritis, 318
Glycophorin A, 161
Gold, 327
Graft enhancement, 259–262
Graft failure
    cytokines in, 257–259
    primary, 257
    secondary, 221–222, 257
    unrelated donor transplants and,
        225, 226
Graft rejection, 188, 195

Graft-vs.-host disease (GVHD), 87–94,
    131, 132, 153, 187, 388
    acute, see Acute graft-vs.-host
        disease
    allogeneic umbilical cord blood
        transplants and, 190, 192, 193, 194,
        195, 196, 198, 199–200, 207–208,
        212
    autologous, 35, 42–43, 88, 91
    chronic, see Chronic graft-vs.-host
        disease
    classical requirements for, 88
    cytokines and, 75, 90–94, 259, 262,
        268
    donor mononuclear cells and, 67–70,
        76
    gene therapy and, 12, 19–20
    graft-vs.-leukemia effect and, 58, 59,
        67–72, 74
    immunologic background of, 87–88
    leukemia relapse protective effects
        of, 60, 61–62, 63–64, 67–69, 70, 74
    minimal residual disease and,
        108–109
    post-transplant immunotherapy and,
        31–32, 34, 36, 43, 45, 47
    pulmonary complications and, 242
    thalassemia and, 306
    transfusion-associated, 66
    unrelated donor transplants and,
        218, 225
Graft-vs.-leukemia (GVL) effect,
    57–77
    allogeneic bone marrow transplants
        and, 27, 28, 57–58, 62–72
    in animal models, 57–59
    in clinical bone marrow transplants,
        59–62
    cytokines and, 75–76
    of donor mononuclear cells, 63–71,
        74–75
    effector cells responsible for
        reactivity of, 73–75
    gene therapy and, 20
    post-transplant immunotherapy and,
        27, 28, 34, 35–36, 38, 43, 45, 46, 47
    unrelated donor transplants and, 224
Graft-vs.-tumor (GVT) effects
    allogeneic bone marrow transplants
        and, 27
    gene therapy and, 12
    post-transplant immunotherapy and,
        27, 30, 32
Granulocyte colony-stimulating factor

(G-CSF), 255, 256, 263, 264, 265
allogeneic umbilical cord blood
    transplants and, 191, 204, 205
clinical applications of, 280
delayed use after transplant, 279
donor mononuclear cells mobilized
    by, 67
engraftment and, 222
erythropoietin and, 276
ex vivo expansion and, 165, 168, 171,
    174
GM-CSF and, 276–277
graft enhancement and, 259–262
graft failure and, 257–259
interleukin-1 and, 272
interleukin-2 and, 39, 40
interleukin-3 and, 270
interleukin-11 and, 274
peripheral blood progenitor cell
    mobilization with, 146–148, 151
radiolabeled antibodies and, 135
stem cell factor and, 273, 278
thrombopoietin compared with, 275
unrelated donor transplants and, 222
Granulocyte-macrophage colony-
    stimulating factor (GM-CSF), 255,
    256, 263, 264, 265, 268, *see also*
    PIXY 321
allogeneic umbilical cord blood
    transplants and, 187, 191, 207
clinical applications of, 280
economics of using, 383
erythropoietin and, 276
ex vivo expansion and, 165, 168, 174,
    179
G-CSF and, 276–277
gene therapy and, 17
graft enhancement and, 259–262
graft failure and, 257–259
interleukin-1 and, 272
interleukin-2 and, 33, 39
interleukin-3 and, 270, 277–278
interleukin-6 and, 269, 270, 278
peripheral blood progenitor cells
    and, 146–147
PIXY 321 compared with, 271–272
thrombopoietin compared with, 275
Growth factors, 255–281, *see also*
    specific types
cost of, 279–280
delayed use after transplant, 278–279
ex vivo expansion and, 165–168
in graft enhancement, 259, 262
peripheral blood progenitor cell

mobilization with, 146–148
pulmonary complications and,
    232–233
unrelated donor transplants and, 226

Haploidentical donors, 221
Head and neck cancer, 18, 19, 20
Hematopoiesis
allogeneic umbilical cord blood
    transplants and, 187, 188–189, 190,
    191–192, 197–199
cytokines and, 256–257
Ph-negative, *see* Ph-negative
    hematopoietic stem cells
Hematopoietic chemoprotection, 21–22
Hematopoietic growth factors, *see*
    Growth factors
Hemolytic anemia, 318
Hepatitis B virus (HBV), 306, 309, 311,
    312
Hepatitis C virus (HCV), 306, 309, 311
Herpes simplex virus (HSV), 232
Herpes simplex virus (HSV)-thymidine
    kinase gene, *see* Thymidine kinase
    gene
Herpes simplex virus (HSV) vectors,
    11–12
High proliferative potential colony-
    forming cells (HPP-CFCs), 147,
    169
High proliferative potential colony-
    forming unit (HPP-CFU), 161,
    201, 202
Histocompatibility, of unrelated
    donors, 217–218
HLA, *see* Human leukocyte antigen
Hodgkin's disease
autologous bone marrow transplants
    for, 391, 393
cytokines and, 258, 264, 279
gene therapy and, 15
GM-CSF and interleukin-3 for,
    277–278
interleukin-1 and, 273
interleukin-6 and, 269
minimal residual disease and, 101,
    102
post-transplant immunotherapy and,
    34
pulmonary complications and, 239
radiolabeled antibodies in treatment
    of, 129
Human antimouse antibody (HAMA),

125, 126, 127, 136
Human immunodeficiency virus (HIV)
  testing, 210
Human leukocyte antigen (HLA)
  allogeneic umbilical cord blood
    transplants and, 188, 190, 191, 192,
    193, 197, 198, 200, 207, 209, 212
  haploidentical donor transplants and,
    221
  identical donor transplants and, 92,
    187, 217, 221, 223, 224, 262, 306
  interferon-α and, 69
  nonidentical donor transplants and,
    240, 241, 246
  pulmonary complications and, 231
Human leukocyte antigen (HLA)-A
  allogeneic umbilical cord blood
    transplants and, 195, 208
  unrelated donor transplants and,
    217, 218, 220, 222
Human leukocyte antigen (HLA)-B
  allogeneic umbilical cord blood
    transplants and, 195, 208
  unrelated donor transplants and,
    217, 218, 220, 225
Human leukocyte antigen (HLA)-B7,
  17, 206
Human leukocyte antigen (HLA)-C,
  218
Human leukocyte antigen (HLA)-DP,
  222
Human leukocyte antigen (HLA)-DQ,
  222
Human leukocyte antigen (HLA)-DR
  allogeneic umbilical cord blood
    transplants and, 195, 202–203, 206,
    208
  chronic myelogenous leukemia and,
    358, 368
  ex vivo expansion and, 162
  unrelated donor transplants and,
    217, 220, 222
Hunter syndrome, 191
Hurler disease (mucopolysaccharidosis
  I), 219
4-Hydroperoxycyclophosphamide (4-
  HC), 112, 342
Hydroxychloroquine, 327
6-Hydroxydopamine, 338, 342
Hydroxyurea, 363, 365

ICH3, 151
Idarubicin, 365

Idarubicin, cytarabine, and etoposide
  (ICE), 363, 365
Identical sibling donors, 187, 262
  acute graft-vs.-host disease and, 223
  engraftment and, 221
  graft-vs.-host disease and, 92
  histocompatibility of, 217
  relapse and, 224
  thalassemia and, 306
Idiopathic pneumonia syndrome (IPS),
  242
Idioplastic aplastic anemia, 199
Immune ablation, 317–329
Immunoadherent selection of CD34
  cells, 151
Immunoadsorption of CD34 cells,
  152–154
Immunomagnetic selection of CD34
  cells, 150–151
Immunotherapy, see Adoptive
  immunotherapy; Post-bone
  marrow transplant immunotherapy
Incremental cost-effectiveness (ICE)
  ratio, 387
Inflammatory bowel disease, 318, 320,
  328
Interferon (IFN)
  gene therapy and, 16, 17
  interleukin-2 and, 34
  in post-transplant immunotherapy,
    34–35
Interferon-α (IFN-α)
  allogeneic umbilical cord blood
    transplants and, 206
  chronic myelogenous leukemia and,
    63, 69, 363, 365, 370
  graft-vs.-leukemia effect and, 69
  in post-transplant immunotherapy,
    34–35, 43
Interferon-γ (IFN-γ), 27
  chronic myelogenous leukemia and,
    361
  gene therapy and, 17
  graft-vs.-host disease and, 93
  interleukin-2 and, 28
  in post-transplant immunotherapy,
    34, 44
Interleukin-1 (IL-1), 256
  acute graft-vs.-host disease and, 223
  allogeneic umbilical cord blood and,
    205
  clinical applications of, 280
  ex vivo expansion and, 172, 178, 179
  graft-vs.-host disease and, 91, 93, 259

interleukin-6 compared with, 270
   properties of, 272–273
Interleukin-2 (IL-2), 256
   acute graft-vs.-host disease and, 223
   allogeneic umbilical cord blood and,
     206, 207
   chronic myelogenous leukemia and,
     369–370
   clinical applications of, 280
   gene therapy and, 15, 16, 17
   graft-vs.-host disease and, 59, 92, 93
   graft-vs.-leukemia effect and, 59,
     75–76
   with interleukin-2-activated grafts,
     35–43
   lymphokine activated killer cells
     and, 28–34, 36, 39
   in post-transplant immunotherapy,
     28–34, 35–43, 44, 46
   properties of, 275
Interleukin-2 (IL-2) receptors, 28, 206
Interleukin-3 (IL-3), 256, 268, see also
   PIXY 321
   allogeneic umbilical cord blood
     transplants and, 203, 204, 205
   clinical applications of, 280
   ex vivo expansion and, 165–168, 171,
     172, 178, 179
   GM-CSF and, 277–278
   interleukin-1 and, 272
   interleukin-2 and, 33
   interleukin-11 and, 274
   peripheral blood progenitor cell
     mobilization with, 146
   PIXY 321 compared with, 271–272
   properties of, 270–271
Interleukin-4 (IL-4)
   allogeneic umbilical cord blood
     transplants and, 207
   clinical applications of, 280
   gene therapy and, 17
   graft-vs.-host disease and, 93
   interleukin-2 and, 33, 46
Interleukin-5 (IL-5), 207
Interleukin-6 (IL-6), 256
   allogeneic umbilical cord blood
     transplants and, 203, 204, 205, 207
   clinical applications of, 280
   ex vivo expansion and, 165–168, 172,
     179
   GM-CSF and, 278
   graft-vs.-host disease and, 93
   interleukin-2 and, 28, 33
   interleukin-11 and, 274

   properties of, 269–270
Interleukin-7 (IL-7), 17, 46
Interleukin-8 (IL-8), 93
Interleukin-10 (IL-10), 93
Interleukin-11 (IL-11), 165, 256, 274,
   280
Interleukin-12 (IL-12), 17, 46
International Bone Marrow Transplant
   Registry, 324
In vitro assays, 161
In vivo assays, 161–162
In vivo purging, 363–366
Iron overload, 306, 308, 309, 311, 312
Italian Cooperative Group for
   Neuroblastoma (ICGNB), 339
Itraconazole, 224

Juvenile chronic myelogenous
   leukemia (CML), 194, 195, 199

Ketaconzole, 388
Kostman syndrome, 199

LCME1 study, 338
LCME2 study, 338
Lesch-Nyhan syndrome, 199
Leukemia, 121, 323, 348
   acute lymphoblastic, see Acute
     lymphoblastic leukemia
   acute lymphocytic, see Acute
     lymphocytic leukemia
   acute myeloblastic, 13, 14, 391
   acute myelocytic, 199
   acute myelogenous, see Acute
     myelogenous leukemia
   acute myeloid, see Acute myeloid
     leukemia
   acute nonlymphocytic, 35, 60, 388
   chronic granulocytic, 388, 389
   chronic lymphocytic, see Chronic
     lymphocytic leukemia
   chronic myelogenous, see Chronic
     myelogenous leukemia
   chronic myeloid, see Chronic
     myeloid leukemia
   chronic myelomonocytic, 131
   cost measurement of treatment for,
     379
   cytokines and, 258
   minimal residual disease and, 100,
     101

pediatric, 237
peripheral blood progenitor cell
  transplants and, 149
post-bone marrow transplant
  immunotherapy and, 37–38
relapse of, *see* Leukemia relapse
thalassemia and, 305
Leukemia relapse
  allogeneic bone marrow transplants
    and, 62–72
  graft-vs.-host disease protection
    against, 60, 61–62, 63–64, 67–69,
    70, 74
  syngeneic bone marrow transplants
    and, 60–61
Leukocyte adhesion deficiency, 219
Linomide, 370
Lipopolysaccharide (LPS), 93
Liver cancer, 20
Lomestine, 388
Long-term culture initiating cells
  (LTC-ICs)
  allogeneic umbilical cord blood
    transplants and, 202–203, 204, 205
  ex vivo expansion and, 161, 163,
    168–169, 172, 173, 174, 176, 178
Lung cancer
  autologous bone marrow purging
    and, 112
  gene therapy and, 17, 20
  minimal residual disease and, 99
  post-transplant immunotherapy and,
    44
  small cell, 99, 112
Lymphocytes
  of allogeneic umbilical cord blood,
    205–208
  cytotoxic, *see* Cytotoxic T
    lymphocytes
Lymphokine activated killer (LAK)
  cells, 27
  interleukin-2 and, 28–34, 36, 39
Lymphoma, 121, 324
  acute myeloblastic, 391
  autologous bone marrow purging
    and, 111, 112–114
  Burkitt's, 100
  diffuse, 103
  donor mononuclear cells for relapse.
    73
  follicular, 13, 103
  GM-CSF and interleukin-3 for,
    277–278
  Hodgkin's, *see* Hodgkin's disease

minimal residual disease and, 100,
  106–107
non-Hodgkin's, *see* Non-Hodgkin's
  lymphoma
parenchymal, 239
post-transplant immunotherapy and,
  30
undifferentiated, 100
unrelated donor transplants for, 219

Macrophage colony-stimulating factor
  (M-CSF), 256
  clinical applications of, 280
  ex vivo expansion and, 171
  graft enhancement and, 259
  properties of, 267–268
Macrophage inflammatory protein-1α
  (MIP-1α), 168, 369
Mafosfamide, 361
Major histocompatability complex
  (MHC), 46
  gene therapy and, 16
  graft-vs.-leukemia effect and, 58, 74
  interferon-γ and, 34, 44
  interleukin-2 and, 31, 36
Major histocompatability complex
  (MHC) class I, 15–16, 89
Major histocompatability complex
  (MHC) class II, 35, 88–89, 90
M195 antibodies, 130–131
Marginal costs, 382–383
Maroteaux-Lamy syndrome
  (mucopolysaccharidosis VI), 219
MB-1 antibodies, 126
Medicare Cost Report, 381
Medicare Fee Schedule, 381–382
Medicare ratio of cost to charges,
  380–381, 395
Melanoma
  cytokines and, 260
  gene therapy and, 17, 18, 19
  post-transplant immunotherapy and,
    28, 44, 45
Melphalan, 269
  for chronic myelogenous leukemia,
    359
  for Ewing's sarcoma, 345, 346
  for neuroblastoma, 335, 336, 337,
    338, 339, 340, 343
  in OMEC, 336, 339
  for osteosarcoma, 352
  for rhabdomyosarcoma, 347–348, 348
  in VAM-TBI, 337, 340

for Wilms' tumor, 350
Memorial Sloan Kettering Cancer
    Center, 70, 244
Mesothelioma, 18, 19
Methotrexate, 22, 61, 71, 88, 92, 131,
    132, 388
  allogeneic umbilical cord blood
    transplants and, 190, 196
  for osteosarcoma, 352
  pulmonary complications and, 246
  for rheumatoid arthritis, 327
  thalassemia and, 306
  unrelated donor transplants and,
    222, 223
Methylprednisolone, 190, 196, 199, 222
MHC, see Major histocompatability
    complex
Minimal residual disease (MRD),
    99–115
  assays for the detection of, 99–107
  clinical utility of detection, 107–110
Mitoxantrone, 365
Molecular biologic techniques, 101
Monoclonal antibodies, see also
    specific types
  autologous bone marrow purging
    and, 111–112
  to MHC, 88–89
Mononuclear cells, see Donor
    mononuclear cells; Peripheral
    blood mononuclear cell
    transplants
Mucopolysaccharidosis I (Hurler
    disease), 219
Mucopolysaccharidosis VI (Maroteaux-
    Lamy syndrome), 219
Multiple drug resistant (MDR) gene,
    21, 370–371
Multiple myeloma
  CD34 cell selection in treatment of,
    152, 153
  cytokines and, 261, 264, 265, 279
  donor mononuclear cells for relapse,
    73
  gene therapy and, 13, 14
  post-transplant immunotherapy and,
    34
Multiple sclerosis, 319, 320, 322, 324,
    325, 326
Myasthenia gravis, 319, 320, 322, 324,
    325, 327
Myelodysplastic syndrome (MDS), 324
  allogeneic umbilical cord blood
    transplants and, 199

cytokines and, 260, 261, 265
  donor mononuclear cells for relapse,
    73
  post-transplant immunotherapy and,
    32, 43
  radiolabeled antibodies and, 132–134
  unrelated donor transplants for, 219
Myelofibrosis, 258
Myeloma, 149, see also Multiple
    myeloma
  gene therapy and, 15
  minimal residual disease and, 104
  post-transplant immunotherapy and,
    45
  unrelated donor transplants for, 219
Myositis, 319, 321

National Marrow Donor Program
    (NMDP), 194–195, 220–221, 225
National Wilms' Tumor Study Group,
    350–351
Natural killer (NK) cells, 27, 369–370
  in allogeneic umbilical cord blood,
    194, 207
  graft-vs.-host disease and, 91, 94
  graft-vs.-leukemia effect and, 59, 74,
    75
  interferon-γ and, 34
  interleukin-2 and, 33, 36, 38, 75, 76,
    275
Neomycin phosphotransferase gene,
    13–14
Neomycin resistance gene, 341, 368
Nested polymerase chain reaction
    (PCR), 102
Neuroblastoma, 346
  allogeneic umbilical cord blood
    transplants for, 193, 199
  autologous bone marrow transplants
    for, 334–345
  controversies in treatment of,
    341–344
  cytokines and, 258, 260, 264
  gene therapy and, 13, 14, 15, 17
  minimal residual disease and, 99
  peripheral blood progenitor cell
    transplants for, 149
Neutropenia, 159, 173, 233, 256
Neutrophil recovery, 277
  erythropoietin and, 276
  interleukin-1 and, 272
  interleukin-3 and, 271
  PIXY 321 and, 272

New Zealand, 391–392
Non-Hodgkin's lymphoma
  autologous bone marrow purging
    and, 113
  autologous bone marrow transplants
    for, 391, 394–396
  cytokines and, 258, 260, 261, 264,
    265, 279
  donor mononuclear cells for relapse,
    73
  gene therapy and, 14, 15
  interleukin-1 and, 273
  minimal residual disease and, 99,
    100, 101, 103, 104, 114
  peripheral blood progenitor cell
    transplants for, 149
  post-transplant immunotherapy and,
    29, 30, 32, 34, 35
  pulmonary complications and, 239
  radiolabeled antibodies in treatment
    of, 125–128, 135
Nonidentical donors, 240, 241, 246
Nonrandomized (observation) studies,
  382
Nonspecific immunotherapy, 27–44

Opportunistic infections
  allogeneic umbilical cord blood
    transplants and, 195
  pulmonary, 232, 233
  unrelated donor transplants and,
    223–224
Oral mucositis, 232
Osteopetrosis, 199
Osteoporosis, 220
Osteosarcoma, 351–352
Ovarian cancer
  cytokines and, 258, 279
  gene therapy and, 18, 19, 22
  minimal residual disease and, 99
  post-transplant immunotherapy and,
    29, 30
Oxygen tension, in ex vivo expansion,
  169–171

p53, 20
Paclitaxel, 42
Pancreatic cancer, 19
Pancytopenia, 65–67, 232
Parenchymal lymphoma, 239
Pediatric bone marrow transplants,
  240, 245

Pediatric leukemia, 237
Pediatric solid tumors, 333–352, see
  also specific types
D-Penacillamine, 327
Pentoxifylline, 93
Peripheral blood mononuclear cell
  (PBMNC) transplants
  for chronic myelogenous leukemia,
    359–360, 361, 364–366
  ex vivo expansion in, 163
  immunotherapy following, 43–44
Peripheral blood progenitor cell
  (PBPC) harvesting, 143–154, see
  also Peripheral blood progenitor
  cell transplants
  CD34 cell selection in, 144, 149–154
  chemotherapy mobilization of,
    145–146
  growth factor mobilization of,
    146–148
  in steady state, 144–145
  tumor-cell contamination in, 148–149
Peripheral blood progenitor cell
  (PBPC) transplants, see also
  Peripheral blood progenitor cell
  harvesting
  allogeneic umbilical cord, 202–204
  for chronic myelogenous leukemia,
    363
  economics of, 379
  gene therapy and, 13, 14
Peripheral blood stem cell (PBSC)
  transplants
  autologous bone marrow transplants
    vs., 393, 396
  interleukin-2 and, 35–43
  for neuroblastoma, 344–345
  pulmonary complications and,
    232–233
  purged autologous bone marrow vs.,
    110, 113, 114
  radiolabeled antibodies and, 127
Peripheral neuroepithelioma, 346
pH
  adenoviral vectors and, 8
  ex vivo expansion and, 172–173, 176,
    177, 178
Ph-negative hematopoietic stem cells,
  359, 360–361, 363, 364, 366, 368,
  369
  persistence of, 357–358
  remission and, 370–371
Physician's Current Procedural
  Terminology (CPT) classification

system, 382
PIXY 321, 165, 179, 256, 271–272
Platelet recovery, 268–269
  interleukin-1 and, 273
  interleukin-3 and, 271
  interleukin-11 and, 274
  PIXY 321 and, 272
Pneumocystis carinii, 231, 247
Pneumonia
  bacterial, 231
  viral, 232
Pokeweed anti-viral protein, 112
pol protein, 4–5, 6
Polycythemia vera (PV), 43
Polymerase chain reaction (PCR), 358,
  368
  autologous bone marrow purging
    assessed with, 110–114
  in chronic myelogenous leukemia, 64
  competitive (quantitative), 106
  gene therapy and, 14
  minimal residual disease detected
    with, 99, 101–107, 108–110
  nested, 102
  pulmonary complications analyzed
    with, 247
  reverse transcription, 64, 108, 109,
    368
  tumor-cell contamination detected
    with, 149
Post-bone marrow transplant
  immunotherapy, 27–47
  nonspecific, 27–44
  tumor-specific, 44–45
Prednisone, 223
Primary graft failure, 257
Progenitor cells, see Peripheral blood
  progenitor cell harvesting;
  Peripheral blood progenitor cell
  transplants
Prostate cancer, 17
Prostatic-specific antigen (PSA), 16
Psoriasis, 323, 324
Pulmonary complications, 231–250
  diagnostic approaches to, 247–249
  impact of transplant techniques,
    232–233
  incidence and significance of, 231
  noninfectious, 242–247
  predicting outcome of, 240–242
  predicting respiratory failure,
    239–240
  pulmonary function testing for, 233–
    239

  temporal sequence of, 231–232
Pulmonary function testing, 233–239
Pulmonary hemorrhage, 244–245

Q-BEND, 151
Quality Adjusted Life Year (QALY),
  384–385, 392
Quality of life, 224–225

Radiografts, 239
Radiolabeled antibodies, 121–136
  in acute leukemia treatment,
    130–134
  design of trial for, 122–125
  in Hodgkin's disease treatment, 129
  in non-Hodgkin's lymphoma
    treatment, 125–128, 135
Randomized controlled trials, 382
Relapse, see also Leukemia relapse
  donor mononuclear cell
    ineffectiveness in, 72–73
  unrelated donor transplants and, 224
Renal cell carcinoma, 15, 17, 28
REP gene, 10, 11
Replication-incompetent retroviral
  vectors, 5–6
Resource-Based Relative Value Scale
  (RBRVS), 381–382
Respiratory failure, 239–240
Retroviral vectors, 3–7, 160–161
Reverse transcription polymerase
  chain reaction (RT-PCR), 64, 108,
  109, 368
Rhabdomyosarcoma, 346, 347–348
Rheumatoid arthritis, 321, 322, 323,
  324, 325, 326–327
Royal Marsden group, 350

St. Jude Children's Hospital, 112
Sargramostim, 255, see also
  Granulocyte-macrophage colony-
  stimulating factor
Scleroderma, 318, 321, 325, 327
Secondary graft failure, 221–222, 257
Seeding density effects, in ex vivo
  expansion, 172–173
Serum-depleted medium, in ex vivo
  expansion, 171–172
Severe autoimmune diseases (SADS),
  317–329
  animal models of, 318–319

414

bone marrow transplants in animal
models of, 319–323
patient selection for bone marrow
transplant, 326–328
results of bone marrow transplants
in, 323–324
Severe combined immunodeficiency
disease (SCID), 388
retroviral vectors for, 3–4
unrelated donor transplants for, 219
Sibling donors, 190–194, *see also*
Identical sibling donors
Small cell lung cancer, 99, 112
Solid tumors
autologous bone marrow transplants
for pediatric, 333–352
cytokines and, 279
gene therapy for, *see* Gene therapy
Steady state, cell harvesting in,
144–145
Stem cell factor (SCF), 256, 273
allogeneic umbilical cord blood
transplants and, 203, 204, 205
for chronic myelogenous leukemia,
369
clinical applications of, 280
ex vivo expansion and, 165–168, 172,
178, 179
G-CSF and, 278
interleukin-1 and, 272
interleukin-11 and, 274
peripheral blood progenitor cell
mobilization with, 147–148
Steroids, 88, 92, 326–327, 328
Streptavidin, 135
Stroma, 168–169
Suicide genes, 12, 19–20
Survival
allogeneic umbilical cord blood
transplants, 193–194, 198
autologous stem cell transplants and,
366–367
pulmonary complications and,
240–242
unrelated donor transplants and, 225
Syngeneic bone marrow transplants,
57, 60–61, 87, 88
Systemic lupus erythromatosus, 318,
321, 322, 324, 325, 328, 329

t(14;18), 103
Taxol, 22
T-cell depleted transplants, 28, 153, 389

acute graft-vs.-host disease and, 222
engraftment and, 221–222
graft-vs.-leukemia effect and, 74
leukemia relapse and, 62
minimal residual disease and, 108,
109
opportunistic infections and, 223–224
from unrelated donors, 221–222,
223–224, 225, 226
T cells
chronic myelogenous leukemia and,
370
graft-vs.-host disease and, 90–91
graft-vs.-leukemia effect and, 73–74,
75
interleukin-2 and, 32, 34, 275
post-transplant immunotherapy and,
44, 45
severe autoimmune diseases and,
318
Teniposide, 336, 338
Teniposide, doxorubicin, melphalan,
cisplatin, and total body
irradiation (VAM-TBI), 337, 340
Testicular cancer, 99
Thalassemia, 305–314
in adult patients, 312
class I, 306–308
class II, 308–310
class III, 310–312
mortality and causes of death from,
312–314
Thalidomide, 93
Theiler's encephalomyelitis virus
(TEMV), 319
Thiotepa, 222, 226, 349, 351
Thoractomy, 249
Thrombocytopenia, 232, 269
amegakaryocytic, 199
cytokines and, 256, 268
ex vivo expansion and, 159, 173
Thrombopoietin, 256
ex vivo expansion and, 165, 171, 174
properties of, 275
Thymidine kinase gene, 17–18, 19–20,
76
Thymoma, 29
Total body irradiation (TBI), 87
allogeneic umbilical cord blood
transplants and, 195, 196
autologous graft-vs.-host disease
and, 88
for chronic myelogenous leukemia,
358

controversy over, 343–344
engraftment and, 221
for Ewing's sarcoma, 345, 346–347
interleukin-1 and, 272
for neuroblastoma, 335, 336, 337,
  338, 339, 340, 343–344
PIXY 321 and, 271–272
pulmonary complications and, 231
radiolabeled antibodies and, 121,
  124, 128, 130, 132, 133–134
for rhabdomyosarcoma, 348
thalassemia and, 305
in VAM-TBI, 337, 340
Transforming growth factor (TGF),
  280
Transforming growth factor-β (TGF-
  β), 44, 46
allogeneic umbilical cord blood
  transplants and, 204
ex vivo expansion and, 172
gene therapy and, 17
Transfusion-associated graft-vs.-host
  disease (GVHD), 66
Trimethaprim-sulfamethoxazole, 247
Tuberculosis, 239
Tumor-cell contamination, 148–149
Tumor-infiltrating lymphocyte marking
  trials, 13, 15–16
Tumor necrosis factor (TNF), 27
gene therapy and, 16, 17
graft-vs.-host disease and, 259
interleukin-2 and, 34
interleukin-6 compared with, 270
Tumor necrosis factor-α (TNF-α)
allogeneic umbilical cord blood
  transplants and, 206, 207
clinical applications of, 280
graft-vs.-host disease and, 91, 92–93,
  94
Tumor necrosis factor-β (TNF-β), 28
Tumor purging, see Autologous bone
  marrow purging

Tumor-specific immunotherapy, 44–45

Ulcerative colitis, 323, 324, 328
Undifferentiated lymphoma, 100
University of Colorado, 152
University of Minnesota, 195–196, 223,
  224, 241
University of Nebraska Medical
  Center, 112, 113, 244, 245, 391,
  393, 395
Unrelated donors
for allogeneic umbilical cord blood
  transplants, 194–200, 208–209
for bone marrow transplants,
  217–226

Vaccines, cancer, 16, 44, 47
Vincristine, 388
for Ewing's sarcoma, 345
for neuroblastoma, 334, 336, 337,
  338, 340
for osteosarcoma, 352
for rhabdomyosarcoma, 347, 348
Vincristine, melphalan, etoposide, and
  carboplatin (OMEC), 336, 339
Viral pneumonia, 232
Viral vector systems, 3–12
VP-16-213, see Etoposide

Wild-type adeno-associated viruses, 10
Wild-type adenoviruses, 7–8
Wild-type herpes simplex viruses
  (HSV), 12
Wild-type retroviruses, 4–5
Wilms' tumor, 350–351
Wiskott-Aldrich syndrome, 219

Yeast infections, 224